The
Good
Health
Fact
Book

The Good Health Fact Book

A Complete Question-and-Answer Guide to Getting Healthy and Staying Healthy

Reader's Digest

The Reader's Digest Association, Inc., Pleasantville, New York / Montreal

STAFF

Project Editor
Joseph Gonzalez

Project Art Editor
Perri DeFino

Senior Research Editor
Maymay Quey Lin

Senior Associate Editors
Don Earnest
Melanie Hulse
Diana Marsh

Research Editor
Shirley A. Miller

Art Associate
Diane Lemonides

Research Associates
Kathleen Derzipilski
Barbara Guarino Lester

Editorial Assistant
Jean Ryan

Editorial Intern
Melanie Williams

CONTRIBUTORS

Editor
Nancy Shuker

Writers
Gordon Bakoulis Bloch
Jean Callahan
Charlene Canape
Nancy Carothers
Nancy A. De Korp
Linda Hetzer
Guy A. Lester
Wendy Murphy
Serena Stockwell

Artists
AIRBRUSH ILLUSTRATION:
Bonnie Hofkin

PAPER SCULPTURE:
Ellen Rixford

PENCIL ILLUSTRATION:
Ray Skibinski

COMPUTER GRAPHICS:
Robin Storesund

EMERGENCY ILLUSTRATION:
Andrew Aloof
Richard Bonson
Gordon Lawson
Stephen Pointer

Picture Editor
Marion Paone

Copy Editors
Kathleen M. Berger
Sue Heinemann

Researchers
Emily Bradshaw
Donna E. Haupt
Mary Lyn Maiscott
Jozefa Stuart
Joan Walsh

Indexer
Sydney Wolfe Cohen

READER'S DIGEST GENERAL BOOKS

Editor in Chief
John A. Pope, Jr.

Managing Editor
Jane Polley

Executive Editor
Susan J. Wernert

Art Director
David Trooper

Group Editors
Will Bradbury
Norman B. Mack
Kaari Ward

Group Art Editors
Evelyn Bauer
Robert M. Grant
Joel Musler

Chief of Research
Laurel A. Gilbride

Copy Chief
Edward W. Atkinson

Picture Editor
Richard Pasqual

Rights and Permissions
Pat Colomban

Head Librarian
Jo Manning

CONSULTANTS

Chief Consultant
ARTHUR W. FEINBERG, M.D.
Medical Director, Center for Extended
  Care and Rehabilitation
North Shore University Hospital—
  Cornell University Medical College
Professor of Clinical Medicine
Cornell University Medical College

Chapter Consultants
MALINDA H. BELL, M.D.
Clinical Assistant Professor
Truman Medical Center
University of Missouri

NORMAN COHEN, Ph.D.
Professor of Environmental Medicine
Nelson Institute of Environmental
  Medicine
New York University Medical Center

EDWARD COLT, M.D.
Assistant Professor of Clinical Medicine
Columbia University

JOHANNA DWYER, D.Sc.
Director, Frances Stern Nutrition Center
New England Medical Center Hospitals

STEVEN M. FREEDMAN, M.D.
Chief of Family Practice and
  of Patient Education
Kaiser Permanente Medical Center
Fairfield, California

LOUIS HOCHHEISER, M.D.
Chairperson, Department of Family
  Practice
University of Vermont College
  of Medicine

HERBERT H. KRAUSS, Ph.D.
Professor of Psychology
Hunter College
City University of New York

MARC L. RIVO, M.D., M.P.H.
Director, Division of Medicine
Health Resources and Services
  Administration
U.S. Department of Health and
  Human Services

JEAN SCHULTZ, M.D.
Chief, Geriatric Psychiatry
North Shore University Hospital—
  Cornell University Medical College

Contributing Consultants
RONALD S. FEINGOLD, Ph.D.
ARTHUR M. FINKELSTEIN, D.D.S.
PAUL A. HOMOLY, D.D.S.
CYNTHIA MACKAY, M.D.
ROBERT A. SILVER, M.D.
STANLEY SNEGROFF, Ed.D.

Library of Congress Cataloging in Publication Data

The Good health fact book
        p.   cm.
    At head of title: Reader's digest.
    Includes index.
    ISBN 0-89577-416-X
    1. Health—Miscellanea.   I. Reader's Digest Association.
    II. Reader's digest.
    RA776.G645   1992
    613—dc20   91-44169

Printed in the United States of America

Contents

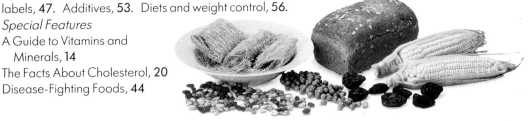

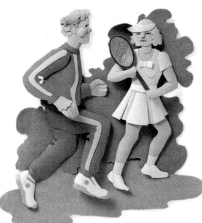

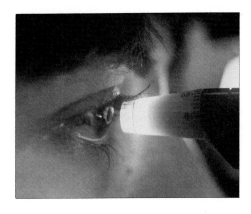

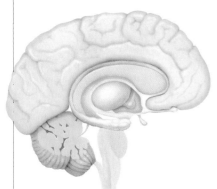

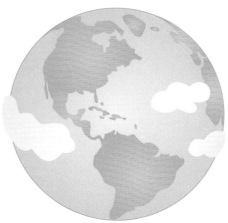

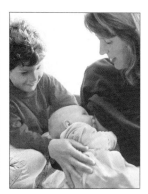

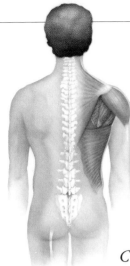

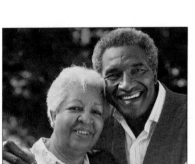

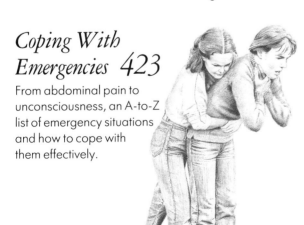

About This Book

Your health is the most precious asset you have. Maintaining and preserving it demand not only good medical care but also sound knowledge and active participation on your part. This book was written to help you become a better participant in your own health care.

The more than 1,000 questions in THE GOOD HEALTH FACT BOOK are questions you would ask if you had the unlimited time and undivided attention of a caring doctor at your beck and call. Written in consultation with leading medical authorities from around the country, the answers provide the facts you need to get healthy, stay healthy, and deal effectively with medical problems when they arise.

Because diet and exercise are such critical factors in maintaining health and living a long life, the book begins with a comprehensive chapter on eating right followed by another equally thorough chapter on staying fit and active at all ages.

The remaining eight chapters deal with such essential health topics as doctor-patient relations and communication, staying mentally healthy, preventive medicine and self-care dos and don'ts, the joys and complications of sex and family life, how the environment affects your health (and what you can do about it), living with chronic illnesses, managing the stresses of middle age, and living well in the later years.

At the back of the book you'll find an A-to-Z guide to coping with emergency medical situations, and an appendix listing the addresses and telephone numbers of the National Institutes of Health, the Centers for Disease Control, and the many professional, government, and service organizations referred to in the text. A detailed index and numerous cross-references within the text will lead you quickly to the precise information you seek.

Each chapter begins with *Personal Stories*, real-life case histories of people making choices and taking action to improve their health and well-being. The case histories are followed by a *Test Your Health I.Q.* quiz designed to get you thinking about the chapter's main topics and how they affect your life.

Throughout the book, *The Facts About...* summaries give you basic information about important, often complex, subjects such as cholesterol, Medicare, 12-step programs, and radon. Shorter *Fact or Fallacy?* features reveal the true stories behind commonly held conceptions and misconceptions about health. Charts and checklists convey essential information in a concise, easy-to-understand way. Diaries outline helpful techniques you can use to reduce your daily calorie intake, set up an exercise program, stop smoking, and monitor your daily medications. Special two-page features will give you new insights about such subjects as Alternative Medicine, Learning to Relax, and Living Alternatives for the Later Years.

Our goal in producing THE GOOD HEALTH FACT BOOK has been to provide the up-to-date, accurate facts you need to make good health-care choices — choices that can make a difference in terms of longer life and better health for you and your family. Our hope is that you'll turn to this book often for information, advice, reassurance, and interesting reading.

— *The Editors*

The information, recommendations, and visual material in this book are for reference and guidance only; they are not intended as a substitute for a physician's diagnosis and care. The editors urge anyone with continuing medical problems or symptoms to consult a qualified physician.

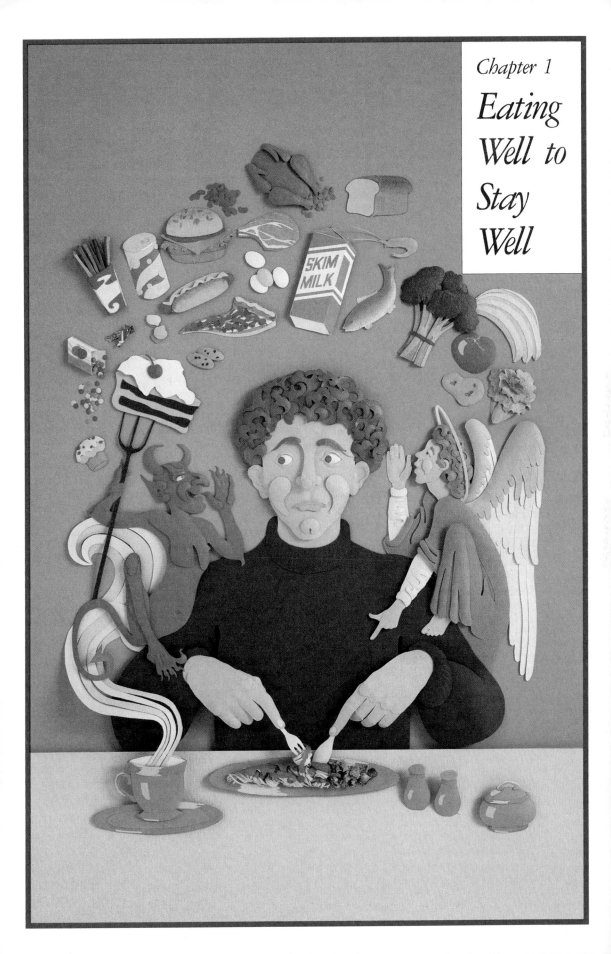

A Change of Habits

achary N., a 66-year-old retired physics professor, had been slim for most of his life. But as he got older, Zachary began putting on weight. By the time he retired Zachary was about 40 pounds over his ideal weight, and his cholesterol level was alarmingly high. During a routine physical one January, Zachary's doctor laid down the law—lose weight and bring down your cholesterol or live with the threat of heart disease hanging over your head. After quizzing Zachary about his eating habits, the doctor also suggested that he consult a registered dietitian.

Even in retirement, Zachary led a busy life, tutoring and doing other volunteer work. Neither he nor his wife, who still worked at a local bank, had much time or inclination to plan or prepare meals. In fact, their idea of a home-cooked meal was anything out of a can or from the freezer that could be popped into the microwave. The dietitian had her work cut out for her.

Her first task was to help Zachary rethink his approach to food. Instead of choosing whatever happened to be available and eating on the run, Zachary had to learn how to plan three balanced meals and two healthy snacks a day. The dietitian taught him how to shop for and prepare meals featuring complex carbohydrates and fresh vegetables, with fish, poultry, or low-fat meat playing a secondary role. She stressed the importance of reading nutrition labels and staying away from processed foods loaded with added fat, sugar, and salt.

Zachary soon became a knowledgeable food shopper and meal planner, and to his wife's delight, he developed a real flair for cooking. At the dietitian's urging, he also began exercising more, riding a stationary bike for 45 minutes every day and taking long walks.

By summer Zachary's new regimen was paying off. He had lost nearly 40 pounds, and his cholesterol was down considerably. Zachary's wife enjoyed coming home to tasty meals she didn't have to prepare herself, and found that her husband's cuisine helped her shed a few unwanted pounds without dieting.

Two years later, Zachary and his wife are trimmer and fitter than they've been in a long while, and Zachary has added cooking to his list of enjoyable retirement activities.

Getting Off the Weight-Loss/Weight-Gain Seesaw

tarvation diets, high-protein diets, liquid diets, single-food diets—Jack S. had tried them all, invariably without success. Each time, he'd lose about 15 pounds, go off the diet, and quickly regain the weight and then some. When not dieting, Jack's eating habits were very irregular. A traveling salesman, Jack would often skip meals and snack on candy bars and doughnuts to alleviate hunger pangs and the boredom of long drives.

At 42, Jack weighed in at 300 pounds—way too much even for a 6 foot 5 inch, large-boned man. Deciding that it was time to seek help, Jack made an appointment with a nutritionist and steeled himself to embark on a strenuous diet. Instead, the nutritionist talked about eating habits. She helped Jack monitor his food intake, plan meals, and control portion sizes. Jack learned that he could make healthy food choices both at home and on the road, even in restaurants. Rather than feeling deprived, as he had on previous diets, Jack discovered that he was rarely hungry. And he solved his boredom problem by listening to tapes in his car instead of eating fattening snacks; now, when he needs something to tide him over, Jacks grabs an apple.

Jack is amazed at how quickly he's lost weight—25 pounds in 3 months—and he's confident that this time he'll reach his goal of 225 pounds and stay there. Just to make sure, Jack intends to join a weight maintenance group to help him keep trim and make sound nutrition a lifelong habit.

TEST YOUR HEALTH I.Q.

How Healthy Is Your Diet?

With each meal you eat and each food item you buy, you're making decisions that affect your health and well-being. Eating habits — both good and bad — are usually learned in childhood and become deeply ingrained. Changing the bad ones isn't always easy, but it can pay off dramatically in terms of better health and longer life. Because diet is so central to good health, this first chapter has been designed to answer two basic questions: What is good nutrition? How can I best achieve it? As an introduction and a test of your nutritional savvy, try picking the phrase or phrases that best complete the statements below.

1 The most important thing you can do to improve your diet is to _____ .

A. eat less fat in general
B. eat less saturated fat in particular
C. eat more protein
D. eat more complex carbohydrates

2 To be usable as fuel, carbohydrates must be broken down into _____ .

A. lactose
B. glucose
C. their constituent amino acids

3 To maintain good health, you need to consume only _____ of polyunsaturated fat a day.

A. 1 teaspoon
B. 1 tablespoon
C. 2 tablespoons

4 High blood levels of _____ cholesterol are associated with a lower risk of heart disease.

A. HDL
B. LDL
C. VLDL

5 New nutrition guidelines place a greater emphasis on _____ .

A. fruits and vegetables
B. dairy products
C. breads, cereals, rice, and pasta
D. meats and meat substitutes

6 Low-fat or skim milk is generally recommended over whole milk except for _____ .

A. nursing mothers
B. children under age 2
C. older people

7 According to the American Heart Association, you should limit your daily salt intake to _____ .

A. 1 tablespoon
B. 1½ teaspoons
C. 2 teaspoons

8 _____ should consider taking a calcium supplement.

A. Women and teenage girls
B. The elderly
C. People with lactose intolerance

9 Factors that determine your ideal weight include _____ .

A. body-fat percentage and distribution
B. race and ethnic background
C. a history of weight-related medical problems

Answers

For more information on any of the quiz topics turn to the pages listed next to the answers.

1. A,B,D, p.12
2. B, p.17
3. B, p.19
4. A, p.20
5. A,C, p.25
6. B, pp.26–27
7. B, pp.33–34
8. A,B,C, p.41
9. A,C, p.57

Planning a healthy diet often sounds complicated. Are there simple rules I can follow?

We seem to be bombarded these days by advice on nutrition. Some of this information is sound; some of it is confusing, contradictory, and on occasion, just plain wrong. But the truth of the matter is that a healthy diet is neither complicated nor restrictive. Easy-to-follow basic rules have been established by major health organizations and federal agencies. One of the clearest, most succinct guides to good nutrition is the *Dietary Guidelines for Americans,* prepared (and revised periodically) by the U.S. Department of Agriculture and the U.S. Department of Health and Human Services. Based on the best available scientific findings on nutrition, these guidelines apply to all healthy Americans age 2 and over:

☐ Eat a variety of foods.
☐ Maintain a healthy weight.
☐ Choose a diet low in total fat, saturated fat, and cholesterol. (See *Controlling Your Fat Intake,* p.18.)
☐ Eat plenty of vegetables, fruits, and grain products.
☐ Use sugars only in moderation.
☐ Use salt and sodium only in moderation.
☐ If you drink alcoholic beverages, do so in moderation.

Two key words in the guidelines are variety and moderation. Be wary of nutritional advice that focuses on a single food or on a few highly fortified foods or supplements, and avoid dietary extremes (both eating too much and eating too little can be harmful). The most important thing you can do to improve your diet is to eat less fat in general, less saturated fat in particular, and more complex carbohydrates (fiber and starchy foods).

What makes a food nutritious?

The components of food that the body uses to sustain itself are known as nutrients (see *The Staff of Life,* facing page). Nutrients are divided into two broad categories: the macronutrients (proteins, carbohydrates, and fats), substantial quantities of which are needed for energy and growth, and the micronutrients (vitamins and minerals), needed in small amounts for growth and to facilitate vital body processes. Although not usually included in lists of nutrients, water and dietary fiber are key elements of a healthy diet, too.

The human body has the ability to synthesize certain nutrients on its own. Those that it cannot make or cannot make in sufficient quantities (the vast majority) must be supplied by the foods you eat. Such nutrients are known as essential nutrients. If you don't get enough of them in your diet, you'll develop potentially harmful deficiencies.

Foods vary in the amounts and types of nutrients they supply. A potato, for example, is more nutritious than a slice of watermelon because it has more protein, complex carbohydrates, vitamins, and minerals. However, no single type of food provides all the nutrients required for good health. For peak nutrition you need to eat a wide variety of foods. By the same token, a food lacking in certain nutrients can still be part of a nutritious diet if you balance it with foods that provide the missing nutrients.

What are RDA's?

The initials RDA stand for *R*ecommended *D*ietary *A*llowance. RDA's are guidelines set by the Food and Nutrition Board of the National Research Council for the amounts of protein, vitamins, and minerals that healthy people should consume daily to maintain good nutrition. Because nutrient needs depend on age and sex (as well as on weight, activity level, and general health), RDA's have been set for men, women, and children of different ages, as well as for pregnant and lactating women. For example, the RDA for vitamin A is 800 milligrams for women 25 to 50 years of age, but 1,000 milligrams for a man of the same age.

RDA's are safe and adequate amounts of a given nutrient for healthy people in a specific age and sex group. As a safety factor, RDA's are set slightly above the actual needs of most individuals within a group. For certain essential nutrients, there isn't enough information to set RDA's. In such cases, the Food and Nutrition Board provides an estimate of safe and adequate intake levels. RDA's do not apply to people with special nutritional needs due to such factors as chronic diseases, metabolic disorders, or nutrient deficiencies.

The initials U.S. RDA on food labels do not mean the same thing as RDA. Set by the U.S. Food and Drug Administration (FDA), U.S. RDA's (*U*nited *S*tates *R*ecommended *D*aily *A*llowances) are a standard for labeling the nutrient content of food products. The U.S. RDA is usually the highest RDA for a given nutrient. A nutrition label lists the percentage of the U.S. RDA of protein and seven vitamins and minerals contained in a single serving of the product. According to proposed changes in food labeling scheduled to go into effect in May 1993, U.S. RDA's will be replaced by Reference Daily Intakes (RDI's), expressed in grams or in percentages of Daily Values. (See *Deciphering Food Labels,* p. 47.)

THE STAFF OF LIFE

The nutrients in food fuel the body and provide the materials needed for growth, for tissue maintenance and repair, and for the regulation of physiological processes. When food is oxidized (burned) in the body, the result is energy, measured in kilocalories (the prefix "kilo" is usually dropped in nontechnical usage). Carbohydrates and fats are the body's main sources of energy, providing 4 and 9 calories per gram respectively. Protein also yields 4 calories per gram but is used as fuel only when energy from other sources is scarce. Vitamins and minerals are essential for body functioning, although they cannot be burned as fuel. Strictly speaking, water and fiber are not nutrients, but water is vital to life and fiber plays an important role in elimination.

A staple in almost every culture, bread is an apt symbol for nutritious food. The nutrient and calorie contents of a slice of whole-wheat bread are listed below.

Carbohydrate. 13 gr (52 Cal). Sources: whole-wheat flour, soy flour, honey, whey.

Protein. 3 gr (12 Cal). Sources: whole-wheat flour, soy flour, gluten, whey.

Fat. 1 gr (9 Cal). Sources: canola oil, soybean oil, wheat germ.

Water. Thirty-eight percent of the bread consists of water.

Fiber. 2 gr. Sources: whole-wheat flour, soy flour.

Vitamins: thiamine (0.10 mg), riboflavin (0.06 mg), niacin (1.1 mg); A and C (traces).

Minerals: calcium (20 mg), iron (1.0 mg), sodium (180 mg), traces of other minerals.

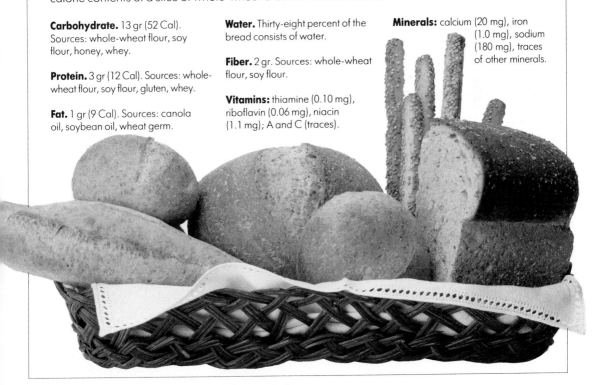

How do I know whether my diet meets all of the RDA's?

As long as you are basically healthy and eat a balanced diet with adequate calories from all the food groups (p.24), you should have no trouble meeting the RDA's for your age group. Although RDA's are recommendations for daily intake, they are not minimum daily requirements. Even if the quality of your diet varies, your body is re-markably adaptable and can store nutrients for varying periods. This means that you can achieve nutritional balance over a period of days, rather than in one day.

When I was growing up, "getting enough protein" was a major concern. How important is protein in the diet?

It's vitally important, but for most Americans today, getting enough protein isn't a problem. Rather, it's our tendency to eat too much protein from high-fat animal sources that worries many nutrition experts.

Proteins are made up of amino acids. When you eat protein, whether from animal or plant sources, your body breaks it down into its constituent amino acids and then uses them (along with other amino acids recycled from worn-out tissue) to manufacture proteins of its own. These proteins play a variety of key roles in the body. They are

A GUIDE TO VITAMINS AND MINERALS

The 13 vitamins and 16 minerals listed here are all important for your health. If your diet is varied, balanced, and has adequate calories, you probably don't need to worry about meeting your vitamin and mineral needs. If you have a chronic illness or other condition or are following a special diet, however, you may need to take supplements (pp.40–43). Consult your doctor or a registered dietitian.

Fat-soluble vitamins are found mainly in oil- and fat-containing foods. Since the body stores these vitamins in its fatty tissues, you don't need to eat them every day. Overdosage can be toxic.

Vitamin	Main role	Good food source
A (retinol)	Needed for maintenance of skin, mucous membranes, bones, teeth and hair; vision; and reproduction.	Liver, eggs, milk, milk products, dark green leafy vegetables, carrots.
D (calciferol)	Helps absorb calcium; needed for bone growth and maintenance.	Fortified milk, dairy products, margarine, liver, cod-liver oil, eggs, oily fish.
E (tocopherol)	Helps form red blood cells; acts as an antioxidant (p.45).	Vegetable oils, nuts, dark green leafy vegetables, wheat germ, whole-grain foods.
K	Needed for blood clotting.	Eggs, liver, cereals, dark green leafy vegetables.

Water-soluble vitamins are found in a variety of plant and animal foods. Because the body stores them in small amounts and quickly excretes excesses, they need to be part of your diet nearly every day.

Vitamin	Main role	Good food source
Thiamine (B_1)	Needed for nervous system function; helps release energy from carbohydrates.	Pork, liver, kidney, whole-grain cereals, enriched breads and cereals, seeds, nuts, legumes, brewer's yeast.
Riboflavin (B_2)	Helps release energy from foods.	Liver, milk, milk products, meat, poultry, fish, enriched breads and cereals, dark green leafy vegetables.
Niacin, or nicotinic acid (B_3)	Needed for nervous and digestive system functions; helps release energy from foods.	Liver, meat, poultry, fish, enriched bread and cereals, peanuts, legumes.
Pantothenic acid (B_5)	Helps metabolize nutrients.	Liver, kidney, whole-grain cereals, legumes, eggs, dark green leafy vegetables, milk.
B_6 (pyridoxine)	Needed for metabolism; helps form red blood cells.	Liver, kidney, pork, poultry, fish, whole-grain foods, potatoes, bananas, enriched cereals, peanuts, walnuts.
B_{12} (cobalamin)	Helps form red blood cells and operate nervous system.	Liver, kidney, meat, fish, seafood, eggs, milk, milk products.
Biotin	Helps form fatty acids and release energy from carbohydrates and amino acids.	Liver, eggs, cereals, yeast.
Folacin (folic acid)	Helps form red blood cells and genetic material.	Liver, dark green leafy vegetables, orange juice, whole-grain breads and cereals, enriched cereals, legumes.
C (ascorbic acid)	Promotes growth, formation and maintenance of bones and teeth, repair of tissues, resistance to infection.	Many fruits and vegetables, including citrus fruits and dark green leafy vegetables.

Major minerals (also known as macrominerals) are needed by the body in relatively large amounts.

Mineral	Main role	Good food source
Calcium	Needed for bone and teeth formation and bone maintenance; plays a role in muscle contraction and blood clotting.	Milk, milk products, canned salmon and sardines with bones, dark green leafy vegetables.
Chloride	Regulates fluid and electrolyte balances; forms part of gastric juice.	Salt, processed foods.
Magnesium	Needed for bone and teeth formation; aids in release of energy, nerve and muscle function.	Dark green leafy vegetables, nuts, seeds, whole-grain foods, legumes, milk.
Phosphorus	Builds and strengthens bones; helps release energy from nutrients.	Milk, cheese, meat, fish, poultry, eggs, whole grains, legumes, nuts.
Potassium	Helps to transmit nerve impulses, control muscle contraction, and maintain proper blood pressure.	Many fruits and vegetables; cereals, legumes, meat.
Sodium	Regulates fluid and acid-base balance.	Salt, processed foods.
Sulfur	Needed to make hair, nails, and cartilage.	Meat, fish, eggs, legumes.

Trace minerals are needed by the body in much smaller amounts, but are no less important for its functioning than the major minerals.

Mineral	Main role	Good food source
Chromium	Helps insulin work efficiently in glucose metabolism.	Brewer's yeast, calf's liver, whole-grain cereals, peanuts, American cheese, wheat germ.
Copper	Needed for iron absorption and metabolism; helps form red blood cells and nerve fibers.	Liver, kidney, seafood, nuts, seeds, tap water.
Fluoride	Contributes to bone and teeth maintenance.	Fluoridated tap water, tea, sardines with bones.
Iodine	Needed to form thyroid hormones.	Iodized salt, seafood, saltwater fish, dairy products, vegetables.
Iron	Helps transport oxygen in blood and muscles; involved in enzyme activities related to energy use.	Liver, meat, eggs, dark green leafy vegetables, cereals.
Manganese	Needed for bone formation; involved in fat synthesis.	Whole grains, fruits, vegetables, tea, legumes, nuts.
Molybdenum	Aids in metabolism.	Milk, legumes, whole-grain breads and cereals.
Selenium	Works in association with vitamin E as an antioxidant (p.45).	Liver, kidney, seafood, meat, whole grains.
Zinc	Needed for metabolism and digestion; aids in wound healing, growth, tissue repair, and sexual development.	Liver, seafood, meat, eggs, poultry, fish, whole-grain cereals.

the main components of muscles and other body tissues and organs. They are needed for the growth, repair, and maintenance of cells and for the synthesis of enzymes and hormones. Some proteins act as antibodies, fighting off disease organisms; others help to digest food, clot blood, transmit nerve impulses, and regulate the fluid balance of cells. Although carbohydrates and fats are considered better sources of energy, proteins provide energy too.

What does the term complete protein mean?

To make its various proteins, the body requires about 22 different amino acids, nine of which it cannot synthesize on its own and must derive entirely from food sources. A food is considered a complete, or high-quality, protein source if it contains adequate amounts of all nine essential amino acids and a good variety of the nonessential ones. Incomplete proteins lack an adequate quantity of at least one essential amino acid. Proteins from animal sources—meat, poultry, seafood, eggs, milk, and milk products—are generally complete, and proteins from plant sources are incomplete. However, as vegetarians well know, one plant food can supply the amino acids that another is missing to provide complete protein. A dairy product or meat eaten with a plant food can also supply the missing amino acids (see *Combining Foods for Complete Protein*, p. 29).

How much protein does the body really need?

Not as much as most Americans consume. The Recommended Dietary Allowance for protein is 0.8 grams for every kilogram (2.2 pounds) of body weight. For

FACT OR FALLACY?

Eating large amounts of protein builds bigger, stronger muscles

Fallacy. Although one of protein's functions in the body is to create muscle tissue, eating a lot of protein doesn't automatically create larger, better muscles. The way to increase muscle size and strength is through exercise (p.81). Be wary of the body-building claims made for high-protein liquids or amino acid supplements. Such products are costly and potentially dangerous. (For more on amino acid supplements, see page 41.) Extra protein, ironically, is more likely to add fat to your body rather than muscle if you don't cut calories elsewhere to compensate for the additional protein calories.

Athletes and very active people need more protein than the average American normally eats

Fallacy. Some athletes— and other adults who regularly engage in serious aerobic exercise—may need to eat more than the recommended daily allowance for protein, according to a recent study at Tufts University. However, the extra protein needed— 50 percent over the RDA— is easily met by a typical American diet, which usually exceeds the RDA for protein by 50 to 75 percent.

a woman weighing 121 pounds (55 kilograms), for example, the RDA would be 44 grams of protein. She could easily meet this allowance by eating just 3½ ounces of roasted chicken (about 24 grams of protein), a half cup of cottage cheese (14 grams), and two slices of whole-wheat bread (6 grams) during the course of a day.

Not eating enough protein can cause a number of serious health problems, including anemia in women of childbearing years and stunted growth in children, but such deficiencies are very rare in developed countries. Indeed, most Americans exceed the RDA for protein by 50 to 75 percent. In a person with kidney disease, a high-protein diet can cause problems. (Filtering out the nitrogen left over from the breakdown of protein taxes already damaged kidneys and further impairs their function.) However, for a healthy person, protein by itself does not seem to be harmful, even at U.S. consumption levels. The problem is that much of the protein Americans consume is derived from meat and milk products that are high in fat and cholesterol. In addition, when you eat more protein than your body can use, the excess is stored as fat.

In keeping with the *Dietary Guidelines for Americans,* nutrition experts are recommending a rethinking of protein sources in the diet, with a greater emphasis on such low-fat foods as poultry, fish, low-fat milk products, and properly combined grains, beans, and vegetables.

What's the role of carbohydrates in the diet?

Carbohydrates are the body's main fuel source. Although fats and, to a lesser extent, protein also provide energy, most of the daily energy needs of the body are best met with carbohydrates. There are three basic types of carbohydrates. The simplest are the monosaccharides, consisting of a single sugar molecule; these include glucose (also called dextrose, corn sugar, or grape sugar), fructose (found in fruits, vegetables, and honey), and galactose (a component of the milk sugar lactose). Disaccharides are the double sugar molecules: sucrose, from sugarcane and sugar beets; maltose, from grain; and lactose. Taken together, monosaccharides and disaccharides are known as simple carbohydrates, or sugars.

The third type of carbohydrates are the polysaccharides, also known as complex carbohydrates, which consist of long chains of many sugar molecules. Complex carbohydrates, which include starches and indigestible dietary fiber, are found in foods of plant origin: fruits, vegetables, legumes, and grains.

To be usable as fuel, carbohydrates must be broken down into glucose. Digestive enzymes in saliva begin the process of converting di- and polysaccharides into monosaccharides. Carbohydrate breakdown continues in the stomach and small intestine. Dietary fiber, however, passes through the body largely unaffected by digestive enzymes (for more on fiber, see pages 31–32).

From the small intestine, the simple sugars glucose, galactose, and fructose pass into the bloodstream. Glucose in the blood can be burned as needed for energy. Galactose and fructose must be converted into glucose by the liver before they can be used as fuel. Excess glucose is stored primarily in the liver and muscles in the form of glycogen (animal starch), which can be converted back to glucose; some excess glucose is also stored as fat.

FACT OR FALLACY?

Starchy foods such as potatoes, bread, rice, and pasta are fattening

Fallacy. Starchy foods actually help you lose weight by filling you up with fewer calories than comparable amounts of fatty foods would. Since starches are carbohydrates, they supply 4 calories per gram, as opposed to the 9 calories in a gram of fat. A 3-ounce hamburger, for example, contains 245 calories, nearly twice the calories in a 5-ounce baked potato. Starchy foods acquired their reputation for being fattening because of the rich sauces that often accompany them. To keep starches low-calorie, serve them with small portions of sauce or with low-fat substitutes (for example, top a baked potato with yogurt instead of sour cream or season rice with herbs instead of butter).

I hear a lot these days about the virtues of complex carbohydrates. Why are they so good?

The health benefits of complex carbohydrates are well established. As long as they are not overly processed or refined, starchy foods such as potatoes, pasta, grains, beans, corn, peas, and other vegetables and fruits are not only excellent fuel sources, they are usually low in fat and rich in other nutrients— supplying vitamins, minerals, some protein, and a lot of fiber.

Besides being good for you, starchy foods are tasty, filling, and generally less expensive than high-protein animal foods.

Not all carbohydrates are created equal, however. Simple carbohydrates may originate in healthful fruits or vegetables, but they are usually consumed in refined or processed foods that have few nutrients besides sugar. Because concentrated sweets such as candies, syrup, gelatin desserts, sugary soft drinks, and, of course, table sugar provide energy and little else, their calories are considered "empty." (Alcohol, which is even higher in calories than sugar, falls into the same empty-calorie category.) Other sweets, such as cakes, cookies, custards, and ice cream, do provide other nutrients, but they usually contain high levels of saturated fat and cholesterol.

Although an RDA has not been set for complex carbohydrates, the *Dietary Guidelines for Americans* emphasizes the importance of vegetables, fruits, and grain products in the diet. Such groups as the National Research Council and the American Heart Association recommend that the calories derived from carbohydrates in general be increased from today's average of about 45 percent to more than 50 percent, with a greater emphasis placed on complex carbohydrates.

Everybody talks about polyunsaturated, monounsaturated, and saturated fats, but I'm still confused. What's the difference?

Most of the fats in your body as well as in the food you eat are made up of fatty acids. These are essentially chains of carbon atoms, which may or may not be chemically bound to hydrogen atoms. A fatty acid is said to be

CONTROLLING YOUR FAT INTAKE

To keep calories derived from fat under 30 percent of your daily calorie total (and saturated fats and polyunsaturated fats each under 10 percent) may require changes in how you eat, shop, and cook. Follow these tips for reducing the fat content of your diet:

☐ Eat lean meats and poultry (see *Foods to Choose: Lean Meats*, p.25) and low-fat dairy products (see *The Fat in Milk and Milk Products*, p.26).

☐ Don't fry or sauté foods in fat; use a non-stick pan with broth or try baking, broiling, poaching, roasting, or steaming instead.

☐ If you do cook or season foods with oil, choose among those oils that are lowest in saturated fat (see chart below). Avoid palm and coconut oils, which are highly saturated.

☐ Cook meat, fish, or poultry on a rack so that fat drips away; baste with fat-free wine, fruit juices, or broth. Don't serve drippings.

☐ Trim fat from meat and trim skin and fat from poultry before cooking.

☐ Cook stews and soups ahead of time and chill. Remove the congealed fat and reheat.

☐ Cut down on peanut butter, avocados, coconut meat, and olives.

☐ Read food labels carefully; avoid foods with high levels of fat, particularly saturated or hydrogenated fats.

☐ Cut down on high-fat snacks such as buttered popcorn, chips, cookies, pastries, chocolate candy, and cakes. If you must nibble, try raw vegetables, air-popped popcorn, or fresh fruit.

☐ Try low-fat or fat-free versions of normally high-fat foods like salad dressings, sour cream, mayonnaise, and whipped cream.

☐ Substitute fruit ices, which have no fat, for ice creams, which have a great deal of fat.

Calculating your daily fat quotas and interpreting the fat-content information found on food labels can be difficult. Here are two useful formulas:

☐ To figure the maximum number of calories you should derive from fat per day, multiply your total daily calorie intake by 30 percent (0.3); divide the result by 9 (calories per gram of fat) for your maximum daily quota of fat in grams. A third of this figure is your limit for saturated fats and for polyunsaturated fats. An active man who consumes 2,800 calories a day should restrict his daily fat intake to under 840 fat calories (2,800 × 0.3), or 93 grams of fat (840 ÷ 9). His intake of saturated fat and of polyunsaturated fat should not exceed 280 calories (31 grams) each.

☐ To figure the percentage of fat calories in a food, multiply the grams of fat in a serving by 9, then divide the result by the total calories per serving. For example, a cup of whole milk contains 8 grams of fat and 150 calories, 48 percent of which come from fat (8 × 9 ÷ 150 = 0.48).

	Saturated
	Polyunsaturated
	Monounsaturated

COMPARISON OF FATS IN VEGETABLE OILS

Oil	Saturated	Polyunsaturated	Monounsaturated
Canola	6%	32%	62%
Safflower	10%	78%	12%
Sunflower	11%	69%	20%
Corn	13%	61%	26%
Olive	14%	9%	77%
Soybean	15%	61%	24%
Peanut	18%	33%	49%
Cottonseed	27%	54%	19%
Palm	52%	9%	39%
Coconut	92%	2%	6%

saturated if it contains as many hydrogen atoms as is chemically possible. If one or more pairs of carbon atoms are free, that is, not fully bound to hydrogen atoms, the fatty acid is unsaturated—monounsaturated, if it has only one pair of free carbon atoms; polyunsaturated, if it contains many such pairs.

All the fats found naturally in foods contain varying amounts of saturated, monounsaturated, and polyunsaturated fats. In general, fats in animal foods such as beef, lamb, pork, chicken, eggs, milk, and milk products are highly saturated and solid at room temperature. (An exception is fish oil, which is high in polyunsaturated fatty acids.) Vegetable oils tend to be unsaturated to various degrees and liquid at room temperature: olive, peanut, and canola oils are mostly monounsaturated; corn, cottonseed, safflower, soy, and sunflower oils are mostly polyunsaturated. Although derived from plant sources, the tropical oils, palm and coconut, are highly saturated.

What is so harmful about fats?

Fats in themselves are not harmful; it's the high-fat diet typical of many developed countries that can cause problems.

Dietary fat is the body's most concentrated source of energy, supplying more than twice as many calories per gram (9) as carbohydrates (4) or proteins (4). Most of the fats in food are triglycerides, combinations of three fatty acids and glycerol (an oily alcohol); in addition, animal foods contain small amounts of the fatlike substance cholesterol (see *The Facts About Cholesterol,* pp. 20–21.) Triglycerides are broken down in the small intestine into glycerol and fatty acids. As fatty acids are absorbed from the intestine via the lymphatic system into the bloodstream, they facilitate the absorption of the fat-soluble vitamins A, D, E, and K. In addition, fatty acids from certain polyunsaturated fats are required for the growth and maintenance of body tissues and other vital functions.

Aside from its nutritional importance, fat enhances the texture and flavor of foods and creates a pleasant feeling of fullness. In other words, people like fat and tend to eat too much of it.

To maintain good health, however, you need only about 1 tablespoon of polyunsaturated fat a day and you don't need any saturated or monounsaturated fat. Unfortunately, most people consume much more than a tablespoon of fat a day, a habit that can have serious health consequences.

Protein, carbohydrates, and fat can all be converted into body fat, which is simply the form in which the body stores excess energy. But since dietary fat is such a concentrated source of energy, it is potentially the most fattening of the macronutrients. Dietary fat has also been implicated in two of our deadliest diseases: cancer and heart disease. Diets high in total fat have been linked with an increased risk of cancer of the colon, rectum, breast, or prostate, while diets high in saturated fat are associated with high levels of blood cholesterol, clogged arteries, and coronary heart disease.

Does this mean I have to limit my fat intake to a tablespoon of poly-unsaturated oil a day?

No. Major health organizations such as the National Cholesterol Education Program and the American Heart Association, as well as the *Dietary Guidelines for Americans,* recommend that you reduce your fat intake so that you derive less than 30 percent of your total calories from fat with less than 10 percent of your total calories coming from saturated fat. A combination of poly- and monounsaturated fats can supply up to 20 percent of your total calories, but polyunsaturated fats should supply no more than 10 percent of your caloric intake. In a typical American diet, about 37 percent of the calories come from fat, often at the expense of complex carbohydrates.

Some health professionals say that even lower levels of fat intake are needed to significantly reduce heart disease and cancer risk. They recommend that you get at most 20 to 25 percent of your calories from total fat with 6 to 8 percent from saturated fat. Others go so far as to recommend a diet in which less than 10 percent of calories are derived from fat. While the figures may differ, the consensus is clear: consume less fat in general and less saturated fat in particular.

Won't I lose important nutrients if I cut back on high-fat but nutrient-rich foods such as red meat and milk?

Some people worry that by reducing their intake of high-fat foods, they may be shortchanging themselves of nutrients found in those foods, such as the iron and B vitamins in meat and the calcium in milk. However, as long as a reduced-fat diet is varied and balanced, it carries little risk of nutritional deficiencies. If you are still worried, it may help you to know that many of the nutrients found in high-fat foods can also be obtained from low-fat or nonfat sources. Beans, grains, and leafy green vegetables, for example, are good sources of iron, if they are eaten with a food

THE FACTS ABOUT CHOLESTEROL

A white, waxy, fatlike substance, cholesterol is a naturally occurring component of cell membranes and nerve sheaths. It also plays a role in the manufacture of bile acids, steroid hormones, and vitamin D, and it helps transport fats in the bloodstream. Most of the cholesterol in the blood is made by the liver; some is absorbed directly from the cholesterol in food (eggs, shrimp, and organ meats are especially rich sources of dietary cholesterol). Whatever its source, cholesterol journeys through the bloodstream as part of "packages" called lipoproteins that also contain protein and triglyceride, the main form of body fat.

The dangers of cholesterol. When too much cholesterol is present in the blood, fatty deposits containing cholesterol tend to build up in artery walls, narrowing the blood vessels and restricting blood flow. When this process, known as atherosclerosis, occurs in an artery in the brain, the result can be a stroke; blockage in the coronary arteries may cause angina (chest pain) or a heart attack.

The lipoproteins that carry cholesterol in the blood come in several forms. Low-density lipoproteins (LDL's) contain large amounts of cholesterol. This is the "bad" cholesterol that helps to clog arteries and increases heart-disease risk. High-density lipoproteins (HDL's), by contrast, contain relatively small amounts of cholesterol and have the ability to remove cholesterol from cells. High HDL levels are linked to lower heart-disease rates.

Lowering cholesterol. Genes and diet both influence cholesterol levels. You can't alter your genetic heritage, but in most cases, a diet low in saturated fat and cholesterol will help keep your blood cholesterol levels down. Although eating too much cholesterol-rich food does raise blood cholesterol levels, the main culprit is saturated fat (pp.17–19). The specifics of a cholesterol-lowering diet vary, but in general, you should restrict fat intake to less than 30 percent of total daily calories; saturated fat, to less than 10 percent of total calories; polyunsaturated fat, to no more than 10 percent of total calories; and cholesterol, to less than 300 milligrams per day. (To calculate your daily fat quotas, see *Controlling Your Fat Intake,* p.18; for the role of exercise in lowering cholesterol, see p.102).

If your blood cholesterol levels are very high or if dieting does not lead to improvement within 3 months, your doctor may suggest a further reduction in your saturated fat intake to less than 7 percent of total calories and in your cholesterol intake to less than 200 mg daily. If this more restrictive diet fails to lower your blood cholesterol levels after 3 to 6 months, a cholesterol-lowering drug may also be prescribed. Although such drugs are effective, people taking them still have to stick to their diet.

Whatever it takes, bringing down high cholesterol levels is well worth the effort. Every 1-percent decrease in blood cholesterol results in a 2-percent drop in heart-disease risk. Even if your blood cholesterol levels are not elevated, following a diet low in saturated fat and cholesterol is still in the best interest of your heart and your general health.

ASSESSING CHOLESTEROL LEVELS

To help identify individuals at increased risk for heart disease, the National Cholesterol Education Program of the National Heart, Lung, and Blood Institute has classified levels of total cholesterol (measured in milligrams per deciliter of blood) as follows:
☐ Desirable, under 200 mg/dl
☐ Borderline high, 200–239 mg/dl
☐ High, 240 mg/dl and over.
   LDL levels are similarly classified:
☐ Desirable, under 130 mg/dl
☐ Borderline-high risk, 130–159 mg/dl
☐ High risk, 160 mg/dl and over.
   HDL levels under 35 mg/dl are also linked with increased heart-disease risk, as are unfavorable ratios of total cholesterol to HDL cholesterol. People with a total to HDL ratio below 3.5 have the lowest risk of heart disease. About 4.5 suggests an average risk; above 4.5, a greater-than-average risk.
   Although triglyceride's role in heart disease is still unclear, high blood levels of triglyceride often coincide with high LDL and low HDL levels. Borderline-high (250–500 mg/dl) and high (over 500 mg/dl) levels may also signal liver disease, diabetes, or alcohol abuse.
   Have your blood cholesterol levels tested regularly (see *Checking Your Cholesterol Levels,* p.23). If your numbers are borderline high or high, discuss with your doctor the lifestyle and dietary changes you need to make to bring down your cholesterol levels.

KEY

VLDL

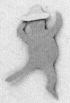

LDL

HDL

Triglyceride

Cholesterol

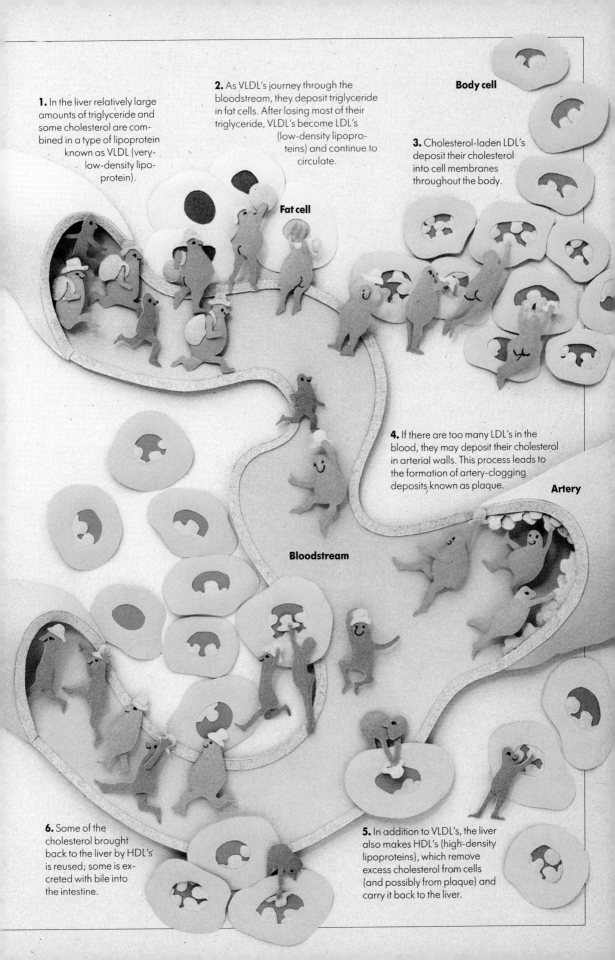

1. In the liver relatively large amounts of triglyceride and some cholesterol are combined in a type of lipoprotein known as VLDL (very-low-density lipoprotein).

2. As VLDL's journey through the bloodstream, they deposit triglyceride in fat cells. After losing most of their triglyceride, VLDL's become LDL's (low-density lipoproteins) and continue to circulate.

Body cell

3. Cholesterol-laden LDL's deposit their cholesterol into cell membranes throughout the body.

Fat cell

4. If there are too many LDL's in the blood, they may deposit their cholesterol in arterial walls. This process leads to the formation of artery-clogging deposits known as plaque.

Artery

Bloodstream

6. Some of the cholesterol brought back to the liver by HDL's is reused; some is excreted with bile into the intestine.

5. In addition to VLDL's, the liver also makes HDL's (high-density lipoproteins), which remove excess cholesterol from cells (and possibly from plaque) and carry it back to the liver.

rich in vitamin C to enhance iron absorption. Whole grains are good sources of B vitamins (except for vitamin B_{12}, which you can get from reduced-fat milk products). Skim milk has about the same amount of calcium—and protein—as whole milk.

Cutting back on fat does not mean doing without meat, milk, or other whole categories of food. Indeed, vegetarian and other diets that eliminate certain foods must be carefully planned and followed in order to avoid nutritional deficiencies (pp. 28–29).

Will quitting smoking help reduce my cholesterol levels?

It's very likely. Compared with people who don't smoke, smokers under age 60 tend to have higher levels of total cholesterol. And the more people smoke (or chew tobacco), the higher their cholesterol levels are. Smokers also have less desirable cholesterol ratios, with higher levels of triglycerides, low-density lipoproteins (LDL's) and very-low-density lipoproteins (VLDL's) and lower levels of high-density lipoprotein (HDL) cholesterol (see *The Facts About Cholesterol*, pp. 20–21).

Once smokers stop smoking, however, their total cholesterol levels begin to drop to the levels of nonsmokers. The HDL cholesterol levels of former smokers also rise slightly, improving their cholesterol ratios.

Scientists believe that nicotine somehow indirectly stimulates the liver to secrete VLDL cholesterol and triglycerides—yet another reason, if you needed one, to give up smoking.

Parents should note, too, that exposure to secondhand smoke at home has been shown to have adverse effects on children's cholesterol ratios.

FACT OR FALLACY?

If a food is labeled "cholesterol free," it can't raise your cholesterol level

Fallacy. Ads and labels can be misleading. While it is important to limit the amount of cholesterol in your diet, the major culprit in raising blood cholesterol levels is saturated fat (p. 17). Since only foods of animal origin contain dietary cholesterol, any food derived from plants by definition is cholesterol free. The trap is that some plant foods—the oils made from coconuts and palm kernels, for example—are high in saturated fat. Such tropical oils are often used in prepared foods because they are cheap and have a long shelf life. Foods containing tropical oils may be labeled "cholesterol free," but their high saturated fat content makes them undesirable in a low-fat diet. It pays to look beyond the hype and check food labels carefully for ingredients high in saturated fat.

My wife says shrimp, oysters, and other shellfish are high in cholesterol. Is this true? Should we avoid them?

Shellfish were once thought to have a high cholesterol content, but new methods of screening foods for cholesterol content indicate that the most commonly eaten mollusks—oysters, clams, scallops, and mussels—contain less cholesterol than red

meats do. Squid, conch, and periwinkle, however, do have high cholesterol contents. Among crustaceans, crabs are low in cholesterol; shrimp, lobster, and crayfish are high.

All shellfish, however, even those that are high in cholesterol, are low in saturated fat, and it's the saturated fat in a food rather than its cholesterol content that has the greater impact on blood cholesterol levels. (Shellfish are also a source of omega-3 fatty acids, which are thought to have a beneficial effect on cardiovascular health.)

To be prudent, limit your intake of shrimp and lobster to one serving per week. When planning menus, however, keep in mind that your blood cholesterol levels are influenced not so much by a single food or food category, but by your total diet, as well as by other factors such as your age, weight, and heredity.

Is it true that omega-3's in fish oils can lower cholesterol levels?

A number of health benefits have been associated with eating more omega-3 fatty acids, a type of polyunsaturated fat found mainly in fish, shellfish, and marine mammals. Among these benefits are reduced levels of triglycerides and VLDL cholesterol and a reduced tendency for platelets in the blood to clot, all of which translates into a lower risk of cardiovascular disease.

However, scientists are not sure whether the cardiovascular benefits attributed to omega-3 fatty acids actually result from the omega-3's themselves or from some other substance in fish. While the jury is still out on omega-3's, the benefits of eating fish are well established. Fish is an excellent low-fat source of protein, and the American Heart

Association recommends that you eat two to three servings of it a week. The fish with the highest omega-3 content include such commonly available species as mackerel, herring, salmon, albacore tuna, bluefin tuna, bluefish, and anchovy.

I'm not much of a fish eater. Should I take fish oil supplements?

Most medical experts question the long-term safety of consuming fish oil in the concentrated dose of a supplement. Although the blood-thinning property of omega-3 fatty acids may have cardiovascular benefits, too much fish oil can cause excessive bruising and bleeding. High doses of fish oil may also interfere with the metabolism of certain essential fatty acids and increase your need for vitamin E, an antioxidant (p.45). Some supplements contain added vitamins A and D, both of which can build up to hazardous levels in the body if too much is consumed. In addition, supplements are expensive, high in calories, and may contain cholesterol and possibly pesticides and toxins, which become concentrated in fish oils. For now, the best advice is to skip the pills and try to eat more fish.

I've heard that eating polyunsaturated and monounsaturated fats can reduce cholesterol levels. But shouldn't I be eating less fat?

You should definitely reduce your fat intake so that less than 10 percent of your calories come from saturated fat and less than 30 percent of calories come from the total fat in your diet. Your main goal, however, should be to reduce your consumption of saturated fat, the kind found pri-

CHECKING YOUR CHOLESTEROL LEVELS

First screening. Everyone age 20 and over and children over the age of 2 with a parent who has high blood cholesterol should have a blood test for cholesterol at least once every 5 years. (Anyone with a family history of heart disease should skip the screening test and have a lipoprotein analysis as described below.) If a simple blood test shows a total cholesterol count of 200 milligrams per deciliter of blood (mg/dl) or more, the borderline danger level, a doctor should arrange further tests a month or two later to confirm the reading and discuss treatment. Two readings give a truer picture than a single test because cholesterol levels in an individual fluctuate from week to week and can be skewed by viral infections, medications, pregnancy, or recent surgery, among other things. Another variable may be the lab work; not all laboratories meet the standards set by the Centers for Disease Control for analyzing blood samples.

Lipoprotein count. If your total cholesterol level measures above 200 mg/dl on two tests, or if you have a family history of premature (under age 55) heart disease, your doctor will probably order a lipoprotein profile to calculate low-density lipoprotein (LDL), high-density lipoprotein (HDL), and triglyceride levels in the blood (see *The Facts About Cholesterol*, pp.20–21). Blood for this test is drawn from a vein after you have fasted for 12 hours. (The test is often scheduled for early morning; eat dinner the night before and postpone breakfast until afterward.) If your LDL cholesterol is 130 mg/dl or more, and your risk for heart disease is high from heredity or obesity, for example, your doctor may recommend a low-fat diet as treatment. If your LDL reading is more than 160, drugs may also be considered. Keep records of your cholesterol measurements. Patterns over time are the best index of cholesterol levels and the best way to evaluate if diet changes are working.

marily in meat, eggs, and milk products. Some people accomplish this by replacing saturated fats with vegetable fats, which consist mostly of mono- and poly-unsaturated fats (pp.17–19). In diets in which the total calories derived from fat are kept the same, but mono- and polyunsaturated fats replace most saturated fats, blood levels of total and LDL cholesterol fall, thereby lowering the risk of heart disease. This may be why you've heard that adding unsaturated

fats to the diet is good for you. But the benefits of this tactic actually come from lowering the intake of saturated fat, not from increasing the consumption of unsaturated fats.

Another common myth about fat is that monounsaturated fats have a greater cholesterol-lowering effect than polyunsaturated fats, or vice versa. The advantage that either type of fat has over the other seems to be slight, and some studies suggest that there is no difference at all.

But there is evidence that consuming too much polyunsaturated fat (more than 10 percent of the total calories in your diet) increases your cancer risk.

If you want to reduce your fat intake, replace the saturated fats in your diet not with other fats but with complex carbohydrates.

The first thing I learned about nutrition was to eat from the "four basic food groups." Is this still recommended today?

The decades-old advice to eat from a variety of food groups is still valid. The only difference

is that the number of basic food groups, which has fluctuated over the years, is now five. Defined by the U.S. Department of Agriculture and the U.S. Department of Health and Human Services, the current food groups (shown below) represent the basic categories of food that

FOODS FOR A HEALTHY DIET

The five basic food groups are shown here along with the number of daily servings you should eat from each and, in parentheses, the recommended serving sizes. A sixth category is comprised of foods that should play only a restricted role in a healthy diet.

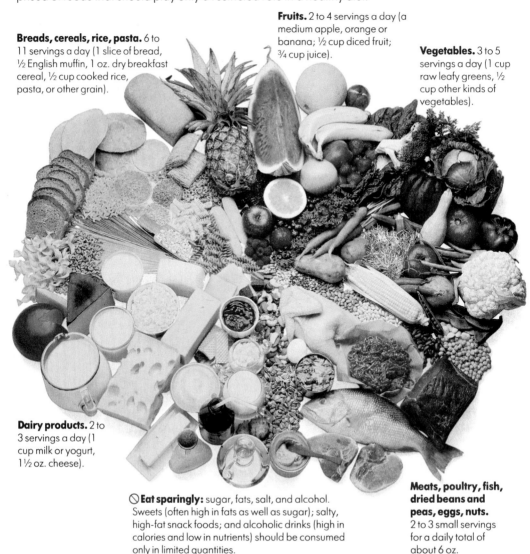

Breads, cereals, rice, pasta. 6 to 11 servings a day (1 slice of bread, ½ English muffin, 1 oz. dry breakfast cereal, ½ cup cooked rice, pasta, or other grain).

Fruits. 2 to 4 servings a day (a medium apple, orange or banana; ½ cup diced fruit; ¾ cup juice).

Vegetables. 3 to 5 servings a day (1 cup raw leafy greens, ½ cup other kinds of vegetables).

Dairy products. 2 to 3 servings a day (1 cup milk or yogurt, 1½ oz. cheese).

⊘ **Eat sparingly:** sugar, fats, salt, and alcohol. Sweets (often high in fats as well as sugar); salty, high-fat snack foods; and alcoholic drinks (high in calories and low in nutrients) should be consumed only in limited quantities.

Meats, poultry, fish, dried beans and peas, eggs, nuts. 2 to 3 small servings for a daily total of about 6 oz.

FOODS TO CHOOSE: LEAN MEATS

The U.S. Department of Agriculture classifies beef into three grades, based on its overall fat content. *Prime* has the most fat, *choice* is in the middle, and *select* has the least. Veal and lamb grades are the same except that the least fatty grade is called *good* rather than *select*. (The USDA inspects pork and poultry but doesn't grade their fat content.) Grading is voluntary, so nearly half of retail meat isn't graded. Inspect meat yourself (the white marbling in red meat is fat). All values below are based on a 3-ounce portion.

Type of meat	Total fat (grams)	Saturated fat (grams)	Cholesterol (milligrams)	Total calories
Beef and lamb				
Broiled beef tenderloin	8.5	3.2	71	179
Broiled beef top round	4.2	1.4	71	153
Roasted top round veal	2.9	1.0	88	127
Roasted lamb leg	6.6	2.3	78	162
Pork				
Broiled pork loin chop	6.9	2.5	70	165
Roasted pork loin roast	6.4	2.4	66	160
Broiled pork sirloin chop	5.7	1.5	78	156
Roasted pork tenderloin	4.1	1.4	67	133
Poultry (skinless)				
Roasted chicken breast	3.0	0.9	72	140
Roasted chicken thigh	9.3	2.6	81	178
Roasted turkey breast	2.7	0.9	59	133
Roasted turkey thigh	6.1	2.1	72	159

healthy people should eat every day for a balanced diet. The groups are vegetables, fruits, grain products, milk and milk products, and meat and meat alternates such as eggs, nuts, and dried beans. Eating adequate quantities from all these food groups ensures that you'll get all the nutrients you need for health.

The number of servings that a healthy person should eat every day from each of the food groups, according to the *Dietary Guidelines for Americans,* is also listed on the facing page. At first, the number of recommended servings may seem like an enormous quantity of food. But a serving as defined by the guidelines may be much smaller than your usual helping. It is not difficult to eat 3 to 5 servings of vegetables when a modest mixed green salad, several slices of tomato, or an ear of corn each constitutes a single serving.

The emphasis in the new guidelines is clearly on fruits, vegetables, and grains rather than on meat and dairy products. The serving suggestions are meant as a guide rather than a prescription. Skipping one group entirely for a day or so shouldn't be harmful if your overall diet is a healthy one. If you are concerned about whether your diet includes adequate amounts of food from each of the different food groups, keep a record of what you eat for 3 or 4 days, and then make changes accordingly.

I eat red meat four to five times a week. Is this unhealthy?

If you are in good health and if the rest of your diet is low in saturated fat, four or five small servings of lean red meat over the course of a week are probably not excessive. Concerns over

red meat (beef, lamb, pork, and game) stem from the fact that it contains a lot of saturated fat and cholesterol, which can raise your blood cholesterol levels. But red meat also supplies important nutrients, notably iron, zinc, complete protein, vitamin B_6, and vitamin B_{12}. As long as it's eaten in moderation, red meat can definitely contribute to a nutritious diet.

When buying meats, choose lean, trimmed cuts and grades (see chart, above). If you want to reduce your red meat consumption, try not to eat it every day. Substitute servings of skinless poultry, fish, or dried beans or peas for red meat on a regular basis. When you do serve meat, keep the portions small. Try to limit your daily intake of meat and meat alternates to the recommended 6 ounces. (A 3-ounce serving of lean red meat is about the size of a deck of cards.) Better yet, use meat as a side dish or a condiment, not as the main focus of a meal. For example, instead of steak accompanied by potatoes and salad, serve a pasta or vegetable dish containing a few ounces of beef or pork. Cut meat consumption slowly. This way, you'll be less likely to miss the meat.

I like dark meat on chicken. My husband prefers light meat. Which is better?

The only notable nutritional difference between light and dark meat on chicken is their fat content. The darker the meat, the higher its fat content, which also means that it is higher in calories. The dark meat on chicken thighs, drumsticks, and wings has more fat and calories than does the light meat on the breast. But even the dark meat on chicken, if served skinless, has less fat and fewer calories than many cuts of red meat.

Here are some tips for keeping the fat and calories low in chicken and other poultry dishes:
☐ Poultry skin is very fatty. Remove it before cooking or eating.
☐ Stick to the leanest types of poultry—broilers, fryers, Cornish game hens, and young turkeys. Eat fattier poultry—older birds (roasters, stewing hens, capons), domesticated duck, and goose—only occasionally.
☐ Look for free-range chickens at specialty meat stores and farmers' markets. Allowed to run free, they cost more but have less fat (and more flavor) than mass-produced chickens.
☐ A good way to reduce your intake of fat and calories is to substitute ground chicken or turkey for ground beef, pork or veal. Ground poultry that does not include dark meat or skin has even fewer calories and less fat.

THE FAT IN MILK AND MILK PRODUCTS

Food	Serving size	Fat (grams)	Total calories
Milk			
Whole (3.3% fat)	8 oz.	8.2	150
Low-fat (2% fat)	8 oz.	4.7	120
Low-fat (1% fat)	8 oz.	2.6	102
Skim (less than 0.5% fat)	8 oz.	trace	86
Buttermilk	8 oz.	2.2	99
Butter and cheeses			
Butter	1 pat	4	36
American process	1 oz.	9	105
Blue	1 oz.	8.7	105
Cheddar	1 oz.	9	115
Cottage (creamed)	4 oz.	5	117
Cottage (dry-curd)	4 oz.	4	97
Cottage (low-fat)	4 oz.	2	82
Cream	1 oz.	10	100
Mozzarella (part-skim)	1 oz.	5	72
Mozzarella (whole-milk)	1 oz.	6	80
Muenster	1 oz.	8.3	105
Parmesan	1 tsp.	1.4	23
Ricotta (part-skim)	4 oz.	10	158
Ricotta (whole-milk)	4 oz.	15	200
Swiss	1 oz.	8	106
Swiss process	1 oz.	7	95
Frozen desserts			
Ice cream (vanilla)	½ cup	12	175
Ice milk (vanilla)	½ cup	3	95
Frozen yogurt (vanilla)	½ cup	4	114
Yogurt			
Whole-milk (3.2% fat; plain)	8 oz.	7	140
Low-fat (1.5% fat; plain)	8 oz.	3.5	144
Nonfat (0.2% fat; plain)	8 oz.	0.4	127

I like the taste of whole milk better than that of skim or low-fat milk. Do I really need to switch?

Substituting low-fat or, even better, skim milk for whole milk is one way to cut your intake of calories, saturated fat, and cholesterol without losing the healthful nutrients that milk contains. The amount of milkfat required in milk is set by the FDA and ranges from at least 3.25 percent in whole milk to less than 0.5 percent in skim milk. Regardless of their fat content, all milks are good sources of calcium, protein, and riboflavin. Most milks are fortified with vitamin D, and reduced-fat milk has vitamin A added. These are good reasons to continue drinking milk.

You may find it easier to adjust to reduced-fat milk if you do it gradually, shifting from whole milk to 2 percent low-fat milk, then to 1 percent, and finally to skim. Note that 2 percent low-fat milk is sometimes called 98 percent fat free and 1 percent low-fat milk, 99 percent fat free. Adding a teaspoon of instant non-fat dry milk to a glass of skim milk improves flavor without significantly raising calorie and fat content. You can also substitute reduced-fat milk for whole milk in recipes, usually without any change in flavor or texture.

In changing your family's milk-drinking habits, however, keep in mind that children need whole milk until age 2; after that, give them low-fat milk, not skim. (For more information on children's nutritional needs, see page 43.)

What types of cheese are the lowest in fat?

With few exceptions, cheeses are high in fat, especially saturated fat. Depending on the particular type, half to three-quarters of the calories in cheese come from fat, approximately half of which is saturated. But cheese is also a concentrated source of protein, riboflavin, and, except for cottage cheese, calcium.

Cheese is made from milk heated with an enzyme or rennet to separate the milk solids from the liquid, or whey. The milk solids are usually salted and pressed, and if the cheese is to be ripened (aged), bacteria or molds are introduced. Among unripened cheeses, dry-curd cottage cheese has the least fat, less than even low-fat cottage cheese. Cream cheese, on the other hand, is very high in fat; when making spreads and dips, consider substituting lower-fat alternatives such as farmer or hoop cheese for cream cheese. But be careful when using part-skim ricotta and part-skim mozzarella; they are only about one-third lower in fat and one-tenth lower in calories than their whole-milk counterparts.

Most hard, ripened cheeses, such as cheddar, Swiss, and Parmesan, have a high fat content and should be eaten sparingly. The same is true of the pasteurized process cheeses, such as American or Swiss process cheese, which are blends of several cheeses. Pasteurized process cheese foods are also cheese blends, but they include other milk products and possibly emulsifiers and other additives. Process cheese foods have somewhat less fat than natural cheeses, but the level is still high.

From a nutritional standpoint, are all yogurts created equal?

No, they are not. Yogurt is widely considered a healthy food, but the nutritive value of the commercial products varies widely. In the United States, plain yogurt is made from whole, low-fat, or nonfat milk that has been cultured with the bacteria *Lactobacillus bulgaricus* and *Streptococcus thermophilus*. Some brands also contain the bacterium *Lactobacillus acidophilus*. These bacteria are harmless and, if alive, may even be beneficial. *Lactobacillus acidophilus,* for instance, is able to thrive in the intestine, where it seems to limit the growth of harmful bacteria. However, the other bacteria used in yogurt cultures rarely survive the passage through the stomach to the intestine.

Yogurt has essentially the same nutrients as the milk from which it is made. Whole-milk yogurt has about the same fat content as whole milk, while low-fat yogurt has less and nonfat yogurt practically none. To reduce tartness and add body, nonfat milk solids are often added to low-fat or nonfat yogurt, boosting the yogurt's calorie, protein, and mineral content. Yogurt sold with sugar-sweetened fruits or flavors has extra calories. (Adding your own fresh fruit to plain yogurt helps save on calories.) Of course, yogurts that are artificially sweetened contain significantly fewer calories than those sweetened with sugar.

Reading labels can help you find the yogurt you want. Look for the words *live cultures* on the label, and assume that a yogurt not marked low-fat or nonfat is made from whole milk.

Don't equate frozen yogurt with yogurt. Many frozen yogurts contain less fat than ice cream, but they are still high in calories from their sugar content. Most are mainly blends of milk, sweeteners, and stabilizers, and they lack live cultures in significant amounts.

Isn't buttermilk very high in fat?

No, despite its name and thick texture. Traditionally, buttermilk is the liquid left from churning butter. But commercial buttermilk today is low-fat or skim milk to which bacterial cultures are added to produce a thick texture and tangy flavor. Its calorie and fat content is about the same as 1 percent low-fat milk. It may or may not be fortified with vitamins A or D. If you are watching your sodium intake, be aware that buttermilk often has added sodium, about twice the amount found in milk.

Is margarine still considered better for you than butter?

In most cases, yes. Margarines that are made from polyunsaturated vegetable oils have no cholesterol and less saturated fat than butter, and are therefore better than butter for your health. Some margarines, however, are made from highly saturated oils and may contain lard. Even the "good" margarines have caused some concern because they contain polyunsaturated fats that have been hydrogenated, a process that partially saturates and solidifies fats. While studies show that consuming hydrogenated fats raises blood cholesterol levels, margarines do not consist exclusively of hydrogenated fats and thus should not raise cholesterol levels as much as butter does.

Margarine and butter have an equal number of calories (about 100 per tablespoon) and both are at least 80 percent fat (11 grams per tablespoon). Softer margarines are less hydrogenated and have fewer saturated fats. Liquid margarine (the type you squeeze from a bottle) has the least saturated fat, while hard stick margarine has the most.

When buying margarine, check labels and choose margarines made from oils highest in polyunsaturated fats (see *Controlling Your Fat Intake*, p.18); the first ingredient listed on the label should be a liquid oil. Or consider a reduced-calorie margarine, which is diluted with water in order to reduce its fat and calorie content by volume. Margarine may also be whipped with air for the same purpose.

My sister is lactose intolerant. Are there any milk products that she can eat?

Lactose intolerance is a reduced ability to digest the milk sugar lactose, due to a shortage of the enzyme lactase in the small intestine. The condition usually develops in early childhood and may get worse with age. An estimated 70 percent of people worldwide, primarily those of Asian, African, Mediterranean, and American Indian descent, are lactose intolerant. Symptoms include abdominal pain, gas, bloating, and diarrhea after drinking milk or eating other milk products that contain lactose. Some people who are lactose intolerant cannot consume any lactose at all, but most can eat moderate amounts of milk products with few or no problems. Lactose intolerance is not the same as being allergic to the protein in milk, a rare condition.

The simplest way to avoid the effects of lactose intolerance is not to drink milk or eat milk products. But because milk and its derivatives are a major part of the American diet and are good sources of calcium, vitamins A and D, and protein, there is an advantage in being able to consume them. Many individuals with lactose intolerance find that they can tolerate milk products in which bacteria have broken down most of the lactose; these include yogurt with live cultures and firm, ripened (aged) cheeses (but not buttermilk). Some people can tolerate milk products when they eat them in small amounts and with other foods. If you are lactose intolerant, you may want to try various milk products in small amounts to see which you tolerate best.

Most lactose-intolerant people can safely enjoy lactose-reduced milk, cottage cheese, and process cheese, which are sold in supermarkets and health food stores. Another way to overcome lactose intolerance is to add the enzyme lactase to milk or to take it as a tablet before consuming milk or its derivatives. Products such as Lactaid and Dairy Ease, which contain lactase in liquid or tablet form, are sold at pharmacies and health food stores.

I am thinking of becoming a vegetarian. How can I make sure that my meals are nutritionally sound?

As long as you plan your meals carefully, you can probably get all the nutrients you need from a meatless diet. How much planning and juggling of foods you'll need to do depends on the specific type of vegetarian diet you choose—and whether or not you stop eating eggs and milk products. There are three basic types of vegetarian diets:
☐ The strictest is the vegan diet, which eliminates not only meat but all foods that come from animals, such as eggs, milk, and milk products.
☐ A lacto-vegetarian diet includes milk and milk products in addition to foods that come from plant sources.
☐ A lacto-ovo-vegetarian diet includes milk products and eggs as well as plant foods.

Instead of becoming full-fledged vegetarians, many people are semivegetarians, occasionally eating fish and poultry but generally avoiding red meat.

As a vegetarian, you must make sure that you are getting complete protein. Unlike most animal proteins, plant proteins are incomplete, lacking one or more of the amino acids that your body needs to make and utilize proteins (pp.13,16). But you can overcome this problem by eating the right combinations of plant protein foods (see *Combining Foods for Complete Protein*, facing page).

If you eat few or no foods from animal sources, you also have to guard against iron deficiency. The body absorbs the iron in meat and other animal products more efficiently than it does the iron derived from plants or iron-fortified breads and cereals. You can increase the amount of iron that your body absorbs from a plant source by eating a food containing vitamin C at the same meal (see *A Guide to Vitamins and Minerals*, pp. 14–15). Vegetarian women of childbearing age and teenagers of both sexes should be especially careful about getting enough iron in their diets.

Only a small percentage of American vegetarians follow a strict vegan diet, but if you do, you need to guard against deficiencies of other vitamins and minerals usually derived from foods of animal origin. A lack of vitamin B_{12}, found only in animal sources, can seriously interfere with the production of red blood cells in the bone marrow, causing pernicious anemia. Vegans are often advised to take a vitamin B_{12} supplement or to eat soy products fortified with the vitamin. To make up for the lack of milk products, vegans should eat plenty of calcium-rich or calcium-fortified plant foods or take calcium supplements (p. 41). A vegan who does not get much sunshine may also develop a vitamin D deficiency, which can interfere with the body's ability to absorb calcium. A strict vegan diet can also result in low levels of zinc, a mineral the body needs for synthesizing protein.

Even if you do become a vegetarian, you still have to watch your fat intake, limiting it to less than 30 percent of total calories and keeping calories from saturated fat below 10 percent. This means restricting your intake of such high-fat foods as whole milk, cheese, eggs, nuts, and vegetable oils.

If you are worried about a lack of nutrients or a lack of balance in your vegetarian diet, see your doctor or a registered dietitian (p. 61). If you eat few or no animal foods, consider a blood test for iron deficiency or anemia.

COMBINING FOODS FOR COMPLETE PROTEIN

Plant foods by themselves provide incomplete protein that the body can't fully use, but when combined with a little meat, cheese, or milk—or with another plant food with complementary amino acids—plant foods pack protein as complete as that in steak. Some complete protein combinations are traditional in ethnic cuisines (like beans and rice in many Latin American countries). Although researchers say that adults can consume complementary amino acids within several hours of each other and not necessarily at the same meal, many such protein combinations are too tasty to split up.

- ☐ Beans (dried, cooked) and rice (white or brown)
- ☐ Lentils and rice
- ☐ Beans and corn tortillas
- ☐ Hummus (mashed chick peas and sesame paste) served on whole-wheat pita bread
- ☐ Peanut butter on whole-wheat bread
- ☐ Peanut butter on sesame bread or crackers
- ☐ Corn and lima beans
- ☐ Cereal with milk
- ☐ Macaroni and cheese
- ☐ Cheese sandwich
- ☐ Tofu (bean curd) and vegetables with rice
- ☐ Pasta and tomato sauce, with Parmesan cheese
- ☐ Cheese-stuffed pasta (ravioli or tortellini)
- ☐ Meatless chili with cheese
- ☐ Baked potato with yogurt
- ☐ Potato and egg salad
- ☐ Split-pea soup with whole-grain crackers
- ☐ Rice pudding

My wife and I follow a vegetarian diet. Can she safely stay on it while she's pregnant? Can we raise our children as vegetarians?

Although most people can safely eat a vegetarian diet, extra care is advised for children and pregnant or breast-feeding women, especially if their diet excludes most or all animal products.

Pregnancy and lactation increase a woman's need for calories and many nutrients (p. 42). In most cases, a pregnant or breast-feeding woman can meet these needs on a well-planned vegetarian diet, but she should consult her doctor about the best ways to ensure good nutrition.

Babies and young children need more protein per pound of body weight and more vitamins and minerals per calorie consumed than adults. Because plant foods are high in bulk and low in fat and calories, it may be difficult for vegan children to get enough calories and nutrients to meet their needs. Many experts urge vegan parents to give their children some animal foods, such as milk products or eggs. A child's vegan diet should be planned and supervised by a registered dietitian or pediatrician. Less-restrictive vegetarian diets have been shown to be healthy for children of all ages. Just make sure that a teenager's vegetarian diet supplies the extra calories and nutrients—protein, iron, calcium, and zinc—needed during this period of fast growth.

A GUIDE TO GRAINS

The seeds of cultivated cereal grasses, grains are a mainstay of human nutrition. They're naturally high in complex carbohydrates and fiber and low in sodium and sugar. Most are also low in fat and a good source of niacin, thiamin, riboflavin, vitamin B$_6$, and some minerals. Although grains do provide protein, it's incomplete protein (p.16), lacking certain essential amino acids.

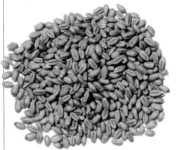
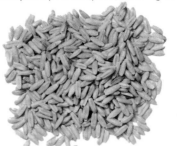
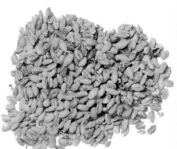

Wheat, the most widely cultivated grain, is sold in many forms including wheat berries, cracked wheat, bulgur, couscous, wheat germ, breakfast cereals, and the flour used to make bread, pastry, and pasta.

Oats are high in soluble fiber and contain better quality protein than wheat. A hearty breakfast food and ingredient in baked goods, oats are sold as whole kernels (groats), rolled oats (oatmeal), flour, and bran.

Barley is fermented to make beer and whiskey. Pearled (polished) barley is used in soups, salads, and side dishes; whole hulled barley is nutritionally richer than pearled barley, but is harder to find.

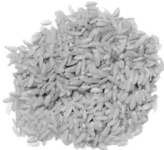
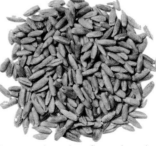
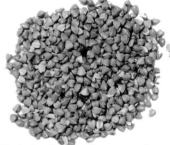

Rice is the staple food of more than half the world's people. Unpolished brown rice is more nutritious than white rice; converted white rice is treated to preserve nutrients. Instant rice is the least nutritious form of rice.

Rye is used mainly as flour in breads and crackers. Whole rye is nutritionally richer than rye from which the bran has been removed, but is harder to find. In general, the darker the rye flour, the more nutritious it is.

Buckwheat, an excellent source of protein, is not a true grain but is used as such. Unroasted buckwheat groats are ground into flour for breads and pancakes. Roasted groats (kasha) are used in soups, stuffings, pilafs.

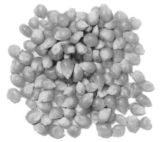
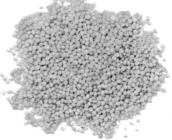
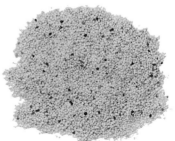

Corn is a New World gift to the global larder. Sweet corn is eaten as a vegetable. Field corn yields cornmeal, cornstarch, flour, hominy, corn syrup, cooking oil, and fodder. Unbuttered popcorn is a healthy snack.

Millet is used mainly as fodder and birdseed in the U.S.; it's also sold (usually in specialty food stores) either whole or cracked for use in soups and as a rice substitute. It's especially high in phosphorus, iron, and B vitamins.

Amaranth is a grainlike food native to Mesoamerica. It has more and better quality protein than most true grains, and is very rich in iron. It is sold in some health food stores as flour, whole grain, or breakfast cereal.

Are whole grains really healthier than other types of grains?

Whole grains are indeed a better choice than refined grain products, and to understand why, you need to look at the composition of grains. Grains—the seeds of cereal grasses—consist of three parts: the bran, or layered outer coating; the germ, the embryo of the new plant; and the endosperm, which feeds the germ. Each section contains different nutrients. The bran contains B vitamins, minerals, protein, and most of a grain's dietary fiber. The germ has fats, B vitamins, minerals, and protein. The endosperm, the largest section of a grain, is mostly starch, with some protein. A whole-grain product contains all the components of the grain. A refined-grain product consists mainly of the starchy endosperm. In removing the bran and germ, the refining process strips away most of the valuable vitamins, minerals, protein, and fiber in grains. Many people think that the grain's taste and texture deteriorate as well.

White flour and other refined-grain products are often enriched, a process that restores a few of the lost nutrients but not the fiber. Some grain products are labeled "fortified," meaning that they've had nutrients added to them which were not there to begin with. A fortified breakfast cereal, for example, contains added vitamins and minerals.

Is fiber as good for you as the media make it out to be? Or is it just another health fad?

It isn't just another food fad. A diet high in fiber—what our grandmothers called roughage—may help reduce cholesterol levels and prevent colon cancer (see *Disease-Fighting Foods,* pp. 44–45). Since fiber provides bulk and a feeling of fullness without excess calories, it can also help control weight. Eating too little fiber, on the other hand, may result in constipation, hemorrhoids, and intestinal disorders such as diverticulosis. A low-fiber diet tends to be high in refined carbohydrates and fats, promoting weight gain and heart disease.

The term *dietary fiber* does not refer to any single substance but rather to all the edible but largely indigestible parts of grains, fruits, vegetables, and legumes (dried beans, lentils, and peas). Fiber is resistant to human digestive enzymes and passes through the stomach and small intestine without being entirely broken down.

There are two principal types of fiber: soluble and insoluble. Most plant foods contain both, with proportions varying from food to food. Although a sure method of analyzing the fiber components of food has not yet been devised, oat bran, barley, beans, peas, apples, and citrus fruits are known to be good sources of soluble fiber (see *Foods to Choose: High-Fiber Sources,* p. 32). Soluble fiber does break down to a certain extent in the digestive tract, forming, among other by-products, fatty acids that are absorbed into the bloodstream and appear to play a role in lowering cholesterol levels. In addition, soluble fiber helps diabetics maintain lower blood glucose (sugar) levels.

Good sources of insoluble fiber include wheat bran, whole grains, vegetables, and fruits. Although insoluble fiber is not broken down at all as it passes through the digestive tract, it does have the ability to absorb large quantities of water—up to 15 times its own weight. This water adds bulk to fecal matter, helps it move through the digestive tract more quickly, and results in softer, easier-to-pass stools. It is the insoluble component of fiber that helps prevent or control intestinal problems. In addition, some experts believe that by reducing the amount of time fecal matter remains in contact with the intestinal lining, insoluble fiber plays a role in preventing colon cancer. However, there is no consensus on which fiber components (or other factors in a high-fiber diet) are responsible for the apparent cancer-preventive properties of fiber.

How much fiber should I be eating? What are some good ways to add more fiber to my family's diet?

The average American consumes about 12 grams of fiber a day, which most nutritionists agree is too little. The National Cancer Institute recommends that you eat about double that amount, from 20 to 30 grams of fiber each day. Building up the fiber content of your diet, however, takes a little planning. Start slowly; increasing your fiber intake too quickly can cause excess gas, bloating, and other intestinal problems. Also, since fiber absorbs water, remember to increase your fluid intake in order to prevent constipation.

Before you actually start adding fiber to your diet, you need to familiarize yourself with foods that are high in fiber (for examples, see *Foods to Choose: High-Fiber Sources,* p. 32). Then begin finding high-fiber alternatives for the foods that you already eat. For instance, substitute shredded-wheat cereal for puffed rice, whole-wheat bread for white bread, lentil soup for chicken noodle soup, and fresh, whole fruit for cooked fruit and fruit

FOODS TO CHOOSE: HIGH-FIBER SOURCES

To get a good mix of both soluble and insoluble fiber as well as a wide range of nutrients, eat fiber from a variety of sources—fruits, vegetables, and grain products. Experts recommend that you try to eat about 30 grams of fiber a day, but it's important to increase your intake of fiber gradually to avoid digestive problems.

Food	Serving size	Fiber (grams)
Cereals		
40 percent bran	1 oz.	5.3
100 percent bran	1 oz.	9.8
Oat bran	1 oz.	4.5
Rolled oats (dry)	1 oz.	2.9
Shredded wheat	2 biscuits	6.1
Other grain products		
Noodles (spinach)	1 cup	13.8
Popcorn	2 cups	2.4
Pumpernickel bread	2 slices	3.8
Rye bread	2 slices	3.1
Whole-wheat bread	2 slices	3.7
Fruits		
Apple (with peel)	1 medium	4.6
Apricots (dried)	3 whole	8.3
Dates (dried)	5 medium	3.1
Figs (dried)	3 medium	5.3
Nectarine	1 medium	2.2
Orange	1 medium	3.5
Pear (with skin)	1 large	5.2
Prunes (uncooked)	4–5 medium	3.5
Raspberries (fresh)	½ cup	4.4
Strawberries (fresh)	⅔ cup	2.9
Vegetables and dried beans		
Black-eyed peas (cooked)	½ cup	7.9
Broccoli (raw)	1 cup	4.3
Cabbage (cooked)	1 cup	4.0
Carrots (raw)	1 medium	2.3
Corn (cooked)	½ cup	3.1
Green peas (boiled)	½ cup	2.4
Kidney beans (cooked)	½ cup	13.0
Lima beans (cooked)	½ cup	6.1
Lentils (cooked)	½ cup	8.1
Potato (baked with skin)	1 medium	5.6
Spinach (cooked)	½ cup	2.0
Winter squash (cooked)	½ cup	2.8
Yam (baked with skin)	1 medium	3.5
Nuts and seeds		
Almonds (oil roasted)	1 oz.	3.1
Peanut butter	2 tablespoons	2.4
Peanuts (dry roasted)	¼ cup	2.9
Pistachio nuts	1 oz.	3.0

juice. In general, choose whole-grain, fresh, and unrefined foods instead of highly processed ones.

Here are some easy ways to increase the fiber content of your favorite recipes:

☐ Add wheat germ or bran to stews, soups, and casseroles.

☐ Use whole-wheat flour for part of the white flour in recipes.

☐ Bind meat loaves with oatmeal instead of white bread crumbs.

☐ When possible, eat the skins of fruits and vegetables.

☐ Add dried fruit and nuts to muffin and cookie recipes.

☐ Include cooked beans in salads and soups that you make.

☐ Occasionally substitute bean dishes for meat.

If fiber is so beneficial, should I start taking fiber supplements?

It's probably not a good idea for several reasons. Fiber pills and powdered supplements are widely sold as bulk laxatives or diet aids. However, not enough is known about the fiber components of food and how they work to be able to say with any certainty that you can get the health benefits of a fiber-rich diet from the concentrated and relatively pure fiber in a supplement. And while fiber may be good for you, it is possible to make too much of a good thing. In addition to causing gas and other intestinal problems, excessive amounts of dietary fiber can prevent your body from absorbing adequate amounts of some essential minerals. Because high-fiber foods tend to be bulky and filling, you're not likely to eat them in amounts that can cause mineral absorption problems. The same cannot be said for supplements.

The best way to get your fiber is from a diet that's low in fat and high in complex carbohydrates, not from pills or powders.

I have a problem with foods like broccoli, beans, and cabbage: flatulence. Any suggestions?

Flatulence—and sometimes bloating and diarrhea—is a common problem for people who aren't used to eating fruits, vegetables, dried beans, and other gas-inducing high-fiber foods. Gas in the large intestine is produced by bacterial fermentation of undigested food matter—often complex carbohydrates and sugars that the body can't digest because it lacks the enzymes needed to break them down. Not all high-fiber foods cause gas, nor is everyone affected by the same foods. And those who are troubled by a certain food may not be affected to the same degree.

If you want to increase your fiber consumption without developing a flatulence problem, add gas-inducing foods to your diet gradually. This gives intestinal bacteria time to adjust—a process that can take a few days. Instead of avoiding nutritious foods like broccoli, beans, and cabbage, try eating them in small amounts. You may digest dried beans more easily if you drain off the water they were soaked in and then boil them in fresh water. Discard the liquid canned beans are packed in.

There are a number of over-the-counter products designed to relieve intestinal gas, but their effectiveness varies from person to person. One such product contains an enzyme that digests some of the gas-making sugars in beans. Simethicone tablets appear to break up gas bubbles in food. Another option is activated-charcoal tablets taken with and after a meal.

Remember that excessive intestinal gas may also be a sign of lactose intolerance (p. 28).

HOW MUCH SODIUM DOES IT CONTAIN?

Food	Serving size	Sodium (mg)
Breakfast foods		
Biscuits (from mix)	1	262
Cornflakes	1 oz.	287
Pancakes (from mix)	3	480
Condiments		
Ketchup	1 tablespoon	156
Mustard	1 teaspoon	63
Salad dressing	1 oz.	171–598
Dairy products		
Cheddar cheese	1½ oz.	300
Cottage cheese	3½ oz.	229
Milk, low-fat (1%)	1 cup	128
Desserts		
Cherry pie	3½ oz.	304
Chocolate pudding (instant)	½ cup	440
Devil's food cake (frozen)	3½ oz.	420
Meats and fish		
Beef, corned	3½ oz.	1,740
Bologna	3½ oz.	540
Canadian bacon	3½ oz.	2,555
Frankfurter (raw)	3½ oz.	1,100
Tuna (canned in oil)	3½ oz.	800
Snack foods		
Mixed nuts (salted, dry roasted)	1 oz.	190
Potato chips	1 oz.	130–285
Pretzels	1 oz.	480–900
Vegetables and vegetable dishes		
Canned vegetables	3½ oz.	230–600
Dill pickle	1 medium	928
Vegetable juice cocktail (canned)	1 cup	883

How much salt is needed in the diet? Do I really have to watch my salt intake if my blood pressure is normal?

Common table salt, known chemically as sodium chloride, is the main source of sodium in our diets. Sodium is an essential nutrient required by the body to help regulate its fluid balance, maintain heart rhythm, conduct nerve impulses, and contract muscles. Although there is no Recommended Dietary Allowance (RDA) for sodium, the Food and Nutrition Board of the National Academy of Sciences has estimated that a safe minimum is 500 milligrams of sodium—about the amount in a quarter teaspoon of table salt. But given the American taste for salt and the prevalence of heavily salted processed foods in our diets, getting enough sodium is rarely a real problem. The average American consumes as much as 7,200 milligrams of sodium a day, far more than the body needs and more than twice the daily maximum recommended by the American Heart Association, which is only 3,000 milligrams of sodium—the amount contained in a teaspoon and a half of salt.

The relationship between salt intake and hypertension (high blood pressure) is complex and not fully understood. A number of studies have demonstrated a direct relationship between sodium consumption and the incidence of high blood pressure. In the majority of people, however, salt intake apparently has no effect on blood pressure. Only about 10 to 15 percent of people are actually "sodium-sensitive," meaning that consuming too much salt directly elevates their blood pressure.

Limiting salt intake is generally one of the lifestyle changes recommended for people with high blood pressure (for more on the treatment of hypertension, see pages 326–327). Many doctors, as well as the *Dietary Guidelines for Americans,* recommend that even people with normal blood pressure use salt only in moderation. Since hypertension is a major risk factor for cardiovascular disease and since there's no way to predict who will develop sodium-induced hypertension and who will benefit from a low-salt diet, it's better to be safe than sorry when it comes to eating salt.

My husband always salts his food before he even tastes it. Should I urge him to stop?

It's worth a try. First, salting food without tasting it is an insult to the cook, who may have given careful attention to the seasoning of the meal. And while many people can eat more than the recommended amount of sodium without developing high blood

FACT OR FALLACY?

Honey is a healthier sweetener than sugar

Fallacy. Honey contains potassium, calcium, and phosphorus, as advocates of the sweetener will tell you, but the amounts are insignificant. To meet the RDA for phosphorus, for example, you'd have to eat 40 cups of honey a day; for calcium, 47 cups; and for potassium, more than 5 cups for a man or 8 cups for a woman. Honey's main ingredients are fructose, glucose, and other sugars. To the body, there is no difference between these sugars and sucrose (table sugar). Honey delivers more calories per tablespoon (65) than white sugar (45) or brown sugar (50). It may also contain bacterial spores that can cause a potentially life-threatening case of infant botulism. For this reason, babies under a year old should not be given honey.

pressure, it's impossible to predict who will develop salt-induced hypertension. Certainly if your husband already suffers from high blood pressure, he should reduce his use of salt.

Only about 10 percent of the salt most people eat occurs naturally in foods; the rest is added during processing and manufacturing (75 percent) and during cooking or at the table (15 percent). The Diet and Health Committee of the National Research Council recommends eating fewer highly processed salty

foods, limiting the amount of salt added in cooking, and not adding salt at the table. Many people find that by gradually cutting back on salt they don't miss it, and in time they may even find heavily salted foods distasteful.

Table salt is basically a flavor enhancer. Lemon, vinegar, parsley, and a variety of other seasonings can play a similar role in the diet. Experiment with different herbs and spices in cooking and at the table to see which ones you and your husband prefer. But be aware that such flavorings as soy sauce, prepared mustard, and Worcestershire sauce are poor salt substitutes because they contain high amounts of sodium. Check the labels of condiments before buying them.

Commercial salt substitutes are safe as long as they are used in moderation. Consumed in excess, those containing potassium chloride can dangerously raise potassium levels in the blood, causing severe muscle weakness and even cardiac arrest; they can also be risky for people with kidney problems and some endocrine diseases. If you plan to use salt substitutes on a regular basis, check with your doctor first.

I'd like to reduce the amount of sugar I eat. What are some good ways of doing this?

You are right in wanting to limit your sugar consumption. When eaten in moderation as part of a balanced diet, sugar provides pleasure for the palate. On the negative side, however, sugar not only promotes tooth decay (p. 228), but when it is eaten in excess, the empty calories that sugar supplies can take the place of important nutrients in the diet. (For more on the dietary role of carbohydrates and sugars, see pages 16–17.)

Here are some tips on how to cut back on your sugar intake:

☐ Educate yourself about which foods contain large amounts of sugar and eat less of them, either by having them less often or by eating smaller portions.

☐ Read food labels carefully to find hidden sources of sugar. Avoid foods that list a sugar first or list a variety of different caloric sweeteners, such as corn syrup or fructose. (See *Deciphering Food Labels*, p.47.)

☐ Choose unsweetened breakfast cereals, and eat them with fresh fruit rather than sugar.

☐ Eliminate or cut back on sugared soft drinks. Substitute seltzer, club soda, unsweetened juices, or plain water.

☐ Serve fresh fruit or canned fruit packed in its own juice instead of dried fruit or canned fruit packed in syrup, which are both much higher in sugar.

☐ Save pastries and rich cakes for occasional treats only.

☐ Prepare sauces, puddings, cookies, cakes, pies, and other potentially sugary foods from scratch instead of buying commercial varieties or using mixes. In many cases, you can significantly reduce the amount of sugar and other caloric sweeteners in such foods without compromising on taste or texture. Experiment with spices and herbs such as vanilla, cinnamon, nutmeg, and ginger to retain flavor without adding lots of extra calories. Instead of frosting a cake, sprinkle a little powdered sugar on it.

☐ Gradually reduce the amount of sugar or honey that you put in coffee and tea.

☐ Don't keep candy and sweets around the house to nibble on.

☐ Don't reward children with sweets, and ask friends and relatives to respect your policy.

For a discussion of artificial sweeteners, see pages 53–56.

HOW MUCH SUGAR DOES IT CONTAIN?

Americans get a whopping 20 to 25 percent of their calories from sugar sources, including sugar, honey, and syrups added to food at the table; sweeteners used in processed foods; and naturally occurring sugars in fruit, vegetables, and milk. This chart compares the sugar content (in teaspoons) of a variety of foods; a teaspoon of sugar contains 18 calories.

Food	Serving size	Sugar (tsp.)
Angel food cake	2 oz.	6
Brownie (with nuts)	2" x 2" x ¾"	2
Doughnut (plain)	1	2
Pie (apple, cherry, pumpkin)	⅙ of a 9" pie	10–12
Chocolate bar	1 oz.	4
Chocolate fudge	1½" square	7
Chocolate milk	8 oz.	3
Eggnog	8 oz.	8
Thick milkshake	10 oz.	13
Ice cream	½ cup	4–5
Sherbet	½ cup	6–8
Frozen yogurt	½ cup	4
Yogurt (flavored, low-fat)	1 cup	4
Yogurt (with fruit, low-fat)	1 cup	9
Yogurt (plain, low-fat)	1 cup	3
Apple juice (unsweetened)	8 oz.	7
Apricots (dried)	4–6 halves	2–4
Dates	5	7
Figs	2	6
Fruit cocktail	½ cup	5
Orange	1 medium	3
Orange juice	8 oz.	6
Peaches (canned, in syrup)	2 halves	4
Prunes	5 medium	5
Raisins	¼ cup	6
Soft drink (carbonated, cola)	12 oz.	6–10
Soft drink (powdered)	8 oz.	4
Honey	1 tablespoon	4
Jam	1 tablespoon	3
Maple syrup	1 tablespoon	3
Tomato ketchup	1 tablespoon	1½

Do I really have to drink eight glasses of water a day to be healthy?

Water is essential to sustaining human life. Virtually every bodily function, from digestion and circulation to muscle contractions, depends on water. Without it, you could die within days. Water is also the body's most plentiful component. It makes up 75 to 85 percent of the body weight of an infant, about two-thirds that of an average young adult, and about half that of an elderly person.

The body's water level is regulated by sodium in the blood. In a healthy person, a rise in blood sodium levels triggers a sensation of thirst. It's possible, however, to satisfy a feeling of thirst long before the body's fluid needs are met. And even partial dehydration (lack of sufficient water) causes most body systems to function below peak levels. That's why health experts recommend that adults drink between six and eight 8-ounce glasses of water a day. Nursing women, athletes, and the obese may require more. And everyone's need for water increases in hot, dry weather.

If you're not used to drinking so much liquid, consider a gradual increase. Drinking more water is especially advisable if you urinate fewer than four to six times every 24 hours (unless the volume of urine each time is unusually large). An increased intake is also in order if your urine is sparse or dark-colored or if you have kidney stones. When you reach the level of water you need, the extra liquid will simply be excreted as urine.

You don't have to meet your fluid quota with water alone. Fruit and vegetable juices, non-caffeinated carbonated beverages, mineral waters, and low-fat milk are all good alternatives. Just be

FACT OR FALLACY?

Hot, spicy foods harm the stomach

Fallacy. There is no evidence that eating hot, spicy foods permanently harms the digestive tract. Hot peppers (cayenne, chili, jalapeño, and the like) contain a substance called capsaicin that makes the mouth burn, the eyes water, and the nose run. But studies in which animal and human stomachs and intestines were observed after ingestion of capsaicin showed no damage to the organ walls.

Countries like Mexico, Thailand, and India, where people traditionally eat a lot of hot peppers and spices, don't have higher ulcer rates than countries where hot peppers are not a staple of the diet. Research in India, for example, shows that members of households that consume lots of spices are no more likely to suffer from gastritis than members of families who don't.

sure to include their calories and nutrients in your overall diet counts; nondiet sodas and many fruit juices, for example, contain significant amounts of sugar. (Water has no calories.) Drinks with alcohol and caffeine are of limited value; they are diuretics that flush fluids from the body.

Severe dehydration can be life-threatening and requires immediate medical attention. Heatstroke (p. 443) and even death can result if as little as 10 percent of body fluids are lost and not re-

placed orally or through intravenous rehydration. Most at risk are babies, who need proportionally more fluid than adults and cannot communicate their thirst; the elderly, with their lower percentage of body water; people who are suffering from acute vomiting, diarrhea, or fever; and exercisers who perspire heavily.

Is it possible to drink too much water? What are the effects?

Under normal circumstances, fluids the body doesn't need are simply excreted. However, if this mechanism is impeded, or if your kidneys for some reason can't keep up with the demands placed on them, you can develop water intoxication. Excess fluid in the body dilutes the concentration of the electrolytes (sodium, potassium, and chloride) in the blood, preventing proper cell function and disturbing a variety of body processes. Symptoms are lethargy, weakness, and confusion, followed by convulsions, coma, and even death if the condition is not treated right away.

Water intoxication is rare. Candidates for the condition include anyone on a weight-loss diet that calls for a massive intake of water and other fluids.

How can I be sure my children are getting enough fluoride in our drinking water? Are there other sources?

Despite fluoridation's benefits to teeth (p. 291), an estimated 40 percent of the American water supply still receives what health experts consider inadequate fluoridation. The American Dental Association (ADA) suggests a range of water fluoridation from 0.7 to 1.2 parts per million (ppm) to protect against cavities. This level can be achieved either naturally (fluoride is a mineral present in small amounts in water and soil) or by adding fluoride to the water supply.

To find out the fluoride content of your water, contact your local water department or board of health. Then ask your dentist whether your children should take fluoride supplements, which are available at pharmacies.

According to the ADA, children age 13 and under who drink water with less than 0.7 ppm of fluoride may need supplements. Other sources of extra fluoride are fluoride toothpastes and dental rinses.

To protect against fluoride overdose (generally a harmless condition, although it may cause mottling of the teeth), the U.S. Public Health Service recommends that parents encourage children to use a small amount of toothpaste, not to swallow toothpaste, and to rinse carefully after brushing their teeth.

I think I'm drinking too much coffee. What's a safe caffeine limit?

It's hard to give a definitive answer, because the effects of caffeine on individuals vary; so does the caffeine content of foods (even from one cup of coffee to another). Caffeine is a central nervous system stimulant found in more than 60 plants, with coffee beans, cocoa beans, tea leaves, and the kola nut being the major dietary sources. In addition to occurring naturally in coffee, tea, cocoa, and chocolate, caffeine is added to many soft drinks and over-the-counter and prescription medications.

Caffeine is absorbed quickly and distributed throughout the body, reaching peak levels in the blood within 15 to 45 minutes. In most people, it increases alert-

HOW MUCH CAFFEINE DOES IT CONTAIN?

The caffeine content of a cup of coffee depends on the type of bean and how it was processed and brewed. Tea's caffeine content increases the longer it steeps. Besides the food items below, over-the-counter drugs (cold remedies, weight-loss drugs, and painkillers) are a common source of caffeine, containing up to 200 milligrams per pill; check their labels.

Item	Caffeine (mg)
Coffee (5-oz. cup)	
Regular, drip	60–180
Regular, percolated	40–170
Regular, instant	30–120
Decaffeinated, brewed	2–5
Decaffeinated, instant	1–5
Tea (5-oz. cup)	
Brewed, imported brands	25–110
Brewed, major U.S. brands	20–90
Iced (12-oz. glass)	67–76
Instant	25–50
Cola drinks and chocolate	
Cola drinks (12-oz.)	30–60
Baker's chocolate (1 oz.)	26
Chocolate-flavored syrup (1 oz.)	4
Chocolate milk (8 oz.)	2–7
Cocoa (5 oz. cup)	2–20
Milk chocolate (1 oz.)	1–15
Semisweet chocolate (1 oz.)	5–35

ness and reduces fatigue. Scientists believe that caffeine works by blocking adenosine, a compound that, in the brain, acts as a brake on stimulants. Caffeine perks you up by reversing the effects of adenosine.

In people who are sensitive to it or ingest a lot of it, caffeine can cause restlessness, anxiety, jitters, tremors, sleep disturbances, headaches, a temporary rise in blood pressure, rapid or irregular heartbeat, increased production of urine, upset stomach, or other unpleasant symptoms. Most people develop a tolerance to caffeine. Someone who normally doesn't take caffeine may become anxious and jittery after a single cup of coffee, while

a six-mug-a-day coffee drinker may feel no adverse effects. The current average daily level of caffeine consumption is about 200 milligrams (two to three 5-ounce cups of coffee, depending on the brewing method). The consensus among experts is that this level of caffeine intake is not harmful for healthy adults.

Judge your own caffeine tolerance by its impact on you. If you drink coffee or cola sodas and are restless, anxious, shaky, or have trouble falling asleep, it may be time to cut back on caffeine or eliminate it altogether. Reduce your intake gradually over a week or two to avoid withdrawal symptoms, such as headaches, lethargy, and drowsiness.

Coffee upsets my stomach. Would it help to drink decaf?

Unfortunately, switching to de-caffeinated coffee won't bring you relief. Coffee—with or without caffeine—triggers the secretion of gastric acid, which can cause stomach discomfort. Both coffee and tea (regular or decaf) also induce heartburn in some people and may irritate ulcers.

To minimize stomach upset caused by drinking coffee or tea, try eating some food with the beverage or adding milk to it. Most perked and instant coffees contain less acid and other irritants than coffee made by a drip process. To lower the acid content of tea, just reduce the time that you steep it.

Is it true that some decaf coffees contain harmful chemical residues?

Decaffeinated coffee does not contain chemical residues in appreciable amounts. One solvent used to remove caffeine from coffee, methylene chloride, caused some concern in the early 1980's when laboratory mice developed cancer after inhaling very large doses of the chemical for long periods of time. Methylene chloride is rarely used today to decaffeinate coffee, but the Food and Drug Administration still approves its use because virtually no solvent remains after decaffeinization. This is also true of ethyl acetate, an evidently risk-free solvent that has largely replaced methylene chloride.

If the thought of solvent in your decaf still bothers you, look for coffee decaffeinated by the patented Swiss Water Process, which does not involve the use of solvents. Decaf coffees labeled simply "water process," however, are made using solvent.

FACT OR FALLACY?

Coffee helps you sober up and can cure a hangover

Fallacy. Drinking coffee (or any caffeinated beverage) after imbibing may make you feel less tired and sleepy at first, but it won't alter how much alcohol is in your blood or the alcohol's effect on your nervous system. Your alertness, reaction time, and motor coordination may all be impaired until your body metabolizes the alcohol. Caffeine exacerbates the fatigue, upset stomach, and dehydration of a hangover. It postpones the sleep you need, aggravates indigestion, and acts as a diuretic, drawing needed fluids out of your system. To combat a hangover, water, juice, and milk are better choices than coffee.

Cutting caffeine out of your diet can cause headaches

Fact. If you're used to consuming a regular amount of caffeine from coffee, tea, or cola, your body may react to the sudden absence of the stimulant with withdrawal symptoms such as nausea, irritability, lethargy, and headache. Doctors believe that the headache that strikes many patients after surgery is due to caffeine withdrawal rather than to the anesthetic or the operation. If you want to cut back on caffeine, do it gradually.

I enjoy drinking herbal teas. Are there any health risks?

In most cases, no. Although many of the compounds in herbs have not been extensively tested for safety, most packaged herbal teas are unlikely to be harmful if they come from a reputable food manufacturer and are consumed in moderation—about one or two cups a day.

The Food and Drug Administration has banned the sale of a few dangerous herbs as food or food additives. These herbs are coumarin from tonka beans, sweet flag (calamus), and sassafras. Some other commonly available herbs are best avoided in teas. Coltsfoot and comfrey may be carcinogenic if taken in large amounts over a long time. Drinking too much European pennyroyal tea may cause convulsions. In large doses, goldenseal can be poisonous and senna, buckthorn, and aloe can have a strong laxative effect. Chamomile and yarrow may produce an allergic reaction in people who are allergic to ragweed, goldenrod, and chrysanthemum.

When trying a new herbal tea, start with a small amount of a weak brew and wait a few days to see if you have a reaction before increasing your intake or the strength of the brew. Unless you know herbs well, never collect herbs for tea yourself; some toxic plants closely resemble common herbs. Don't use herbal teas as a substitute for medical care, and never drink herbal teas if you are taking medications.

Can I safely consume any alcohol if I'm going to be driving?

It's not safe to drink before you drive or while you drive—not even beer or wine. In most states, you are legally drunk if your blood alcohol content is measured at 0.1 percent (1 part alcohol for every 1,000 parts blood) or more. There is no simple standard for safe drinking because so many factors influence how quickly alcohol gets into your bloodstream, including your sex, weight, body-fat composition, prior drinking experience, and the amount of food in your stomach. A 200-pound man who drinks regularly and has just eaten a full meal might be able to have a beer without becoming intoxicated, whereas a 110-pound woman with little or no prior drinking experience who hadn't eaten in 6 hours probably could not. In addition, the effects of alcohol on reaction time, judgment, and other factors affecting safe driving vary among individuals. Studies have shown impairments at blood alcohol levels of 0.04 percent and less.

If you have been drinking and need to get somewhere by car, do not drive. Have someone else do the driving, call a cab, or take public transportation.

Is nonalcoholic beer a safe alternative for pregnant women and recovering alcoholics?

Not necessarily. Legally, only products labeled "alcohol free" are required to contain no alcohol at all. Nonalcoholic beverages may contain up to 0.5 percent alcohol. By comparison, most domestic beer contains about 4.5 percent alcohol by volume, and wine about 12 percent.

For most people, 0.5 percent alcohol is a negligible amount, and it is unlikely that the traces of alcohol in nonalcoholic beer could harm a fetus. (Natural fermentation in bread can bring its alcohol level up to 0.5 percent.) However, since the results

FACT OR FALLACY?

Chocolate has special mood-altering powers

Fallacy. Links between chocolate and emotion have been suspected for centuries but remain unproven. Researchers in the mid-1980's studied people who claimed to use chocolate and other sweets to lift their spirits. Although the subjects were found to share certain personality traits—they were moody, quick to fall in love, and dependent on the approval of others—the study did not actually test chocolate's mood-altering powers.

Chocolate contains a substance called phenylethylamine (PEA), which also occurs naturally in the brain and may play a role in emotional arousal. Some experts speculate that it's the PEA in chocolate that causes certain people to crave it when a romance ends. However, it has not been proven that the PEA in chocolate actually reaches the brain. Chocolate also contains caffeine but not enough of it to affect most people. Another stimulant in chocolate, theobromine, may elevate mood, but only mildly. The carbohydrates in chocolate foods may have a calming effect on some people, while others find chocolate soothing simply because it's a comfort food, associated with happy childhood memories.

of studies on safe alcohol consumption during pregnancy have been inconclusive, pregnant women may want to refrain from drinking even such a small amount of alcohol.

Recovering alcoholics should definitely exercise caution with nonalcoholic wines and beers. Some experts feel that a product that mimics the taste and other appeals of alcoholic beverages can lead a recovering alcoholic back to drinking, and that he or she would be better off sticking to fruit and vegetable juices, soft drinks, and water.

Can drinking increase my risk of cancer? Is there a safe level for alcohol consumption?

Chronic heavy drinking is linked with an increased risk of cancer of the mouth, throat, esophagus, liver, pancreas, and rectum. The risk of mouth, throat, or esophagus cancer is heightened if a heavy drinker also smokes. But scientists have not established a level of alcohol consumption that increases cancer risk significantly, nor do they know whether alcohol causes cancer directly.

Several studies have suggested that women who consume alcohol even moderately (according to one study, as few as three drinks a week) have a higher risk of developing breast cancer than women who don't drink, but other studies don't fully agree with these findings and no clear cause-and-effect relationship between breast cancer and alcohol consumption has been found. Women who have had breast cancer or have a family history of it should consider avoiding or at least limiting their consumption of alcohol.

For more on the potential impact of heavy drinking, see *Alcohol and Your Health,* p.163.

Is it true that moderate drinking guards against heart disease?

Various studies have suggested that healthy men and women who drink moderately have a lower risk of developing heart disease and dying from a heart attack than abstainers. Two of the most important studies on this subject were conducted at the Harvard School of Public Health. In a 5-year survey of 50,000 men, 40 to 75 years old, those who drank more than 5 grams but less than 30 grams of alcohol a day lowered their heart disease risk by about 25 percent compared with men who drank less than 5 grams or drank nothing. (A drink generally contains from 11 to 15 grams of alcohol, so 5 to 30 grams represents from a half drink to two or three drinks.) The other Harvard study showed similar results in women who consumed three to nine drinks a week. Keep in mind, however, that having more than two or three drinks a day is not healthy for most people's hearts and may raise blood pressure.

Does alcohol have any nutritional value?

Alcohol contains traces of vitamins and minerals, but its nutritional contribution to the diet is negligible. Beer, for example, is a relatively poor source of carbohydrates compared with fruit juice. And wine contains small amounts of niacin, riboflavin, iron, calcium, and potassium, but richer sources of these nutrients are found in foods.

Because of its low nutritional content, alcohol is often described as providing "empty" calories, but this doesn't mean they are few in number. Pure alcohol contains 7 calories per gram— fewer than fat but more than car-

bohydrates and protein. You can calculate the approximate caloric content of a hard liquor drink by multiplying the proof by the number of ounces and then by 0.8 (thus 2 ounces of 80-proof hard liquor contains about 128 calories). For wine and beer, multiply the alcohol percentage by the number of ounces and then by 1.6 (6 ounces of 12 percent wine contains about 115 calories). Mixers such as nondiet ginger ale add more calories. If you are trying to control your weight, consider that for the same 150 calories in a can of beer, you could eat a medium-size baked potato, about 2½ ounces of broiled, trimmed sirloin steak, or 2 slices of whole-grain bread.

I've heard that drinking can block absorption of nutrients. How does this happen, and which ones are blocked?

Alcohol consumption may impair the absorption of some nutrients, but there is no evidence that people who drink moderately have a poorer nutritional status than those who don't drink. Most moderate drinkers do not replace nutrient-rich foods with alcohol. A moderate drinker who wants to lose weight, however, risks a nutritional problem if he sharply reduces his food intake but continues to drink. A much better plan would be to give up alcohol altogether for the duration of the diet or limit consumption to an occasional drink.

Chronic heavy drinking, on the other hand, does have a serious impact on how the body absorbs, uses, and stores food. Alcohol is metabolized by the liver, a process that takes precedence over other liver functions and interferes with that organ's effectiveness in processing nutrients. For example, in a chronic heavy

drinker, fat is stored in the liver instead of being metabolized efficiently. As a result, the liver grows larger and its ability to metabolize many vitamins and minerals is impaired. Damage to the pancreas, stomach, and gastrointestinal tract due to chronic heavy drinking may also hinder the absorption of nutrients.

Vitamin and mineral deficiencies—particularly of magnesium, calcium, phosphorus, zinc, pyridoxine, thiamine, riboflavin, niacin, folic acid, and vitamins A, C, and D—have been noted in alcoholics. In most cases, such deficiencies result from a combination of poor nutrition and alcohol-related problems with metabolism and nutrient absorption. Special high-calorie, nutrient-rich diets, along with nutritional counseling, are usually part of alcoholism recovery programs.

Many people I know take vitamin pills. Are such supplements really necessary?

According to nutrition experts, people who eat a balanced, varied diet with adequate calories do not need supplements. Exceptions to this rule are pregnant women and nursing mothers, who may be counseled to take a vitamin and mineral supplement, and infants, who may need additional iron, vitamin D, or fluoride. Even though nutritional deficiencies are rare in the United States, surveys show that about 40 percent of American adults regularly take supplements "just in case" their diets lack anything. In doses less than the U.S. Recommended Daily Allowances, supplements aren't harmful and may help protect against deficiencies in children, teenage girls, the elderly, dieters, certain vegetarians, smokers, heavy drinkers, people with low incomes, and others whose diets may sometimes fall short of optimum nutrition.

Even if you are in one of the higher-risk groups, however, your first line of defense against deficiencies should be improving your diet rather than relying on supplements. If you do choose to take supplements, look for a multivitamin and a multimineral product with a variety of nutrients. A pill containing just a few vitamins won't benefit you if what your diet chiefly lacks is potassium or some other mineral. In addition, keep these facts in mind:

□ Supplements are just what their name implies. They are not intended to replace an adequate diet. People who rely on pills to supply their nutritional needs may develop deficiencies anyway, since supplements do not deliver all the nutrients or calories contained in foods.

□ Taking too many supplements can be a health hazard. High doses of some vitamins and minerals can interfere with the absorption and utilization of others. The fat-soluble vitamins A, D, and E, which accumulate in body fat, can reach toxic levels if consumed in excessive amounts; the result can be a wide range of symptoms, including headache, irritability, dizziness, nausea, and vomiting. Some other vitamins and most minerals are potentially harmful when taken in multiples of their U.S. RDA. For example, women who take large amounts of vitamin B_6 to relieve premenstrual discomfort have suffered nerve damage and numbness in their hands and feet. If a supplement causes unusual symptoms, discontinue using it and notify your doctor.

□ Supplements can put a dent in your budget, yet unless you have a deficiency, they may be of little benefit to your health. The high levels of vitamins and minerals in

some supplements are poorly absorbed, and if a vitamin or mineral is water soluble, your body will simply excrete whatever it does not need.

□ More expensive "natural" supplements (derived from plant and animal sources) are no better than synthetic ones; in fact, your body can't tell the difference between the two types.

My brother is taking amino acid supplements to build his muscles. I'm concerned because I've read that they can be harmful. Are they?

The Food and Drug Administration removed amino acid supplements from its list of substances that are "generally recognized as safe" in 1974 because of potentially harmful side effects. In 1990, the manufacturers of supplements of the amino acid L-tryptophan, taken to treat premenstrual symptoms, insomnia, and depression, voluntarily withdrew these products from the market after they were linked to hundreds of cases of eosinophilia myalgia, a sometimes fatal blood disorder. But other amino acids are still available, as single supplements and in protein compounds sold as muscle-builders.

The body needs amino acids in certain proportions in order to make proteins (p.13). By taking a dietary supplement of a single amino acid, you disturb this balance, making it difficult for your body to utilize amino acids from food sources. In addition, pure amino acids have been known to drastically lower blood pressure and blood sugar levels, and they react adversely with certain medications. Amino acid supplements are expensive, and even those that don't cause harm do not seem to confer any health benefits.

Prescription drugs containing amino acids do have legitimate medical uses—for example, to supplement the special nutritional needs of people with liver or kidney disease. Such drugs are legal only if prescribed by a doctor.

Should all women, even young ones, take calcium supplements?

Women, in particular, are at risk of developing osteoporosis, or loss of bone mass, later in life if they don't get enough calcium beginning in their formative years. Although it's better to get calcium from milk, milk products, and other food sources rather than from supplements, surveys indicate that the diets of many people—especially teenage girls, women, and the elderly—are lacking in calcium.

The Recommended Dietary Allowance for calcium for women aged 25 and over is 800 milligrams; the National Institutes of Health and other health organizations recommend an even higher intake: about 1,000 milligrams a day for premenopausal women; about 1,500 milligrams a day for postmenopausal women. Yet according to a national survey by the U.S. Department of Agriculture, most women consume only about 600 milligrams of calcium per day. Unfortunately, a calcium deficiency may not be detected until osteoporosis has reached an advanced stage. Anyone who is not getting sufficient dietary calcium—especially women and people who are lactose-intolerant (p.28)—should consider taking a calcium supplement. For a comparison of the different types of calcium supplements available, see *The Facts About Osteoporosis*, pp.378–379. For good food sources of calcium, see *A Guide to Vitamins and Minerals*, pp.14–15. Although consuming an excessive amount of calcium is not a problem for most people, do not take calcium supplements if you have a tendency to develop kidney stones or if your blood levels of calcium are abnormally high.

A friend of mine takes a daily iron supplement to give him "pep," he says. How much iron do we need, and is it a good idea to take a daily supplement?

The Recommended Dietary Allowance for iron is 10 milligrams for adult men, 15 milligrams for women 50 years and younger, and 10 milligrams for women 51 years and older. For most people, a balanced, varied diet provides more than enough iron, and supplements are neither necessary nor recommended. However, iron-deficiency anemia is one of the few nutritional deficiencies still seen in the United States (for good food sources of iron, see *A Guide to Vitamins and Minerals,* pp.14–15). The individuals most at risk are infants, children, adolescents, vegetarians, and women who are pregnant or who menstruate heavily. For these groups and others who may not be able to meet their iron needs through diet alone, iron supplements may be advisable.

Supplements should be taken only on a doctor's recommendation. Self-supplementing without a diagnosis of iron deficiency or iron-deficiency anemia is unwise because the underlying causes of a person's symptoms (your friend's lack of "pep," for instance) may go untreated. Although consuming up to 75 milligrams of iron a day is usually not harmful to healthy adults, higher doses can be dangerous, and children can be poisoned or

die if they take iron supplements intended for adults. In some people, iron supplements cause diarrhea or constipation. For some 1 million Americans who have hemochromatosis, a genetic disease in which the body absorbs too much iron, taking iron supplements can lead to severe damage of the liver and pancreas, arrhythmia, and heart failure.

Even if you are taking iron supplements, don't neglect dietary methods of increasing your iron intake: eat foods rich in iron, cook in cast-iron cookware, and accompany iron-rich foods with a source of vitamin C (vitamin C facilitates iron absorption). Several different ferrous compounds are sold as iron supplements. They do not differ significantly in terms of absorbability or side effects.

I've just become pregnant. Should I start "eating for two"?

You don't need to double your food intake, but you do need to consume more calories and gain weight. Most obstetricians recommend that a woman of normal weight carrying one baby gain between 25 and 35 pounds over the course of the pregnancy: 2 to 4 pounds during the first trimester and about a pound a week during the second and third trimesters. You will need to gain more weight if you are underweight and less if you are overweight; ask your doctor or midwife what weight gain would be most appropriate for you. Insufficient weight gain during pregnancy is associated with low birth weight in the infant, who may have long-term health problems and reduced mental abilities as a result.

To gain weight during pregnancy, you will need to increase your normal food intake by about

300 calories a day (especially during the second and third trimesters). But rather than trying to gain a certain amount of weight, your goal should be to eat healthily throughout the pregnancy. It's important to eat a varied, nutrient-rich diet to meet the nutritional demands of your developing child as well as your own increased requirements during pregnancy. You don't need any special foods, but take care not to skip meals or restrict your fluid and salt intake.

The American College of Obstetricians and Gynecologists recommends that pregnant women eat the following every day (for serving sizes, see *Foods for a Healthy Diet,* p.24):
☐ Four or more servings of fruits and vegetables.
☐ Four or more servings of whole-grain or enriched breads, cereals, or other grain products.
☐ Four or more servings of milk and milk products.
☐ Three or more servings of meat, poultry, fish, eggs, nuts, or dried beans and peas.

Healthy eating during pregnancy also prepares you for the demands of breast-feeding, when your needs for calories, fluid, and many nutrients are even greater than during pregnancy. Your doctor or a registered dietitian can give you more specific recommendations on what foods to eat while you're pregnant or breast-feeding. (For more on staying healthy during pregnancy, childbirth, and the postpartum period, see pp.258–265.)

My friend says smokers need more vitamin C. Is this true?

Getting enough vitamin C seems to be a special problem for smokers. Regardless of age, sex, and other characteristics, smokers have lower levels of vitamin

GETTING CHILDREN TO EAT RIGHT

To foster good eating habits in your children, make meals pleasant and well balanced, keep nutritious snacks in the house, and don't use food as a bribe or a substitute for attention. Parents sometimes create eating problems in their children because they fail to understand the eating patterns of children at various ages. The guidelines below can help you lay the groundwork for a lifetime of healthy eating.

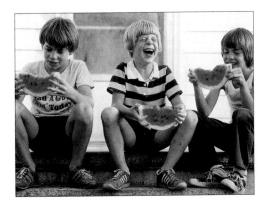

Preschoolers who are offered a variety of nutritious foods will, over the course of a week, take in all the calories and nutrients needed for healthy growth—as long as meals haven't become a battleground. Try not to make an issue of a toddler's picky eating habits. Have young children eat (or not eat, as the case may be) with the family, but don't insist that they finish anything they don't like.

If your child's weight concerns you, consult your pediatrician. To avoid weight problems, some parents give toddlers too few calories and too little fat. Children under age 2 need proportionally more fat than adults; at age 2, a diet that limits calories from fat to 30 percent of total calories (see *Controlling Your Fat Intake,* p.18) can be phased in gradually.

Snacks can be a good source of nutrients for young children. Time healthy snacks (p.61) to supplement, not replace, meals.

Busy teenagers often miss meals and then fill up on high-fat snacks. Encourage older children to eat with the family by being flexible about meal schedules. Stock the pantry with healthy snacks they can take with them. Some teens skip meals because they become obsessed about losing weight and are drawn to fad diets. In rare cases, a preoccupation with weight loss can lead to eating disorders (p.177). Parents can help by taking their child's concerns about weight seriously and offering healthy, low-calorie meals.

Weight control. Children should diet to lose weight only under medical supervision. Growing preteens rarely need to lose weight; at most they may have to be placed on a program to control weight gain. Overweight teenagers may benefit from a doctor's objective advice about choosing low-fat foods and burning more calories through exercise. Parents should be alert to a child's use of food to meet emotional needs. When food becomes a psychological crutch, professional counseling may be in order.

C in their blood than do nonsmokers. This may be due in part to smokers' eating habits. Some studies show that smokers consume less vitamin C than do nonsmokers. However, even when a smoker's vitamin C intake is the same as that of a nonsmoker, the smoker still ends up with less vitamin C in his blood; why this happens is not fully understood. Smokers whose vitamin C intake is low may even risk developing a vitamin C deficiency.

As a result of such findings, the National Research Council recommends that smokers get at least 100 milligrams of vitamin C a day, more than the Recommended Dietary Allowance of 60 milligrams for adults. A 1991 study suggests that smokers need more than 200 milligrams daily to prevent signs of deficiency.

Smokers also tend to consume less beta carotene (which is converted to vitamin A) than do nonsmokers—a disadvantage since diets low in beta carotene are associated with a higher incidence of lung cancer (see *Disease-Fighting Foods,* pp.44–45).

By far, the best way to overcome a vitamin shortage associated with smoking is to quit. Taking a vitamin supplement isn't going to compensate for the harmful effects of smoking. But if you can't quit, then eating more foods rich in vitamin C and beta carotene and possibly taking a supplement may be in order.

DISEASE-FIGHTING FOODS

Although it is only one of many factors, diet may affect your chances of getting cancer or coronary heart disease. The diet typical of the United States and other industrialized nations has virtually eliminated diseases caused by nutritional deficiencies, but the high saturated-fat content of that diet is known to have detrimental effects on health. While eating a varied, balanced diet does not guarantee that you will never develop cancer or heart disease, it may well cut your risk. Certain categories of food, such as cruciferous vegetables and foods rich in beta carotene, have an especially strong protective effect.

EATING TO REDUCE YOUR CANCER RISK

By some estimates, about one-third of cancer deaths may be related to diet. The following recommendations, based on those of the American Cancer Society and the National Cancer Institute, may help to reduce your risk:

☐ Avoid obesity. It's associated with an increased risk for cancers of the uterus, ovary, gallbladder, kidney, colon, and breast.

☐ Cut total fat consumption (see *Controlling Your Fat Intake,* p.18). Excess fat intake may raise the risk of breast, colon, and prostate cancer.

☐ Eat more high-fiber foods (see *Foods to Choose: High-Fiber Sources,* p.32).

☐ Eat a variety of vegetables and fruits, especially cruciferous vegetables and foods rich in beta carotene and vitamin C.

☐ Limit your intake of salt-cured, nitrite-cured, and smoked foods. Nitrites and nitrates in cured foods can be converted into carcinogenic nitrosamines during cooking or in the body. The incidence of stomach and esophageal cancers is higher in countries where cured foods are eaten regularly.

☐ Moderate your alcohol consumption. Heavy drinking increases smokers' cancer risk; among both smokers and nonsmokers, heavy drinking is associated with a higher risk of cancers of the mouth, throat, esophagus, liver, and possibly breast.

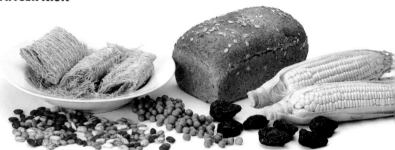

Fiber. Populations whose diets are high in fiber generally have a low incidence of cancer, particularly colon cancer. Insoluble fiber (p.31) is considered especially anticarcinogenic because it adds bulk to the stool and helps speed its passage through the bowel, thereby reducing the colon's exposure to potentially harmful substances in the stool. Whole grains, dried beans, and many vegetables are good sources of fiber.

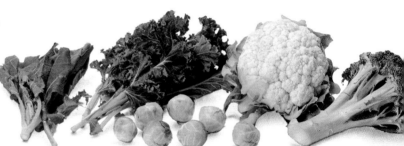

Cruciferous vegetables. Named for the characteristic cross made by the four petals in their flowers, these cabbage family vegetables include broccoli, brussels sprouts, cauliflower, collard greens, kale, kohlrabi, and mustard greens, as well as cabbage. They contain compounds called indoles, isothiocyanates, and flavones that seem to offer protection against lung, gastrointestinal, and other cancers.

ANTICANCER COOKING

The high temperatures used to fry, broil, or grill meat produce potentially cancer-causing substances called heterocyclic aromatic amines, or HAA's. The longer meat (or fish or poultry) is cooked, the more heterocyclic aromatic amines are created. Roasting and baking produce fewer HAA's; microwaving and lower-temperature, moist-cooking techniques such as poaching and boiling produce practically none at all.

Fat that drips onto hot coals, stones, or coils when meat is grilled can also produce potential carcinogens known as polycyclic aromatic hydrocarbons, or PAH's; smoke rising from the heat source deposits PAH's on your food. To minimize your exposure to PAH's, choose lean cuts of meat, trim visible fat, and don't use fatty marinades or basting liquids. Cover the grill with foil; punch holes in it to let fat drip out. To reduce grilling time, precook meat by poaching or microwaving it for a few minutes. Protect fish and vegetables from smoke by wrapping them in foil.

EATING FOR A HEALTHY HEART

To cut your heart-disease risk, you need to control your blood cholesterol levels through low-saturated-fat, low-cholesterol eating. The guidelines below are based on American Heart Association recommendations and closely parallel the *Dietary Guidelines for Americans* (p.12):

☐ Keep your total fat intake to less than 30 percent of your total daily calories.

☐ Keep your saturated fat intake to less than 10 percent of total calories.

☐ Limit your polyunsaturated fat intake to 10 percent of your calories; monounsaturated fat should supply the rest of your fat calories.

☐ Limit cholesterol to 300 milligrams per day.

☐ At least half of your daily calories should come from carbohydrates, preferably complex ones.

☐ Protein should provide the remainder of the calories in your diet.

☐ Limit sodium to 3 grams a day.

☐ Limit your alcohol consumption to 1 or 2 ounces of pure alcohol per day. Two 12-ounce beers, an 8-ounce glass of wine, or 2½ ounces of 80-proof liquor contain 1 ounce of pure alcohol.

☐ Don't eat more than needed to maintain your recommended body weight.

☐ Eat a wide variety of foods.

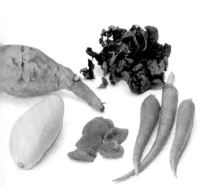

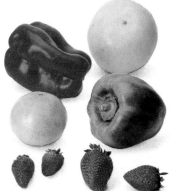

Beta carotene. A form of vitamin A, beta carotene acts as an antioxidant (see below), offering protection against lung cancer and reducing heart disease and stroke risk. Unlike vitamin A, beta carotene isn't toxic in high doses. Good sources are orange, yellow, and dark green vegetables and fruits, including apricots, broccoli, cantaloupe, carrots, kale, spinach, sweet potatoes, and winter squash.

Vitamin C. In addition to acting as an antioxidant, this vitamin may help to prevent the development of cancer, especially cancers of the esophagus and stomach, by blocking the formation of cancer-causing nitrosamines (see facing page) in the digestive tract. Rich sources of vitamin C are citrus fruits, strawberries, broccoli, brussels sprouts, guavas, black currants, and bell peppers.

UNDER REVIEW

Research continues on the possible benefits of other nutrients and foods in preventing disease. Here are some promising leads.

Garlic can help reduce blood cholesterol and triglyceride levels and may be anticarcinogenic.

Onions contain substances that prevent blood clots and raise HDL-cholesterol levels.

Selenium, a trace mineral, may reduce cancer incidence, possibly by acting as an antioxidant. Seafood is a good source of selenium.

Vitamin E may cut cancer and heart attack risk by acting as an antioxidant. Wheat germ and whole grains are good food sources.

Omega-3 fatty acids from fish have an anti-inflammatory effect and may help control blood pressure and cholesterol levels.

Phytochemicals found in fruits and vegetables may protect against cancer and heart disease.

ANTIOXIDANTS VS. FREE RADICALS

Oxygen, and the countless chemical reactions with oxygen that take place in the body's cells, are essential to life. These oxidation reactions create as by-products highly unstable molecules called free radicals, which combine with other molecules in reactions that release even more free radicals. Although free radicals are generated naturally in the body, exposure to cigarette smoke and other environmental pollutants can also trigger oxidation and the release of free radicals. Reactions involving free radicals not only can damage cell membranes, they alter genetic material within the cell nucleus, potentially promoting the formation of cancer cells. In addition, there is evidence that low-density lipoproteins (LDL's) damaged by free radicals contribute to the buildup of fatty deposits in arterial walls and eventually to the development of coronary heart disease. Antioxidants, such as beta carotene and vitamins C and E appear to block the action of free radicals before cell damage can take place.

What is a food allergy? How is it different from a food intolerance?

A food allergy (or food hypersensitivity) is an abnormal reaction of the immune system to a food. The allergic reaction can occur immediately—or hours—after eating the food. Consuming (or in rare cases, just smelling or touching) the food causes the immune system to make antibodies that attack the offending substance. This reaction in turn triggers the release of histamine, which is responsible for the various symptoms of a food allergy. These include abdominal pain, nausea, diarrhea, vomiting, hives, flushing, eczema, swelling of the lips or throat, or red, itchy, tearing eyes. The severity depends on the victim's sensitivity and how much of the offending food, or allergen, was eaten. A serious allergic reaction, called anaphylaxis, may cause swelling of the face, lips, or tongue, difficulty breathing, stomach or uterine pain, diarrhea, and vomiting. In extreme cases, the victim may experience anaphylactic shock—swelling and constriction of the throat and air passages of the lungs, rapid pulse, and an extreme drop in blood pressure. If not promptly treated (usually with an injection of the hormone epinephrine), the condition can, in rare cases, cause death. A less severe allergic reaction is often treated with antihistamines.

Among the foods that commonly cause allergic reactions are egg whites, cow's milk, wheat, nuts, peanuts, soybeans, fish, and shrimp, lobster, and other crustaceans. It is estimated that no more than 7.5 percent of children and fewer than 1 percent of adults are affected by food allergies. Allergies may develop at any time but are most common among children and often disappear in adulthood. The tendency to develop food allergies is partly inherited.

If you suspect you have a food allergy, consult a doctor who specializes in allergies and is certified by the American Board of Allergy and Immunology (see Appendix). The usual treatment consists of identifying and avoiding the offending food.

A food intolerance is also an abnormal response to a food, but unlike an allergy, it doesn't involve the immune system. A common cause of food intolerance is the lack of an enzyme needed to digest the food. For example, lactose intolerance is caused by insufficient lactase, the lactose-digesting enzyme (p. 28). A person may be intolerant of certain substances in food; for example, vasoactive amines, chemicals found in beer, wine, and cheese, cause headaches in some people prone to migraines.

Do canned and frozen fruits and vegetables lose some of their nutritional value during processing?

Yes, but the amounts and types of nutrients lost vary widely. Frozen fruits and vegetables are more nutritious than canned, and they can even be more nutritious than fresh produce. Many items are frozen very soon after they are picked and therefore retain vitamins and minerals in their near-fresh state. The nutrients in some fresh produce may decline during the days or weeks between their harvesting and their arrival in the store.

Canned fruits and vegetables are generally less nutritious than fresh or frozen, because the high temperatures involved in canning destroy nutrients. Processed foods are also more likely to have added sugar, salt, and other additives. However, if produce in the store looks old, or if you don't plan to eat it right away, then consider buying canned or frozen products instead.

All frozen foods lose some of their nutritional value over time. To retain nutrients longest, store foods at or below 0° F. Date the packages and use those dated earliest first. It's not a good idea to keep frozen foods in the freezer for more than a couple of months. The vitamins in canned goods also deteriorate in storage. To retain nutrients longest, keep canned foods between 50° and 65° F; vitamin losses tend to increase at higher temperatures.

Is there any way to be sure that canned food is safe to eat?

Commercial canned foods are safe to eat for up to a year (and often longer) if they are stored properly. A dented can is generally safe as long as the surface isn't broken. But a leaky or corroded can is defective and should be discarded.

It's a good idea to date canned goods and use older ones first. Wipe dust from the tops before opening. Once a can is opened, transfer unused food (especially acidic foods, such as tomatoes or citrus juices) to a nonmetallic container and refrigerate it; if food is left in the can, lead and other metals in the can may leach into the food. Avoid lead-soldered cans (pp. 298–299).

Never buy or use food in swelling or bulging cans (or in glass containers with bulging lids); this may be a sign of botulism, a rare but potentially fatal type of food poisoning (p. 50). Other signs of botulism in canned goods include discoloration, spurting when the can is opened, and clouding of normally clear liquids.

DECIPHERING FOOD LABELS

In proposals issued in 1991 and scheduled to take effect in mid-1993, the Food and Drug Administration and the U.S. Department of Agriculture moved to make the often confusing nutritional information on food packages a thing of the past. Chief among the proposed rules are strict definitions of terms used to describe foods (see below). Here are the other major requirements:

Mandatory uniform labeling. Virtually all packaged foods must display a uniform label. The label must give the amount per serving of total calories, calories from fat, total fat, saturated fat, cholesterol, total carbohydrates, complex carbohydrates, sugars, dietary fiber, protein, sodium, vitamins A and C, calcium, and iron. Ingredients must be listed in descending order by weight. All sweeteners—including corn syrup, dextrin, dextrose, fructose, glucose, honey, lactose, maltose, mannitol, maple syrup, molasses, sorbitol, sugar (sucrose), and xylitol—are considered one collective ingredient. (Previous rules allowed each to be listed separately.) Ingredients that some people are allergic to (milk products, sulfites, monosodium glutamate) must be clearly listed.

Defined serving sizes. Only standardized serving sizes can be used, and they must be given in common household measures, such as 1 cup, as well as in metric. The sizes are set by the FDA and USDA, based on the amounts an average person ordinarily consumes.

Health claims. Only health benefits supported by solid scientific evidence can be claimed. The FDA is initially allowing food manufacturers to address only the following relationships: between calcium and osteoporosis, sodium and hypertension, fat and cardiovascular disease, and fat and cancer.

Produce and meats. Retailers have been asked to voluntarily post nutritional information for the most common types of raw fruits, vegetables, meat, poultry, and fish.

THE LANGUAGE OF FOOD LABELS

The FDA has defined these nine key terms used on food packaging:

Free. Contains an amount unlikely to affect the body. Specific limits are set for foods called calorie free, fat free, sugar free, sodium free, and cholesterol free.

Fresh. Raw food that hasn't been processed, frozen, or preserved.

High. A serving provides 20 percent or more of the recommended daily intake for the nutrient.

Less. Has at least 25 percent less of a nutrient than an identified comparable food.

Light. Has one-third fewer calories than an identified comparable food. (Does not apply to beer or wine.)

Low. Won't exceed the dietary guidelines for a nutrient if eaten frequently. Specific limits are set for foods termed low calorie, low and very low sodium, low fat, low in saturated fat, and low in cholesterol.

More. Contains at least 10 percent more of a nutrient than an identified comparable food.

Reduced. A reduced sodium, fat, or cholesterol food has no more than half the amount in an identified comparable food; a reduced calorie food must have one-third fewer calories than a comparable food.

Source of. A serving contains 10 to 19 percent of the recommended daily intake for the nutrient.

Is it safe to use a pot or pan that has a badly scratched or chipped nonstick coating?

Swallowing a few particles of a nonstick coating along with your food may not sound very appealing, but it won't hurt you, according to experts at the Food and Drug Administration, which approved the coating as a cooking surface in 1960. Nonstick coatings, such as Teflon, which is made from a fluorocarbon resin, can chip or flake with age, especially if they are scratched by utensils or in cleaning. However, FDA officials assert that coating particles cause no damage because they pass undigested through the body.

For health-conscious individuals who want to control their fat intake and cholesterol levels, nonstick coatings have a distinct advantage: the coatings reduce the amount of fat needed for cooking. The cookware is also easier to clean. To avoid scratching and chipping, use only plastic or wooden utensils and avoid scouring pads and cleansers.

PRESERVING NUTRIENTS

Foods lose nutritive value during storage and cooking. Exposure to air, light, heat, and water speeds the process. (Even freezing does not preserve nutrients indefinitely; to minimize nutritional loss, frozen foods should be kept at 0° F.) Follow these guidelines to preserve the vitamins and minerals in foods:

Meat, poultry, and fish. Cook meats and fish thoroughly to kill harmful microorganisms (see *Handling Food Safely,* p.50), but don't overcook them. In general, roasting, baking, stir-frying, steaming (fish), and broiling retain more nutrients than braising or stewing (unless you also serve the defatted juices). Microwave cooking helps preserve nutrients by cutting cooking time. The cooking liquid from meat and poultry is a rich source of B vitamins; after skimming off the fat, serve it with the meat or use it to make gravy or soup.

Vegetables and fruits. Produce that is soaked or boiled in water, exposed to air, or stored for long periods loses nutrients, particularly B-complex and C vitamins. Refrigerate ripe produce and consume it quickly. Handle fruits and vegetables carefully to avoid bruising, which hastens vitamin-C loss. Delay cutting up produce (and don't cut off the tops of berries) until just before use. The outer leaves of vegetables are the most nutritious; discard as few as possible. Nutrients are often concentrated in or just below the skin; if possible, eat unpeeled fruits and vegetables, or don't peel them too deeply.

Produce is most nutritious served raw. The best cooking methods for vegetables are quick and use little or no water; these include steaming, blanching, stir-frying, pressure-cooking, and microwaving. If you must boil vegetables, leave them whole (with skins on, if possible) or cut them into big pieces. Use a small amount of water in a pot with a tight-fitting lid, remove the vegetables when they're tender-crisp, and serve right away. Use the cooking liquid for soup, stock, or gravy.

Refrigerate cooked produce in airtight containers and use within 2 to 3 days. Refrigerate fruit juice in small containers so that less surface area is exposed.

Cereals and grains. Store cereal and grain products in opaque containers to avoid exposure to light, which destroys riboflavin and vitamin E. Don't wash rice before cooking; cook it in just enough water so that you don't need to drain any off when the rice is done. Cook pasta quickly in plenty of fully boiling water, drain, and serve right away. Nutrients leach out when pasta is overcooked or rinsed. In hot weather, refrigerate breads and other whole-grain foods to avoid spoilage.

Milk and milk products. To block light and prevent the breakdown of vitamin A and riboflavin, store dairy products in opaque containers.

I always cook chicken well done to kill any salmonella. Should I do the same with meat?

Both red meat and poultry should be cooked to a temperature high enough to kill any harmful organisms that may have contaminated the meat during raising, processing, shipping, storage, or preparation. This precaution is necessary because the contamination of raw poultry and meat with disease-causing organisms is far from uncommon.

The surest way to test the doneness of meat and poultry is by using a meat thermometer; cooking time or appearance is not a reliable gauge. Chicken or turkey is done when a meat thermometer inserted in the thick part of the inner thigh muscle (away from the bone) registers 180° to 185° F. When you poke this section with a long-tined fork, the juices should run clear—not pink or red; the leg should move easily and the hip joint should give readily.

Pork, beef, and lamb should register a temperature of 160° F in the meat's thickest part. Temperature this high kills all bacteria as well as trichina larvae in pork, which can cause trichinosis, a potentially serious illness. It's safest to avoid eating even slightly pink pork. Beef and lamb, however, may still be slightly pink in the middle when done; even rare beef and lamb may be safe to eat as long as internal temperatures reach at least 140° F, a point at which bacteria will survive but not multiply. Ground beef, however, should be heated to 160° F all the way through. Because ground meat is handled more and has greater surface exposure, it is more easily tainted. (For more on keeping meat and poultry safe, see *Handling Food Safely,* p.50.)

SAFE MICROWAVING

Microwaves are safe if used as directed (p.301) and can be a health boon. Dishes don't need as much fat, and reduced cooking times help preserve nutrients. Follow microwaving directions from the oven manufacturer as well as on food packages and in recipes. Use these tips to keep microwaved food safe:

☐ Adhere to recommended cooking and standing times to allow food to heat fully. Cover dishes with microwavable ceramic or glass to promote thorough, even cooking.

☐ When microwaving a large casserole, take thermometer readings in several places to make sure the dish is thoroughly cooked.

☐ Cook turkeys and large roasts in cooking bags to promote even heating. Don't microwave stuffed poultry.

☐ Don't let plastic wrap (even if labeled microwave-safe) and plasticized packaging touch food in the oven; the plastic may contain toxic chemicals that could contaminate food. Never microwave plastic containers such as sour-cream cups or margarine tubs.

☐ Shallow, wide dishes heat foods more evenly than deep, narrow ones. For the same reason, round or oval dishes are better than square or rectangular ones. In newer microwave ovens, you can prevent overcooking in the corners of a square or rectangular dish by covering corners with foil (don't let foil touch oven walls).

☐ If your oven does not have a revolving carousel, turn food several times during cooking to heat it evenly. Stirring dishes during and after cooking also distributes heat.

☐ Don't use heat susceptors (thin pieces of reflective plasticized metal that come with some microwavable foods to make them crispy). Some contain harmful chemicals that break down at high temperatures.

```
10:51
SENSOR  TEMP
1  2  3
4  5  6
7  8  9
CLOCK  0  TIMER
LOW  MED LOW  MED
MED HIGH  HIGH
STOP/ CLEAR  COOK
OPEN DOOR
```

How can I be sure the fish and shellfish I'm buying are fresh?

Since only a small sample of all the seafood that goes on the market is inspected, you are right to be concerned about the freshness of the fish you buy. Always purchase seafood from a reputable dealer, and make sure it is displayed on ice. Whole fish may lie directly on the ice, but cut fish and shellfish (in or out of the shell) should be kept on trays or on paper or plastic wrap.

Fish should smell fresh, clean, and slightly sweet, not ammonia-like, sour, rancid, or what is commonly referred to as fishy. When you press the flesh, it should spring back. Fillets and steaks should feel moist, not slimy, and have a glistening shine. Avoid pieces that are lying in juice, which encourages spoilage and is a sign of age. On whole fish, look for clear eyes that bulge slightly (however, cloudy, sunken eyes aren't always a sign of staleness; a fish's eyes may cloud from contact with ice and they may be sunken if the fish came from deep water). The skin should be moist and shiny without dry or flaky scales; gills should be bright red or pink, not brown, green, or gray. There should be few or no traces of blood.

When buying fresh shrimp, look for translucent shells colored light pink, pinkish-tan, or gray-green. (Be aware that to prevent discoloration shrimp may be treated with sulfites, which can cause allergic reactions, especially in people with asthma.) When buying oysters, mussels, and clams in the shell, select only live ones (a live mollusk's shell is tightly closed or will close when tapped). When buying shucked mollusks, look for plump ones in clear liquid that smell fresh. Buy lively crabs and lobsters; a lobster should tuck its tail under when you pick it up.

Fresh fish and shellfish are highly perishable. Unless you plan to cook them immediately, refrigerate them as soon as possible, keeping the temperature as close to 32° F as you can. (If necessary, put the fish in a waterproof bag and keep it packed in ice in the refrigerator.) Refrigerate live shellfish in a well-ventilated container, and discard any that die before you cook

HANDLING FOOD SAFELY

The key to avoiding food poisoning is to keep cold foods cold (below 40° F) and hot foods hot (above 140° F). Foods kept between 40° F and 140° F eventually become breeding grounds for bacteria and other microorganisms. Some cause illness directly; others, by secreting heat-resistant toxins. To keep food safe, follow the guidelines listed below. For more information on food safety, call the USDA Meat and Poultry Hotline or the National Fisheries Institute (see Appendix).

Buying. Shop at reputable stores. Check dates on foods that have a limited shelf life. Pick perishable items last; if you won't be home in an hour, store them in an ice chest. Be sure that meat, poultry, and fish are well wrapped so that juices can't leak out.

Storing. Set your refrigerator at 40° F or below (use a thermometer to check); set the freezer at 0° F or lower. Refrigerate or freeze perishables immediately. Rewrap frozen items only if the packaging is torn or loose. Freeze raw meat and poultry that you don't plan to use within a few days (2 days for poultry; 3 to 5 days for meats); otherwise refrigerate meat and poultry in the meat-keeper or near the freezing unit. (For advice on storing fish, see page 49.) Freezing keeps meat, poultry, and fish safe for a year or more but flavor and texture begin to deteriorate after a few months.

Defrosting. Thaw frozen food in a refrigerator, catching the juices in a pan so they don't taint other foods. A 5-pound roast takes 3 to 5 hours per pound; a 16- to 20-pound turkey takes 3 to 4 days. You can also thaw meat, poultry, and fish in cold water (wrap the item and change water every 30 minutes) or in a microwave. Cook thawed foods immediately.

Preparing. Wash hands with hot soapy water before handling food. To avoid cross contamination, wash hands and work surfaces thoroughly with hot soapy water after each preparation step, especially after touching raw or undercooked egg, poultry, meat, or fish. Use a clean utensil each time you taste food you're cooking. Keep your kitchen clean. Launder kitchen linens often; replace sponges every few weeks. Cover cuts, sores, or rashes on your hands (use adhesive bandages or wear rubber gloves).

Serving. Chafing dishes or warming trays may not be hot enough to prevent bacterial growth, especially in large amounts of food. Divide food into smaller portions; discard foods that have been warmed for more than 2 hours. Keep cold foods refrigerated or iced until ready to serve.

Leftovers. Discard any meat, fish, poultry, egg, or dairy dish that has been left standing at 40° F to 140° F for 2 hours or longer. Refrigerate or freeze leftovers in clean, shallow containers. Store stuffing separately from meat. Reheat leftovers fully to 165° F, bringing liquids to a full boil and covering dishes in order to retain heat.

COMMON CAUSES OF FOOD POISONING

One of the most serious forms of food poisoning, botulism (p.46), caused by a spore-produced toxin, is quite rare. More common causes of food poisoning are listed below.

Typical food-poisoning symptoms are unpleasant, but short-lived. They include nausea, vomiting, diarrhea, and abdominal cramps. Headaches, fever, and muscle weakness may also occur. For mild cases, drink fluids to avoid dehydration. Call a doctor when symptoms are severe or occur in young children, the chronically ill, or the elderly.

Salmonella bacteria, the most common cause of food poisoning, are found mainly in meat, poultry and eggs (see *Egg Safety*, p.51). Symptoms begin 12–24 hrs. after contaminated food is eaten.

Staphylococcus aureus bacteria occur naturally in skin and nasal passages and are passed to food via dirty hands, coughing, and sneezing. Toxin-producing staph germs multiply rapidly, especially in cream or egg sauces, custards, starchy salads, and meats left too long between 40° F and 140° F. Symptoms begin 1–8 hrs. after tainted food is eaten.

Campylobacter jejuni can taint raw milk, poultry, or meat during processing or handling. Symptoms begin 2–5 days after tainted food is eaten.

Clostridium perfringens taints meat and other high-protein foods that are undercooked or left to stand too long between 40° F and 140° F (on steam tables, for example). Symptoms begin 6–24 hrs. after tainted food is eaten.

them. Unless you are sure they are very fresh, use fish and shellfish within 2 days of purchase. Remember that by the time you buy a fish, it is probably already a week to 10 days old. Oily, fatty fish, such as bluefish, salmon, and mackerel, tend to spoil faster than do less fatty fish, such as whiting and flounder.

Commercially frozen fish is usually quick-frozen within a few hours of being caught and, if kept solidly frozen, is comparable to fresh fish in taste and texture. Frozen fish should feel solid when you buy it; the package should be intact with little or no frost.

I love raw oysters and clams, but periodically I hear warnings against eating them. What are the real health risks?

Eating raw and undercooked mollusks puts you at risk of contracting a variety of bacterial and viral infections, including hepatitis A (see *The Facts About Hepatitis*, p.349). Symptoms of infection can range from relatively mild abdominal cramps and nausea to diarrhea, vomiting, and fever. People with liver problems, cancer, diabetes, or a compromised immune system are especially urged not to eat raw or undercooked shellfish. For such people, infection with *Vibrio vulnificus*, a bacterium common in oysters, can be fatal.

Mussels, oysters, and clams filter gallons of water each day. If they live in waters containing raw or undertreated sewage, they can accumulate harmful levels of viruses and bacteria found in human waste. State agencies participating in the National Shellfish Sanitation Program carefully monitor the waters where mollusks are harvested for signs of sewage contamination and keep most tainted mollusks off

☐ Buy only grade AA or A eggs that have been kept under refrigeration and show no cracks.

☐ A fresh egg sinks when submerged (unbroken, uncooked) in cold water. Eggs that float are usually safe to eat if thoroughly cooked, although some experts suggest that you discard them.

EGG SAFETY

A sharp increase in salmonella contamination (p.50) of eggs in recent years poses a particular danger for the elderly and the ill. To reduce the risk, follow these guidelines for buying, storing, and cooking eggs.

☐ Wash hands and all work surfaces and utensils with hot soapy water before and after contact with raw eggs. Toss out egg-containing foods that are left standing at room temperature for over 2 hours.

☐ Refrigerate eggs in their carton to reduce handling. Keep them inside the refrigerator, not on the door.

☐ Avoid foods prepared with raw or undercooked eggs, including Caesar salad; some mousses and meringues; homemade eggnog, mayonnaise, and hollandaise and béarnaise sauces; most homemade ice creams; uncooked egg-containing pie fillings; French toast; and any eggs that are soft or runny.

☐ To cook thoroughly, scramble 1 or 2 eggs for 1 minute over medium heat; prepare scrambled eggs for a crowd in batches no larger than 3 quarts and keep at 140° F until ready to serve (but no longer than 30 minutes); fry over-easy eggs 3 minutes on one side, 2 on the other, over low or medium heat (don't fry eggs sunny-side up); poach eggs in boiling water for 5 minutes; boil for 7 minutes.

the market. But it's still best to avoid any risk by steaming clams, oysters, or mussels for at least 4 to 6 minutes, which kills all viruses and bacteria. Lightly steaming mollusks until they open isn't enough.

How dangerous is it to eat raw fish in sushi?

If you eat raw fish in sushi or sashimi, there's a slight possibility that you'll ingest parasites—especially the roundworm anisaki, which can cause abdominal pain,

nausea, and diarrhea, among other symptoms. Although this problem is not common, take care to eat sushi or sashimi only at a reputable restaurant; a well-trained sushi chef can spot and remove the anisaki worm.

In general, raw fish that has been frozen at -4° F for 72 hours is safe to eat. But marinating raw fish in lime juice, as is done with seviche, will not kill any parasites nor most microorganisms. Neither will cold-smoking or salt-curing fish kill all parasites or microorganisms.

SEAFOOD SAFETY

A healthful, low-fat source of protein, seafood is becoming a popular staple in the American diet. People who eat a lot of it, however, may be troubled by reports of waterborne pollutants, such as lead and mercury, contaminating fish and shellfish. In general, offshore fish are less likely to be tainted than fish caught closer to shore or than freshwater fish. To limit your exposure to pollutants in fish, follow the guidelines listed below.

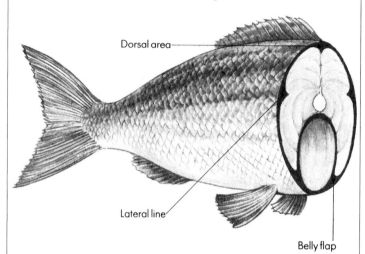

Dorsal area

Lateral line

Belly flap

Contaminants in fish tend to collect in fatty areas. To reduce your risk, remove the skin and the layer of fat beneath it, as well as the dark-colored streaks of fatty tissue shown above.

☐ Buy fish from a reputable dealer, not from local sport fishermen. (Commercially harvested fish tend to come from deeper, less polluted offshore waters.)

☐ Vary the types of fish you eat (freshwater, deep sea, farm bred) to limit contamination from a single source.

☐ Choose younger, smaller fish, which will have accumulated fewer contaminants.

☐ Avoid raw shellfish.

☐ Trim off fat and discard innards and gills from fish. Do not eat the green tomalley (liver) in lobster or the "mustard" in blue crabs.

☐ Before eating their catch, recreational fishermen should check on its safety (through local health or environmental agencies or where fishing licenses are sold).

☐ Children and pregnant or nursing women should avoid fish that are likely to contain high levels of methyl mercury, which has been linked to adult and fetal neurological damage. Saltwater species that often contain methyl mercury are swordfish, shark, and halibut; freshwater species include brook and brown trouts, smallmouth and largemouth bass, walleyed and northern pikes, yellow perch, and pumpkinseed sunfish.

I recently read an article about the dangers of antibiotics and hormones in meat and milk. How serious a problem is this?

There may be small amounts of these veterinary drugs in your food, but they almost certainly won't hurt you. Low levels of antibiotics (mainly penicillin and tetracycline) are added to the feed of most food animals to prevent illness and stimulate growth. Some food animals are also given steroids and other hormones to promote growth. The Food and Drug Administration sets the period of time required for a drug to clear from an animal before it can be slaughtered or milk drawn from it can be sold; it also sets acceptable levels of these chemicals in meat and milk. The U.S. Department of Agriculture monitors the amounts of drug residues in meat; state agencies monitor the residues in milk.

The major concern about the regular use of antibiotics in livestock is that it can lead to the development of antibiotic-resistant strains of bacteria and outbreaks of difficult-to-control infections in animals or people. But so far, the use of antibiotics in animals has not been shown to be harmful to humans. In some rare cases, antibiotic residues in food may trigger an allergic reaction, but usually only in extremely sensitive individuals.

Steroids, which are legally given only to beef cattle and sheep, pose no health risks to humans because the residues in meat are insignificant compared with the amounts humans produce themselves. To avoid concentrations of steroids in edible parts of an animal, the time-release hormone pellet is implanted behind the animal's ear.

A genetically-engineered hormone, known as bovine growth hormone, or bovine somatotropin, has been tested on some dairy cows to make them produce more milk. But the use of this hormone is still limited to experimental herds and has not yet received FDA approval. However, all indications are that the milk and meat from cows treated with the hormone are safe for human consumption.

As long as they are used legally and correctly, veterinary drugs seem to pose no health threats to human beings. However, abuses can and do occur. If you are worried about antibiotic residues or hormones in your meat, it is possible to reduce your exposure by simply trimming fat from meat and poultry and avoiding liver, kidneys, and other organ meats (residues of veterinary drugs tend to concentrate in fat tissue and organ meats). If you are willing to pay the higher price, consider buying meat and poultry produced without antibiotics, hormones, or feed additives.

How can I reduce my chances of exposure to pesticides in fruits and vegetables?

Pesticide is an umbrella term for any chemical used to kill insects, weeds, fungi, mold, and other pests or prevent them from harming crops, livestock, or feed. Pesticides are usually sprayed or dusted on crops and sometimes applied to the soil. Their use is so widespread that small amounts in food are nearly impossible to avoid. The types of pesticides and allowable levels of residues—called tolerances—are set by the Environmental Protection Agency. The levels in produce are monitored by the Food and Drug Administration.

Concern over pesticide residues stems largely from the possibility that long-term exposure to even small amounts can increase the risk of cancer. Over the years some pesticides found to be or suspected of being carcinogenic have been banned or voluntarily taken off the market in this country; some farmers have reduced their use of pesticides on their own initiative.

The EPA maintains that pesticide residues at legal levels are not a health risk. Other sources disagree. What risks, if any, there may be are far outweighed by the health benefits of eating plenty of fruits and vegetables. Take these steps to limit your exposure to pesticide residues:

☐ Eat a variety of different fruits and vegetables. Consuming too much of one particular kind might lead to a build-up in your system of residues of the pesticide typically used on that food.

☐ Wash fruits and vegetables with warm water and scrub them with a food brush when possible. This helps remove some pesticide residues. For a more thorough cleaning, wash produce in a very mild soapy water solution, then rinse well.

☐ Peeling produce ensures that all surface residues are removed but will not eliminate systemic pesticides—those within the plant. Peeling removes the wax applied to some produce—and the fungicide it usually contains. Unfortunately, peeling also reduces the nutrient and fiber content of some produce.

☐ Discard the outer leaves of leafy vegetables, and wash the inner leaves.

☐ Be aware that imported foods may not be subject to the same pesticide restrictions as domestically grown produce.

☐ Shop for food that is grown and shipped without pesticides (see *Organic Food,* p.54).

More and more foods seem to contain artificial sweeteners these days. Are they safe?

Noncaloric (or non-nutritive) sweeteners must undergo extensive testing before they can be sold commercially. Nonetheless, questions have been raised (and in some cases continue to be raised) about the safety and possible cancer-causing potential of artificial sweeteners. Those currently available include:

☐ Aspartame. Marketed as Equal (a tabletop sweetener) or NutraSweet (an ingredient in a wide variety of food products), aspartame is the most commonly used artificial sweetener. Some users have complained of such side effects as headaches and gastrointestinal upset. After investigating hundreds of health complaints thought to be aspartame-related, the Centers for Disease Control concluded that the sweetener did not cause serious, widespread, adverse health effects. A possible link between aspartame and behavioral disorders and brain cancer has also caused concern. But studies have found no consistent link between aspartame and behavioral or learning problems, and a cancer connection seems to be very unlikely. Some individuals may be sensitive to aspartame and should avoid it. People with the genetic disorder phenylketonuria (PKU) cannot metabolize one of the components of aspartame (the amino acid phenylalanine) and therefore should not consume it.

☐ Saccharin. Some studies have shown that saccharin can cause bladder tumors in laboratory rats. But the doses given to the rats were extremely high—at times the human equivalent of 850 cans of diet soda a day. In addition, the incidence of bladder

ORGANIC FOOD: PROS AND CONS

Eating organically grown foods has gone from being an exclusive concern of a few health faddists to an appealing alternative for an environmentally sensitive, health-conscious general public. Until recent years, there was no universal definition of *organic* and the term was used quite freely to label everything from bona fide pesticide-free apples to "organically mined salt." As a result, both health and food experts routinely warned consumers not to waste money on organic products, which are usually more expensive than comparable conventionally grown foods. Now, however, the federal government has stepped in to define and regulate organic foods.

What is organic food? In general, food is said to be organic when it is produced without manmade chemicals. This means fruits, vegetables, and grains grown without synthetic fertilizers, pesticides, or herbicides, as well as poultry and livestock raised without growth hormones or antibiotics. Organic farmers fertilize their soil with organic waste and mineral-bearing rocks. They control pests by planting early, using pest-resistant plant strains, and rotating their crops.

A federal law passed in 1990 called for the establishment of national standards for growing and processing organic foods. The new regulations, which take effect in late 1993, are expected to stipulate not only that foods labeled *organic* must be produced without the use of synthetic chemicals, but that the soil in which such produce is grown must not have been treated with chemicals for 3 years. In addition, food producers will have to meet rigid, uniform standards and keep careful records. If a state has more stringent requirements governing organic foods (almost half of the states have regulations), state standards apply.

Are organic foods healthier? This is a controversial issue. According to the Food and Drug Administration, there is no evidence that organic food is safer or more nutritious than nonorganic food. Proponents of organic foods argue that products raised without synthetic chemicals are safer for the environment, for farm workers, and for consumers, even if they are no more nutritious. They believe that the limits imposed by the federal government on the use of pesticides and other chemicals in ordinary food production are inadequate. On the other hand, organic foods are more perishable than chemically treated foods. Unless organic foods are harvested and marketed quickly, they are more likely to be contaminated by potentially harmful bacteria, molds, and toxins.

Cosmetics for consumers. Proponents of organic food point out that many of the chemicals sprayed on produce are used simply to enhance the food's appearance and not to preserve or protect its nutrients. The now-banned pesticide Alar, for example, was used primarily to enhance the color and firmness of apples. The reasons for this emphasis on appearance are simple: consumers are reluctant to buy mottled-looking produce and producers know that they can charge more for perfectly formed, blemish-free items. Appearance is also one of the U.S Department of Agriculture's criteria for grading many types of produce.

Buying organic products. Until national standards take effect, look for state-certified organic produce in health food stores and produce markets. In season, farmers' markets are often a good source of organic produce. Even if not grown organically, fruits and vegetables from farmers' markets are likely to be fresh and free of wax and fungicides.

The outlook for organic farming. Although they still represent only a tiny percentage of all food sold, sales of organic food in the United States have risen dramatically in recent decades, increasing sevenfold in the 1980's. As the demand for organic products increases and as many nonorganic farmers voluntarily reduce their reliance on pesticides and begin adopting other techniques of organic farming, it's likely that the number of chemical-laden items in the American food basket will decline in the future.

cancer in humans does not reflect the increase in saccharin use since 1950. When the FDA decided to ban saccharin in 1977, public and industry outcry prompted Congress to postpone the ban. Saccharin is still available today, but products containing it must carry a label noting the link to cancer in animals.

☐ Acesulfame-K. Sold as Sunette and Sweet One, acesulfame-K is used, like aspartame, to sweeten many different products. Unlike aspartame, it can also be used in cooking. Although the FDA has declared the sweetener to be safe, the Center for Science in the Public Interest, an advocacy group, claims that the studies on which the FDA bases its judgments on additives are inadequate and that acesulfame-K's safety is still in doubt.

Another noncaloric sweetener, cyclamate, was banned by the FDA in 1969 because of test results linking it to bladder cancer in animals. However, cyclamate is still used in Canada and other countries, and may be an ingredient in products purchased overseas. In 1985 the National Research Council cited evidence that cyclamate does not in itself cause cancer, and the FDA is considering lifting the ban.

Will artificial sweeteners help me lose weight?

Artificial sweeteners would seem to be a dieter's dream, adding sweetness but few or no calories to food. However, it's unclear whether they really help people lose weight or at least avoid gaining it. The average weight of Americans has not dropped in proportion to the increased use of noncaloric sweeteners; this suggests that people do not use artificial sweeteners to replace sugar, but rather use them in addition to the sugar already in

THE FACTS ABOUT FOOD ADDITIVES

What are they? Food additives are substances that make foods last longer, taste better, look more appetizing, and have a smoother consistency; some even enhance the nutritional value of food. The Food and Drug Administration estimates that at least 2,800 additives are used in the U.S. food industry. The most common are salt, sugar, and corn sweeteners.

Additives are divided into several different categories. Preservatives, for example, include antioxidants, which retard rancidity in fats and oils, and antimicrobial agents, which inhibit the growth of microorganisms. Flavorings and flavor enhancers may be natural substances such as salt, sugar, and spices or synthetics such as ethyl vanillin (a vanilla substitute). Food colorings give foods a more appealing and consistent appearance. Stabilizers, thickeners, and emulsifiers ensure smooth consistency and keep ingredients from separating.

Are additives dangerous? Most aren't. Since 1958, federal law has prohibited food producers from adding potentially carcinogenic substances to foods. Exempted from this ruling were about 700 additives in long use and "generally recognized as safe" (GRAS). In 1970, the FDA began a review of the items on the GRAS list and since then has found nearly 80 percent of them to be safe. Some GRAS substances, such as red dye no. 2, a suspected carcinogen, have been banned. Among the items still under review are the antioxidants butylated hydroxyanisole (BHA) and butylated hydroxytoluene (BHT), used singly or in combination to prolong the shelf life of baked goods and many other food products. Both chemicals have been linked with cancer in lab animals.

Critics of the FDA claim that many of the additives it has declared safe have not been adequately tested. The list of controversial additives includes artificial sweeteners (p.53); the few remaining artificial food dyes; sulfite, a preservative added to wine and dried fruit, which may cause allergic reactions, especially among asthmatics; sodium nitrite and sodium nitrate (see *Disease-Fighting Foods*, pp.44–45); and the flavor-enhancer monosodium glutamate (MSG), which may also cause allergic reactions in certain people. Concern about the safety of additives has led some food processors to find safer substitutes for questionable additives.

Limiting your intake of additives. Choose fresh or minimally processed foods over additive-laden products. Eat a variety of foods to avoid ingesting too much of any single additive. Read food labels carefully (see *Deciphering Food Labels*, p.47). Restrict your intake of foods containing artificial colors. And to keep matters in perspective, remember that too much fat or salt in your diet can be far more damaging to your health than any of the synthetic additives currently approved for use in our food.

their diet. One study showed that when sugar was secretly replaced with aspartame in the diets of 24 people, the subjects ate less food during a 12-day period. However, an analysis of data on more than 78,000 women revealed that those who reported using artificial sweeteners gained more weight in a year than non-users. It has been suggested that artificial sweeteners actually increase appetite and stimulate the taste for sweet foods, but studies trying to prove this have yielded inconclusive results.

If you're trying to lose weight, remember that artificially sweetened foods may still be high in fat and that fat contains more than twice the number of calories per gram as does sugar.

Why is it unhealthy to be overweight or underweight?

Although it is possible to be overweight or underweight and never develop a major disease, too much deviation from the recommended range may indicate an underlying health problem (especially if your diet is a sound one). Being naturally a bit underweight does not seem to carry any health risks. On the other hand, obesity (generally defined as being 20 percent or more over the acceptable weight range for your height and age) has been associated with cardiovascular disease, hypertension, atherosclerosis, osteoarthritis, gallbladder disease, adult-onset diabetes, menstrual irregularities, sleep apnea, and certain cancers, including those of the breast, endometrium, prostate, and colon.

How being overweight causes health problems is still not fully understood. Part of the answer may be that an obese person is likely to have higher triglyceride and, to a lesser extent,

cholesterol levels than someone who isn't overweight. Many obese people also have larger-than-normal fat cells. Such cells interfere with the action of the hormone insulin, which regulates blood sugar (glucose) levels (pp. 342–345). This may explain why adult-onset diabetes is more common among the obese, and why for them losing weight may help to control the disease. In some overweight people, weight reduction also brings down cholesterol, triglyceride, and blood-pressure levels, even if their weight never makes it into the recommended range.

As hazardous as obesity can be, repeatedly losing and gaining weight, the so-called yo-yo syndrome, may be even more dangerous. A study of more than 3,000 men and women found that those who put on and took off pounds over and over again were significantly more likely to die of heart disease than people whose weight remained stable. It may actually be healthier to maintain a weight a bit above the one recommended for you than to lose and regain extra poundage in an endless—and stressful—cycle. Certainly the dangers of yo-yo dieting make it clear why learning to *maintain* a weight loss through better eating habits should be part of any weight-loss program.

What causes a person to become obese?

The causes of obesity are varied, complex, and still not fully understood. A tendency to become obese does seem to run in families, but some people gain excess weight by a variety of means, including overeating and not exercising enough, taking certain medications, and repeatedly losing weight and gaining even more back.

Obesity sneaks up on some adults who gain just a few pounds a year over a long period. People with sedentary jobs may gradually gain significant amounts of weight, and women may put on pounds as a result of having children. The loss of lean body mass with age may contribute to obesity in some older people. Although overeating can cause obesity, studies have shown that not all obese people overeat.

An obese person may have too many fat cells (hyperplastic obesity), cells that are too big (hypertrophic obesity), or both. Some researchers believe that while fat cells can shrink, they never disappear, which may be one reason why obese people, despite valiant efforts, often have a hard time losing weight and maintaining the loss. This theory suggests that many obese children will find it extremely difficult to avoid being overweight in adulthood. While some studies have shown hyperplastic obesity to be more stubborn than hypertrophic obesity, other research has shown no differences.

It's not clear why obesity tends to run in families, although both genetic and environmental factors are probably involved. The children of obese parents may not only grow up eating more and exercising less than kids in thin families, they may also have an inborn tendency to hoard pounds. Despite popular belief, glandular or hormonal problems seem to cause relatively few cases of obesity.

Experts agree that anyone whose excess weight is a health risk should try to reduce through a sensible diet and exercise program under medical supervision. Because of their genetic heritage, some obese people may never become thin, but many can lose enough weight to significantly improve their health.

SUGGESTED WEIGHTS FOR ADULTS

These weight ranges were developed as part of the *Dietary Guidelines for Americans* (p.12) and are likely to change as research in this area continues. Unlike many weight charts, this one allows for a small increase in weight as you age (p.364). The higher weight in each range applies to people with more muscle and bone (generally men); the lower weight usually applies to women.

Being in the right range does not guarantee that your weight is healthy. Other factors are body-fat percentage and distribution (p.68) and whether you have a personal or family history of weight-related medical problems. Consult your doctor for a more accurate assessment of your ideal weight.

Height (no shoes)	Weight in pounds (no clothes)	
	Age 19 to 34	Over age 34
5'0"	97–128	108–138
5'1"	101–132	111–143
5'2"	104–137	115–148
5'3"	107–141	119–152
5'4"	111–146	122–157
5'5"	114–150	126–162
5'6"	118–155	130–167
5'7"	121–160	134–172
5'8"	125–164	138–178
5'9"	129–169	142–183
5'10"	132–174	146–188
5'11"	136–179	151–194
6'0"	140–184	155–199
6'1"	144–189	159–205
6'2"	148–195	164–210
6'3"	152–200	168–216

If I want to lose weight, are there certain foods I should give up?

Eating a varied, balanced diet is essential to getting all the nutrients you need for good health—whether you are trying to lose weight or not. Your weight-loss diet should include foods from all the main food groups (see *Foods for a Healthy Diet,* p.24). Eliminating certain types of foods can lead to nutritional deficiencies.

Labeling a favorite high-fat, high-calorie food off-limits may seem to make a weight-loss diet easier to follow, but it can also backfire. Promising yourself never to eat, say, chocolate cake again may create such feelings of deprivation that eventually you may wind up binging—if not on chocolate cake, then on some other "sinful" treat.

A better strategy for most people is to establish a pattern of healthy, balanced low-fat eating and moderate, consistent exercise that you can maintain for the rest of your life. This plan can, and indeed should, include all your favorite foods. Those that are high in fat (especially saturated fat), cholesterol, sugar, sodium, and alcohol should simply be eaten in moderation—a rule that applies to any healthy eating plan. (For more information on strategies for losing weight and diets to avoid, see *A Weight-Loss Diary,* p.58–59.)

Is skipping meals an effective way to lose weight? What about grazing, or eating a number of small meals throughout the day?

The only way to lose weight is to consume fewer calories than you use up in activity. Although skipping meals may seem like a convenient way to reduce food intake, you may actually end up getting the missed calories at other times during the day. For example, if you skip breakfast and lunch, you may feel free to eat a huge dinner and snack during the evening, which can compensate (and then some) for the calories saved earlier.

Skipping meals may also slow your metabolism. After a time without sufficient nourishment, your body reacts to what it perceives as a starving state by lowering the rate at which it burns calories, making it more difficult for you to lose weight.

Some diet authorities advocate grazing, or eating small meals throughout the day, as a way to control weight. A few early studies seemed to show a link between increasing the number of meals per day and lowering body fat. In some of these studies, the grazers consumed fewer total daily calories; in others, the two groups ate the same amount of calories, but the grazers still lost weight, suggesting that food eaten in large servings is more readily stored as fat. However, a more recent study by the U.S. Department of Agriculture found that the rate at which people burned calories was the same whether they consumed equal amounts of food in two large daily meals or in several small ones.

Grazing may not be a good weight-control strategy for people who tend to overeat without thinking or have trouble limiting

Continued on page 60

A Weight-Loss Diary

To lose weight, you need to consume fewer calories than you burn up in your daily activities. But this does not have to involve a drastic reduction in your food intake. As these diary entries show, what matters is replacing calorie-rich fatty and sugary items with complex carbohydrates that are filling and nutritious, yet low in calories. Changing your eating habits and maintaining those changes after your diet will ensure that the weight you've lost will stay off. When you diet, make sure to eat at least 1,200 calories a day, and don't aim to lose more than 2 pounds a week. If you have a serious health problem, consult your doctor before starting a diet.

Diets to Avoid

Unbalanced diets usually fail to keep weight off and can be dangerous to your health. Here are some to avoid:

Crash diets. Severe calorie restriction can lead to loss of muscle tissue. The body may also adapt to a drop in calories by slowing the rate at which it burns calories, making weight loss even more difficult. Repeated or prolonged crash dieting may also cause nutritional deficiencies.

Fad diets. Some plans focus on a single food; others encourage eating mostly protein or fat and drastically cutting carbohydrates. Followed for long periods, such diets may cause nutrient deficiencies, kidney problems, and other complications.

Fasts. Not eating for more than a few days causes toxins to accumulate in the bloodstream, burdening the kidneys. Long-term fasting causes muscles and organs to lose protein, depletes essential minerals, and can result in heart-rhythm abnormalities and drops in blood pressure. Fasters may feel dizzy, weak, tired, and depressed.

Diet pills. Over-the-counter appetite suppressants stimulate the nervous system, speed up the heart, and raise blood pressure. They may cause headaches, jitteriness, and other symptoms; prescription versions can be addictive. Water pills (diuretics) can dangerously dehydrate the body. Fiber pills may cause gastrointestinal and other problems.

Very-low-calorie diets (VLCD's). For most people, consuming fewer than 1,200 calories a day can be dangerous. Very-low-calorie liquid-formula diets provide as few as 400 calories a day and should not be undertaken unless you are more than 20 to 30 percent over the recommended weight for your height and are under medical supervision. Common side effects of VLCD's include fatigue, headache, gallstones, and gastrointestinal disorders.

Vomiting; laxatives. Self-induced vomiting and chronic use of laxatives to control weight are signs of an unhealthy relationship to food and eating. Frequent vomiting can also cause tooth and gum decay, and long-term laxative use can permanently affect bowel function. (For more on eating disorders, see page 177.)

At breakfast, just switching 1 percent fat milk for whole milk saved 25 calories. The change from orange juice to a sliced orange eliminated another 35. Thus the day started with 60 fewer calories.

Substituting a half bagel with jelly for a Danish cut 245 calories while drinking 1 percent milk instead of a cola dropped 45 more. That's 290 fewer calories than at previous coffee breaks.

A chicken salad on rye saved 100 calories over a cheeseburger. An apple has 135 fewer calories than french fries, and even with some sugar, an iced tea has 120 fewer calories than a cola. All told, 355 calories were eliminated at lunch.

Snacks are often where the calories pile up. Making the change from cake and milk to crackers and seltzer and eliminating an after-work beer and nuts resulted in a whopping 880-calorie saving.

The diet dinner actually starts with an extra course: an appetite-taming cup of soup with crackers. But still the meal's soup-and-salad preliminaries contain 50 fewer calories than the regular salad, thanks to the substitution of herb-flavored lemon juice for french dressing and the elimination of bacon-flavored bits from the salad. A main course of pasta with tomato sauce and grated cheese rather than fried chicken and fries cut another 564 calories. Serving steamed broccoli rather than peas in sauce eliminated 124 calories while drinking no-calorie seltzer instead of a cola knocked out 145 calories. For dessert, replacing 1 cup of ice cream with ½ cup of sorbet cut 260 calories. Total calories eliminated at dinner: 1,143.

When the evening munchies set in, popcorn and a diet cola provided satisfaction with 542 fewer calories than the usual corn chips and regular cola. And at bedtime, substituting 1 percent milk for whole milk saved another 100 calories. Altogether nearly 3,300 calories were eliminated for the day by switching to a filling, low-fat diet.

Pre-diet menu
(4,625 cal.)

Food	Amount	Calories
BREAKFAST		
Cereal with		
whole milk		
Orange juice		
Coffee		
with sugar		
COFFEE BREAK		
Danish roll		
Cola		
LUNCH		
Cheeseburger		
French fries		
Cola		
SNACK		
Pound cake		
Whole milk		
AFTER WORK		
Beer		
Peanuts		
DINNER		
Salad		
French dressing		
Frozen fried chicken		
French fries		
Peas (frozen in sauce)		
Cola		
Ice cream		
Coffee		
with sugar		
WATCHING TV		
Corn chips	3 ounces	450
Cola	1 can	145
BEDTIME		
Whole milk	1 cup	150
	Total	4,625

Weight-loss diet
(1,336 cal.)

Food	Amount	Calories
BREAKFAST		150
Cereal with	1 cup	50
1 percent fat milk	½ cup	75
Sliced orange	1 medium	0
Coffee (black)	1 cup	16
with sugar	1 teaspoon	
COFFEE BREAK		80
Bagel with	half	25
low-calorie grape jelly	1 tablespoon	100
1 percent fat milk	1 cup	
LUNCH		125
Chicken salad	½ cup	80
on rye bread	2 slices	85
Apple	1 medium	1
Iced tea with lemon	large glass	24
and sugar	1½ teaspoon	
SNACK		35
Wheat crackers	4 small	0
Seltzer	1 glass	
DINNER		50
Vegetable soup	1 cup	25
Soda crackers	two	30
Green salad with	1 cup	10
lemon juice and herbs	2 tablespoons	150
Macaroni with	1 cup	35
tomato sauce and	½ cup	25
grated Parmesan	1 tablespoon	26
Steamed broccoli with lemon	½ cup	0
Seltzer	1 glass	40
Sorbet	½ cup	0
Coffee (black)	1 cup	16
with sugar	1 teaspoon	
WATCHING TV		30
Popcorn, air-popped	1 cup	3
Diet cola	1 can	
BEDTIME		50
1 percent fat milk	½ cup	
	Total	1,336

themselves to small portions. Such people can end up eating more food throughout the day by uncontrolled grazing than by limiting themselves to three reasonably sized sitdown meals.

You may find yourself grazing not to lose weight but because you lack the time or inclination to eat regular meals. This practice is not unhealthy as long as the food choices you make result in balanced nutrition and a reasonable calorie total. For people who use up a lot of energy—children, teenagers, and athletes, for example—judicious grazing may be an excellent way to ensure that they get all the calories and nutrients they need.

I've never been much of a breakfast eater. Is this meal as important as it's made out to be?

It is unclear whether a person who always or sometimes skips breakfast is less healthy than a regular breakfast eater. Most studies on the effects of not eating breakfast have been carried out on schoolchildren. According to many (but not all) of these studies, children who don't eat breakfast tend to perform less well on mental tasks, a finding that researchers attribute to hunger, fatigue, and the low blood sugar levels that result after a night- and morning-long fast. Breakfast skippers also tend to get less nutrients in their diet.

The Iowa Breakfast Studies—conducted on both children and adults from 1949 to 1961 and the first to focus attention on the effects of eating a morning meal—found that adults who ate breakfast could perform physical and mental tasks in the late morning more efficiently, with faster reaction times and less neuromuscular tremor than those who skipped breakfast. But other studies show that breakfast eaters and skippers perform about equally well on mental tasks.

While the importance of eating breakfast remains a matter of some debate, many nutritionists do recommend that you spread your caloric intake throughout the day and suggest that your breakfast supply about one-fourth of your total calories for a day. Such a breakfast should include a variety of foods that provide carbohydrates both simple (fruit or juice, for example) and complex (whole-grain bread or cereal), protein (low-fat milk or yogurt), and a little fat (already contained in the whole-grain foods and milk products).

HEALTHY EATING AT FAST-FOOD RESTAURANTS

Fast food is appreciated for its convenience, low price, variety, and predictability. And these days, it can even be nutritious—if you make the right choices. The guidelines listed here can help you limit fat, salt, sugar, and calories in fast foods:

☐ Keep it simple. Order food without mayonnaise, sauces, or dressings, or remove them yourself. A plain burger, for example, has much less fat, calories, and salt than one with cheese and bacon. Topping a baked potato with butter, sour cream, or cheese adds fat and can double calories. Choose unbreaded chicken or fish that is baked or broiled, or remove the breading. Order pizza plain or with vegetable toppings.

☐ Think small. A "whopper" or "jumbo" item may wipe out much of a day's fat and calorie allotment. Small fries and shakes can save hundreds of calories over their larger counterparts; cones usually have less fat and fewer calories than sundaes.

☐ Visit the salad bar. Your best bets are vegetables and beans (*not* seasoned with oil-based dressings) and fresh fruit. Don't load up on high-fat, high-calorie, sodium-packed salad bar staples such as bacon bits, cheese, croutons, nuts, olives, eggs, and whole-milk cottage cheese. Avoid chicken, shrimp, and tuna salads; coleslaw; and pasta, potato and rice salads, all of which usually contain large amounts of salt and mayonnaise. **Caution.** Salad bars can be dangerous sources of food-borne disease if the management doesn't watch the bar (to keep customers from touching the food), install plastic sneeze guards, keep cold dishes on ice and hot dishes hot, and provide a frequent fresh supply of cut fruits and vegetables.

☐ Get the facts. Fast-food restaurant chains respond to consumer preferences. For example, some chains that once prepared fries in highly saturated beef fat now use vegetable oil, and shakes and dessert items may be lower in fat and calories than in the past. Some places offer nutrition information. What you learn may surprise you: extra-crispy chicken, for example, has more fat and calories than regular fried chicken.

☐ Make eating at fast-food restaurants a treat. Consider limiting fast-food meals to once a week or less. Frequent fast-food eaters should vary their choices.

How can I find a professional to advise me on my diet?

There are three types of professionals in the field of nutrition: registered dietitians, nutritionists who are physicians, and nutritionists with academic degrees. A registered dietitian (look for the initials R.D. after the name) has earned, at the least, an undergraduate college degree in nutrition, food science, food service management, or a related field; in addition, an R.D. will have undergone a supervised internship and passed a national certification exam. A nutritionist may be a medical doctor with training in nutrition or a Ph.D. who specialized in nutrition or a related area. Ideally, a nutritionist should be a member of The American Society for Clinical Nutrition or be certified by the American Board of Nutrition.

Credentials are important, because many states have no training, licensing, or certification requirements for nutritionists or dietitians—anyone can hang up a shingle and charge for nutrition advice. Some "nutritionists" are more interested in selling expensive supplements than in providing accurate dietary advice.

Get a referral to a registered dietitian or a nutritionist from your doctor, the local hospital, the nutrition or dietetics department of a local university, or the American Dietetic Association (see Appendix).

The cost of seeing a nutritionist varies; call first to find out how much both an initial consultation and subsequent visits will cost. These fees may or may not be covered by your health insurance. Know what you want before you select a nutrition expert—a diet to lose weight, for example, or to manage diabetes or lower blood cholesterol levels.

HEALTHY SNACKS

Watching your weight does not mean that you must give up between-meal eating. In fact, healthy, well-timed snacks can help control your weight by curbing mealtime hunger and overeating. Snack in moderate, measured amounts. To avoid turning a light snack into a caloric feast, measure out snack foods into a dish, rather than eating them right from the package. Make trade-offs: a mid-afternoon snack, for example, might replace dessert later on. The variety of snack foods is enormous. Here are some healthful choices:

☐ Angel food cake
☐ Bread (whole grain)
☐ Bread sticks
☐ Cereal (low-fat; unsweetened)
☐ Cheese (low-fat)
☐ Cocoa (made with skim or low-fat milk)
☐ Cookies and crackers (whole grain, low-fat)
☐ Frozen fruit bars
☐ Fruit (fresh, dried, unsweetened canned)
☐ Fruit juice (unsweetened)
☐ Ice milk
☐ Milk (skim or low-fat)
☐ Muffins (low-fat)
☐ Popcorn (made with little oil or salt; unbuttered)
☐ Pretzels (low-salt)
☐ Pudding pops (low-fat)
☐ Rice cakes
☐ Scandinavian crisp bread
☐ Seltzer (plain or flavored)
☐ Sherbet or sorbet
☐ Tortilla chips (baked)
☐ Vegetables (fresh, juices)
☐ Yogurt (low-fat or nonfat)

Having clear objectives before you begin your search may help to steer you toward someone with expertise in the area that concerns you.

At the first visit you may be asked to keep a diary of everything you eat for a few days or longer; the nutritionist or R.D. will analyze and discuss this record with you. A complete physical examination by a doctor may be recommended. A nutritionist who is not an M.D. should refer you to a physician for treatment of any medical problems.

Beware of so-called nutritionists who promise too much. In spite of too-good-to-be-true promises in the popular media, no diet will cure major diseases, turn you into a star athlete, or help you lose large amounts of fat in a matter of days.

Avoid practitioners who push hair, nail, or saliva analyses, or other such unproven tests for nutrient deficiencies and those who sell nutritional supplements or special foods in the office or give you a prescription for supplements that can be filled only by a certain pharmacist.

I enjoy eating out, but I can't seem to stick to my diet at restaurants. Any suggestions?

Apply the same strategies you use at home to cut intake of fat, saturated fat, sugar, and alcohol. These guidelines can help:
☐ Learn the language of menus. Certain terms provide clues to a dish's fat and calorie content. Items listed as baked, broiled, fresh, in wine or juice, poached, roasted, steamed, or stir-fried tend to be lower in fat and calories than those described as au gratin, basted, braised, breaded, buttered, creamed, creamy, crispy, fried, marinated in oil, rich, sautéed, or scalloped

(escalloped). Any food cooked in pastry or with cheese or served with a sauce or gravy is also likely to be high in fat and calories. Try to select less fatty cuts of meats (see *Foods to Choose: Lean Meats,* p.25).

☐ Explore ethnic cuisines, which often feature dishes that are low in calories and fat and taste delicious. Follow the principle of choosing simply prepared foods that emphasize vegetables and grains cooked without a lot of fat.

☐ Ask the waiter how a dish is prepared and what changes or substitutions are possible. For example, sauces, gravies, and dressings sometimes can be eliminated or served on the side.

☐ When you've had enough to eat, let the waiter clear your plate; if you wish, have leftovers wrapped up to take home.

Is there any polite way to stick to a diet when you're dining in someone else's home?

Being a guest takes away some of your control over food choices. Here are ways to cope:

☐ If you know the host well, explain in advance that you are trying to control your weight. The host may or may not serve a low-calorie meal but will at least understand why you are taking small portions and passing up the high-calorie foods.

☐ If the meal is served buffet-style, make low-fat choices and take small servings.

☐ Limit alcoholic drinks. Besides being high in calories, alcohol stimulates the appetite.

☐ Don't feel you must eat everything on your plate, no matter what everyone else does or what you may have been taught about being polite.

☐ Don't give up if you slip on occasion. It's the total diet that counts. One high-calorie meal won't undermine all your other efforts. Just return to your healthy eating habits and try to eat more carefully the next time you eat out.

I seem to balloon around the holidays. How can I avoid this?

The parties and feasts that are a holiday tradition don't have to doom your diet. Here are some ideas for healthy holiday eating:

☐ Host a party or holiday meal yourself and serve plenty of low-calorie options for dieters like yourself. Just be sure to control the urge to nibble while you are in the kitchen.

☐ Choose lower-fat, lower-calorie entrées—fish or turkey breast rather than roast beef or duck. Go easy on (or avoid) high-fat, high-calorie accompaniments. If you are still hungry, fill up on low-fat, high-carbohydrate foods such as bread, potatoes, salad, vegetables, and fruit.

☐ At a buffet, use a small plate if you have a choice. It's much too easy to load up a large one.

☐ Watch your alcohol intake.

☐ Pace yourself. Eating too fast can make you overeat because it takes time for the brain to recognize that hunger is satisfied.

☐ Don't center holiday fun on food. Outdoor activities, games, and good conversation away from the table can add to the merriment as much as food can.

☐ Select only the high-calorie foods you really want. For example, you might pass up your cousin's cheese appetizers so you can enjoy a slice of Uncle Ralph's irresistible pumpkin pie.

☐ If you are trying to lose weight, consider shifting to a goal of weight maintenance for the holidays. Even if you eat more than usual and work out less, continue to choose mainly high-carbohydrate, low-fat foods and keep on exercising. Hitting a plateau doesn't mean you'll never lose more weight. By maintaining healthy habits, you'll be able to return easily to your weight-loss regimen after the holidays.

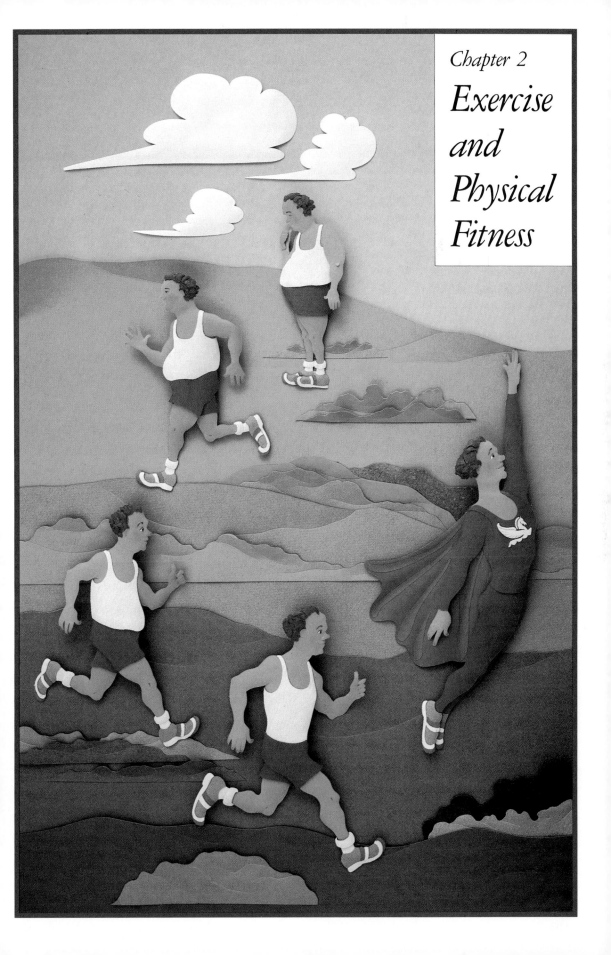

Chapter 2
Exercise and Physical Fitness

Too Much, Too Soon

Charles M., age 32, was a hard-driving business executive who smoked and drank more than he should. He was at least 30 pounds overweight and got no regular exercise. When his father suddenly died of a heart attack at age 60, Charles took drastic measures. All at once he stopped smoking and drinking, went on a crash 600-calorie-a-day diet, and started running up to 2 miles a day. A week later he felt so terrible he called his doctor.

After giving Charles a thorough physical examination, the doctor told him that while he wasn't in any immediate danger of suffering a heart attack, he had plenty of serious risk factors to contend with. The doctor recommended a program of moderate aerobic exercise and a low-fat, low-cholesterol diet.

He also advised Charles to join a support group for people trying to give up smoking.

Charles gave his aching knees and muscles a week off to recuperate, then began an easy walk-jog program. Over the next 6 months, he worked up to jogging 25 miles a week and kept to a 1,500-calorie-a-day diet. He dropped the 30 pounds he had to (and then some) and brought his cholesterol level down to near normal. A year later, Charles still jogs 25 miles a week. Thanks to his own willpower and the help of the support group, he doesn't smoke and rarely has more than a drink a day. Although his job is as demanding as ever, Charles considers the time he spends exercising a worthwhile investment: for every hour he works out, he feels he gets back 2 hours of productive activity.

Unfit Beginnings

Will B., 35, had been sedentary and overweight as a child. By his sophomore year of college, he weighed 237 pounds. With his social life heading nowhere, Will went on a crash diet. After living exclusively (and unhealthily) on high-protein foods and lots of water for 6 months, Will was down to a slim but flabby 160.

Over the next decade, Will struggled to maintain his weight, allowing it to creep up to as much as 200 pounds on several occasions before going on yet another diet. All along he had refused to exercise (it was too boring,

he claimed). Finally, as Will approached his thirtieth birthday (and 200 pounds once again), a girlfriend dared him to take an aerobics class. Will agreed, and to his surprise, enjoyed it very much. Soon he was taking three classes a week, eating less, and working out with weights at home to strengthen his newly trim body.

Five years later, Will's weight has stabilized at about 175 pounds, and exercise is as much a part of his life as brushing his teeth. He eats what he wants, within reason, without dieting or feeling deprived.

Taking the Right Steps

Barbara L., 52, was basically healthy and not overweight, but she'd begun to feel some joint stiffness, and had added a few inches to her hips. She figured she'd start simply, walking a mile home from work instead of taking the bus.

At first, Barbara did her walking in old tennis shoes, but when her ankles began to hurt,

she decided to invest in new walking shoes. Barbara's walk takes only minutes longer than the bus ride. She gets home feeling refreshed and invigorated. The stiffness is gone, she's lost weight, and her body is more toned. More important, she's cut her risk of developing heart disease — even if she adds no more exercise to her life.

TEST YOUR HEALTH I.Q.

What Does It Mean to Be Physically Fit?

Which exercises are best for achieving fitness? What does the term "aerobic" really mean? Is it ever too late to start an exercise program? Aside from toning your body, what are the other benefits of engaging in a regular exercise program? Are there any drawbacks? Physical activity seems to be on a lot of people's minds these days, but how much do you really know about what it takes to get and stay fit? This True/False quiz will help you find out.

1 It is possible to have a "healthy" weight and still be carrying too much fat on your body.

_____ True _____ False

2 To maintain cardiovascular fitness, you need to work out at least 20 minutes every day.

_____ True _____ False

3 People who are over age 65 or who have chronic conditions such as arthritis should avoid all types of aerobic exercise.

_____ True _____ False

4 An aerobic exercise is considered to be low impact if it's performed upright, with one foot always touching the ground.

_____ True _____ False

5 Unlike most other exercises, cross-country skiing works every major muscle in the body.

_____ True _____ False

6 People who exercise regularly should eat a high-protein diet to keep up their strength.

_____ True _____ False

7 Stretching is the most efficient way to warm up before you begin an exercise routine.

_____ True _____ False

8 A well-rounded fitness program does not have to include resistance training.

_____ True _____ False

9 Jumping rope ranks high on the list of effective aerobic exercises.

_____ True _____ False

10 Raking leaves, scrubbing floors, and making love all burn more calories per hour than bowling.

_____ True _____ False

11 To be on the safe side, women should always give up jogging during pregnancy.

_____ True _____ False

Answers

For more information on any of the quiz topics turn to the pages listed next to the answers.

1. True, p.68	5. True, p.75	9. True, p.92
2. False, p.71	6. False, p.81	10. True,
3. False, p.72	7. False, p.83	pp.104, 66
4. True, p.74	8. False, p.85	11. False, p.105

I'd like to lose weight. Will dieting alone be enough, or do I really have to exercise too?

No matter how good a diet may be, exercise is an important part of any safe, gradual weight-loss plan. To lose weight effectively, you need to do two things: decrease your calorie intake and speed up your metabolism (the rate at which your body burns calories) through exercise. If you diet without exercising, your metabolism may actually *slow down* as your body tries to conserve all the fat it can from the few calories it's getting. Dieting alone may cause you to lose muscle tissue, whereas regular exercise burns off fat while minimizing muscle loss. A diet too low in calories and nutrients may make you tired and lethargic; a good workout is both energizing and relaxing. You are also much less likely to eat out of boredom or nervous tension after exercising.

To lose weight and keep it off, exercise regularly—at least three times a week—and keep working out even after you meet your weight-loss goal.

What kinds of exercise are best for taking off weight?

Brisk walking, jogging, swimming, aerobic dancing, cycling, rowing, rope jumping, and cross-country skiing are good choices. To take off weight, an exercise must work the large muscle groups (legs, arms, torso), get the heart pumping at 70 percent to 85 percent of its maximum capacity (this is known as your *training zone*), and be performed for at least 20 minutes.

It's important to do something you enjoy so that you'll keep at it even after you've lost weight.

BENEFITS OF YOUR FAVORITE SPORT OR EXERCISE

The American College of Sports Medicine lists six basic components of physical fitness: body composition (fat to lean ratio), cardiovascular efficiency (how much oxygen the heart and lungs deliver to working muscles), muscular strength (the ability of a muscle to exert force for a brief period), muscular endurance (the ability of a muscle to apply

Sport	Weight control Calories per hour	Cardiovascular efficiency
Aerobic dancing	360–480	excellent
Basketball	360–660	good–excellent
Bicycling (12 mph)	600	excellent
Bowling	240	fair
Calisthenics	360–600	fair–good
Golf (walking and carrying clubs)	300–360	fair
Handball / racquetball / squash	660	good–excellent
Ice skating (figure)	420	good
Jogging (5 mph)	600	excellent
Roller skating (rapid)	700	good
Rope jumping (60 jumps/min.)	800	excellent
Rowing	840	excellent
Skiing (cross-country)	700 (5 mph) 1,020 (8 mph)	excellent
Skiing (downhill)	500–600	fair–good
Softball (pitcher)	450	fair
Swimming (front and back crawl)	360–750	excellent
Tennis (singles)	480	good
Walking (3 mph)	300	good–excellent
Walking (5 mph)	480	good–excellent
Weight lifting	480	fair

Don't exhaust yourself, but do keep a steady pace. Choose more than one activity in order to give your program variety.

Activities such as bowling, tennis, or weight training—which don't keep your heart rate consistently high—can be part of a total fitness plan but probably won't help you shed pounds if they're your only exercise.

Won't exercise increase my appetite?

It may, but even if you eat more, exercise will help burn off the calories and develop a trimmer figure. You may also find that you aren't hungry for an hour or more after exercising. This can help you lose weight by controlling the urge to snack.

continuing force), flexibility (the ability to move joints and use muscles through their full range of motion), and coordination (the ability to shift smoothly between positions). While a fit person should do well in all areas, cardiovascular fitness is the most important health factor. This chart rates popular sports or exercises for all the major fitness components. An activity's effects on body composition is expressed in the "Weight Control" column as the average number of calories burned per hour. When a range of ratings is given, the activity's benefit depends on the intensity with which it's done and on the performer's fitness level.

Muscular strength	Muscular endurance	Flexibility	Coordination
good	excellent	excellent	excellent
good	good–excellent	good	excellent
good	excellent	good	good
good	fair	fair	excellent
excellent	excellent	excellent	fair–good
fair–good	fair–good	fair	good
excellent	good–excellent	good	excellent
good	good	good	excellent
good	excellent	fair	fair
good	good–excellent	good	excellent
good	excellent	fair	excellent
good–excellent	excellent	good	fair
good	excellent	good	excellent
good	good	good	excellent
good	fair	good	excellent
good	excellent	excellent	good
good	good–excellent	excellent	excellent
good	good	good	fair–good
good	good–excellent	good	fair–good
excellent	good–excellent	good	good

After exercising for 3 weeks, I've lost only a pound! What can I do to lose faster?

Don't make that a goal. Most nutritionists recommend shedding 1 to 2 pounds a week for safe weight loss. Weight that's lost rapidly seldom stays off, and trying to lose weight quickly can cause dizziness, nausea, nutritional deficiencies, and other potentially dangerous side effects.

Dieters often lose several pounds of water in the first few days but gain them back later when water and mineral levels stabilize. To lose fat, you have to burn off 3,500 calories for every pound you want to drop. This means that if you take up walking at a rate of 3 mph (an average pace) for 45 minutes four times a week, you stand to burn 900 calories per week, or the equivalent of 13 pounds over the course of a year *without* dieting. If you eat less, you'll lose even more.

A smaller number on the scale isn't the only sign that your body is changing. Tune in to how you look and feel as you continue to work out and eat sensibly. Are your clothes looser? Do your muscles feel tighter? Do you have more energy and sleep better? Exercise builds muscle, which weighs more than fat; so you may even *gain* weight yet still be leaner and healthier than before you started. These benefits will stay with you as long as you keep exercising.

Excess weight seems to run in my family. Am I "destined" never to be thin and fit?

Genetics plays a real role in how we adapt to exercise. Studies have shown that two people on the same eating and exercise program can end up with completely different results. However, virtually everyone can improve fitness, lose fat, and feel better by exercising. If it bothers you that you have to work harder than others to get fit and control your weight, consider working out alone or joining a class or program with others in the same situation. Focus on your own goals and progress; there will always be *someone* out there doing better, and someone else struggling along behind you.

How can I find out what my "ideal" weight is?

This is still not an easy question to answer. Recommended weight charts have changed considerably over the years and are still being refined, as researchers develop more precise methods of describing healthy weight (see *Suggested Weights for Adults*, p.57). Use the chart on page 57 as a starting point to help you assess your weight status. If you weigh more than the upper limit of your recommended range, you may be endangering your health. See your doctor to discuss your

weight and formulate an appropriate weight-loss plan. Weighing less than the lower limit of your recommended range may actually be healthy if you are small-boned, but it can also be a sign of a problem, especially if you have lost weight suddenly.

Even if your weight does fall within a recommended healthy range for your age, height, and sex, other factors help determine whether this is actually the "ideal" or healthiest weight for you. These factors include how much of your weight is fat, how the fat is distributed throughout your body, and whether you already have heart or other weight-associated health problems or a family history of such problems.

Another helpful tool in evaluating your weight is the Body Mass Index, a measure of fat tissue in the body that is calculated by dividing your body weight in kilograms by the square of your height in meters.

An even better health index than weight is body-fat percentage–the ratio of fat to lean tissue. For example, a 6-foot, 200-pound man, considered overweight on standard weight charts, may be perfectly healthy if he carries a lot of muscle and relatively little fat. On the other hand, a 5-foot woman who weighs 120 pounds may be carrying a greater percentage of body fat than is good for her, even though she falls within her recommended weight range.

What is a healthy body-fat percentage?

Doctors haven't set strict guidelines, but the consensus is about 25 percent or less for women, 15 percent or less for men. An easy way to determine whether your body-fat percentage is too high is the pinch test. Pinch a

fold of skin at the back of your arm halfway between shoulder and elbow. If you can pinch more than ½ inch, it may be time to start losing fat.

A more accurate way of gauging body fat percentage is with a skinfold caliper (see facing page), a device that measures fat at various spots on the body. You can get a skinfold caliper test at many teaching hospitals or university exercise science labs for a small fee. More sophisticated tests, such as underwater weighing, have not proven to be any more effective than the relatively simple skinfold test.

Why is body-fat distribution so important in determining a person's ideal weight?

New research indicates that where fat is located in your body does have an impact on your health. Pear-shaped people– heavy in the hips and thighs– are thought to be at lower risk for heart disease than those with extra abdominal padding. The reason, say experts, is that abdominal fat is associated with higher blood levels of LDL cholesterol, the type that raises heart-disease risk (see *The Facts About Cholesterol*, pp.20–21).

The simplest way to assess your body shape is to take an honest look at yourself unclothed in a full-length mirror. Although the experience can be sobering, it will quickly reveal whether you're carrying a health risk around your waist in the form of excess fat.

A more scientific method of determining your body-fat distribution is to calculate your waist-to-hip ratio:

☐ While standing relaxed, not pulling in your stomach, measure around your waist where it is smallest.

☐ Measure around your hips where they are largest (around the buttocks).

☐ Divide the waist measurement by the hip measurement to get your waist-to-hip ratio.

Research indicates that ratios above 0.80 for women and above 0.95 for men are associated with a greater risk for heart and other diseases.

If you are overweight, have an unfavorable waist-to-hip ratio, or have a personal or family history of weight-related medical problems, consult your doctor about making changes in your diet and exercise regimen.

Is it safe for a very heavy person to exercise?

If you are more than 20 percent over your ideal weight, see a doctor before starting any kind of diet and exercise program. He or she will tell you if it is safe to start, what to look out for, and whether you need a stress test.

As a general rule, start with moderate activities that don't stress the joints, such as swimming, walking, and low-impact aerobics. (Swimming, especially, may be easier for an overweight person, because fat increases buoyancy in the water.) As you lose weight and gain fitness, you can slowly adopt a more vigorous, varied program.

I smoke but I'd like to start exercising. Are there any activities I should avoid?

Smoking makes aerobic exercise tougher by reducing the ability of the respiratory system to provide oxygen to working muscles. You are more likely to tire and get short of breath than someone of your age and general fitness level who doesn't smoke.

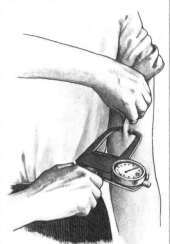

A skinfold caliper gives a precise measurement of the thickness of a fold of skin and is thus a more scientific estimate of body fat percentage than the pinch test. Caliper measurements are taken at the back of the arm, side of the waist, inner thigh, and below the shoulder blade.

As a smoker, you are at increased risk for heart attack and stroke, so it's a good idea to see your doctor (and possibly have a stress test) before you start an exercise program to determine if any activities are off-limits. Remember, exercise doesn't have to be strenuous to provide cardiovascular benefit. Walking, dancing, swimming, even yardwork are all good choices.

A friend of mine claims that exercise helped her stop smoking. Is there anything to this?

Former smokers often cite exercise as one of the things that helped them to give up smoking and resist the temptation to start again. There are a number of reasons for this. Since both exercise and quitting smoking are health-promoting activities, success in one area can keep you motivated in the other. Exercise

can reduce the stress and burn off the excess energy that quitting smoking may produce. It also distracts you and occupies your time. You can take a walk instead of lighting up after a meal, for example. And exercise helps control the snacking and weight gain that are often a side effect of giving up cigarettes.

Do I need to take any special medical tests before I start an exercise program?

If you are under 35, don't smoke, aren't overweight, and have no known heart problems, the answer is no—although you may still want to check with your doctor. If you are over 35, do consult your doctor first (see *Before You Start*, p.73). If you have a heart problem or are thought to be at risk, your doctor will probably suggest a *stress test*—also called a graded-exercise test or an exercise-tolerance test—to measure your heart's ability to handle aerobic exercise.

To perform the test, you walk or jog on a treadmill while hooked up to an electrocardiogram (ECG), a device designed to detect heart abnormalities. Blood pressure is tracked, and the doctor asks you to report any dizziness, breathlessness, or chest pain. If the stress test reveals a problem, more tests are done to determine treatment. As with most sophisticated medical tests, a stress test can yield false positive results (indicating disease in a healthy person) as well as false negative results.

Is there a simple way to gauge cardiovascular fitness at home?

Your resting pulse rate—best taken in the morning before you engage in any physical activity—is a good indicator of cardiovascular fitness. As you become fitter, your resting pulse becomes slower, stronger, and more regular. For a man in his twenties, a good range is between 60 and 69 beats per minute (under 60 is excellent), rising to between 68 and 75 for a man over 50. The comparable figures for a woman are 72 to 77 and 77 to 83 beats per minute.

To assess your tolerance for exercise and your general fitness level, take this simple "step test," which measures your heart rate after moderate activity. All you need are comfortable clothes and shoes, a watch that measures seconds, and a low bench or bottom stair about 8 inches high.

Take the test in a room that's not very hot or very cool. You should feel relaxed and not have eaten for at least an hour, exercised vigorously, or had any caffeine for several hours beforehand (check medicine labels for the presence of caffeine).
Caution. If you can't climb three flights of stairs (15 to 20 steps each) without pausing for breath, don't take this test. If you feel faint, dizzy, or nauseated during the test, stop immediately.

Start the watch and step onto the stair with the right foot followed by the left; step off the stair, one foot at a time. Make 24 complete steps per minute for 3 minutes (either use a metronome or have someone count). Rest for 15 seconds, then take your pulse. (This is known as your recovery pulse rate).

A good rate is between 74 and 84 beats per minute for a man in his twenties, rising to between 83 and 90 for a man over 50. The comparable ranges for a woman are 86 to 92 and 90 to 98. You should start an aerobic fitness program *now* if your recovery rate is poor: over 100 for men and 112 for women under 45

years; over 102 for men and 116 for women over 45 (see *Before You Start,* p.73). Take the step test again after a few weeks of exercising aerobically to see if your recovery rate has improved.

Some health clubs offer fitness testing (a few require it as part of membership), and tests may also be available, for a fee, through hospital-based sports exercise departments. However, fitness testing usually isn't needed before you start to work out.

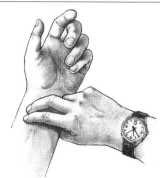

Find your pulse by pressing two fingers (not the thumb) of one hand against the other wrist just below the base of the thumb. Using a wristwatch with a second hand, count the beats for a set period (10 seconds for an exercise pulse; 15 seconds for a resting or recovery pulse). Then multiply (by 6 or by 4 in the examples given) to determine the number of beats per minute.

How does a heart-rate monitor work, and who needs one?

The proliferation of high-tech fitness devices has led to the widespread use of gadgets that measure pulse rate or record heartbeats during exercise. Sometimes these monitors are built into exercise machines. Separate, hand-held devices are designed to clip onto a fingertip or earlobe. Some monitors have electrodes that attach to the chest to directly

record heartbeats; others can be programmed to beep when you start exercising above or below your training zone (see *Aerobic training,* opposite).

Unfortunately, heart-rate monitors, even the ones that directly measure heartbeats, aren't always accurate. They can be expensive—up to several hundred dollars—and some people find them cumbersome. In general, unless you have a heart condition that makes it dangerous to exercise beyond a certain level, you probably don't need one. You can get a pretty good idea of your heart rate by taking your pulse manually or taking the "talk test": when exercising in your training range, you should be able to talk (but not sing or whistle) without gasping for air.

I already feel tired and run-down. Won't exercise make me even more tired?

No. Aerobic exercise should give you more energy throughout the day, since it causes the brain to release various chemicals—endorphins and other neurotransmitters—that induce feelings of well-being, vigor, and calm. You'll find it easier to handle your daily physical demands—walking to the bus stop, preparing a report, folding the laundry, chasing your 3-year-old, watering the lawn, even making love—with energy to burn.

The wiped-out feeling you have at the end of a long day is different from the pleasurable fatigue that follows a good workout. Exercisers report an improved ability to concentrate as well as deeper, more restful sleep, which can counter fatigue. Finally, exercise tends to impart a sense of accomplishment that carries over into other areas of your life.

THE FACTS ABOUT AEROBICS

What does it mean? The word *aerobic* literally means "with oxygen." It refers to activities that increase the efficiency of the body's oxygen-delivery system. Aerobic exercises, such as jogging, raise heart rate and quicken breathing through continous, rhythmical movement of the torso, arms, and legs. As a result, more blood—and with it oxygen and fuel—is pumped to working muscles. Quick, high-intensity bursts of activity, such as sprints, in which heart and lungs can't meet the muscles' oxygen needs, are called *anaerobic* (without oxygen).

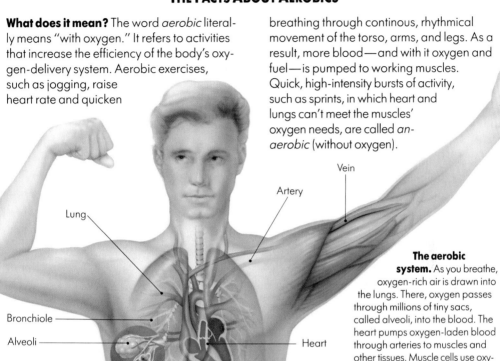

Lung

Bronchiole

Alveoli

Vein

Artery

Heart

The aerobic system. As you breathe, oxygen-rich air is drawn into the lungs. There, oxygen passes through millions of tiny sacs, called alveoli, into the blood. The heart pumps oxygen-laden blood through arteries to muscles and other tissues. Muscle cells use oxygen to turn fuel—mainly carbohydrates and fat—into energy. The by-product of this process, carbon dioxide, is carried by the blood through veins to the heart and on to the lungs for expulsion.

Aerobic training. The most important benefit of aerobic exercise is improved cardiovascular fitness, which translates into a reduced risk of heart and arterial disease. To maintain cardiovascular fitness, you should exercise continuously for 20 to 30 minutes at least three times a week with your heart rate in what is known as your *training zone*. This is a level between 70 and 85 percent of your body's maximum capacity to consume oxygen. To calculate your training zone, subtract your age from 220; multiply the result by 70 percent and by 85 percent. Your pulse rate during exercise should fall within this range. For example, if you're 40 years old, your training range is between 126 and 153 ($220-40 \times .7$ and $220-40 \times .85$). If your pulse during exercise is below 126, you're not working aerobically. If it's above 153, slow down.

Aerobic exercises. Any activity in which you move the large skeletal muscles continuously for a period of time so that you breathe harder and break out into a sweat is aerobic. Brisk walking, jogging or running, swimming, rowing, bicycling, rope jumping, and cross-country skiing are all excellent aerobic exercises. Aerobic dancing, commonly called "aerobics," is a combination of rhythmic movements set to music and designed to provide a complete aerobic workout. Best learned from a qualified instructor in a studio (p.77), aerobic dancing rivals or exceeds many other exercises in promoting balanced fitness (that is, strength, endurance, and flexibility as well as cardiovascular efficiency). Because aerobics is performed to music in a social context, many consider it the most enjoyable way to exercise.

If I don't feel better with regular exercise, is there something wrong with me?

If your workouts leave you truly exhausted, you may be overdoing it. It takes only 20 to 30 minutes of aerobic activity every other day to maintain physical fitness. If fatigue persists even after you have scaled back your routine and you can't pinpoint another cause, you should seek your doctor's advice.

Someone suffering from fatigue due to tension will feel better after a good workout. But if the fatigue is caused by a physical disorder, exercise may make it worse. Some doctors use exercise as a test when they want to establish the cause of persistent fatigue.

I have arthritis. Does that mean I can't exercise?

It used to be thought that exercise caused arthritis, but the latest evidence suggests that moderate activity does not make healthy joints more susceptible to the disease. In one study, runners logging an average of 27 miles a week were no more likely than sedentary people to develop early signs of osteoarthritis in their knees and hips (osteoarthritis is the most common kind of arthritis, usually caused by years of wear and tear on the cartilage, or connective tissue, that cushions the joints).

Ask your doctor whether you would benefit from moderate activities, such as swimming, walking, biking, and low-impact aerobics. More and more, sports-medicine specialists are encouraging people with arthritis to take up such activities to help relieve the pain and joint stiffness associated with the disease.

Although moderate exercise can be beneficial for an arthritis sufferer, certain types of exercise may predispose previously injured joints to arthritis. Activities that subject joints to repeated pounding, such as jogging, high-impact aerobics, and contact sports, can cause joint inflammation and swelling: if the activity is continued, the condition may become chronic. If you have persistent joint pain and stiffness, especially if you have a family history of osteoarthritis, your doctor will probably advise you to avoid high-impact exercises. A sports-medicine specialist or orthopedist can design a safe, effective program for you.

My 65-year-old father wants to take up exercising. Is it safe and worthwhile for him to do so at his age?

The evidence is overwhelming that people can safely start exercising at any age and achieve great health and fitness benefits. Like other active individuals, older people who exercise regularly feel less tense, sleep better, suffer from less depression, and have better diets than their sedentary friends. Aerobic fitness cuts their risk of developing cardiovascular problems and provides more energy and strength for daily activities; exercise also improves balance, coordination, and flexibility (balance is especially important for older people because it helps prevent falls).

Before beginning an exercise program, your father should see his doctor to rule out any underlying health problems and define safe exercise limits (see *Before You Start*, facing page). If he has been sedentary for a long while, he should start slowly and build fitness gradually to avoid overfatigue and injury.

A program of regular moderate aerobic exercise should strengthen your father's cardiovascular system and lower his resting heart rate. It's likely he'll feel more energetic and relaxed, and reduce his body fat whether he diets or not.

Numerous studies have shown that men and women age 65 and over improve their aerobic fitness dramatically within a few weeks of starting an aerobic exercise program. Many could walk farther and faster, take longer strides, and get out of chairs more easily. In one study, men and women whose average age was *90* increased their thigh muscle area by 10 percent!

What specific exercises would be the most beneficial for my father?

The best exercises are aerobic activities that get his heart pumping in its training range for at least 20 minutes, three times a week. Brisk walking, jogging, swimming, cycling, rowing, and aerobic dancing would all be good for him. Many local Y's, health clubs, and community centers have aerobics classes geared for seniors. Of course, he should choose activities he thinks he would enjoy.

One of the best choices for an older person is walking, either alone or in a group. Many communities have walking clubs; the National Organization of Mall Walkers (see Appendix) can tell you if there are such clubs in your area. Swimming is another nonstressful, low-impact fitness activity; it's especially good for people with arthritis and other joint problems because it doesn't stress the joints. Studies also show that older people can improve their strength, balance, and coordination by lifting weights regularly.

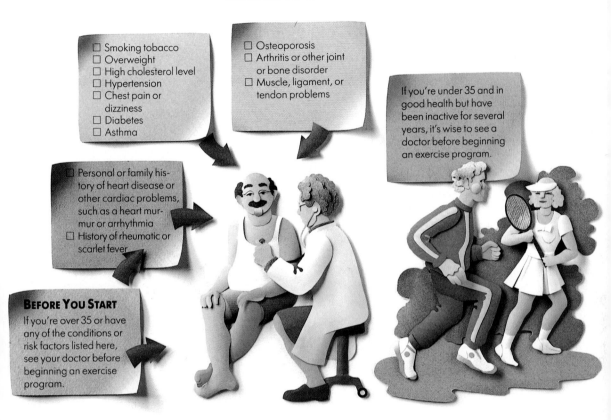

☐ Smoking tobacco
☐ Overweight
☐ High cholesterol level
☐ Hypertension
☐ Chest pain or
dizziness
☐ Diabetes
☐ Asthma

☐ Osteoporosis
☐ Arthritis or other joint
or bone disorder
☐ Muscle, ligament, or
tendon problems

If you're under 35 and in good health but have been inactive for several years, it's wise to see a doctor before beginning an exercise program.

☐ Personal or family history of heart disease or other cardiac problems, such as a heart murmur or arrhythmia
☐ History of rheumatic or scarlet fever

BEFORE YOU START

If you're over 35 or have any of the conditions or risk factors listed here, see your doctor before beginning an exercise program.

Last month I decided to get in shape by running 4 miles a day. After 3 days of this I was so sore I could barely walk. How can I do better next time?

If you have been sedentary for a while, starting with 4 miles of running a day is way too much—even if you were the star of your high school track team 20 years ago. A better strategy would be to start with 20 minutes of light aerobic activity, such as brisk walking, alternated jogging and walking, slow cycling, or slow swimming, every other day, preceded by a warmup and stretching routine and followed by gentle stretching and a cooldown. The program may feel too easy, but by sticking with it you'll reduce your risk of injury to muscles, joints, and bones and keep yourself hungry for more vigor-

ous activity when your body is ready to handle it. It's normal for muscles to feel slightly sore when you begin to exercise, but the pain should diminish during workouts. If you feel any sharp pain, stop right away, massage the area, elevate it, and apply ice. Take a day off, then resume workouts cautiously.

Few people can exercise every day without injury. Every other day is plenty for basic fitness. If you want to do more, that's fine, but make sure to take at least one day a week off from your exercise routine.

I stopped exercising for a month. Can I pick up where I left off, or should I start back at square one?

A month without any exercise will probably decondition all but the most seasoned athlete. A

good rule of thumb: Aim to work back to your previous level over a period equal to the time that you took off.

Start where you began in the first place, making sure to include a good warmup, gentle stretching, and a cooldown with each session. Scale back the intensity of your exercise—say, from jogging to brisk walking or from high-impact to low-impact aerobics. You may be able to build up more quickly than before, but monitor your progress (this is a good time to start an exercise diary; see p. 76), and cut back if you experience dizziness, breathlessness, nausea, or pain in your muscles or joints.

If you stopped exercising because of an injury or illness—particularly if you required bed rest—you may have to start even more modestly than before, and work up to your previous exercise level more slowly.

Jogging makes my knees hurt. Am I doing something wrong?

Jogging, ballet, jumping rope, and some aerobic dance routines are all high-impact activities, in which your feet strike the ground with a force equal to three or four times your body weight. The knees bear the brunt of that impact, and beginners, who haven't developed strong leg muscles to take the pounding, are especially vulnerable.

If you have a preexisting knee injury, high-impact exercise may not be a good idea. If you've experienced some soreness, but it hasn't been incapacitating, here are some things you can do to minimize the problem:

☐ Wear proper shoes. They should be designed for the activity, and you should replace them every 6 months or 500 miles. Don't wait until the tread is worn-out—most shoes lose their cushioning long before that.

☐ Choose soft surfaces. If possible, work out on grass, dirt, or an all-weather track rather than blacktop, concrete, or wood.

☐ Strengthen your leg muscles with alternative activities. Substitute swimming, skiing, rowing, or biking for your high-impact activity a couple of days a week. If your knees still hurt, you may have to drop high-impact exercise altogether.

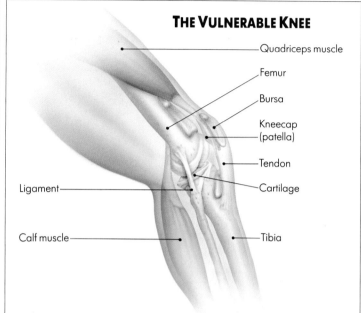

THE VULNERABLE KNEE

Quadriceps muscle
Femur
Bursa
Kneecap (patella)
Tendon
Cartilage
Ligament
Calf muscle
Tibia

The bane of athletes, the knee is subject to injury in at least five places: the cartilages that cushion it, the ligaments that support it, the muscles that control it, the kneecap that protects it, and the kneecap tendons. In addition, the bursae, fluid-filled sacs around the kneecap and behind the knee, can become inflamed. (See *Sports Injuries: Causes and Prevention,* p. 108.)

What's the difference between high-impact and low-impact aerobics?

Activities that are performed upright with one foot always on the ground, such as walking and some aerobic dances, are called low-impact aerobic exercises. Low-impact aerobics are good for beginners because they put less stress on knees, ankles, and hips. No-impact exercises such as swimming, rowing, and biking, in which the feet never touch the ground, are also good choices for beginners.

In high-impact aerobic exercises, such as jogging, running, and some aerobic dancing, both feet leave the ground at once. The forces generated with each foot-strike are greater than in low-impact activities; thus knee and ankle injuries are more common.

I'm bored with jogging and I don't feel comfortable in aerobics classes. What are some alternatives?

Picking an activity you enjoy is crucial to the success of any fitness program. Two of the most popular exercises today are walking and swimming. Both are aerobic yet easy on the joints. One of walking's biggest advantages is that you can do it almost anywhere, alone or with others (just make sure you walk quickly enough to work up a sweat and breathe hard). The only equipment you need is a good pair of walking shoes. Swimming is an all-round conditioner that can be particularly effective for elderly, overweight, and disabled people. The only requirement is easy access to a pool.

I have a busy schedule. How can I fit walking into my life?

Here are some tips for gaining the benefits of walking without turning your life upside-down.

☐ Walk to and from work. If the distance is too great, get off the bus a few stops early or park your car several blocks from the office and walk the rest of the way.

☐ Walk at work. Take the stairs rather than an elevator or escalator (unless you have knee problems). Use your coffee break to take a walk rather than eat a calorie-laden snack. Walk during your lunch hour. Bring your lunch to work so you can eat at your desk, then follow up with a healthy walk.

☐ Walk your dog, if you have one, and increase the length of time you're out so that both of you get more exercise.

☐ Walk instead of waiting. If you're early for an appointment or if someone you're meeting is behind schedule, walk around the block instead of sitting in the waiting room reading magazines.

☐ Walk after dinner. It's relaxing, and you may cut back on the number of times you have dessert or indulge in evening snacks.

Does any single exercise provide total fitness?

While all aerobic exercises strengthen the heart, only cross-country skiing works every major muscle in the body. Swimming uses most major muscles, but it doesn't seem to strengthen bones—which protects against osteoporosis—as well as weight-bearing exercises, such as running and walking.

To broaden the benefits of exercise while avoiding boredom, injury, and burnout, consider *cross training*, in which different activities are combined into a total exercise plan. For example, you might swim on Monday, run on Wednesday, lift weights

EXERCISES FOR THE DISABLED

Maintaining muscle tone is especially important for anyone forced into a sedentary life by a disability. These stretching and toning exercises can be done by a person with upper-body mobility; for a more complete program tailored to your needs, consult your doctor or physical therapist. Check with your doctor before starting an exercise program. When exercising, lock your wheelchair in place; don't overdo it. For more information on exercises for the disabled, see Appendix.

Elbow-arm extensions.
For neck rotation, shoulder and elbow mobility. Place right hand on chair seat, left hand across chest on right shoulder; turn head to right. Extend left arm beyond left shoulder, as you turn head to left. Return to starting position. Do up to 8 repetitions with each arm.

Elbow-shoulder stretches. To stretch and strengthen chest and shoulder muscles. Clasp hands behind neck with elbows together in front of chin. Keeping elbows at chin-level, bring them back as far as possible. Repeat up to 12 times.

Hand-trunk stretches.
To stretch lower back and increase shoulder mobility. Put feet on footrests; hold right armrest or back of seat with right hand. Sit up, then bend forward from waist, reaching down with left hand as far as you can. Hold for 6 counts without bouncing; then sit up again. Repeat 4 times with each arm.

Wheelchair push-ups.
For triceps, abdominal, back, and wrist muscles. Place hands on wheel rims or armrests; straighten elbows to lift body out of chair. Lower body to count of 3. Repeat 4 times. To strengthen side abdominals, lift body slightly out of chair; swing hips to right, then left, before sitting back down.

BEGINNER'S EXERCISE DIARY

To monitor your progress, write down your exercises each day in a small notebook or looseleaf binder. Over the months you'll be able to see how far you've come and take pride in your efforts. You can also use the log to determine whether you're doing too much or too little or ignoring certain fitness components (like flexibility, for example). For stretches and light calisthenics, see pages 82–83 and 88–89.

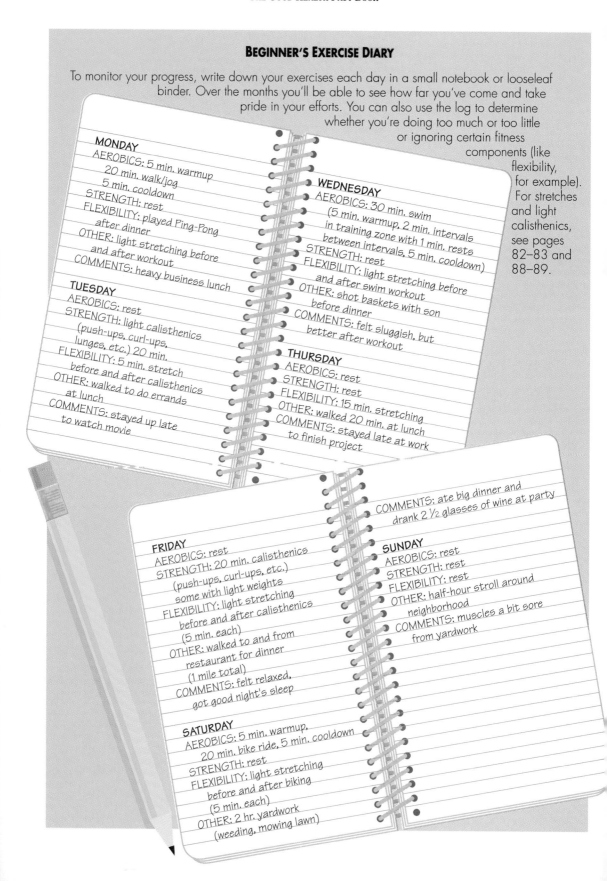

MONDAY
AEROBICS: 5 min. warmup
   20 min. walk/jog
   5 min. cooldown
STRENGTH: rest
FLEXIBILITY: played Ping-Pong
   after dinner
OTHER: light stretching before
   and after workout
COMMENTS: heavy business lunch

TUESDAY
AEROBICS: rest
STRENGTH: light calisthenics
   (push-ups, curl-ups,
   lunges, etc.) 20 min.
FLEXIBILITY: 5 min. stretch
   before and after calisthenics
OTHER: walked to do errands
   at lunch
COMMENTS: stayed up late
   to watch movie

WEDNESDAY
AEROBICS: 30 min. swim
   (5 min. warmup, 2 min. intervals
   in training zone with 1 min. rests
   between intervals, 5 min. cooldown)
STRENGTH: rest
FLEXIBILITY: light stretching before
   and after swim workout
OTHER: shot baskets with son
   before dinner
COMMENTS: felt sluggish, but
   better after workout

THURSDAY
AEROBICS: rest
STRENGTH: rest
FLEXIBILITY: 15 min. stretching
OTHER: walked 20 min. at lunch
COMMENTS: stayed late at work
   to finish project

FRIDAY
AEROBICS: rest
STRENGTH: 20 min. calisthenics
   (push-ups, curl-ups, etc.)
   some with light weights
FLEXIBILITY: light stretching
   before and after calisthenics
   (5 min. each)
OTHER: walked to and from
   restaurant for dinner
   (1 mile total)
COMMENTS: felt relaxed,
   got good night's sleep

SATURDAY
AEROBICS: 5 min. warmup,
   20 min. bike ride, 5 min. cooldown
STRENGTH: rest
FLEXIBILITY: light stretching
   before and after biking
   (5 min. each)
OTHER: 2 hr. yardwork
   (weeding, mowing lawn)
COMMENTS: ate big dinner and
   drank 2 ½ glasses of wine at party

SUNDAY
AEROBICS: rest
STRENGTH: rest
FLEXIBILITY: rest
OTHER: half-hour stroll around
   neighborhood
COMMENTS: muscles a bit sore
   from yardwork

on Thursday, and bike on Saturday for a week's worth of varied activity. Gentle stretching before and after workouts may enhance flexibility, but be careful—vigorous stretching and bouncing can tear muscles. Use moderation with stretching as with exercise in general.

An advantage of cross training is that it balances muscle strength, thereby lessening the risk of injury and ensuring that you don't neglect important areas of your body. For example, runners often have weak abdominal muscles, which can contribute to back problems. These athletes can benefit from rowing and swimming, which strengthen the abdominals.

Ask a fitness professional at a health club to help you design an effective cross-training program, and pick activities you enjoy so that you'll stick with them.

Is it better to exercise alone or with others?

It's really up to you. Working out alone is fine, and some people report that solo workouts are calming. For them, exercise is their only "me" time, and they treasure the solitude.

Exercising alone is also a good idea if you tend to be very competitive, even in recreational situations. Strong competitiveness can push people to the point of stress and, eventually, injury. If there are others around, you can still capture a sense of aloneness by tuning in to your body and avoiding conversation. Although wearing headphones during exercise is generally not advisable (see *Exercising Safely*, p.107), if you feel you must wear them to get the message across, turn the sound off for safety's sake.

Even if you usually prefer to exercise alone, you may want to plan group workouts every so often to socialize and vary your routine.

If I decide to work out alone, are there any special precautions I should take?

Just follow these simple commonsense rules:
☐ Don't walk, run, or cycle by yourself in a deserted spot where you could easily become a crime victim (see *Avoiding attacks*, p. 107).
☐ Don't swim alone in an unguarded area.
☐ Don't lift heavy weights without a spotter—someone standing next to you who knows how to steady or catch the weight if you lose control of it.
☐ Don't exercise alone in extreme heat or cold. You could be in serious trouble if you have an accident.
☐ Don't engage in a high-risk sport alone. Surfing, white-water rafting, kayaking or canoeing, hang-gliding, rock climbing, and downhill skiing are all examples of high-risk sports.

I'd like to learn aerobic dance. How do I find a good class?

Considering the popularity of aerobics (aerobic dance), finding a class is easy—the hard part may be choosing among the many options. Classes are taught in health and sports clubs, Y's, community centers, traditional dancing schools, and university and school settings. Some health club memberships include unlimited access to classes; others require a fee for each session or block of classes.

It's important to find a class that matches your fitness level and interests, and is convenient, accessible, and affordable. Look for a program with beginner, intermediate, and advanced levels so that you can move up as you gain fitness. If you aren't sure of your level, ask the program director or an instructor; if possible, sample a class before making a long-term commitment.

Aerobics classes are either high impact, in which both feet may leave the floor at once, or low impact, in which one foot is on the floor at all times. Because low-impact classes are gentler on knees and ankles, they are often recommended for beginners or anyone prone to injury. No matter which type you take, wear shoes designed for aerobics rather than for another activity, such as jogging. Make sure the studio has an appropriate floor surface. Hardwood over a cushion of air is best; avoid concrete floors, even if they are carpeted.

Before signing up for a class, check the qualifications of the instructor. The American College of Sports Medicine, The Institute for Aerobics Research, and the IDEA Foundation (see Appendix) certify aerobic-dance instructors. Working with a certified instructor ensures that he or she has passed a written test of fitness and aerobic-dance knowledge, nutrition, and motivational and teaching skills.

What should I expect from an aerobics class?

Most aerobics (aerobic dance) classes emphasize choreographed, rhythmic body movements set to lively dance music. The class is led by an instructor who demonstrates and explains the moves in front of the group and watches to see that members do them safely and effectively. Although such classes are noncompetitive, you're expected to keep up to the best of your ability, and you'll be encouraged to seek another class if the one you're attending is too easy or too hard.

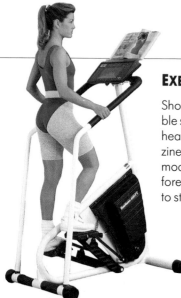

EXERCISE EQUIPMENT

Shop around before investing in exercise equipment. Visit a reputable sporting-goods outlet, seek recommendations from friends and health-club personnel, and check ads in sports and fitness magazines. Machines for home use are usually cheaper than health-club models, but can still cost several hundred dollars. If possible, try before you buy, and remember that you don't need fancy equipment to stay in shape.

Rowers give a vigorous aerobic workout that doesn't pound joints. With a piston rower (shown) you pull and push two long rods while sitting on a sliding seat. More expensive fly-wheel models, in which you pull on a bar attached to a chain, more closely simulate on-the-water rowing motions. To avoid injury, start with low resistance and build up gradually.

Climbers work leg and buttock muscles and quickly get the heart pumping in or above the training zone. Resistance, step height, and speed can be adjusted on many models; some keep track of pace, time, and number of steps. Climbers are not recommended for beginners.

Ski machines mimic outdoor cross-country skiing, though even experienced skiers have difficulty finding their balance on them at first. Feet are held in place on sliding platforms, and hands grip either push-and-pull, polelike levers or handles attached to a rope-and-pulley system.

Cycles run the gamut from simple resistance trainers that attach to outdoor bikes to whisper-quiet, air-resistant ergometers that give both arms and legs a workout. A good performance feature: Clips or straps to hold feet in place, so that legs pull up as well as push down on the pedals, working more muscles.

Treadmills allow you to jog or run indoors. The safest models have handrails and let you adjust speed gradually so that you won't stumble or fly off the back of the moving belt. Manual (non-electric) models cost considerably less than the sophisticated electronic versions, with programmable intervals, "hills," and video screens.

A good class works all the major muscles of the upper and lower body, and includes a warm-up to raise your heart rate gradually, and a cooldown period of slow movements and stretching. For the most part, you stay in one place (or move around a small area), moving your arms, legs, and trunk in a vigorous but controlled manner, so that you sweat, breathe hard, and feel your muscles working. Try to find an instructor who demonstrates moves before you perform them, and who can answer questions about what the exercises do, how they should feel, and how they can be modified.

If aerobic dance is to be your only aerobic activity, you should find a class that meets at least 3 times a week and includes work that gets your heart rate into your training range for at least 20 consecutive minutes. You can take classes less often if you combine them with a program of walking, jogging, swimming, or other aerobic activity.

I'd rather do aerobics at home. How can I find a good exercise video?

There are many good aerobics videos on the market—and plenty of bad ones. Rent several from your local library or video-rental store and try them out. Check the instructor's qualifications on the video jacket. Instructors should be certified by the American College of Sports Medicine, the IDEA Foundation, or The Institute for Aerobics Research.

The tape should explain why you're doing each move or group of moves, and why they're in the particular order given, how they should feel as you do them, and what muscles are involved. There should be a progression from simple to more involved movements. And as you complete

---

SELECTING A HEALTH CLUB

Know what you want. Some clubs focus on group instruction, others on the individual exerciser. You'll find clubs with a dance emphasis; others cater to body builders, or take a "mind-body" approach, offering meditation, yoga, and massage. If you're a beginner but plan to get into top shape, make sure a club offers advanced classes and adjustable machines.

Visit the club at a time of day when you'd be likely to work out so you can note crowdedness, client type, and classes offered. Don't let high-pressure salesmen get you to sign a contract on the spot or pay for a lifetime membership. Visit all facilities, looking for equipment in working order, roominess, well-lit and well-ventilated areas, and cleanliness. Workout flooring should be hardwood with an airspace beneath—never concrete or anything, including wood, carpet, or rubber, laid directly on concrete. Ask whether instructors are certified by the IDEA Foundation, the American College of Sports Medicine, or The Institute for Aerobics Research.

Ask about membership terms. Some clubs will suspend your membership for a time so you can take a break without losing money if you're injured, busy, or out of town. A club may also have an arrangement that allows you to use other clubs either locally or out of town when you travel.

Look for an established facility. The health-club industry is volatile, and some clubs have closed without refunding members' money. Get a report from the Better Business Bureau about a club you're considering; make sure the club is bonded so that you can get a refund if it goes under. Take the club's contract home. Read it carefully and check policies on refunds and transferring memberships before you sign or pay any money.

---

a step, the instructor should be cuing you about the next one.

Rent videos geared for beginners at first. If you have been sedentary, you should build up slowly; if a routine seems too strenuous or fast, pick another. At most, the video workout should be done every other day.

What are the advantages of joining a health club?

A health club membership can be a good motivator. The setting puts you with other people whose goals are similar to yours. Classes, open fitness areas, and locker rooms encourage social interaction, which can motivate you to keep coming. Paying the membership fee may help you take your commitment seriously.

Many clubs have on-site trainers whose job is to help members design fitness programs, instruct them in the use of weights and machines, and in some cases give advice on injuries, nutrition, and other concerns. For those who prefer same-sex workouts, most YWCA's offer women-only classes, and all-female clubs are opening in more and more cities. (Health spas, too, are often separated by sex.)

As much as all these things can help, joining a health club does not guarantee fitness. *You still have to do the work.* A sizable proportion of people who join health clubs drop out each year. If possible, try to establish a commitment to a regular exercise routine first by walking, jogging, or working out at home, rather than depending on a health club. It helps to find a facility that's close to your home or office, with hours that fit your schedule. Look for workout options that interest you.

What does a personal trainer do?

If classes, videos, and workout partners can't keep you motivated, and you have a relatively generous fitness budget, the answer may be a personal trainer. The trainer's job is to increase your motivation, improve technique, and keep workouts varied and fun. He or she should be able to answer questions about fitness, nutrition, and lifestyle, and help you work on problem areas—say, a weak upper body or flabby thighs. The trainer either comes to your home or works with you at a health club.

What should I look for if I want to hire a trainer?

Trainers can be expensive. Before you hire one, the two of you should discuss your fitness level, goals, weaknesses, injuries, likes and dislikes, lifestyle, medical and nutritional history, and any other concerns you have. Get a sense of the trainer's style and approach to fitness. Ask about his or her training in physical education, exercise physiology, and nutrition.

Check credentials too. Personal trainers should be certified by the IDEA Foundation. The American College of Sports Medicine's health fitness instructors or The Institute for Aerobics Research's physical fitness specialists are also qualified to do one-to-one training.

FACT OR FALLACY ?

You can sweat off weight

Fact. But only to a degree. The weight you lose by sweating is water, not fat, which is what really counts. The only way to lose fat is to burn off more calories than you take in; the best way to do that is through a combination of exercise and diet. Failing to replace the water you lose through perspiration can cause cramps, dizziness, headaches, constipation, kidney problems, and other complications. Drink water during and after exercise and whenever you take a sauna or steam bath.

Is a stay in a spa a good way to get fit fast?

A week or two at a spa can get you started on a lifelong fitness program or help you to improve on what you're already doing, but it is not an instant fix for an out-of-shape body. Spas can be expensive; it pays to know what you want and what to expect in advance so that you can get the most from the experience. Here are some tips:
☐ Pick your type of spa. Are you a gung-ho fitness fan or more into pampering and relaxation?

Do you prefer solitude or mingling? Would you like a body-mind approach, emphasizing meditation, biofeedback, hypnosis, stress management, and the new "mind-fitness" techniques? Do you have weight and nutritional concerns? Read brochures carefully and talk with representatives who can answer your questions about what's offered and emphasized.
☐ Tell the staff about yourself. The more they know about your fitness level, lifestyle, stresses, and goals, the more they can help you.
☐ Think long term. If you're out of shape, it's a good idea to precondition your body by eating sensibly (limit caffeine, alcohol, sugar, salt, and fat) and exercising regularly for 2 weeks or so before you go. Once you get to the spa, don't engage in so many activities that you exhaust or injure yourself. And make sure to apply what you learn after you get home.

An alternative to a spa is a fitness vacation or sports camp. Fitness vacations are usually group packages stressing physical activity—hiking, cycling, skiing, canoeing, mountain climbing, and the like, often in a remote area. There are camps for walkers, runners, rowers, tennis players, golfers, aerobic dancers, weight lifters, and other enthusiasts, from the beginner to the advanced level.

The sauna in my health club is very popular. How beneficial is it?

Although sauna, the practice of surrounding the body with hot air for health purposes, is more than 1,000 years old, its health benefits are unclear. In Finland, where the practice is a national tradition, people gather in saunas to relax, socialize, and do business. There's no question that lounging in a warm room can relieve stress; heat soothes muscle stiffness and joint pain by relaxing fibrous connective tissue and triggering the release of natural painkillers in the body.

But however pleasant a sauna may feel, it doesn't provide the benefits of aerobic exercise. Although the heat does raise heart rate, it lowers blood pressure, so that the heart's overall work load increases very little. A sauna also does nothing to strengthen muscles, burn calories, or promote fat loss.

As for the cleansing properties of a sauna, you should take such claims with a grain of salt. Regular bathing is all that's needed to keep the skin free of dirt and dead cells, and we perspire enough throughout a normal day to keep our pores and sweat ducts clear of impurities. In fact, saunas may aggravate skin problems such as acne and dermatitis.

Caution. In order to sauna safely, take the following steps:
☐ Set the timer for 15 minutes maximum; leave earlier if you feel dizzy, faint, or nauseated.
☐ Drink water before and after a sauna to replace fluid lost through perspiration. Do not attempt to lose weight by perspiring.
☐ Don't take a sauna after drinking alcohol or eating. Sweating profusely while digesting food diverts blood from the brain; you may faint. Alcohol has a dehydrating effect and dulls senses and reflexes; you might accidentally stay in too long, fall asleep, or even stumble into the stove.
☐ Sit on a towel or mat to protect yourself against infections; some bacteria tolerate high heat.
☐ Check with your doctor before taking a sauna if you are pregnant; have heart disease, epilepsy, hypertension, or diabetes; or if you take such medications as antibiotics or tranquilizers.

Do I need to eat a special diet if I exercise?

The consensus among nutritionists is that a balanced diet (as outlined in Chapter 1) is desirable whether you exercise or not. With the possible exception of iron, active people seem to have no unusual nutritional needs. Of course, if you don't always eat well, exercise performance may suffer as a result. The following nutrition tips apply to anyone, not just athletes.
☐ Eat plenty of complex carbohydrates. Pasta, cereal, whole-grain breads, vegetables, and fruit are all good choices. Complex carbohydrates are easily converted to glycogen, which fuels muscle activity. Proteins and fats are more difficult to convert to usable muscle fuel.
☐ Eat enough calories. Eating too little can make you light-headed when you exercise and cause serious nutritional deficiencies in the long run.
☐ Don't eat too much protein. Once touted as an energy enhancer and strength builder, protein is actually a poor choice for active people. It puts extra strain on the liver and kidneys, which must excrete protein that isn't used; it causes calcium loss, which can increase the risk of osteoporosis; and it's often found in foods high in fat.
☐ Drink lots of water or other fluids before, during, and after a workout. If you don't, you may feel light-headed, develop headaches and muscle cramps, and become dangerously dehydrated. Don't wait until you're thirsty, and don't worry about stomach cramps—they are seldom caused by drinking too much water.
☐ Make sure you get enough iron and calcium. If iron stores in your muscles are low (which may not show up in a blood test),

you'll tire more easily during workouts. Eat plenty of iron-rich foods; ask your doctor about taking an iron supplement.

Some studies suggest that running may cause mild iron deficiency, possibly because of the destruction of red blood cells caused by pounding on the feet and increased blood (and therefore iron) loss from the kidneys, bowels, and in sweat. The condition doesn't seem to improve when runners take iron supplements.

Exercisers don't seem to need extra calcium; however, women who exercise so much that they stop menstruating (p. 105) and who don't take in enough calcium appear to be at increased risk for osteoporosis. If you're concerned about your diet, consider seeing a registered dietician or nutritionist for an evaluation.

Is it necessary to drink "sports drinks" during and after a workout?

No drink has been shown to be superior to water. So-called thirst quenchers, such as Gatorade or 10-K, contain electrolytes (sodium, potassium, and other minerals), which sweating depletes. But the loss of electrolytes doesn't immediately affect the body, and you can compensate by eating bread, bananas, oranges, potatoes, or canned soup at your first post-workout meal.

Sports drinks also contain carbohydrate (in the form of sugar), which fuels working muscles. However, studies show that it takes such drinks 90 minutes after ingestion to get into the bloodstream and to your muscles. So unless you work out at least that long, sports drinks won't help your performance.

It *is* essential to replace fluids when you sweat, but water or any nonalcoholic, noncaffeinated beverage will do the trick.

STRETCHING EXERCISES

Although not a substitute for a warmup, these stretches can help prepare your body for exercise; they can also provide a soothing workout on their own. Do them gently (after a warmup). Don't arch your back, bounce, or stretch to the point where you feel pain. Stop if you feel any discomfort.

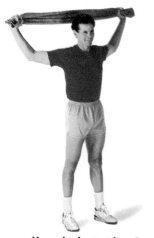

Neck stretches. Sit or stand upright, arms and shoulders relaxed. Slowly let head fall toward right shoulder, then toward left. Use a continuous, relaxed motion. Don't hunch shoulders. Repeat 5 times in each direction.

Side bends. Stand with feet 24 in. apart, left hand raised above head, right hand resting on right leg. Stretch left arm up; bend body to right, sliding right hand down right leg. Hold for 10 counts; straighten up slowly. Do reverse bend. Repeat 10 times in each direction.

Forward lunges. Standing with feet together, step forward as far as possible on right foot. Bending right knee, lower yourself as far as is comfortable keeping spine and left leg in a straight line. Use hands for balance. Hold for 10 counts. Stand up and repeat on left leg. Repeat 5 times on each leg.

Upper body stretches. Stand with feet shoulder-width apart. Hold a rolled bath towel firmly at both ends behind neck. While pulling on towel, lift it overhead as high as you can; hold for 5 counts, then lower towel behind neck. Repeat 5 times.

Drinks containing more than 8 percent sugar, such as non-diet soft drinks and fruit juices, should be diluted with water for faster absorption.

Is it all right to have a beer right after exercising?

Hold off for a while. Your first concern should be to replace fluids lost through sweating. If you drink alcohol right after a workout, when you are very thirsty, you may drink too much too quickly and wind up dizzy, disoriented, or with a headache. Although it may quench your thirst for the moment, a beer or other alcoholic beverage actually dehydrates the body even more; until you start replacing lost fluid, you are likely to experience nausea and muscle cramps. A good strategy is to drink two glasses

of water right after exercising, then have an alcoholic drink later on if you wish.

Drinking alcohol before or during exercise is never a good idea because it impairs coordination, reaction time, and perception, and can intensify fatigue. Wait at least 2 hours after your last drink before you start exercising. And if you do drink, always do it moderately—no more than two drinks a day, if any at all.

I've seen packets of pure oxygen for sale as a pick-me-up during exercise. Is this needed? Is it safe?

You may *think* you feel better after taking a shot of oxygen, but doctors say it has no impact at all on health or athletic performance. Breathing pure oxygen raises the level of oxygen in the

blood only slightly, and the effect disappears after a minute or two of breathing normal air. Although considered safe for healthy people, inhaling pure oxygen may be harmful to anyone with cardiovascular illness or chronic lung disease.

Is it necessary to warm up before exercising?

Warming up is thought to improve your range of motion and prevent soreness. It's generally recommended, although there is some question as to whether warming up actually reduces the risk of muscle injury.

Warming up means loosening muscles and raising body temperature and heart rate gradually to prepare the body for exercise. The best warmup is a slow, gentle version of the exercise you'll be doing—runners can walk or jog

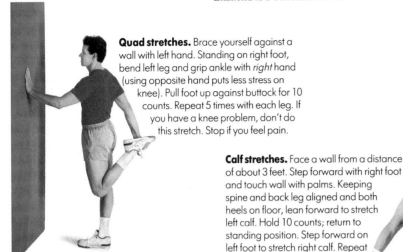

Quad stretches. Brace yourself against a wall with left hand. Standing on right foot, bend left leg and grip ankle with *right* hand (using opposite hand puts less stress on knee). Pull foot up against buttock for 10 counts. Repeat 5 times with each leg. If you have a knee problem, don't do this stretch. Stop if you feel pain.

Calf stretches. Face a wall from a distance of about 3 feet. Step forward with right foot and touch wall with palms. Keeping spine and back leg aligned and both heels on floor, lean forward to stretch left calf. Hold 10 counts; return to standing position. Step forward on left foot to stretch right calf. Repeat 2 to 3 times for each leg.

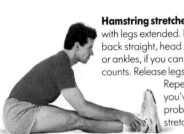

Hamstring stretches. Sit on floor with legs extended. Bend forward, back straight, head up. Grip calves or ankles, if you can; pull gently for 5 counts. Release legs; sit up again. Repeat 5 times. If you've had hamstring problems, do this stretch gently.

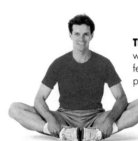

Thigh stretches. Sit on floor with knees bent and soles of feet touching. Grasp shins and place elbows on inside of knees. Gently press knees to floor as far as you comfortably can; hold for 10 counts. Repeat 2 or 3 times.

slowly, for example. Warm up until you're breathing harder than normal or sweating lightly (usually in about 5 to 10 minutes).

A cooldown is the opposite of a warmup. After vigorous activity (in or above your training zone) you continue the activity *slowly* for 5 to 10 minutes to allow the body to return gradually to its resting state. The harder the workout, the more important a cooldown is.

Taking a cold shower after exercise can stress the heart. Instead, shower in water that's close to body temperature.

Is stretching a good way to warm up?

Contrary to what many people think, warmup and stretching aren't the same thing. In fact, the value of stretching in exercise has not been established. Be-

cause flexibility is so varied and hard to measure, it's difficult to prove that stretching makes muscles and joints more flexible and improves performance. Although most people find that stretching before and after vigorous exercise makes the exercise more comfortable and helps prevent soreness, it's not a substitute for a good warmup. In fact, you shouldn't stretch before a warmup when your muscles are completely cold. If you stretch before a workout, do your normal warmup, then stretch the muscles you will be using for support and movement (see above), plus those of the abdomen and lower back.

How you stretch is very important. The most effective and safest stretches are gentle and static—that is, they're performed without straining or bouncing. Rather, you get into a

position where you can feel a stretch but no pain, and hold it for 5 to 30 seconds, depending on the stretch. Relax; then repeat the stretch, if you wish.

Stretching after exercise feels good because the muscles are warm and pliable. Some people enjoy stretching in the morning to prepare for the day's activities, and at bedtime, to relax.

What exercises are good for building upper-body strength?

Upper-body muscles are neglected in many aerobic routines and are not strengthened during everyday activities, such as walking. Simple calisthenic and weight exercises, such as those described on pages 88–89, are a good way for a beginner to strengthen arms, shoulders, and upper back. If you're interested

WORKING YOUR MUSCLES

Muscles and performance. Skeletal muscles, which hold your bones together and enable you to move, are made up of two different types of fibers: fast-twitch fibers, responsible for speed and strength, and slow-twitch, for endurance. The ratio of fast- to slow-twitch muscles varies with the individual and may determine athletic ability. Top marathon runners, for example, tend to have a high proportion of slow-twitch fibers; sprinters have the reverse.

Building endurance and strength. Low-resistance exercise, in which you stress muscles against a relatively light weight for many repetitions, builds endurance. High-resistance exercise, in which you stress muscles against heavier loads for a limited number of repetitions, builds strength. For best results, work a muscle "to near exhaustion," until you can barely contract it again.

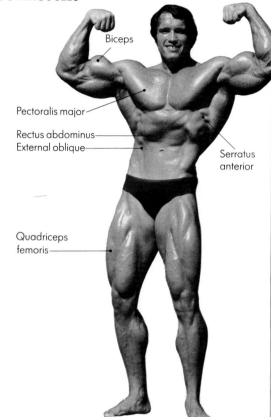

Biceps

Pectoralis major

Rectus abdominus

External oblique

Serratus anterior

Quadriceps femoris

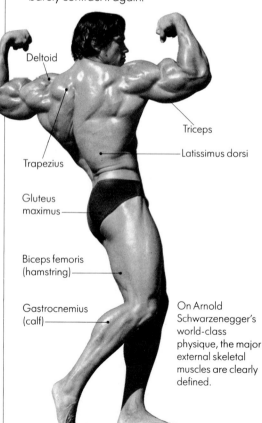

Deltoid

Triceps

Trapezius

Latissimus dorsi

Gluteus maximus

Biceps femoris (hamstring)

Gastrocnemius (calf)

On Arnold Schwarzenegger's world-class physique, the major external skeletal muscles are clearly defined.

Three types of exercises are used to build muscle strength and endurance:

In *isometric exercise,* muscles work against a static resistance. (An example is pressing your hands palm to palm.) Isometric exercises build strength without harming muscles or joints and can be done anywhere, but because they tend to elevate blood pressure, they may pose a danger to people with hypertension, heart disease, and stroke risk factors.

In *isotonic exercise,* muscles contract at varying speeds against a constant resistance. Free-weight and most weight-machine exercises are isotonic. In calisthenics, such as push-ups, the resistance is supplied by your own body weight.

Isokinetic exercise, in which muscles move at constant speed against a variable resistance, is a highly effective way to strengthen them, but the sophisticated equipment needed is not widely available.

in more serious weight training, talk to a qualified trainer about designing a safe, effective program. Swimming, rowing, and cross-country skiing are also good ways to build strength and endurance in the upper body.

Is weight training essential for fitness?

You do not need to lift weights to be fit, but some form of resistance training, either calisthenics or working with free weights or weight machines, is essential for building muscle strength and endurance and should be a part of a well-rounded fitness program. Whether a joint functions well depends mainly on the health and strength of the muscles that surround it. Strong muscles make everyday tasks easier. Flexible, conditioned muscles improve posture and balance, prevent injury, and enhance sports performance.

The American College of Sports Medicine recommends working each major muscle group at least twice a week; for each group, do at least one set of 8 to 12 repetitions to near exhaustion (see *Working Your Muscles,* facing page).

Do I really need a trainer if I want to start lifting weights?

To be effective, a weight-training program should be designed by a professional trainer or coach. Weight training requires considerable technique, and beginners should get expert advice if they are to avoid injury. Even if you're not interested in building bulk and brute strength, you should work out a plan and learn technique from a qualified instructor at a health club, school, or community center or with a personal trainer.

Are weight machines better than free weights?

Both weight machines and free weights (such as barbells and dumbbells) will help you get and stay strong. One advantage of free weights is that they also help you develop coordination and balance (the weight will tilt if you use more effort on one side than on the other). Another advantage is that with free weights you can generally do more exercises per muscle group than you can on machines.

On the other hand, free weights can be difficult for a beginner to control—you may drop them, try to lift too much, or strain muscles and connective tissues by using improper form. If possible, start your training

with weight machines. Once you learn the technique and build up your strength, you can switch to free weights if you wish.

Whichever method you use, be careful not to lift too much.

Does a weight-training routine provide aerobic benefits?

Not significantly. Although you may breathe hard at times during weight-training workouts, the aerobic effect is not consistent enough to help your heart.

There is an advanced techique called circuit training, which involves lifting weights quickly enough to get your heart rate into its training zone and doing aerobic work, such as jogging, cycling, or rope jumping,

---

CHECKLIST FOR A SAFE WORKOUT

☐ Warm up before your workout; cool down afterward.

☐ Make sure barbells have collars or clips at the ends to keep the weights in place.

☐ Start easy. For each exercise, pick a weight you can lift about 8 times. Do the sequence once (or, in gym jargon, do 1 set of 8 repetitions, or reps). As you gain strength, you may want to do 2 or 3 sets of 8 to 12 reps; rest a minute or so between sets.

☐ Don't lift too much weight. (If you can't lift a weight 6 times, you're lifting too much.) Try to work out with a spotter (p.77).

☐ Lift and lower weights in a slow, controlled manner; never fling them. Make sure your body is properly aligned with the weight you're lifting. Don't lock your elbows or knees, or arch your back.

☐ Breathe evenly; don't hold your breath. Exhale with the effort (generally, as you lift a weight); inhale with the release.

☐ Work through your range of motion. That means fully extending and contracting the muscles you're working.

☐ To avoid strain, work opposing muscle groups, such as biceps and triceps; work large muscle groups first, then smaller ones.

☐ Increase weight gradually. Add reps until you can do 12 per set to near exhaustion, then increase the load by no more than 5 percent and go back to 8 reps per set. Keep a progress log.

☐ Don't work the same muscles on consecutive days. Muscles need 48 hours to recover. Don't lift weights if muscles are injured.

THE FACTS ABOUT STEROIDS

What are they? Steroids are a group of natural and synthetic hormones with a variety of medical applications. *Anabolic steroids* are used illegally by many athletes to increase muscle size and strength and enhance sports performance. Steroid use has been banned by most major sports organizations, including the International Olympic Committee, not only because of the unfair advantage they give an athlete but because of their potentially dangerous side effects. Random testing of blood and urine for steroids has resulted in the barring of several prominent athletes from competition. Despite the risks, steroid use is rising among professional and many young amateur athletes.

What do they do? Anabolic steroids stimulate the buildup of muscle tissue. They also strengthen bones and help muscles recover after an injury.

The degree of muscularity an individual can achieve normally depends on genetic makeup, age, and training. Anabolic steroids provide a shortcut to developing the bigger, stronger, leaner muscles that can make the difference between a winning and losing athletic performance.

What are the side effects? Steroid use can lead to jaundice, liver damage, hypertension, lower levels of HDL cholesterol (the "good," heart-protective type), and damage to the heart muscle. The side effects may reverse themselves after steroid use is discontinued, but in a few cases they have been fatal.

Because anabolic steroids are closely related to the male sex hormone testosterone, they also affect the male and female reproductive systems and secondary sex characteristics. Steroids may lower testosterone production in men and interfere with a woman's menstrual cycle. Some women develop male sex characteristics, such as deepening of the voice, growth of facial and chest hair, and reduced breast size; some men develop breast tissue. These changes may or may not disappear after steroid use stops.

Other side effects can include mood swings, aggressive behavior, loss of muscle coordination (ataxia), stunted growth in young people, increased oiliness of the skin in women, changes in fat distribution, changes in body hair growth patterns, and hair loss. Unfortunately, there's no way to predict how a certain type of steroid will affect an individual.

spine. This can be an important safety factor when heavy loads are lifted. However, a belt is probably not a good idea for beginners because it keeps some abdominal muscles from doing any work. You may hurt your back if you train with a belt and then try to carry a bag of groceries without one. A better strategy: Include abdominal exercises in your fitness routine.

Gloves protect the hands from blisters and calluses. Most are made of leather, with open fingers for a better grip, and can be purchased at sporting-goods stores. (Rubbing chalk on your hands helps your grip too. Many weight rooms will have pieces lying around; ask a trainer or manager if you don't see any.)

Won't my muscles "bulk up" if I lift weights?

Weight training can increase muscle size (bulk), strength, and endurance; what happens to you depends on how you design your program. To really increase bulk requires a great deal of effort and the right set of genes. With a regular weight-training program (see *Checklist for a Safe Workout,* p.85) you have little reason to worry about building huge muscles. With their relatively small supply of the muscle-building male sex hormone testosterone, women are less likely than men to bulk up.

Are there good exercises for trimming waist, hips, and thighs?

Exercise can't alter your basic body type, and only bodywide weight loss will get rid of fat. However, any aerobic or resistance exercise involving the leg muscles can help tone thighs. Exercise combined with a low-fat, high-carbohydrate diet will

between sets. If you're a novice, circuit training isn't recommended because it can keep you from using proper form. You should, however, complement weight training with aerobic workouts to keep your heart healthy.

Do I need to use a weight belt and gloves?

Some weight lifters wear a special wide leather belt that compresses the abdominal muscles and so helps support the

promote overall weight loss, and in the process trim fat from hips and waist. The abdominal and lower-body exercises on pages 88–89 won't "shrink" your waist, hips, and thighs, but they'll tone muscles and help make those problem spots look trimmer.

I travel a lot. How can I stay fit on the road?

Thanks to the continuing fitness craze, more and more hotels have gyms, pools, and other fitness facilities. When you or your travel agent book your reservation, look for a hotel with a pool, health club, sauna, tennis courts, exercise classes, or jogging paths.

If your hotel doesn't have a gym or pool, you don't have to miss workouts. You can jog or take a brisk walk from the hotel—just ask the front desk or concierge to recommend the safest, least congested route; there may even be a map of the area, so you don't get lost.

If the neighborhood is too busy or dangerous, or if walking and jogging don't appeal to you, consider climbing the hotel stairs. Even at a moderate pace, this will raise your heart rate within a few minutes. (Warm up first and cool down afterward.)

Exercising right in your hotel room is another option; many travelers stay fit this way, and it takes little or no equipment. Here are some possibilities:

☐ Jumping rope (p. 92) is a vigorous aerobic workout that can burn significantly more calories than jogging. Make sure you have adequate ceiling space and good ventilation. Wear sturdy, properly fitting shoes; aerobic or tennis shoes are best. If you aren't used to jumping, practice without a rope first. Warm up and cool down with a few minutes of slow jogging in place, and gently stretch the muscles in your ankles, calves, hips, and lower back before and after your jumping workout.

☐ Stretching. You can do a complete stretching routine, such as the one described on pages 82–83. Sitting and lying-down exercises can be done on the floor (use a folded bath towel or a blanket as a cushion) or even on a bed with a firm mattress.

☐ Calisthenics. Any of the exercises in the full-body routine shown on pages 88–89 can be done right in your hotel room. If you're traveling light, look in sporting-goods stores for a set of plastic weights that can be filled with sand or water. A folded blanket can be used in place of an exercise mat.

☐ Exercise bands. Sporting-goods stores sell rubber bands in various lengths and thicknesses that you can use for bodywide stretching and strengthening. They're great to take on the road because they're lightweight, durable, and can be stashed anywhere. Many sets come with suggested routines.

☐ Other easy-to-pack workout aids include

A small rubber ball that you can squeeze between your knees while lying on your back with your knees bent, to strengthen inner-thigh muscles.

A hand-held grip strengthener to work hand, wrist, and forearm muscles. Use it while watching TV, reading, even at lectures and in meetings.

A small wooden foot massager soothes tired, aching feet at the end of the day, providing the perfect post-workout reward.

I'd like to take up jogging. How do I go about it?

Check with your doctor before starting a jogging program if you meet any of the conditions listed in *Before You Start* on page 73.

If you've never jogged before, it's a good idea to begin with a walking-jogging program. The New York Road Runners Club's beginner classes start by alternating a minute of walking with a minute of jogging for 20 minutes. After a week the classes alternate 2 minutes of jogging with a minute of walking, again for 20 minutes, and build up to jogging for 20 minutes nonstop after 10 weeks. Performed three times a week with your heart rate in its training zone, this program will maintain basic fitness. You should warm up first and cool down afterwards with a few minutes of walking, and stretch before and after if it makes you feel more comfortable.

Although you can jog virtually anywhere, smooth, stable surfaces are best: sidewalks, grass, dirt paths, tracks, and roads (jog in the reverse direction of the traffic on your side). If roads are slanted to allow for runoff, change your direction periodically so that one foot isn't always higher than the other. When surfaces are icy, consider jogging indoors on a treadmill or an indoor track.

Keep in mind that a jogging program shouldn't be an end in itself, but a means to getting and staying fit and healthy. Don't overdo it, and don't run if you're in pain. Pay special attention to pain in the knees and ankles. Many people are more comfortable when they combine jogging with less stressful activities, such as walking, swimming, and low-impact aerobics.

How can I avoid cramps when I jog?

Side cramps, or "stitches," are common among joggers. They have many causes, among them improper breathing, weak abdominal muscles, and food in the

Continued on page 90

Firming and Toning Exercises

This simple exercise routine has been designed to strengthen and tone you from top to bottom. Always begin your routine with a warmup and, if you like, a few stretches (pp.82–83). For starters, use dumbbells weighing 3 to 10 pounds or more, depending on how strong you are. Do floor exercises on a folded bath towel or exercise mat. Breathe evenly, inhaling to prepare for a movement, exhaling with the effort; pay special attention to form (see *Checklist for a Safe Workout*, p.85).

Upper body

Backstrokes. With one arm extended forward, the other behind you, slowly rotate your arms from your shoulder backward (as if doing the backstroke in a pool). Do not arch your back; keep knees slightly bent. Do this exercise 1 to 2 minutes in each direction. Backstrokes are a good warmup exercise.

Easy push-ups. Start with your hands and knees on the floor, arms straight and shoulder-width apart. Bend elbows to lower upper body to floor. Straighten arms to return to original position. Keep back straight throughout exercise; don't tilt head back or drop hips. Repeat 8 to 12 times.

Dumbbell push-ups. Lie on floor, with lower legs on a bench or bed. Hold dumbbells with palms facing, elbows bent, arms held close to body. Push dumbbells up by straightening arms smoothly. Return to starting position. Repeat 8 to 10 times.

Abdominals

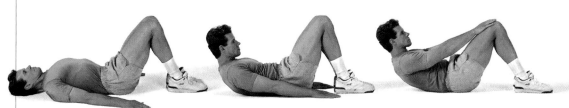

Tummy holds. Lie on your back, feet together, knees bent. Exhale, then hold your breath as you pull stomach in and up toward rib cage. Hold for 3 counts, then inhale and relax. Repeat 5 times.

Head and shoulder curls. Lie on your back with knees bent. Lift head and shoulders so that upper back is rounded and abdominal muscles contract. Hold for 5 counts. Repeat 10 times.

Curl-ups. Lie on your back, knees bent, hands on thighs. Curl head, shoulders, and upper back off floor as hands reach toward knees. Lower back stays on floor. Roll back slowly. Repeat 10 times.

Lower body

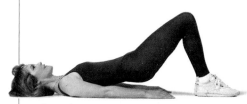

Buttock squeezes. Lie on your back, knees bent, feet together and flat on floor. Raise your hips slightly, leaving your upper back on the floor. Squeeze thighs and buttocks tightly. Hold for a count of 5; slowly return to starting position. Repeat 5 to 10 times.

Side tucks. Lie on your side, head resting on arm, lower knee bent, top leg straight. Raise top leg to hip level (leg should be parallel to floor). Gently bend knee toward chest, then straighten leg again. Repeat 8 times without lowering top leg. Repeat 8 times on other side.

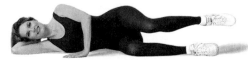

Donkey kicks. Kneel and place hands and lower arms on floor. Extend one leg out behind you, toes touching floor. With back straight and abdomen pulled in, raise leg to hip level (no higher), then lower to floor. Repeat 8 times for each leg. Avoid donkey kicks if you have back problems.

When doing exercises that require you to lie on your back, keep your lower back pressed against the floor. Don't arch your back when doing *push-ups, donkey kicks, knee bends,* and standing exercises.

Work out at least three times a week, starting with the larger muscles of the lower body and ending with upper-body work. Pick and choose among these exercises to vary your routines or find the one that's most comfortable for you. A typical workout, lasting about 30 minutes, might include *buttock squeezes, side tucks,* and *leg lifts; crunches* and *twists;* and *backstrokes, push-ups,* and *lateral raises.*

Floor flies. Lie on floor, lower legs on a bench or bed. Hold dumbbells in your hands, palms up, arms extended at shoulder level. Slowly raise arms, with elbows slightly bent, until dumbbells just touch. Slowly lower arms to starting position. Repeat 5 to 10 times.

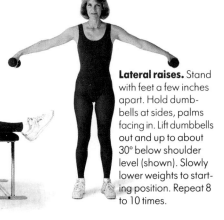

Lateral raises. Stand with feet a few inches apart. Hold dumbbells at sides, palms facing in. Lift dumbbells out and up to about 30° below shoulder level (shown). Slowly lower weights to starting position. Repeat 8 to 10 times.

Biceps curls. Sit at end of bench or chair. Hold dumbbell in right hand. Prop right elbow against inside of right thigh, forearm parallel to floor. Rest left hand on left thigh. Raise dumbbell toward chin as shown, using only arm muscles; don't start lift by pulling back with your torso. Slowly lower weight. Repeat 8 to 10 times on each side.

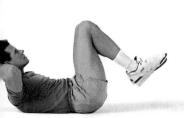

Crunches. Lie on back, hands clasped behind head, knees bent, feet flat on floor. Lift head, shoulders, and feet off floor, bringing knees and chin toward each other and pulling abdominals in tight. Return to starting position. Repeat 10 times.

Knee lifts. Sit holding the edge of a bench or sturdy chair for support. Raise bent knees to chest, then return feet to the floor slowly. Start with 8 repetitions. Work up to 20 reps, then if desired add ankle weights for greater resistance.

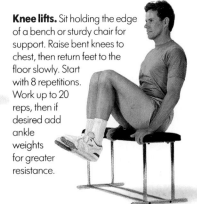

Twists. Put an old broom handle across your shoulders and rest hands on the ends. Rotate upper body from side to side gently without rotating hips. This exercise can be done sitting down to keep hips from rotating. Work up to 40 or more repetitions.

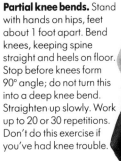

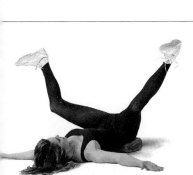

Frogs. Lie on floor with two rolled bath towels or firm pillow under buttocks. Extend arms to shoulder level. Bend knees over chest as in *crunches.* Slowly spread legs until they're wide apart. Return to starting position. Repeat 8 to 10 times.

Horizontal leg lifts. Lie on one side with body slightly bent forward at waist; partially support weight on arm, hold stomach in. Lift leg as shown, then slowly lower it to starting position. Repeat 10 times for each leg.

Partial knee bends. Stand with hands on hips, feet about 1 foot apart. Bend knees, keeping spine straight and heels on floor. Stop before knees form 90° angle; do not turn this into a deep knee bend. Straighten up slowly. Work up to 20 or 30 repetitions. Don't do this exercise if you've had knee trouble.

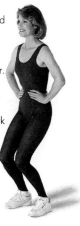

stomach and intestine. A good strategy for avoiding cramps is to jog before breakfast or lunch. Relax and start off slowly to avoid straining the diaphragm, the muscle that controls breathing.

If you get a stitch, breathe slowly and rhythmically and slow your pace. If that doesn't work, knead the area gently with your fingers. You might have to stop for a moment, lean over to relax the muscles, then walk a bit, breathing slowly and rhythmically. Most cramps go away with these simple treatments.

Foot and leg cramps can be caused by starting too quickly and pushing too hard, and sometimes by dehydration. If a cramp doesn't go away promptly, stop and massage the area, elevate and ice it, and take a day off from jogging. The problem is usually short-lived and is unlikely to recur if you warm up properly, drink enough fluids, and run at a reasonable pace.

What's the value of using hand and ankle weights in a workout?

Carrying light hand-held weights (1–3 pounds) is thought to raise heart rate and burn more calories when you walk, run, and do aerobics. In one study, subjects with hand and ankle weights burned only 58 more calories in an hour of running—too little to matter in weight loss. However, hand weights can enhance an aerobic-dance workout if you hold them correctly and don't overextend your movements, particularly of the arms.

Some experts discourage the use of hand weights for running because they upset the bio-mechanics of the activity. Ankle weights can put undue strain on the muscles in the front of the leg, which can lead to sore knees and other problems.

If you are determined to try hand weights, swing your arms so that you strengthen the muscles of the shoulders, arms, and upper back. (Simply holding the hand weights as you walk or jog doesn't make a bit of difference.) If you develop shoulder, arm, back, or hip pain, it's probably a good idea to leave the weights at home.

What are orthotics?

Orthotics are shoe inserts designed to reduce impact and compensate for imbalances, weaknesses, and other leg and foot problems. They can be slid into athletic shoes or other shoes that have backs. Made of leather, fiberglass, polyurethane, graphite, or other lightweight material, these inserts weigh only a few ounces. They are tapered at the edges to avoid irritating the feet. Orthotics can be quite expensive—up to several hundred dollars. Some shoe stores and mail-order houses sell ready-made orthotics. But since everyone's feet are different, it's often better to get custom-made ones from a knowledgeable podiatrist or from a specialist, called an orthotist.

Who benefits most from wearing orthotics? Are they more important for some sports than for others?

Although most often prescribed for people who run more than 25 miles a week, orthotics can prevent or relieve many problems—including knee pain, shin splints, hip problems, and foot injuries—caused by participation in

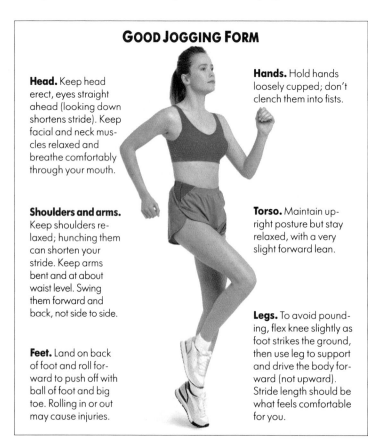

GOOD JOGGING FORM

Head. Keep head erect, eyes straight ahead (looking down shortens stride). Keep facial and neck muscles relaxed and breathe comfortably through your mouth.

Shoulders and arms. Keep shoulders relaxed; hunching them can shorten your stride. Keep arms bent and at about waist level. Swing them forward and back, not side to side.

Feet. Land on back of foot and roll forward to push off with ball of foot and big toe. Rolling in or out may cause injuries.

Hands. Hold hands loosely cupped; don't clench them into fists.

Torso. Maintain upright posture but stay relaxed, with a very slight forward lean.

Legs. To avoid pounding, flex knee slightly as foot strikes the ground, then use leg to support and drive the body forward (not upward). Stride length should be what feels comfortable for you.

WHAT TO LOOK FOR IN A WALKING SHOE

No matter what your sport or activity, the right footwear is essential. Buy comfortable, well-fitting shoes designed specifically for your activity. Shown here are the features to look for in a good walking shoe.

Upper. For breathability and wear, leather or leather-and-mesh are best.

Tongue. Should be padded and fit securely under laces without sliding.

Ankle collar. Padding ensures comfort and secure fit; collar may be notched in back to avoid hurting Achilles' tendon.

Toe box. Should give toes enough room to wiggle while protecting them from stubbing; some shoes have a toe "wrap" for extra durability.

Insole (not visible). A pliable liner, usually removable, provides extra cushioning.

Midsole (not visible). The shoe's main cushioning and shock-absorbing part.

Heel counter (not visible). A hard, cuplike device inside the shoe to stabilize heel and prevent slippage.

Outsole. Durable rubber provides stability and traction. Look for flexibility across ball of foot so that foot can bend naturally as you walk.

Arch. An internal rubber arch cushion (not visible) adds support; snug fit helps prevent foot fatigue.

---

high-impact sports. Using orthotics may cause you to lose a bit of elasticity, but if you are prone to injury, the gain in protection can be well worth it.

Orthotics, however, are not the only way to prevent sports-related pain and injuries. It's best to see a physician and consider other solutions—new shoes, stretching, reduced mileage and intensity, exercising on soft surfaces, and avoiding hills—before trying expensive orthotics.

Is there a proper walking technique?

Believe it or not, there are right ways and wrong ways to walk, especially if you want a good aerobic workout. The most important thing is to direct all motion forward. Walk tall and look straight ahead. Relax your shoulders. Keep your arms bent and at about waist level. Your hands should be loosely cupped, not clenched into tight fists. Swing your arms back and forth, not side to side across the chest. Relax your hips (some pre-walk stretching may help) and take comfortable strides; overstriding can strain leg and buttock muscles. Shorten your stride going up hills; lengthen it slightly coming down.

Your feet should contact the ground heel first; then roll across the ball of the foot as you step through, pushing off with the toes. The feet should move in two parallel lines about hip-width apart. This should feel natural and is probably something you don't have to think about. As you walk faster, the parallel lines should move closer together.

Brisk walking can be as effective as jogging in raising your heart rate into the training zone, the level at which activity strengthens the heart and lungs. While walking, check your pulse (p. 70) periodically to make sure you're staying within the zone.

What's the difference between race walking and fitness walking?

Walking is divided into categories based on speed, purpose, and technique. Select the type of walking best suited to your fitness level and goals:

☐ Leisure walking. A stroll: You cover ground at speeds under 3 mph, or at a pace that doesn't get the heart beating in its training zone. Some studies suggest that even at this level, walking may add years to your life. It also burns calories and works leg and buttock muscles.

☐ Fitness walking (or health walking). At speeds between 3 and 5 mph, most people will raise

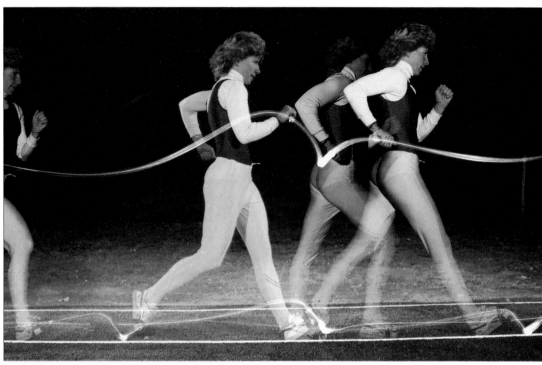

A champion race walker shows proper race-walking form, with its unusual hip wobble. Hold head level, chin up. Step forward with left leg, locking left knee as the heel hits the ground; simultaneously swing right arm forward forcefully, with elbow at right angle. Immediately push off with right foot and swing it forward, close to the ground, while you swing left arm forward and right arm back. Lock right knee as right foot hits the ground and left foot pushes off. Keep placing feet on a straight line in front of you, always keeping rear foot on the ground as long as possible before pushing off.

their heart rates into the training zone and perspire lightly. This burns calories (roughly 300–500 per hour, depending on exact speed, fitness level, and body size), strengthens leg and buttock muscles, and improves cardiovascular fitness. It's best to begin fitness walking on a smooth, level surface in an area where you won't have to make frequent stops for traffic lights, stop signs, and people.

□ Hiking. This is a general term for walking in a natural setting, often with a destination and over an extended period. Terrain may vary and you may carry a pack. Speed depends on fitness level, terrain, and distance, but hikers should be in good physical shape before setting out on a trip of more than a few hours.

□ Race walking. This is a competitive sport with strict rules regarding technique. Race walkers must keep one foot on the ground at all times and straighten each leg as the body passes over it. The resulting up-and-down rotating motion of the hips makes the race walk look like a fast waddle. Competitive race walkers move at speeds of up to 8 mph— faster than most people can run! Because it uses more muscles in the abdomen, buttocks, arms, and shoulders than running does, race walking burns more calories per hour. But because it's easier on the joints, it leads to fewer injuries.

How does jumping rope rate as an aerobic exercise?

It's one of the best aerobic activities you can do. Jumping rope raises heart rate, builds strength and endurance in the legs, develops the forearms, improves balance and coordination, and can be done almost anywhere. It's a vigorous workout, however. If you're starting to exercise for the first time or after a long layoff, get in shape first with a few weeks of walking or light jogging.

If you don't have a jump rope, clothesline will do (ask for No. 10 sash cord in a hardware store). It should be long enough to reach to your armpits when you run it under both feet and up each side of your body (with extra rope, if you wish, to loop around your hands). Some people prefer ropes with handles. The best models have ball bearings that allow the rope to swing smoothly.

Wear comfortable, lightweight clothes. Work out in a well-ventilated area on a level, resilient surface (hardwood flooring with

JOGGER'S/RUNNER'S DIARY

As with any exercise program, it's a good idea to monitor your progress, writing down how far, how fast, and how often you run. These sample diaries are meant only as a guide; don't feel you have to follow them to the letter. For example, you may want to add light stretching after each warmup and cooldown. Other useful things to record are how you feel during and after a run as well as notes on diet, sleep patterns, and any illnesses or special stresses.

Beginner

MONDAY: 5 min. walking warmup
Walk/jog 20 min. (1 mile)
5 min. walking cooldown
TUESDAY: No jogging
15 min. calisthenics and stretching
WEDNESDAY: 5 min. walking warmup
Walk/jog 20 min. (1 mile)
5 min. walking cooldown
THURSDAY: No jogging
15 min. calisthenics and stretching
FRIDAY: No jogging
15 min. calisthenics and stretching
SATURDAY: 5 min. walking warmup
Walk/jog 30 min. (1 ½ miles)
5 min. walking cooldown
SUNDAY: No jogging
30 min. walk

Intermediate

MONDAY: 5 min. warmup
Jog 25 min. (2 ½ miles)
5 min. cooldown
TUESDAY: No jogging
20 min. calisthenics and stretching
WEDNESDAY: 10 min. jogging warmup
Run 3 intervals of 440 yds. each,
all at a fast (anaerobic) pace,
with 2 ½ min. rests
between intervals
10 min. cooldown
THURSDAY: No jogging
20 min. calisthenics and stretching
FRIDAY: 5 min. warmup
Jog 30 min. (3 miles)
5 min. cooldown
SATURDAY: No jogging
30 min. bike ride or swim
at an easy pace
SUNDAY: 5 min. warmup
Jog 25 min. (2 ½ miles)
5 min. cooldown

Advanced

MONDAY: 5 min warmup
Run 30 min. (3 ½–4 miles)
5 min. cooldown
Light calisthenics and stretching
TUESDAY: 10 min. jogging warmup
Run 4 intervals: 440 yd.,
880 yd., 880 yd., 440 yd., at a
fast (anaerobic) pace, with
2 ½ min. rests between intervals
10 min. cooldown
WEDNESDAY: No running
30 min. bike or swim
at easy pace

THURSDAY: 5 min. jogging warmup
Run 30 min. (3 ½–4 miles)
5 min. cooldown
Light calisthenics and stretching
FRIDAY: 5 min. warmup
Run 40 min. (4 ½–5 miles)
5 min. cooldown
SATURDAY: No running
20 min. calisthenics and stretching
SUNDAY: 5 min. warmup
Run 50 min. (6–6 ½ miles)
5 min. cooldown

THE CRAWL

The most popular swim stroke, the crawl, is also the easiest to master. In the standard crawl, the arms move alternately in a smooth, circular motion: one arm recovers above the water, while the other pulls straight down beneath the water alongside your body. In the more powerful and efficient S-pull

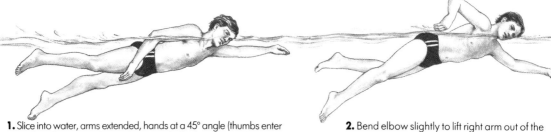

1. Slice into water, arms extended, hands at a 45° angle (thumbs enter water first), fingers together. Pull one arm (right shown here) down and back, bending elbow so that hand traces an S as it passes beneath torso. Straighten arm to complete pull at hip or upper thigh.

2. Bend elbow slightly to lift right arm out of the water. Increase elbow bend as hand clears the water and arm swings forward. Simultaneously begin pulling action with left arm.

an airspace beneath is best; never jump on a concrete surface, even if carpeted). Wear aerobic-dance or tennis shoes; running shoes are not a good choice because they chiefly protect the heel. If you develop soreness, especially in the ankles, calves, or knees, make sure your shoes have adequate cushioning and support (see *What to Look for in a Walking Shoe*, p.91). If necessary, cut back on the frequency or intensity of your workouts.

How do I design a rope-jumping program?

First, try jumping without a rope. Keep your feet together, knees slightly bent, and jump 1 to 3 inches off the ground. You should be able to jump 100 times without getting breathless. Adding the rope may take practice (even if you were the champ back in third grade), so be patient and proceed slowly, at a rate of about one jump per second. Don't worry if you miss—your heart rate will stay up for the time it takes to get going again.

Start by jumping 60 or 70 turns per minute for 1 or 2 minutes, rest 30 seconds (or longer if your heart rate is still at the high end of your training zone),

then jump for another minute or two. Take your pulse after each set of jumps, and if you're above your training zone, cut back on the intensity. When you can do five or six sets comfortably, increase their length to 2 to 3 minutes (with 30-second rest periods). After a month or so of every-other-day jumping, you should be able to jump 5 minutes nonstop. When that feels comfortable, try increasing your speed to 100 jumps per minute. If you can do four 5-minute sets, with 30-second rest periods, you've become an accomplished jumper!

Warm up with a few minutes of walking or jogging in place, and cool down afterward in the same way. It's a good idea to stretch your ankle, calf, hamstring, quadriceps, hip, and lower-back muscles before and after you work out. Since jumping doesn't condition the abdominals and upper body (except forearms), balance your workouts with rowing, swimming, calisthenics, or weight training.

I'd like to swim to get in shape. How do I start?

Swimming is an excellent aerobic exercise that works all the major muscle groups and involves

little risk of injury. If you have never learned to swim, sign up for a beginner class at a local pool, Y, community center, or health club. (Intermediates may want to brush up on their technique too.) Most people easily master the crawl, the most efficient stroke.

Once you've learned the mechanics, you can achieve basic fitness by swimming laps at a steady pace, working up to a 20-minute continuous workout three times a week. As with land-based exercise, build up slowly to condition the heart gradually and avoid soreness in your muscles and connective tissue. The most common swimming injury is shoulder soreness. Don't ignore or push yourself through excessive pain. To keep your shoulders strong, consider supplementing your swimming program with regular weight-training exercises (calisthenics or working out with weights).

Begin your program by swimming 100 yards (four laps of a 25-yard pool) with a 1-minute rest between each lap. After a few weeks you should be able to swim 150 yards in three 50-yard intervals, resting a minute between each. Because of such factors as water pressure and the variation, the pulling arm bends in order to trace an S-curve as it passes beneath your body.

Do about three flutter kicks for every arm stroke. Breathe by pivoting your head to the right or the left, whichever side feels more comfortable. Inhale about three-quarters of the way through the pull (Figure 1, below); exhale into the water as the arm on the breathing side recovers.

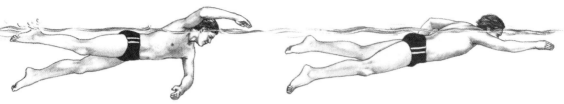

3. Continue recovery by extending right arm forward; it should be nearly straight as it enters the water. As right arm completes recovery, left arm passes beneath torso with elbow bent about 90°.

4. To do the flutter kick, move legs alternately up and down 12 to 18 inches, keeping your feet just below the surface. Knees should be straight but not locked, ankles loose, toes almost pointed. Churn the water instead of splashing it.

cooling effect of water on the body, your heart will beat at least 10 fewer times per minute when you swim. Adjust your training zone accordingly by subtracting 10 from your normal upper and lower range. And remember, you are sweating, even though you are in water and can't feel it, so drink plenty of fluids after swimming to replace what you have lost.

I'm 68 years old and never learned how to swim. Is it too late to start now?

Swimming is an excellent exercise for people of all ages, and an older person who has checked with his or her doctor can start swimming just as easily as a younger person can. Because it's gentle on the joints, swimming (and other aquatic exercise) is a great workout for people with arthritis. Keep in mind, however, that swimming does less than weight-bearing activities, such as walking or jogging, to strengthen bones, which can help prevent osteoporosis. Beginner swim classes are open to people of all ages, so don't let the fact that you've never worked out in the water hold you back.

The pool at my health club is so crowded that I often wind up bumping into people. Any suggestions for avoiding this problem?

Ask the lifeguard or pool manager at your health club if there's a policy on passing slower swimmers. Some facilities use the "toe tapping" rule: If you want to pass a swimmer, tap her toe as a signal to move over. In order to minimize passing, some health clubs designate lanes for slow, medium, and fast swimmers. If there is no passing policy at your pool, you might suggest implementing one (perhaps passing might be permitted only at the end of a lane).

If possible, avoid swimming at peak hours—usually before and after work. If the pool is crowded, pick a stroke that allows you to see other swimmers, such as the crawl or breaststroke, rather than the backstroke or butterfly. Keep alert to avoid potentially dangerous head-on collisions with swimmers or divers. Finally, it's a good idea to count the number of strokes you take in an average lap, so that you'll always know when you're getting near the wall.

What swim stroke gives the best workout?

For aerobic conditioning, pick the crawl. It requires constant, steady movement without the gliding intervals characteristic of the breaststroke and sidestroke or the energy bursts and difficult technique of the butterfly. Some people find the backstroke (also called the back crawl) easier than the regular front crawl because with the backstroke they don't have to coordinate breathing and arm movement; both strokes provide a similar workout. If you develop shoulder soreness, alternate crawl laps with a less strenuous stroke, such as the breaststroke.

What else can I do in the water to get a good aerobic workout?

Water-based walking, running, aerobic dancing, and other sports are gaining popularity. They are easier on joints than landed versions, because your body is buoyant and less vulnerable to weight-bearing stress. And since water offers greater resistance than air, a water workout can be better at building muscles and burning calories. Walking at 3 mph

WATER SAFETY

☐ Don't go into the water alone. Don't fish, sail, row, or canoe solo either.

☐ Don't swim where there's no lifeguard on duty, unless you're a strong swimmer.

☐ Don't swim if you feel full because you could become nauseated in the water. Keep children out of the water for an hour after a meal.

☐ Never jump into water if you can't see the bottom or if it's less than 9 feet deep.

☐ Never drink alcohol before swimming or boating. Do drink nonalcoholic, non-caffeinated fluids to replace those lost through sweating.

☐ Stay away from open water if thunder, lightning, or darkening clouds with a greenish or purplish tint signal an approaching storm.

☐ Don't stay in cold water too long.

☐ Keep life jackets for every person on a boat; children and nonswimmers should wear theirs. Children who cannot swim should wear a jacket whenever they're in or around water.

☐ For emergencies, learn how to float. Lean back with your ears underwater, chest above, and breathe gently. Swallowing a little water won't hurt you. Relax your lower body, extend your arms at shoulder level, and stroke lightly with your hands (propelling yourself toward shore if you can). Keep calm until help arrives or you reach safety on your own.

in thigh-high water, for example, burns up to 175 more calories than doing it "dry." Ask about "hydro aerobics" or "aqua aerobics" classes at local pools, health clubs, and Y's; or contact the Aquatic Exercise Association (see Appendix) for information on classes in your area.

How can I protect my eyes, skin, and hair from chlorine?

The best protection for eyes and hair is to cover up. Wear goggles and a bathing cap. To care for your skin, take a shower or at least rinse off after leaving the pool, if possible, and apply a moisturizing lotion while you're still damp. When you bathe, use a moisturizing soap, and wash and condition your hair to keep it from drying out.

If you swim outdoors, use a water-resistant sunscreen with a sun protection factor (SPF) of 15 or more. Reapply the sunscreen after you dry off if you plan to spend more time in the sun.

What is swimmer's ear?

It's a bacterial or fungal infection that results from water being trapped in the ear canal. Initially, you may experience itching or pain in the ear. The external ear canal may become red and swollen and a discharge may appear. To avoid swimmer's ear, shake water from your ears after you swim, and dry them thoroughly. If an ear does become infected, see your doctor; keep the ear dry until the infection clears.

I enjoy riding a bike. How does this rate as an aerobic activity?

Because it engages many of the large muscles in continuous, repetitive activity, biking is a great

way to build cardiovascular and muscular endurance, provided that you work in your training zone for at least 20 minutes three times a week. If done at this intensity, riding a bicycle compares favorably as a calorie burner and weight reducer with jogging, cross-country skiing, and swimming (see *Benefits of Your Favorite Sport*, p.66).

Riding a bicycle is especially good for developing the quadriceps (front of thigh) muscles, which help protect the knees during high-impact activities, such as jogging. (It's an excellent exercise for people with knee problems because it doesn't involve pounding). If you use toe clips, biking gives your calves and hamstrings a good workout too.

Although biking can serve as your only aerobic activity, many people enjoy it as part of a general exercise program. To help prevent muscle soreness in your neck, shoulders, arms, back, and legs, supplement your biking with a calisthenics or weight-training routine twice a week.

Caution. There are about 1,100 bicycle fatalities a year in the United States, many of which could have been prevented had the victims been wearing helmets. Always wear a snug-fitting helmet when you ride a bicycle; make sure that your children wear them too. When purchasing a helmet, look for a sticker of approval from the Snell Memorial Foundation or the American National Standards Institute (ANSI).

A relatively flat, traffic-free area is best for outdoor bike riding. Remember that stopping time is lengthened when you brake on wet, oily, icy, dusty, gravelly, or downhill surfaces.

If your bike's pedals are equipped with toe clips, practice slipping out of them quickly before you ride in traffic.

WHAT TO LOOK FOR IN A BICYCLE

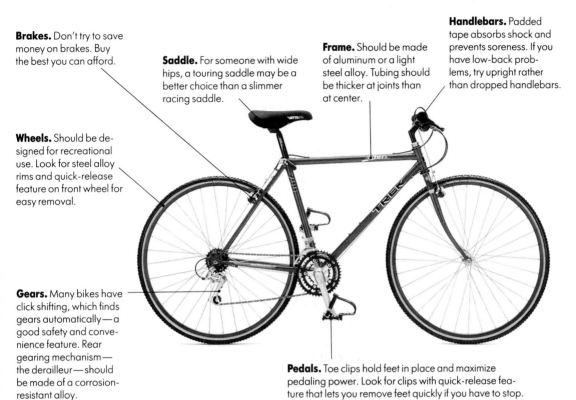

Brakes. Don't try to save money on brakes. Buy the best you can afford.

Saddle. For someone with wide hips, a touring saddle may be a better choice than a slimmer racing saddle.

Frame. Should be made of aluminum or a light steel alloy. Tubing should be thicker at joints than at center.

Handlebars. Padded tape absorbs shock and prevents soreness. If you have low-back problems, try upright rather than dropped handlebars.

Wheels. Should be designed for recreational use. Look for steel alloy rims and quick-release feature on front wheel for easy removal.

Gears. Many bikes have click shifting, which finds gears automatically—a good safety and convenience feature. Rear gearing mechanism— the derailleur—should be made of a corrosion-resistant alloy.

Pedals. Toe clips hold feet in place and maximize pedaling power. Look for clips with quick-release feature that lets you remove feet quickly if you have to stop.

How should I go about buying a bike?

Visit a reputable shop and tell the salesperson how much and under what conditions you plan to ride. The bike's fit is crucial. Riding a bike that's too big or too small is dangerous and can strain muscles and joints. Women and men under 5 feet 4 inches, as well as anyone with a short torso, should consider getting a specially constructed women's bike with a smaller frame and front wheel. Before buying a bike, take it for a test ride to make sure it's comfortable for you. If you find the seat is too narrow, ask to have a wider one installed.

For basic fitness riding, a good choice is a 10- or 12-speed all-purpose recreational bike— sometimes called a road or touring bike. Such bikes are built for safety, comfort, and durability. Unless you actually plan to race, don't buy a racing bike, which is designed for maximum speed, with powerful gears, very thin tires, and little shock absorption.

Designed for use on rough surfaces, a mountain bike (also called an all-terrain bike) has a low center of gravity, a heavy frame, and handlebars that keep the rider sitting upright. Its tires are fatter than those on a recreational bike, with a tread that provides good traction. Some people find that these features make for safer and more comfortable biking on and off the road.

For good maintenance and safety, have your bike's bearings greased and its brakes and gears adjusted at least once a year. Keep tires properly inflated unless you're going to store the bike for an extended period.

Which is better, biking outdoors or exercising on a stationary bike indoors?

You can get a good aerobic workout either way, but for safety and consistency, the stationary bike is better. You have complete control of the pace and length of time you ride; darkness and bad weather needn't deter you; and you do not have to worry about flat tires and other mishaps. But riding an indoor bike can be boring, and people tend to work out on them with less intensity. You can counter boredom by wearing headphones, watching TV, or riding with a friend. Some stationary bikes can be programmed to simulate hills, and even have screens showing scenery and other riders.

If you choose outdoor biking,

stay in a gear that lets you pedal at about 70 to 90 rpm, the most efficient speed for a good workout. Take your pulse or the "talk test" (p. 70) periodically to make sure that you're working in your training zone.

How can I make the most of my rowing machine?

Start with just a few minutes of rowing every other day, preceded by a warmup and followed by a cooldown. Gradually build up to 20- to 30-minute workouts, three times a week. Row at a steady pace until you feel comfortable; later, if you wish, you can add faster intervals. It's a good idea to stretch lower-back and hamstring muscles before beginning a vigorous session.

Most rowing machines have a sliding seat. If the action is done correctly, the legs, buttocks, and abdominals do the initial work, while the back, shoulders, and arms finish off the stroke, for a total body workout. Check your pulse periodically to make sure you're working in your training zone.

Of course, rowing is also an outdoor sport performed on lakes and rivers. Like its indoor counterpart, outdoor rowing is an excellent aerobic exercise, but the logistics and costs involved limit its accessibility. For information on rowing opportunities in your area, contact the United States Rowing Association (see Appendix).

Why is cross-country skiing considered such a good exercise?

Cross-country skiing uses muscles all over the body, burns more calories than just about any other workout, and doesn't pound joints. Its advantages over

downhill skiing are that it's safer and easier to learn, it uses the upper torso, it can be done almost anywhere there's snow, the equipment is less expensive, and there are no lift lines.

Still, it's important to learn technique from a qualified instructor and to use the proper equipment. You'll need cross-country skis, special clip-on boots, poles, and lightweight layers of warm clothing (including mittens, a hat, and face protection for very cold days). If you've never skied, consider renting equipment first and going to a ski area where you can take lessons and work in a controlled environment. The basic movement is step-and-glide, with right arm and left leg moving together and vice versa, as in walking.

Once you have the technique, you'll be able to get your heart rate into its training zone (after warming up) with just 5 to 10 minutes of moderate skiing. Go easy, making sure you don't ski so far from shelter that you exhaust yourself getting back. Skiing can be exhilarating, and many people do too much the first time. Beginners should take frequent breaks to rest, drink fluids (no caffeine or alcohol), and stretch the muscles of the legs, back, shoulders, and arms.

I'm an avid cross-country skier. What's the best way to stay fit during the off season?

You can ski year-round on an indoor machine, or try "skiing" outdoors with in-line skates (see facing page). Walking, jogging, cycling, swimming, or aerobic dancing 3 days a week are other ways to stay fit when you can't ski. To maintain muscle strength, include a twice-weekly calisthenics or weight-training routine in your fitness program.

How does telemark skiing differ from cross-country skiing?

Picture yourself swooshing down hills on long, skinny skis that give you the flexibility in the ankles of cross-country skiing combined with the turning ability afforded by the downhill variety. You glide to the bottom, then dig in and climb up the next hill. That's telemark skiing, and if you love the excitement of downhill but want more of an aerobic workout, you might want to try it.

The telemark ski is a little wider than a cross-country ski and has metal edges, which make it easier to control and turn. You can buy or rent the equipment at ski and sporting-goods stores. Because telemark skiing allows you to turn and negotiate uphills and downhills, you can do it anywhere you can cross-country ski—and beyond. Avid telemarkers are happiest off the trails, skiing through the woods.

Before you hit the telemark trail, build a good fitness base through cross-country skiing or some other aerobic activity. Even if you're already fit, it's a good idea to try cross-country skiing or downhill skiing first. Experienced skiers can learn the basics of telemarking in a few hours. (For more information on telemark skiing, see Appendix).

Is ice skating an effective aerobic exercise?

Not until you get very good at it. Skating builds strong ankle and leg muscles and develops balance and coordination, but to achieve an aerobic benefit you must skate quite vigorously. A beginner would do better to concentrate on learning proper skating technique while getting an aerobic workout from walking, jogging, or swimming.

If you've never skated before, it's best to take skating lessons in a controlled environment, such as a rink. Children shouldn't skate unsupervised. One way to give youngsters their first skating experience (rinks are often crowded and lakes and ponds may be snow-covered, bumpy, and dangerous) is with an inflatable pool filled with a few inches of water and left to freeze overnight.

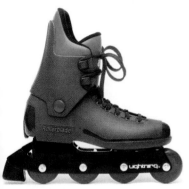

Blades, or in-line skates, are an increasingly common sight in parks and on city streets.

Are the new in-line skates better than conventional roller skates?

In-line skates, popularly known as blades or Rollerblades (a trademark), are faster, smoother, and more maneuverable than regular roller skates. Blades have three to five small wheels arranged in a row rather than in front and back pairs. The wheels are narrow enough to allow the foot to lean from side to side, but they're wider than the blade of an ice skate, providing greater stability. Because its side-to-side motion is similar to that of skiing, roller-blading is a popular off-season activity for both downhill and cross-country skiers.

Blading is not hard to learn, especially if you already know how to skate or ski. And once you get the hang of it, blading provides a very good aerobic workout. Wear elbow and knee pads and plastic wrist guards. Practice in a flat, uncrowded area until you feel comfortable. Other exercises that use the legs, such as jogging or aerobic dancing, are a good preparation for blading; but even if you're already fit, limit your first few workouts to about 10 minutes to avoid ankle soreness. Be careful on downhills; you can reach very high speeds, and blades usually don't have toe stops, as most roller skates do.

Are triathlons and biathlons for superathletes only?

A triathlon is a race in which you swim, then bike, then run; a biathlon leaves out the swimming and sandwiches a bike ride between two running segments. Both sports are reputed to demand extraordinary effort, but in fact their popularity has led to a proliferation of shorter races that can be completed by most moderately fit people. Training isn't effortless, however; if you're thinking of doing a biathlon or triathlon, discuss an appropriate training schedule with someone who's participated in an event or with a fitness professional.

The Triathlon Federation and the U.S. Biathlon Federation (see Appendix) will give you schedules of races across the country. Local health clubs, Y's, running clubs, and cycling clubs may have more information on training and local events.

My company is putting in a fitness parcour. How will I benefit?

A parcour is a series of exercise stations, usually set up in an outdoor space, designed to provide a total-fitness workout. A good parcour will offer aerobic, strength, and flexibility exercises at each station, with instructions on what to do at different levels of fitness. Equipment is simple and weatherproof. For example, you may repeatedly step onto and down from a knee-high platform to raise heart rate, or do chin-ups on a bar to build strength.

Before your first workout, look at all the stations and plan to skip or go easy on any that seem too difficult. If a warmup isn't specified, do one on your own. It's better to begin with too few than with too many repetitions and see how your body feels over the next couple of days.

Most parcours are designed to take between 20 and 30 minutes; jogging or walking briskly between stations keeps your heart rate in its training zone. Give yourself a day to recover between workouts, perhaps taking a walk, a swim, or doing some light stretching on the alternate days.

My only exercise is weekend tennis. What can I do during the week to stay fit?

Tennis and other racquet sports are stop-and-start activities that burn calories, build muscle strength and endurance, and develop balance and coordination. But, for all but the most advanced players, tennis doesn't keep the heart rate consistently in the training zone. The best complementary activities, which should be done every other day during the week, are aerobic exercises that use the muscles you call upon—in the legs, arms, shoulders, and back—to swing your racquet and run around the court. Jogging, walking, rowing, cycling, and cross-country skiing are all good choices. You can also strengthen these muscles by training with weights or doing calisthenics (such as push-ups and crunches) twice a week.

What is the value of exercise classes for infants and toddlers? Do they give kids an edge later on?

The American Academy of Pediatrics states that exercise classes for children under age 6 or 7, though generally harmless, don't do much good, nor is there any evidence that structured exercises will help young children become more athletic. Children less than 7 years of age don't have the motor skills that can improve fitness. Moreover, they may be pushed into activities for which they aren't ready and thereby lose interest in being physically active.

The academy's Committee on Sports Medicine urges parents to provide young children with a safe, stimulating play environment, to touch and hold them often, and to encourage them to have social contact with other children and adults during unstructured play time.

My 8-year-old child has always been chubby. Should she lose weight?

Although children grow at different rates and many shed their "baby fat," some overweight children may have difficulty maintaining a healthy weight as adults. However, it's not a good idea to put children under 18 on a weight-loss plan without consulting a pediatrician. Children of all ages need enough calories to meet daily energy needs and maintain a healthy growth rate. Your pediatrician should be able to tell you if your child needs to lose weight, and to prescribe a safe, effective diet and exercise program. Like adults, children are more likely to remain at a healthy weight if they make a habit of exercising.

PLAYGROUND SAFETY

About 200,000 children in the United States are hurt in playground accidents every year. Here are some features that make play areas safer for children of all ages:

Swings. Look for seats made of canvas, rubber, or plastic; they should be secured to the frame with ball bearings. The area around swings should be soft to minimize the impact of falls. Fencing should be far enough away so that a child won't fall on it, but close enough to discourage traffic into the area. Swings should be located where children engaged in other activities won't run into them.

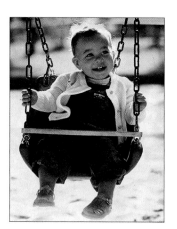

Jungle gyms and **monkey bars.** Surfaces should be easy to grip and slip-resistant. Painting or galvanizing prevents rusting. Look for soft surfaces underneath—not macadam or concrete.

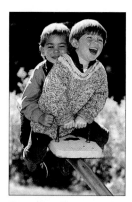

Slides. Make sure there are guardrails and a 10-inch-wide platform on top. The incline should be no more than 30°; the drop to the ground from the bottom, 9 to 15 inches.

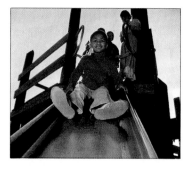

Seesaws. Bury a tire at each end to absorb the impact when the seesaw hits the ground.

Ground surface. The ground under and around every piece of equipment should be rubberized or cushioned with sand, wood chips, or other soft material.

General rules. Keep children away from equipment with protruding bolts, sharp corners, loose nuts and bolts, or rust. (See Appendix for sources of more information on playground safety.)

My son seems rather sedentary and seldom wants to go out to play. Should I worry?

Children who don't exercise not only lose fitness, they establish habits that can compromise their health as adults. Unfortunately, American children are becoming less fit; experts attribute the problem to inadequate physical education programs in schools and communities and to insufficient activity at home. Unfit children may lack energy and tire easily, have poor posture and coordination, and be overweight.

How can I get my child to be more active?

The best way to spark interest in fitness is to set a good example yourself by exercising regularly. Make it clear to your child that exercise is important to you and that you enjoy it. Your fitness program is probably not appropriate for your child, but try to find some time each week for shared activities: walks, jogs, bike rides, active games, and the like. If you ride a bike or jog with your child, go at his pace, not yours. Make the activities feel like play, not work, or most children will lose interest. It's important to strike a balance between encouraging your child to be active and pushing him too hard. The best way to do that is to make it clear that fitness is fun, and that you value the fun too.

Is jogging a suitable exercise for children? What about weight training?

It's fine to expose younger children to jogging in the form of "peewee" and "fun" runs. These are usually noncompetitive events organized by Y's, commu-nity organizations, and running clubs, at distances ranging from 100 yards to several miles. Some allow children as young as 2 to take part. There are no winners or losers, and often everyone gets a ribbon.

It's not a good idea, however, for children of any age to start a structured jogging program without the supervision of an experienced trainer. Excessive, unsupervised running may lead to injuries. Among teenagers treated at the Boston Children's Hospital Sports Medicine Clinic, running accounts for more injuries than any other sport. Overtraining may also delay the onset of a girl's menstrual periods, although this does not seem to have any long-term effects on health or fertility.

Weight training can increase muscle strength or mass in children under the age of puberty, but only minimally. In addition, lifting too much weight can easily injure young bones. Adolescents who wish to start weight training should learn technique from a qualified trainer and stay with a low-weight, high-reps routine until their bodies mature.

Neither jogging nor weight-training programs are necessary for a child to achieve fitness. Performed on a regular basis, calisthenics, rope jumping, sports such as soccer and football, and games like tag that involve lots of running will provide a child with the exercise he or she needs.

My teenage son is on the wrestling team and is always trying to lose weight. Is that healthy?

No, but unfortunately it's a common practice, often encouraged by coaches. Unlike some athletes who try to bulk up to improve performance—and sometimes resort to steroids to do so (see *The Facts About Steroids,* p.86)—wrestlers often try to lose weight in order to compete in a lighter weight class. To "make weight" just before a match, many wrestlers diet and dehydrate themselves by restricting fluid intake, exercising, wearing rubber suits, sitting in saunas and "hot boxes," and using diuretics and laxatives. The process may be repeated 15 to 30 or more times a season.

These routines are unhealthy and can be dangerous. Food restriction and dehydration can cause weakness and fainting, impair heart function, lower aerobic capacity, and cause other changes that can impede a young person's growth and development.

The American College of Sports Medicine (see Appendix) discourages severe dieting and fluid deprivation and urges coaches and school administrators to educate themselves and their wrestlers on the dangers of these practices. If you're concerned about your son's pre-match routine, discuss the matter with him and his coach.

Do physically active people live longer?

Studies have shown that, in general, people who exercise regularly live longer than those who don't. Exercise seems to reduce the risk and severity of various life-threatening conditions: heart disease, hypertension, stroke, and others. It appears that exercise doesn't have to be lengthy or strenuous to make a difference; one well-known study found that men who walked, climbed stairs, and played recreational sports outlived their sedentary counterparts.

Of course, exercise is just one part of the formula for a long, healthy life. Nutrition, stress relief, environment, lifestyle, and genetics all play a role.

What's the relationship between exercise, cholesterol, and heart disease?

It's a complex one that is still not completely understood. The leading cause of heart disease and heart attacks is a buildup of fatty deposits, or plaque, in the arteries, caused in part by high levels of cholesterol in the blood (see *The Facts About Cholesterol,* pp. 20–21). Just by helping you lose weight, exercise plays an important role in improving cardiovascular health and reducing heart disease risk. In addition, exercise raises blood levels of HDL cholesterol (the type thought to protect against plaque buildup), and may reduce blood levels of LDL cholesterol (the plaque-producing type).

The cardiovascular benefits of regular exercise extend even to people with genetically high cholesterol, who despite medical treatment may not be able to bring their cholesterol levels down to normal. In most cases, the combination of a diet low in saturated fat and a regular program of moderate aerobic activity (performed for at least 20 minutes, three times a week) helps improve cholesterol levels within as little as 3 months.

My doctor says I should exercise for my high blood pressure. How will that help?

High blood pressure, or hypertension (p. 326), is a serious health condition that increases your risk of heart attack, kidney disease, and stroke. Because excess weight is a major contributor to hypertension, exercise can be part of the treatment, along with diet and medication. In some people the weight loss brought about by exercise is enough to bring blood pressure within the normal range. Exercise even reduces blood pressure in some people who don't lose weight, although it's not entirely clear how this happens.

Are there any exercises that someone with high blood pressure should avoid doing?

Blood pressure rises temporarily during exercise of any kind, although less during aerobic workouts. If you have high blood pressure, avoid heavy-weight training and isometric exercises (see *Working Your Muscles,* p. 84), which can elevate your blood pressure excessively. A program of moderate aerobic exercise performed for at least 20 minutes three times a week will not only improve your overall cardiovascular fitness but may help lower your blood pressure. Check with your doctor before starting any exercise program.

Can exercise reduce the risk of stroke?

It may. Regular, moderate aerobic exercise helps reduce two major contributing factors to stroke: high blood pressure and high blood cholesterol. Exercise also relieves stress, which is thought to increase stroke risk.

If exercise is good for the heart, how come Jim Fixx died of a heart attack while running?

When runner and best-selling author Fixx died of a heart attack during a run in 1984, skeptics saw it as evidence that aerobic activity did nothing for heart health—or worse, that it could *cause* heart attacks. But the subject of exercise and heart disease is not so simple.

Many factors can predispose a person to heart disease; the most important are male sex, age over 35, family history of heart disease, smoking, high fat and cholesterol blood levels, hypertension, diabetes, and stress. Fixx, who died at age 52, was an ex-smoker whose father died of a heart attack when he was 43. An autopsy revealed extensive plaque buildup in Jim Fixx's heart and arteries. Running may have triggered his attack, but it had probably already added years to his life by strengthening his heart and slowing the buildup of plaque. Jim Fixx did, after all, outlive his father by 9 years. It is also reassuring to note that studies have found only 1 sudden death occurring for every 396,000 hours of jogging.

What Fixx's death does show is that it's possible to be fit yet unhealthy. Exercise is not a panacea for heart problems. But if you have risk factors beyond your control, such as age, sex, and family history, it's especially important to work on those you *can* influence: stress, smoking, high blood pressure, and high cholesterol levels.

Caution. People who have heart attacks while exercising often didn't know they were at risk or ignored signs of a problem (such as chest pain). If you are at risk for heart disease, or have had a heart attack, it's important to establish a safe exercise program with your doctor so that you won't overstress your heart.

Can exercising help prevent colds or does it make you even more susceptible to them?

There hasn't been enough research to give a definitive answer. Many people who exercise moderately report experiencing fewer colds and other infections;

scientists speculate that exercise may shore up the immune system, making the body more resistant to infection. However, one of the signs that a person is exercising too much is an *increased* susceptibility to infection, suggesting that overtraining impairs immunity.

Is it advisable to exercise if I already have a cold?

It really depends on how bad you feel. Exercising when you have a cold can help drain secretions from respiratory passages and relieve congestion; it also promotes relaxation. However, with a bad cold, you may tire quickly or be too tired to exercise at all.

Most doctors recommend not exercising when you have a fever, because your temperature may go up even more, making you feel worse.

My mother has osteoporosis and I'm afraid of getting it too. Can exercise help us?

The osteoporosis seen in women after menopause is associated with low levels of the female hormone estrogen (see *The Facts About Osteoporosis,* p.379). Although the evidence is still inconclusive, it does seem that exercise may help preserve bone mass in women with osteoporosis. Before starting an exercise program, however, your mother should check with her doctor.

In your case, there's considerable evidence that exercising regularly throughout life strengthens bones and may protect against osteoporosis in later years. (Conversely, lack of exercise quickly weakens bones at any age; patients confined to their beds lose bone mass in a matter of weeks.)

Although younger women certainly benefit from exercise, you should avoid overtraining to the point where you become excessively thin and your menstrual periods stop. This condition, known as amenorrhea, is thought to depress estrogen levels and may increase a woman's risk of developing osteoporosis as she gets older.

What activities are best for preserving bone density?

Weight-bearing exercises such as weight-training, jogging, and aerobic dancing are the most beneficial. Although not as effective in preserving bone density, walking is also a good choice, especially for older people. Even non-weight-bearing exercises such as swimming, rowing, and cycling seem to help too, but not as much as weight-bearing exercises. Most experts say that any physical activity is better than none in preserving bone mass, but if a weight-bearing exercise is feasible, it should be the first choice.

I have a demanding, high-stress job, and my doctor thinks I should exercise to reduce tension. What's the best way to do this?

The best exercises for stress relief are activities that are rythmic, mindless, steady, and last for at least 20 minutes. Although aerobic exercises such as walking, running, swimming, rowing, and cycling are ideal, any physical activity will help; choose the ones you most enjoy.

Most people report feeling refreshed, calm, and at peace after a workout. Although the mechanism isn't entirely clear, exercise seems to trigger the release of

chemicals in the brain (endorphins and other neurotransmitters) that control mood. These chemicals interrupt the stress-producing cycle of anxious thoughts. They are thought also to decrease the activity of the sensory receptors in muscles that cause them to contract, thereby easing the tension that can lead to muscle soreness and fatigue.

What is the value of yoga?

The philosophy of yoga, which comprises many forms, has been practiced in the East for more than 1,000 years and in the United States since the early 1900's. One type, known as hatha yoga, teaches posture and breathing exercises designed to stretch and strengthen the body, relieve stress, and improve balance. With its emphasis on the integration of body, mind, and spirit, yoga is an excellent fitness activity by itself or as an adjunct to aerobic and strengthening exercises.

Although advanced yoga postures may appear impossible or dangerous to the novice, most beginning positions feel good and aren't difficult to learn.

The best way to learn yoga is from a qualified instructor; many health clubs, Y's, community centers, and private teachers offer classes. Classes are noncompetitive, and good instructors help participants use concentration, relaxation, and regulated breathing to ease into a pose without discomfort or strain. The only equipment you need is an exercise mat, or a towel on a carpet. Wear comfortable, nonbinding clothing in a breathable material, such as cotton. Bare feet are best for keeping contact with the floor and maintaining balance.

If you can't find a yoga class in your area, a stretching or medi-

CALORIES BURNED BY NONSPORTS ACTIVITIES

Because your body uses calories around the clock, what you do at each moment makes a difference in the number of calories you burn off in a 24-hour period. The chart below lists a variety of routine, nonsports activities and the average number of calories they burn up in an hour. Whether you get regular, formal exercise or not, you can use the information to find ways to incorporate more calorie-burning activities into your life.

Activity	Calories burned per hour
Ballroom dancing	360
Card playing	102
Carpentry	210
Chopping wood	450
Driving a car	168
Eating	96
Gardening/yardwork	220
Heavy housework	250 (vacuuming, mopping)
House painting	210
Light housework	132 (ironing), 150 (dusting), 204 (making a bed)
Lying down	90
Mowing lawn	300 (pushing power mower)
Playing the piano	200
Raking leaves	300
Scrubbing floors	300
Sewing	94 (hand), 183 (machine)
Sexual activity	300
Shoveling snow	420
Sitting	80 (reading), 110 (talking), 120 (writing)
Sleeping	70
Standing	108
Typing/office work	240
Walking downstairs	420
Walking upstairs	800
Washing and dressing	156
Washing dishes	135
Window cleaning	300

tation class may offer similar benefits. In addition, yoga manuals are widely available.

A friend of mine says that since she started exercising she gets by on less sleep. Could exercise have the same effect on me?

It might. Some people who exercise regularly sleep fewer hours; and studies show that regular exercise improves the quality of sleep. By reducing stress levels through exercise, you may fall asleep more easily, sleep more soundly, and awaken less often during the night. Exercise can also counter depression, which is associated with sleep disturbances (either sleeping too little or too much).

Overtraining, on the other hand, can cause depression and its attendant sleep problems. One of the earliest signs of overtraining is insomnia in someone who has previously been sleeping well.

Sleep needs are very individual, so don't worry if you sleep more or less than other people—even if you exercise—unless, of course, you suffer from excessive daytime fatigue or other unexplained symptoms. In that case, see your doctor.

Do sports and fitness activities have any special benefits for women and girls?

They're the same as those for men and boys. Besides building fit, healthy bodies and improving athletic skills, sports and fitness activities can raise confidence and self-esteem, improve social skills, teach values, open career paths, and provide a lot of fun. The problem is that females have traditionally been barred from full participation in sports. Now, thanks to Title IX of the Education Amendments of 1972, which prohibits sex-based discrimination in school sports programs, many more girls and women are enjoying physical activity.

Is it safe for a woman to exercise after she becomes pregnant?

Doctors gave the OK to moderate exercise during pregnancy in 1985, when the American College of Obstetricians and Gynecologists published a report entitled "Exercise During Pregnancy and the Postnatal Period." According to the report, a woman who was exercising regularly before she became pregnant can continue to exercise moderately at least three times a week for 15 minutes at a time unless there is a medical reason not to.

A pregnant woman should not exercise in hot, humid weather and should make sure that her body temperature stays below 100.4°F. To avoid dehydration, she should drink plenty of water before and after workouts (and during exercise if needed). Her exercising heart rate (see *Aerobic training,* p.71) should stay below 140 beats per minute.

A pregnant woman should avoid jarring movements, overextending the joints, and after the fourth month, exercises that are performed lying on the back (which may impede the flow of blood to the fetus).

Regardless of the activities she chooses, it's important that a woman listen to her body and stop exercising if she experiences pain, bleeding, dizziness, shortness of breath, or palpitations. More research on the subject is needed, but until it is complete, the safest course for a pregnant woman who wants to exercise is to follow the ACOG guidelines and consult her doctor.

What are some good exercises for pregnant women?

Swimming is excellent because it keeps body temperature and heart rate under control; many pregnant women find water exercises more comfortable than those done on land. If you were sedentary before becoming pregnant, you should probably not engage in any activity more demanding than walking. If you jogged, you may continue to do so in moderation but will probably need to modify the type and intensity of the exercise as your body changes. You may find it more comfortable to switch to walking, low-impact aerobics, or stationary biking. Health clubs, Y's, and community centers offer special classes for pregnant women.

How soon can I start exercising after having a baby?

Most doctors say you can resume gentle exercise when you feel strong enough and it doesn't cause pain. If you have had an episiotomy (p.262), as many women who deliver vaginally in a hospital do, you'll probably have to wait several weeks until you've healed sufficiently. Postpartum exercise is a very individual matter, so it's best to consult your doctor and listen to your body.

Is it true that exercise can cause a woman to stop menstruating?

Amenorrhea, the loss of regular menstrual periods, occurs among some women engaged in intensive training or activities that demand a low body weight, such as running, gymnastics, and ballet. Girls performing such demanding exercise seem to start menstru-

ating later and may have irregular periods until they put on weight or cut the intensity of their training. Experts aren't sure why this happens, but suspect it's related to low body fat and possibly the emotional and physical stress of competition and performance, which may lead to hormonal changes.

Does amenorrhea affect health and fertility?

A woman with athletic amenorrhea is largely infertile, although this is not a reliable means of birth control. The effect appears to reverse itself when she reduces her level of activity, gains weight, or both. Another concern is that the loss of periods in women with low body weight or little body fat is associated with a lower level of estrogen. Low estrogen levels result in decreased bone mass, which is one reason why the incidence of osteoporosis rises after menopause, when estrogen levels fall (see *The Facts About Osteoporosis,* p.379). While it's not clear that amenorrhea causes an irreversible bone loss, many doctors urge amenorrheic women to decrease the intensity of their exercise or gain weight so that their periods resume. Some even recommend estrogen replacement therapy, especially if a woman has a family history of osteoporosis or other risk factors.

I feel bloated and edgy before my period. Can exercise help relieve those symptoms?

Many women find that regular exercise helps relieve the signs of premenstrual syndrome (PMS) you describe (see *The Facts About PMS,* p.251). Several studies have shown that women with PMS who engage in regular aerobic exercise have fewer symptoms. However, this doesn't mean that exercise will necessarily work for you or that there's something wrong with you if it doesn't.

Your first step should be to keep track of your symptoms to confirm that they're associated with your periods; then talk with your doctor about possible treatments. Changes in diet (reducing fat, alcohol, caffeine, sugar, and salt) have been found helpful in reducing PMS symptoms; some drugs are also effective.

Are there sports women shouldn't do?

Women's remarkable progress in sports and fitness in this century has exploded many of the old myths about what women can and can't do in the exercise arena. They now compete in sports from which women were previously excluded, such as basketball, hockey, marathon running, and race walking (an Olympic medal event for women for the first time in 1992).

Women play separately from men in activities in which their smaller size could endanger them or put them at a competitive disadvantage. But male athletes are similarly divided among themselves. Boxers and wrestlers, for example, compete in different weight classes.

Will women ever be able to beat men in races or other sports events?

Although their endurance is equal or superior to men's, women are generally smaller and have more fat and less muscle for their size than men do; consequently, they are not as strong or as fast as men. It's highly unlikely that women's world records in sprinting, weight lifting,

shot-putting, and other events that rely on strength and speed will ever surpass men's. Even very long races, such as the marathon run (26.2 miles), require speed and strength as well as endurance, so men seem destined to hold an edge.

In events emphasizing pure endurance, however, there's evidence that women and men can compete as equals. A woman holds the world record for swimming the English Channel, for example, and women's and men's times are close in 100-mile endurance runs.

However, most women are less concerned with beating men in sports than with being allowed full participation and having equal attention and money devoted to women's sports.

How does exercise affect sex drive?

Many people who start exercising find that their increased self-esteem, energy, attractiveness, and reduced stress levels have a positive effect on their sex life. One study of swimmers ranging in age from 40 to 80 found that 97 percent were sexually active—a figure much higher than that of the general population. They had sexual relations often, enjoyed it, and considered themselves sexually attractive.

On the other hand, too much exercise may depress sex drive. In one survey, people who swam more than 18 hours a week reported less interest in sex and had sex less often than more moderate swimmers. A study of women runners found that those who ran 10 miles a week had sex more often than those logging up to 45. Intensive training may also lower levels of sex hormones; studies of male competitive runners found decreased levels of the hormone testosterone.

I have a friend who exercises a great deal and seems to be getting thinner all the time. I'm concerned about her health. Could she be anorexic?

It's possible that she's becoming anorexic (p. 177). Excessive exercise by itself is not healthy; it's even more of a problem when associated with extreme thinness, an obsession with food combined with a refusal to eat, or other bizarre eating behaviors, such as eating only certain foods or shifting from one food to another.

Of course, not everyone who exercises a lot and is thin is anorexic. Some competitive athletes must put in what seems like inhuman hours of training and maintain a low body weight in order to succeed. Many recreational exercisers overtrain simply because they are misinformed about the amount and intensity of exercise needed for optimum health. Anorexia has nothing to do with a healthy level of exercise. If your friend has a "never enough" attitude and seems unhealthily thin, chances are she needs help.

Is there anything I can do to help a friend who may be anorexic?

Unfortunately, there's not a great deal you can do. Anorexia is a complex emotional condition, which should be treated by a medical professional.

If you feel concerned enough to confront your friend, be supportive. Listen to her thoughts and concerns—whether they are food- and exercise-related or not. Do not be surprised if she denies having any problem. Above all, suggest that your friend see a therapist.

EXERCISING SAFELY

Avoiding accidents

☐ Dress to be seen. Wear bright colors in the daytime, light colors at dusk. At night, add a reflective vest (available at sporting-goods stores) and carry a small flashlight. Bicycles should have reflectors and a front-mounted lamp.

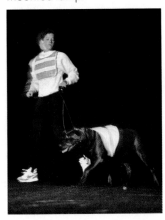

☐ If possible, stay on sidewalks or bike paths. Keep to the right to avoid collisions with pedestrians and cyclists coming in the other direction.

☐ Avoid exercising in heavily trafficked areas.
☐ Obey traffic rules. On roadsides, walkers and joggers should face oncoming traffic; cyclists should ride with traffic and use hand signals to communicate their intention to turn or stop. If you're walking or biking in a group, go single file. Try to make eye contact with motorists before crossing, even if you have the right of way.
☐ Watch parked cars. Be alert for people opening doors suddenly and for pedestrians stepping out from between or behind vehicles.

Avoiding attacks

☐ Exercise in places where there will be other people: a park, a mall, or a residential neighborhood. Pick times when you're likely to have company, such as lunchtime or just before or after work.
☐ Familiarize yourself with the locations of phone booths,

the local police precinct, neighbors who are likely to be home and, in a park, the emergency call boxes.
☐ Carry a whistle to sound if you are threatened. Carrying a weapon or chemical Mace isn't a good idea, because it can be used against you.
☐ Don't wear headphones. They can tune out the sound of an approaching attacker, and they invite theft. Expensive clothing and jewelry are also best left at home.
☐ If you think you're being followed, cross the street. If the person follows you, try stopping and talking to anyone you see. If possible, call the police from a phone booth or emergency call box.
☐ If you are attacked, yell for help if at all possible. If your attacker is armed, however, it may be better to submit to demands to keep quiet and not fight. Try to remain calm and get help as soon as possible afterward.

I live in a large crowded city. What are the hazards of exercising in polluted air? At what time of day is air quality best, and worst?

Unfortunately, pollution from our automobiles and industrial smokestacks can detract from the health benefits of outdoor exercise. Air pollution can cause breathlessness, coughing, a feeling of tightness in the chest, stinging eyes, and irritated nose and throat in healthy people; anyone suffering from heart and respiratory ailments can develop

even more serious problems.

The long-term effects of exercising in polluted air are still unknown, but they may well constitute a significant health hazard. One study of runners found a threefold rise in levels of blood carbon monoxide after 30 minutes of running in rush-hour traffic. (There was even a significant rise in the blood carbon monoxide levels of people who were merely standing around near traffic for the same length of time.)

To minimize the problem, do not exercise outdoors when traffic is at its heaviest, usually during the morning or evening

rush hours. Avoid the mid- to late-afternoon hours, after morning pollution has reacted with sunlight to raise ozone levels. Stay away from highways and well-traveled roads, or if this isn't possible, try to remain upwind of the pollution. When you stop at an intersection, step back from the curb to avoid inhaling exhaust fumes.

Pollution levels tend to rise on hot, humid, windless days. People who are particularly sensitive to polluted air should cut back on the intensity and duration of their workouts at such times, or as a last resort, exercise indoors.

SPORTS INJURIES: CAUSES AND PREVENTION

Conditioning, warmup and cooldown, good form, and a moderate program all reduce your risk of injury. This chart outlines common injuries, tells how to avoid them, and offers a treatment prescription.

Common injuries		How to avoid
Shinsplints, sore knees, pain in Achilles tendon (back of ankle), heel and foot pain; shoulder pain from vigorous arm motion.	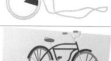 **Aerobics**	Wear aerobics shoes that fit; do extra exercises to strengthen legs, arms, and abdomen; choose a low-impact routine.
Sore muscles in neck, shoulders, and back from leaning over handlebars; tendinitis in knees or ankles; wrist and hand soreness after long rides; sore quadriceps and hamstring muscles; head injuries from falls.	 **Biking**	Make sure bike is right size and tuned; use regular rather than dropped handlebars; stop periodically to rest and stretch; do extra exercises to strengthen legs; wear a helmet.
Foot and lower-leg soreness; tendinitis and stress fractures; sore calf, hamstring, and quadriceps muscles; runner's knee.	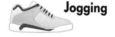 **Jogging**	Wear proper running shoes; run on soft surfaces; do extra exercises to strengthen quadriceps, which supports knee.
Foot, knee, and lower-leg problems from impact of jumping; low-back pain; wrist and forearm soreness from turning rope.	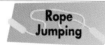 **Rope Jumping**	Stretch calves, ankles, back, arms; wear supportive, well-fitting shoes; increase intensity and duration slowly.
Sore or cramped shoulder, arm, low-back, or quadriceps muscles; pain in wrists and hands after long sessions.	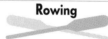 **Rowing**	Increase intensity and duration of workouts slowly; stretch shoulders and arms before and after workouts.
Tendinitis and sore muscles in ankle and lower leg; shinsplints; sprained ankles; sore hamstrings and quadriceps; bruises, scrapes, and head injuries from falls.	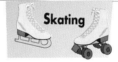 **Skating**	Wear skates that fit and support ankles; wear protective clothing, including pads and a helmet for roller skating; do extra exercises to strengthen ankles and legs.
Muscle soreness. *Downhill:* ankle, knee, and leg sprains; strains and fractures from falls. *Cross-country:* back, shoulder, and arm muscle strain from vigorous poling.	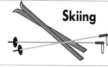 **Skiing**	Keep fit in off season; stretch arms, shoulders, back, legs; have equipment checked for safety and fit; strengthen muscles with extra exercises.
Muscle soreness, tendinitis and bursitis in shoulders and neck; "breast-stroker's knee" (pain along inside of knee).	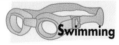 **Swimming**	Stretch shoulder and neck muscles; keep distance and intensity at comfortable level; vary strokes.
Tennis elbow; shoulder and neck soreness; tendinitis and bursitis; ankle sprains; pain in foot and knee; eye injuries.	**Tennis**	Stretch arms and shoulders; wear proper shoes; play on clay or grass courts; wear protective eyewear.
Muscle soreness; low-back pain from excessive weight or improper form; foot injuries from dropped weights.	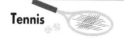 **Weight Training**	Progress gradually; don't lift on consecutive days; don't lift too much weight; train with a spotter.

A Glossary of Injuries

-itis. This suffix indicates inflammation. Tendinitis is inflammation of the tendons, bands of tissue that attach muscles to bones; bursitis is inflammation of the bursae, fluid-filled sacs that cushion joints.

Runner's knee. Pain behind and around the kneecap, often caused by weak quadriceps muscles or ill-fitting running shoes.

Shinsplints. Ache caused by swelling or tiny tears in the muscles along front of lower leg.

Sprain. A partial tear in a ligament, the fibrous band that holds bones together at a joint. A mild sprain causes localized swelling and tenderness. A severe sprain, in which ligaments are completely torn, requires prompt medical attention.

Strain. A "pull" or slight tear in a muscle or tendon. Symptoms range from mild pain and swelling to muscle or joint immobility.

Stress fracture. Hairline cracks in the lower-leg bone, caused by repeated high

Treating Injuries With RICE

See a doctor immediately if you sustain a serious injury. Treat milder injuries with RICE: rest, ice, compression, and elevation.

Rest means immobilizing the injured area and keeping your weight off it until pain and swelling diminish. (If they don't within a few days, see a doctor.) Minor muscle and connective-tissue injuries don't require complete inactivity; just cut back your exercise level until the pain goes away.

Ice an injury several times a day for 15 to 20 minutes at a time in the first 48 hours after you sustain the injury to reduce pain and swelling. Rub ice on the skin for injuries close to the surface; use an ice pack for joint or deep-muscle pain.

Compression usually means wrapping an injured area in an elastic bandage to slow the buildup of fluids that cause swelling. The bandage should be snug, but not tight enough to impede circulation. Unwrap the bandage every half hour to allow blood to circulate freely. Keep the area compressed for the first 2 to 3 hours until pain and swelling have decreased significantly.

Elevating an injured area keeps it from being engorged with blood and fluids. This will keep swelling down, especially in the leg and foot, by utilizing gravity to drain fluids.

impact. Symptoms of a stress fracture are localized pain and tenderness.
Tennis elbow. Pain at the outside of the elbow and in the back of the forearm, caused by using a racquet that's too heavy or too tightly strung, by hitting the ball with a wrist movement, or by employing faulty backhand technique.

What causes muscle cramps? How are they treated?

A cramp is a sudden muscle contraction. The best way to relieve one is by gently stretching the affected muscle.

A severe muscle cramp, often called a spasm, can be excruciatingly painful, but with proper treatment the damage is rarely permanent. Take the weight off the muscle, then slowly, gently ease it into a position in which you feel minimum pain. Gently massage the area to promote blood flow. Over the next few days your best prescription is RICE: *r*est, *i*ce, *c*ompression, and *e*levation (see left). Don't apply heat until any inflammation has subsided— usually after a day or two.

Muscles cramp when they are overstressed, so the best prevention is to warm up before vigorous exercise and avoid sudden increases in your level of activity. And since cramps can also result from dehydration, be sure to drink enough fluids before, during, and after exercise. Minimize muscle soreness by cooling down and gently stretching muscles after you work out.

I gave up skiing because it seemed dangerous, but I hear it's safer now because of advances in equipment design. What are the innovations?

Over the past decade, ski bindings—the device that attaches the boot to the ski—have been improved greatly to help reduce injuries. In the past, accidents often occurred when the bindings either didn't release, which can cause foot, ankle, and leg injuries, or released at inappropriate times, leading to wipeouts. The Snow Skiing Committee of ASTM, a materials standards and testing organization, has established standards for ski shops to check the release function of new bindings. This testing is voluntary, but the six largest binding manufacturers require that it be done on their equipment. Ski rental shops must test bindings in order to obtain insurance protection from the manufacturer.

Today's bindings are also lighter and more flexible than in the past, which makes turning easier. Many are made of light metals and plastics, instead of the all-metal constructions of the past. Bindings that are more than 10 years old probably don't have these features.

Many shops won't test or adjust bindings that are too worn or outdated. If you have old bindings, take them to a ski shop for evaluation. Testing and adjustment, which should be done at least once a year, is usually available at modest cost.

Are there any other precautions I should take before hitting the ski slopes?

Make sure that your boots, skis, and poles are comfortable and fit properly. Skis should also be sharpened periodically. If you are not sure whether a piece of equipment is safe or the right size for you, take it to a retail shop and have a professional evaluate it.

If you haven't skied in a few years (or ever), take lessons before you hit the slopes. Most ski areas offer instruction for beginners to advanced skiers of all ages; some require that a first-timer take a lesson. Knowing what you are doing on the ski slopes can make a big difference in reducing the risk of injury to yourself and others.

Is it dangerous to exercise in the cold?

Cold weather doesn't mean no exercise. If you're adequately dressed, outdoor workouts aren't dangerous and can be invigorating. A rule of thumb for joggers, cross-country skiers, and fitness walkers is to dress as you would for a day 20 degrees warmer; this allows for the heat you generate by exercising. Wind makes a cold day feel colder; knowing the wind-chill factor can help you plan what to wear on breezy days.

On very cold days, stay close to shelter, don't go out alone, and be alert to signs of hypothermia—shivering, sudden unexplained euphoria, drowsiness, disorientation, weakness, loss of coordination and concentration—in yourself and others. Watch for frostbite, too, which is signaled by pallor, numbness, prickling, and itching of the extremities—fingers, toes, nose, and ears. Get inside immediately if signs of frostbite or hypothermia occur. Warm up and cool down indoors, and don't stand around outside after a workout. Consider moving your whole routine inside on particularly cold, wet, windy days. You lose water through perspiration and breathing even in bitter weather, so remember to stay well hydrated.

How should I dress for cold-weather exercise?

You are dressed adequately if you don't feel cold when you are exercising. The most important thing is to keep your head, neck, hands, and feet covered and to avoid hypothermia, a potentially fatal condition that occurs when your core body temperature dips to a dangerously low level. Wear a hat (you lose 30 to 40 percent of your body heat if your

---

FACT OR FALLACY?

No pain, no gain

Fallacy. This is probably the most prevalent exercise myth, and the most damaging, because it keeps so many people from exercising. The best exercise for losing weight, promoting relaxation, and reducing the risk of heart disease is moderate, continuous activity—not stressful, high-intensity workouts. The exercise should feel like work, and you may occasionally experience soreness and fatigue. But if muscle or joint pain, dizziness, nausea, or exhaustion are part of the package, you're probably working harder than you need to.

You can train through the pain

Fallacy. Some pains caused by injury do lessen as you keep exercising, but the continued stress is likely to make the condition worse. If you feel pain during exercise that's more than a mild twinge, decrease your intensity. If the pain continues, stop, then evaluate and treat the condition (see *Sports Injuries*, p.108). Most injuries that are caught early heal within a matter of days or weeks. This lets you resume full activity sooner than if you try to "push through" the pain, which may cause it to become incapacitating.

---

head is bare), gloves, warm socks, and a face mask. Cover your lips with petroleum jelly for extra protection. There are many high-tech fabrics on the market designed to block wind, repel water, and "wick" moisture away from skin. Lock in warmth by dressing in layers—a wicking fabric next to the skin, wool in the middle, a lightweight, wind- and water-resistant shell on top. Layering also allows you to add and remove clothing as needed.

What precautions should I take when I'm exercising in warm weather?

If you aren't careful, exercising in hot weather can bring on heat exhaustion and potentially fatal heat stroke. Problems occur when overexertion and dehydration drive body temperature too high. Here's how to prevent that from happening.

☐ Drink fluids. Having enough water inside you is the only way your body can keep cool in the heat. Drink before, during, and after exercise—at least 8 ounces (a cup) every 15 to 20 minutes. Avoid alcohol and caffeinated beverages, which have a dehydrating effect. Weigh yourself before and after a workout; if you've lost weight, you're not drinking enough.

☐ Avoid the heat of the day. During hot months, exercise in the early morning or evening, when it's coolest. Stay in the shade, and protect your head with a light-colored hat or bandana.

☐ Dress appropriately. Wear loose-fitting clothing that permits free circulation of air, nothing that binds or chafes, and lightweight fabrics in light colors (to reflect the sun). Keep your hair off your neck and use sunscreen on face, shoulders, and back.

☐ Don't overexert yourself.

Even top athletes scale back the intensity of workouts in hot, humid weather. Don't feel you have to go as far or as fast as usual; consider working out indoors or taking the day off during extremely hot, humid spells.

☐ Know when to stop. If you feel dizzy, faint, nauseated, disoriented, excessively fatigued, or you stop sweating, stop exercising immediately. Get into the shade and get cool water in you and on you. If symptoms persist, summon help. Body temperature can rise very suddenly, and a physician may have to administer intravenous fluids to bring the situation under control.

Should I exercise even though I have asthma?

Not only is it possible to exercise with asthma, it appears that being active may reduce your symptoms. Improved aerobic conditioning makes the body more efficient in its use of oxygen, allowing it to get by with less. You may still have attacks of wheezing, coughing, breathlessness, and chest pain, but they are apt to be less frequent, less severe, and of shorter duration.

According to the the American Academy of Allergy and Immunology, however, a small percentage of the population is susceptible to exercise-induced asthma, a condition in which the breathing passages go into spasm during periods of exertion, narrowing so that air can't get in or out. Symptoms are most likely to occur during strenuous bouts of activity that are maintained for 5 minutes or longer, and when the air is cold and dry.

The severity of an attack also depends on other triggers, such as pollutants, dust, pollen, or viral infections. A person's emotional state (being tense or upset) can worsen symptoms too.

CARING FOR THE ACTIVE FOOT

Blisters are caused by friction against the skin. Make sure that shoes fit properly. Socks should act as a cushioning agent (a cotton-acrylic combination is best); wear a clean, dry pair for each workout. Cover any "hot spots" on your feet with petroleum jelly to reduce friction, or protect them with moleskin. Cover small blisters with a sterile gauze pad. Puncture very large ones at the edge with a sterilized needle, clean with antiseptic, blot with sterile gauze, and cover with a gauze pad. Leave the top of the blister on; pulling it off can cause a serious infection.

Calluses and **corns** don't always hurt, but large, hardened ones can be painful under pressure. A podiatrist can file or cut them down, and you can soften callus-prone areas with body lotion. Rubbing corns with pumice stone or the fine side of an emery board after a bath is also effective. Covering the surrounding area with pads or moleskin relieves pressure. Never try to remove corns with a razor blade. Structural abnormalities that cause blisters, calluses, and other problems can be corrected with pads or inserts; see a podiatrist for advice.

Bunions are usually hereditary, but the pounding of vigorous exercise can make these painful bony protrusions worse. People with moderate bunions can get by with shoes that are wide in the forefoot and socks with good cushioning. Most doctors recommend surgery for bunions only if they're very painful.

Nails can become painful if they repeatedly push into the front of your shoe during exercise. There should be at least a quarter inch of space between your longest toe and the shoe. Cut toenails straight across, and long enough to protect the toes. Rounding or picking at the nails can cause them to become ingrown.

Athlete's foot is a fungal growth that can often be prevented. Wash and dry feet thoroughly after exercising or whenever they sweat profusely. Wear shoes of natural materials, such as canvas and leather, that let feet "breathe." Air them (ideally for 2 days) between wearings and sprinkle foot powder inside to promote dryness. Avoid contact with flooring in gyms (wear rubber-thong sandals or the new "aqua sock"–type shoes). Over-the-counter antifungal powder (with tolnaftate) is effective when sprinkled between the toes; for stubborn, painful cases, a dermatologist may prescribe a more potent antifungal cream.

Cramps are a common problem. To minimize them, curl your toes and flex your feet throughout the day. Massaging your feet after a workout or rubbing them over a rolling pin or a ball can ease sore muscles and prevent stiffness. But if you feel sharp pain or see redness or swelling, the muscle may be pulled or sprained. Stay off the foot as much as possible, apply ice, and see a doctor if the pain doesn't diminish within a few days.

If you have asthma, it's particularly important to start your fitness program slowly and work up gradually, so you're less likely to trigger attacks. Some people can exercise through mild episodes by breathing slowly, relaxing, and using a medicated inhaler, which opens the bronchial tubes. However, if breathing becomes increasingly difficult, or coughing and wheezing persist, stop your activity and rest.

Are there any other precautions an asthma sufferer should take when exercising?

Here are a few tips.
☐ Pick exercises with built-in rest periods, since sustained exertion without a break may trigger spasms. Try sports such as tennis, baseball, or softball. Or simply slow the pace of your jogging, rowing, or other aerobic activity every few minutes to catch your breath. Many asthmatics find swimming to be an ex-

cellent activity because the warm temperatures and moist air make breathing easier. But beware of highly chlorinated pools, which can trigger an attack.
☐ Since asthma attacks are more likely to take place in the early morning hours, try to do your exercising after noon.
☐ Warm up properly.
☐ Do regular deep-breathing exercises to increase the volume of air you are able to inhale and exhale. Put your hand on your diaphragm (between your navel and rib cage) and inhale to a count of four, feeling your stomach push against your hand. As you exhale, to a count of eight, feel your stomach retract.
☐ Breathe through your nose during and after exercise to filter and warm the air.
☐ Cool down your lungs after you exercise with 5 to 10 minutes of deep breathing.
☐ Keep your medicated inhaler handy when you exercise.
☐ Wear a scarf or mask over your nose and mouth in cold, dry

weather to warm and moisten the air you breathe.
☐ You may have to avoid outdoor exercise during certain times or in certain settings if your asthma is triggered by pollen or grass.

For more on living with asthma, see pages 338–339.

I've heard of people being allergic to exercise. Is this possible?

Some people actually do sneeze, wheeze, cough, and break out in hives when they engage in vigorous physical activity. The causes of this rare condition, called exercise-induced anaphylaxis, remain unclear. Those who are susceptible seem to be otherwise healthy, although they may have other allergies. Attacks don't necessarily occur at every workout. If you think you have exercise allergy, see your doctor. He or she may prescribe a self-injectable medication, which you can carry with you during your workouts.

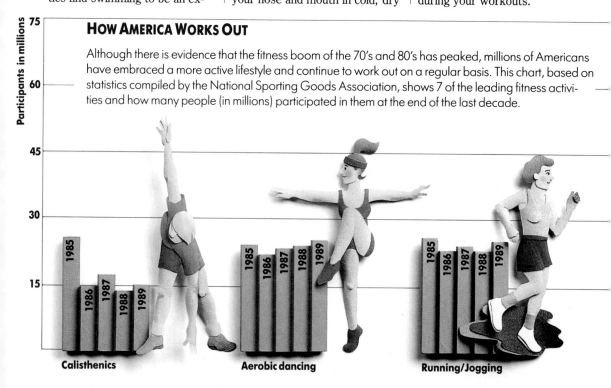

HOW AMERICA WORKS OUT

Although there is evidence that the fitness boom of the 70's and 80's has peaked, millions of Americans have embraced a more active lifestyle and continue to work out on a regular basis. This chart, based on statistics compiled by the National Sporting Goods Association, shows 7 of the leading fitness activities and how many people (in millions) participated in them at the end of the last decade.

Participants in millions
75
60
45
30
15

Calisthenics — 1985, 1986, 1987, 1988, 1989

Aerobic dancing — 1985, 1986, 1987, 1988, 1989

Running/Jogging — 1985, 1986, 1987, 1988, 1989

Exercise allergy should be distinguished from the gasping and breathlessness that take place when anyone starts exercising strenuously without a proper warmup. Such responses are normal and can be avoided by beginning slowly and gradually working the heart rate into its training range (p. 71).

Can a person become addicted to exercise?

It is possible to develop a dependency on exercise similar to an addiction to other behaviors, such as overeating or gambling. People who exercise regularly feel better physically and emotionally; they get a sense of accomplishment from the number of miles jogged or pounds lifted. As their fitness improves, they're able to go farther and heft more. That's fine—up to a point. Exercising more and more and getting hooked on its effects can lead to a dependence that's unhealthy physically and psychologically.

A person who can never get enough exercise, overtrains to the point of injury or constant fatigue, exercises despite injuries, or allows exercise to take precedence over job or family is probably heading toward an exercise addiction. (Other symptoms of overtraining include sleeplessness, weight loss, obsession with weight, digestive and menstrual irregularities, irritability and anxiety.)

There are several ways to overcome exercise addiction. Most exercise-dependents engage in solitary sports, a tendency that can be countered by taking a class or working out with friends. A personal trainer (p. 80) can help clients maintain a sensible schedule. Engaging in different activities can make the escalating goals set for one exercise seem less important.

Some people benefit from psychotherapy designed to get at the underlying reasons for their compulsive behavior. Remember, the value of exercise is its ability

to enhance the rest of your life. It can't do that if it becomes your whole reason for living.

What is "runner's high," and how is it achieved?

When running was becoming popular in the mid-1970's, many people were converted not only by the physical benefits but by the much-touted mental lift. Runners claimed to feel a euphoric "high" as they ran. Pain disappeared, miles flew by, the runner entered a higher state of consciousness. Though such claims were no doubt exaggerated, the lure of "runner's high" endures.

People do tend to feel happier, calmer, more clearheaded and energetic after aerobic activity. One reason for this may be physiological: Exercise triggers the release of chemicals that elevate mood and reduce pain and anxiety. It can also improve mood indirectly by providing time out from a busy day and creating a feeling of accomplishment.

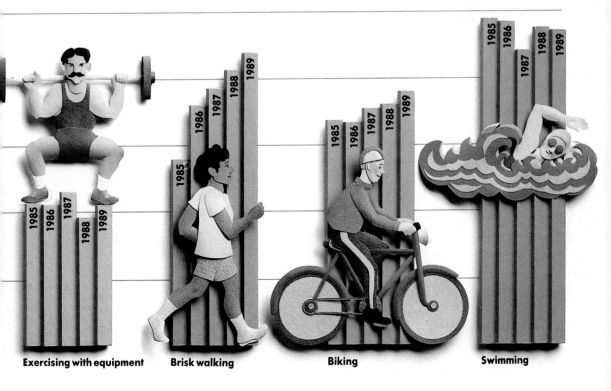

Exercising with equipment   **Brisk walking**   **Biking**   **Swimming**

Most people report that runner's high is more a feeling of calm and satisfaction than an intense euphoria, and that it is sweetest not during exercise but right afterward. You do not have to work to exhaustion; any sustained, moderate aerobic activity—jogging, brisk walking, cycling, swimming—will do the trick. Relaxing, avoiding competitiveness, and choosing activities you enjoy can help give you that happy feeling.

My jogging partner and I occasionally race each other. She always wins. How come?

A large part of athletic ability is determined by our genes. Your friend may simply have been born with stronger, faster legs, more "slow-twitch" muscle fibers (see *Working Your Muscles*, p.84), and a better ability to transport oxygen to muscles. She may always run faster than you no matter how much either of you trained. You shouldn't be concerned about the difference, though, since it doesn't make your friend any healthier or fitter than you are.

I've heard that athletes use "visualization" to improve performance. Does this work for casual exercisers too?

Essentially a form of positive thinking, visualization is an umbrella term for techniques used to perform and feel better in any situation, including exercise. Top-level athletes visualize to gain a competitive edge, but anyone can use visualization to improve performance.

Visualization is the creation of a positive mental picture of an activity, either before or during its performance. For example, a jogger who has trouble reaching the top of a hill without stopping to walk would see herself reaching the tough part, relaxing, concentrating, breathing deeply, and making it to the top at a jog.

There's nothing magical about the technique, and it won't eliminate the effort or occasional discomfort of exercise. Don't use visualization to help you attempt something beyond your capabilities (running a marathon when you've just started jogging, for example), and be willing to experiment to find methods that work best for you. Does visualization work? Studies suggest that it can improve performance, and certainly it can't hurt to try. Here are the basic steps.

☐ Relax. Before you work out, find a quiet, private place to rehearse your activity. Get comfortable (many people lie or sit in a dark room). Breathe deeply, close your eyes, and let your mind settle. During exercise, relax nonworking muscles (your face, your shoulders in jogging or walking).

☐ Get in touch with the moment. Focus your thoughts on the activity you'll be doing. Think about *this* workout—not past ones when you've had trouble, or future ones when you may again. Think about the mechanics —moving your arms and legs, lifting a weight—rather than success or failure (beating a friend in a race, dropping a weight because it's too heavy).

☐ Key in on sensations. Imagine the sights, sounds, smells, and other physical sensations that surround the event, such as the slap of your running shoes on the pavement or the swish of water over your body. The process is

different for everybody: Some people's visualizations are very detailed, while others see snapshotlike pictures. There are no right or wrong images.

Are there other mind tricks I can use to make exercise easier?

Sticking with a fitness program requires mental as well as physical effort. While there's no magic formula, mental techniques can help you deal with the difficulty, fatigue, and boredom you'll inevitably feel at some point. Psychologists have found that exercisers use either *associative* or *disassociative* strategies for getting through the tough spots. Associative strategies are ways of focusing on what's happening here and now: how your body feels, what you see, hear and smell, what others around you are doing. Disassociative strategies "tune out" such signals in an effort to minimize the pain, fatigue, and boredom of the exercise effort.

Studies show that people of average fitness levels who disassociate perform better than those who associate, yet don't perceive themselves as working as hard. There are many ways to disassociate while exercising: talk to a friend, listen to music, look at the scenery, fantasize, make lists, solve problems or write letters in your head. Just don't become so distracted that you put yourself in danger (by overexercising or ignoring traffic, for example). Occasionally, you may find that tuning into the here and now gives you a boost by helping you appreciate your fitness and the positive feelings exercise can bring.

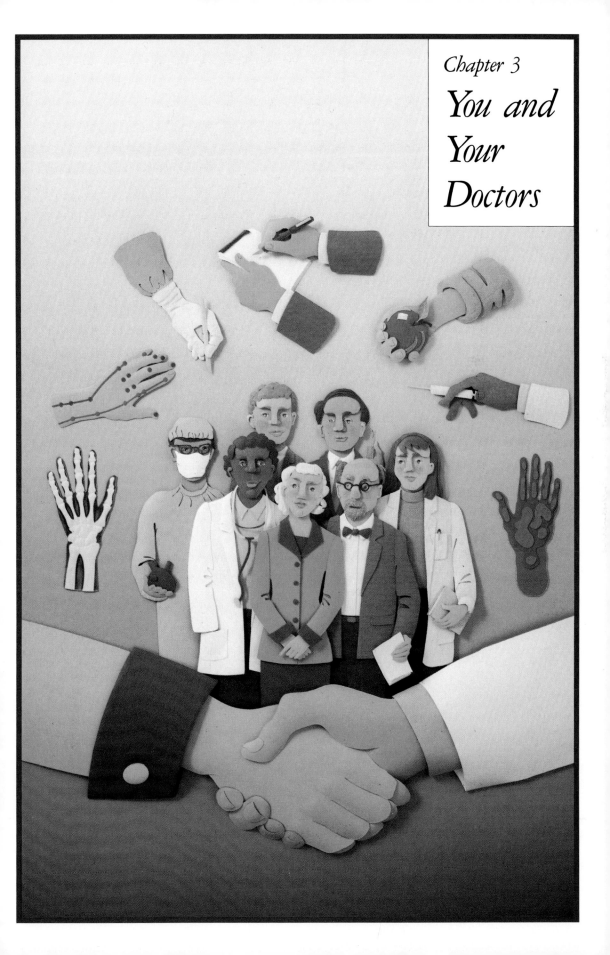

Just in Time

During her annual visit to her gynecologist, Debra B. complained about a dull pain that seemed to come and go on the left side of her abdomen. When a pelvic exam revealed a possible enlargement of the left ovary, the doctor sent Debra for an ultrasound scan. The results were a shock to all. The ovaries, it turned out, were just fine, but clearly visible on the scan was a large tumor on Debra's right kidney. Since the growth was not the likely source of Debra's abdominal pain, it was sheer luck—and Debra's attention to her medical care—that allowed her condition to be detected before it was too late.

Debra went to see a urologist for further testing. The doctor concluded—and a second specialist agreed—that the tumor might be malignant and the kidney should be removed. Fortunately, as Debra learned, it's possible to live a fully normal life with just one kidney.

Less than a month after her visit to the gynecologist, Debra underwent surgery. As was feared, the tumor was malignant, but the cancer had not spread. Two years later, Debra continues going for CT and ultrasound scans every 6 months with no sign of recurrence. Soon, her testing schedule will be reduced to once a year as her prognosis continues to improve.

Pharmacist to the Rescue

For Tammy J., 62, the most frustrating thing about the bronchitis her doctor had diagnosed was that it kept her from taking her daily two-mile walks. Tired and coughing heavily, Tammy wasted no time in filling the tetracycline prescription the doctor had given her. A week later, feeling worse, Tammy had to have the prescription refilled. When she appeared at the pharmacy a third time with a prescription for a stronger antibiotic, the pharmacist became alarmed. Noticing a

bottle of iron supplements in her shopping basket, the pharmacist asked Tammy whether she had been taking the supplements during her illness. "Yes," Tammy replied, "to make me feel less tired." "There's your problem," explained the pharmacist. "The iron is interfering with your body's ability to absorb tetracycline." The pharmacist called Tammy's doctor, and together they decided to try tetracycline again, but without iron supplements. Two weeks later, Tammy was back on her walking routine.

Easing a Sick Child's Fears

Michael D. was scheduled to go into the hospital for a serious hip operation and his parents were worried, about the surgery, of course, but also about the recovery period. Michael, an active 8-year-old, would be immobilized by a body cast for 10 weeks. The parents' concerns lessened considerably, however, when they met Sandy, the hospital's child life specialist. Her job was to make the hospitalization of youngsters like Michael as unfrightening as possible.

Before Michael even entered the hospital, Sandy gave him a tour, explaining what happens where and who does what. Once the boy had settled into his room, Sandy used a doll to explain what the operation would involve. Together she and Michael used real cast material to wrap the doll in a body cast and put it in traction. This exercise helped Michael better understand what was going to happen to him and made him feel much more confident as he was wheeled into the operating room.

Ten long weeks later, when Michael's cast was ready to come off, Sandy was still involved, demonstrating the procedure on the doll first. Today, the boy is doing just great.

TEST YOUR HEALTH I.Q.

Monitoring Family Health

Finding good basic health care for yourself and those who depend on you is not always easy. Communicating with medical experts can be even more difficult. This chapter is designed to help you ask the right questions and get the information you need — whether you are looking for a family doctor, weighing the pros and cons of surgery, buying medical insurance, or just choosing among cold remedies at the pharmacy. For starters, pick the phrase or phrases that most accurately complete the health-care statements below.

1 Healthy adults under age 65 should have a physical exam _____ .

    A. annually
    B. every 2 to 5 years
    C. as needed; it's no longer considered necessary to have a regular physical exam

2 _____ is a technique for detecting internal disorders by tapping the chest or abdomen with the fingers and listening to the sounds produced.

    A. Percussion
    B. Palpation
    C. Auscultation

3 A false positive test result can be caused by _____ .

    A. equipment or technician error
    B. patient error
    C. limited reliability of the test itself

4 A flu shot is about _____ percent effective in preventing influenza.

    A. 50–60
    B. 70–80
    C. 90

5 It's advisable to get a second opinion when _____ .

    A. major surgery is recommended
    B. there is doubt about the accuracy of a primary diagnosis
    C. your doctor diagnoses a rare or serious disease

6 An _____ is a professional qualified to examine eyes and prescribe lenses.

    A. ophthalmologist
    B. optometrist
    C. optician

7 You should schedule your child's first dental visit when _____ .

    A. the first tooth appears
    B. the primary teeth have emerged (usually between ages 2 and $2^1/_2$)
    C. a problem occurs

8 A preferred provider organization is a health insurance plan that is _____ .

    A. based on paying a fee for a service
    B. the same as a health maintenance organization
    C. a cross between a health maintenance organization and traditional health insurance

9 A generic drug _____ .

    A. is always cheaper than its brand-name equivalent
    B. can be interchanged with its brand-name equivalent in all cases
    C. is as potent and pure as its brand-name equivalent

Answers

For more information on any of the quiz topics turn to the pages listed next to the answers.

1. B, p.122	4. B, p.129	7. B, p.137
2. A, p.122	5. A,B,C, p.130	8. C, p.149
3. A,B,C, p.124	6. A,B, p.135	9. C, p.152

I grew up with a general practitioner who was like a family friend. Is it still possible to find someone like him?

Although their numbers have dwindled considerably, there are still some general practitioners around. A G.P. is a nonspecialist who, in most cases, received only 1 year of hospital training after medical school. When looking for a family (or primary-care) doctor today, you usually have to choose between a specialist in internal medicine (an internist) and a specialist in family care (a family practitioner). Like nearly all new M.D.'s now, internists and family practitioners both undergo 3 or more years of hospital training before entering practice.

What is the difference between an internist and a family practitioner?

An internist and a family practitioner are both broadly trained to provide comprehensive medical care. Either can perform routine checkups, advise you on good health habits, diagnose and treat everyday maladies, and recommend specialists for serious complaints. But the training that they receive differs. For internists the emphasis is on ailments of the cardiovascular, respiratory, gastrointestinal, urogenital, and other body systems as well as on infectious and chronic diseases. Most treat only adults and never do surgery. Family practitioners learn many aspects of internal medicine, too, but they are also trained to treat the special needs of women and children, deliver babies, perform minor surgery, and handle emergencies. They treat the entire family and pay special attention to family dynamics and its effects on health and medical care.

A family practitioner is often your only practical choice if you live in a rural area. In urban and suburban areas, where internists are more common, parents often choose an internist as the primary physician for themselves and take their youngsters to a pediatrician—a doctor who specializes in the care and treatment of children from infancy through their teens or later.

Can my gynecologist serve as my primary physician?

A gynecologist is a doctor specially trained in the care and treatment of the female reproductive system. Because most gynecologists are also obstetricians—specialists who provide complete care during pregnancy and birth—they become especially important to women during their reproductive years. As a result, some women use their obstetrician-gynecologists as their primary physicians.

This arrangement can work well if the doctor is willing to function as a primary physician and is accessible for relatively minor complaints and if you're in good health and expect most of your medical problems to be gynecological. It's convenient and often beneficial to have a single doctor who has a thorough knowledge of your medical condition. But a gynecologist is not fully trained in the diagnosis and treatment of other adult medical ailments and might not be as alert as an internist or a family practitioner would be to the subtle early signs of disease. If you have a personal or family history of medical problems not related to your reproductive system, it's certainly advisable to have an internist or a family practitioner or even a specialist serve as your primary-care physician.

What is the best approach to finding a primary doctor?

Ideally you should choose your doctor when you are well, not when you are sick or have a medical emergency. You want a doctor who is pleasant, dependable, and affordable, who is competent and stays up to date, and who will be available to you and get to know you well. The doctor's office should also be easy for you to get to.

Before looking for a doctor, decide what kind you want. Do you need an internist, a family practitioner, a pediatrician? Do you want a doctor who can treat the entire family or just you alone? Would you prefer a man or a woman? Do you want a younger physician just recently trained in the latest techniques or an older doctor with more clinical experience? Do you have a particular health problem, such as chronic emphysema or rheumatoid arthritis? If so, you may want an internist with a subspecialty in that field.

Then ask for recommendations. Ask your friends, relatives, neighbors, and business associates about their doctors and what they do or don't like about them. Ask other doctors, such as your children's pediatrician, your gynecologist, or your dentist. Nurses, pharmacists, and others in health-related fields usually know a lot about the area's doctors. Local hospitals and medical societies are also good sources of physicians' names. If you've moved, your former doctor may be able to recommend a colleague in your new community.

If you belong to a health maintenance organization or other health plan, use the same basic approach to narrow down the list of doctors you are given to choose from.

PERSONAL HEALTH RECORD

A permanent record of each family member's health data can be an invaluable aid. This example is for a woman; a man's record would list dates of prostate exams instead of gynecological and breast exam dates. Keep copies of prescriptions and medical test results with the basic record.

Name _Elizabeth Peters_   Date of Birth _August 18, 1941_   Blood Type _A-_

Name and telephone   _Dr. Robert MacDonald (internist) - (914) 555-5155_

number of doctor(s)   _Dr. Jean Smith (gynecologist) - (914) 555-9246_

Allergies _Hay fever_

Adverse drug reactions _Penicillin (rash)_

Examinations	Date	Comments	Date	Comments
Complete physical	4/4/92			
Blood pressure	4/4/92	120/80		
ECG	4/4/92	attached		
Fecal occult blood test	4/4/92	negative		
Serum cholesterol	4/4/92	170 mg/dl		
X-rays	2/20/90	chest-neg.		
Location of X-rays	Dr. MacDonald's office			
Cervical (Pap) smears	4/92	negative		
Pelvic examination	4/92	negative		
Mammography	4/92	benign cyst, left breast		
Eye test	2/14/92			
Dental checkup	9/20/92			

Medications (Dose, Side effects)	Immunizations	Dates
	Tetanus-diphtheria booster	5/87
	Flu	11/91

Contraceptives

Ovulen-21	1966-1980	
Diaphragm	5/80	

Injuries, illnesses, operations	Date
Lyme disease – mild case;	9/87–1/88
treated with antibiotics	
Twisted right ankle and torn ligaments –	3/21/88
treated in emergency	
Biopsy and removal of cyst	4/11/92
in left breast	

How can I find out about a doctor's qualifications?

The easiest way is to consult medical directories at your local library. Two useful guides are the *Compendium of Certified Medical Specialties* (published by the American Board of Medical Specialties) and the *Directory of Medical Specialists* (published by Marquis Who's Who, Wilmette, Illinois). These directories can tell you not only what a doctor's specialty is but also which medical school he or she attended, whether it was fully accredited, and the name of the hospital where the doctor did postgraduate training. (As a general rule, attending a prestigious medical school is less important as a credential than doing a residency at a well-established teaching hospital, because training usually contributes more to a doctor's skills than medical school.) The directories also show whether doctors are board certified—that is, have completed the required years of residency and passed an examination given by their medical specialty board.

To find out if a doctor is board certified, you can also call the American Board of Medical Specialties (see Appendix).

Is it useful to know a doctor's hospital affiliation?

It's often helpful to know the hospital where a doctor has staff privileges—a piece of information you can find in a directory of medical specialists (see preceding question). The fact that a physician is on the staff of a well-regarded hospital is no guarantee of high qualifications. But the lack of a hospital affiliation should prompt you to check out a doctor more thoroughly. Most hospitals screen staff doctors for personal and legal problems—including a history of malpractice suits—and monitor them for errors that have seriously harmed patients.

Knowing a doctor's hospital affiliation is also of practical importance. If you become very ill, this is the hospital you'd probably go to. And if you need a specialist, you're most likely to be referred to one of its staff members.

How can I find out about a doctor's style of practice without going for a checkup?

Call the doctor's office. Ask about working hours, the doctor's policy on insurance and payments, and whether the doctor sets aside a part of the day to receive and return calls. If you don't already know, ask about

---

FACTS A DOCTOR NEEDS ON YOUR FIRST VISIT

Accurate information about your background greatly enhances a doctor's ability to provide good care. Here are the details that you should be prepared to provide on your first visit:

The specific complaints that may have brought you to the doctor. Describe concisely any fever, congestion, pains, rashes, or other symptoms. When discussing a symptom, tell the doctor how long you've had it, how severe it is, whether you've had anything similar in the past, and what makes the symptom better or worse.

Your personal medical history, including serious childhood and adult illnesses, immunizations, chronic conditions, hospital stays, and any operations or other medical procedures. Bring the name and phone number of any specialist treating you now and of any other doctor who has treated you in recent years.

Your family's medical history, especially ailments that tend to run in families, such as high blood pressure, heart disease, diabetes, and cancer. Include your brothers, sisters, parents, and grandparents, as well as any aunts, uncles, and cousins among whom there's a noticeable pattern of illness.

Any allergies or drug reactions you've had along with a description of your reactions.

Any medications or supplements you are taking. Include over-the-counter products such as aspirin, allergy medicines, and vitamins, as well as prescription drugs. Give the name, dosage, daily frequency, and length of time you have been taking them.

Lifestyle. Be ready to discuss family, job, stress, diet, exercise, sex, smoking, drinking, and other factors that may affect your health.

---

the doctor's specialty, board certification status, and hospital affiliation. Also find out who covers for the doctor when he or she is away and cannot be reached. You want that doctor to be as qualified as your primary physician. Your questions should be answered accurately and courteously. If they are not, it's best to look elsewhere.

If you are satisfied with the information you get, set up a get-acquainted visit to see if you like the doctor. When talking to the doctor, note especially if you feel

you are being rushed and if the doctor takes the time to listen to you and answer your questions clearly and fully. Good communication with your doctor is essential to good health care.

Can a doctor's office tell me anything about the quality of his practice?

Yes. A smooth-running office is usually a sign of an able, well-organized doctor who is concerned about his or her patients. Look for a clean, orderly office with regular hours and a strict no-smoking policy. Is the waiting room uncrowded? Are there magazines or other reading materials for waiting patients? Are the receptionists, nurses, and other staff members helpful and considerate? Do they know where the doctor is and tell you how long you will have to wait? Do they answer the telephone courteously? Do they take care not to discuss one patient in front of another? Is the examining room meticulously clean? Are the examination table cover and patient gown fresh?

What questions should I ask a doctor during a first checkup?

If you're seeing a new doctor for a routine health maintenance exam, find out what the doctor checks for on a regular basis. If you're not sure why a certain exam or test is being done, ask about the doctor's rationale for doing it. Ask what each exam or test reveals and if the results are normal. After the examination (p. 122), ask if all your body's systems are in good order. Ask what you can do to improve your health. If some factor, such as blood pressure, weight, or heart rhythm, is not optimal, ask what you should do and how the doctor will monitor the condition.

What questions should I ask when I visit a doctor because I'm ill?

During an examination for a specific illness, ask the doctor for a clear explanation of the diagnosis. If it is a definitive diagnosis with a known cause, find out what the cause was. Is the condition contagious? How long will it last? How can you prevent a recurrence? How will your progress be monitored? Are tests needed?

Will they help the doctor make a diagnosis or determine the treatment? Do you need to take a medication? Are there any side effects (p. 151)? Is there anything special that you should do or that you should avoid doing?

If the diagnosis and test results are inconclusive, ask what the next step will be. Will the doctor try a different approach, refer you to a specialist, or just wait and see?

I get flustered during a medical exam and leave confused about what the doctor has told me. How can I avoid this?

Feeling flustered at the doctor's office isn't unusual. But if you prepare yourself beforehand, you'll feel more confident and in control.

Start by listing all the symptoms that are bothering you. Are they steady or sporadic? How intense are they? What makes them feel better or worse? Have you had them before and did any treatment help? Make a list of the questions you want to ask the doctor. Consider having a family member or a friend come with you; he or she may make you feel more comfortable and help you to remember what your doctor said.

Tell the doctor frankly that you feel uneasy or have trouble remembering details. Although many patients feel this way, the doctor doesn't always sense it. If you reveal your problem, the doctor is likely to take time and explain both the diagnosis and treatment more thoroughly. If the doctor is unclear, ask for more information. Many doctors are unaware that they have not been understood and appreciate the chance to clarify the facts.

Before leaving the office, ask yourself if you understood what the doctor said. Do you know

what the problem is? Do you know what actions or medicines you are supposed to take? Do you have to call for test results? Do you have to call back if certain symptoms occur? Do you have to return for another visit? Do you know when you might expect to feel better, and what to do if you don't?

If you still have important questions afterward, call the doctor's office to get more information. If you have many questions, or if you are generally uncertain about your diagnosis and treatment plan, make an appointment for another visit.

I recently put off visiting my doctor because I was afraid of what might be found. Is this fear unusual?

Not at all. It's very common to be apprehensive about being examined, undergoing tests, and especially about receiving a diagnosis of a serious disease. But putting off a visit often works to your detriment. Many diseases and conditions are best treated early. People with chest pains, for example, often put off being examined for fear of being told they have heart disease, but they would be much better off seeing a doctor. If they do have heart disease, they can benefit from early treatment. If they don't, they are worrying needlessly. If you have symptoms that are troubling you, see a doctor and have them diagnosed and treated.

My doctor told me to lose weight, but I haven't. Now I don't want to go back to see him. What should I do?

Make an appointment with your doctor. Most doctors confront this situation often, and know how difficult it is for a person to change habits—whether the change involves stopping smoking, remembering to take a medication, getting more exercise, or modifying eating patterns to lower cholesterol or lose weight. Even when people see the value of changing their behavior, as they usually do, they often are unable to do so. In such cases, it's best to discuss the problem with your doctor. Ideally, your doctor should work with you to help you identify obstacles to change in your family, work, and social situations and develop techniques to overcome them.

Do I need to have a full physical examination every year?

While some doctors still strongly recommend a full physical exam every year, most experts now believe that this is too frequent for a healthy adult. And instead of a complete physical, they recommend a more selective (and cost-effective) examination tailored to your age, sex, and risk factors. If you're an adult under the age of 65 with no apparent health problems, it's now considered advisable to have a physical exam every 2 to 5 years. After 65, a yearly checkup is usually recommended.

Of course, you should be examined more often if you have a chronic illness or if you are at risk for a serious disease because of your family history, lifestyle, or working conditions. If breast cancer runs in your family, for example, your doctor will probably want to give you a clinical breast exam every year after the age of 35. If you smoke and have high blood pressure and high cholesterol, an examination every few months may be in order to check for signs of heart disease. Similarly, a doctor may

THE PHYSICAL EXAM

In an age of high-tech medicine, doctors still rely on their senses to detect subtle physical changes that signal disease. During a checkup, your doctor will employ some or all of these techniques.

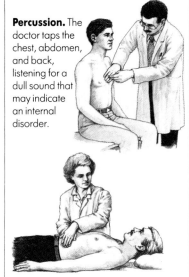

Percussion. The doctor taps the chest, abdomen, and back, listening for a dull sound that may indicate an internal disorder.

Palpation. With the flat of the hand, the doctor presses on the abdomen, neck, or chest, feeling for abnormal masses, enlarged organs, or areas of tenderness.

Auscultation. The doctor listens to the heart, abdomen, and lungs through a stethoscope. Certain diseases produce characteristic sounds.

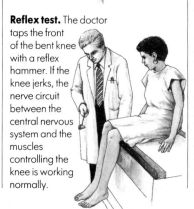

Reflex test. The doctor taps the front of the bent knee with a reflex hammer. If the knee jerks, the nerve circuit between the central nervous system and the muscles controlling the knee is working normally.

want to monitor regularly the liver of a patient who drinks, the kidneys of someone who takes a lot of ibuprofen, or the hearing of someone who works in a noisy environment.

What should I expect during a complete physical examination?

Before examining you for the first time, a doctor will review your personal and family medical history and personal habits that affect your health (see *Facts a Doctor Needs on Your First Visit,* p.120). On later visits, the doctor may simply ask you some follow-up questions. The physical exam itself starts with an overall evaluation of your appearance— your alertness, coordination, body proportion and body symmetry, muscle tone, skin color and quality. Your height, weight, temperature, pulse, and blood pressure are taken.

Then each major part of the body is examined, usually from the top down, with special attention to your complaints and risk factors. The doctor checks the ears and throat and notes the interior and exterior condition of the eyes along with their movement and reaction to light. The neck and underarms are felt for enlarged glands. To check the heart and lungs, the doctor inspects and feels (palpates) the chest, taps (percusses) the chest and back, and listens to (auscultates) both with a stethoscope. To check the other internal organs the abdomen is deeply palpated. With a man, the doctor examines the penis and scrotum and inserts a gloved finger in the rectum to feel the prostate gland and check for growths. During a woman's pelvic exam (p.252), the doctor inspects the exterior and interior of the genitals and palpates the pelvic organs through the vagina and rectum. The doctor also examines your arms, legs, hands, and feet and tests your reflexes, usually by tapping a stretched tendon at the knee.

In addition to the physical exam, the doctor usually takes blood, urine, and feces samples for analysis and performs other routine tests (see *Screening Tests for Healthy Adults,* p.124). For some of these, the doctor may send you to a laboratory.

On subsequent visits, your doctor may give you a more selective examination, omitting some procedures and focusing on areas where the doctor feels he or she may find abnormalities.

When should a child start having checkups?

Even before a baby is born, it's a good idea for parents to visit the pediatrician they've chosen for the child (this is in addition to the mother's regular prenatal exams, pp.260–261). At this visit, the doctor can offer guidance and take a family medical history.

At birth, the newborn is given a battery of tests to detect any congenital defects and assess general well-being. The first visit to the pediatrician usually takes place at the end of the second week. At this time, the doctor records the infant's height, weight, and head circumference, screens vision and hearing, assesses development and behavior, gives the infant a complete physical examination, and discusses any problems with the parents. For a well-cared-for child with no major health problems, the American Academy of Pediatrics recommends that subsequent checkups take place at 2 months (when the vaccination schedule begins, see p.129), 4, 6, 9, 12, 15, 18, and 24 months; yearly to age 6; and every 2 years through adolescence.

IS THIS TEST NECESSARY?

At least $30 billion is spent each year on medical tests in the United States. Half of this expenditure, say critics, is unneeded. To decide whether a test is necessary for you, ask your doctor the following questions.

What do you hope to learn from it? A test is usually indicated only when it will help a doctor find a treatable disease, rule out a disease for which you have some symptom or risk, or monitor an illness and its treatment.

Are there alternatives? If a condition is not serious or is not treatable in the early stages, observing symptoms over a period of time may work just as well as the proposed test. Or another, simpler test may give a result that is almost as accurate.

Are there any risks? A test normally has potential risk only when it involves radiation, usually X-rays, or when it is "invasive," that is, involves introducing something into the body, either an instrument, such as a endoscope, or a substance, such as a drug or a contrast medium.

What will it cost? For some tests, you may pay only a lab fee. Others may require paying a specialist and hospital bills. Most doctors can tell you approximately how much a test will cost, but you will have to contact your insurance company directly to find out if, and to what extent, it covers a particular test's cost.

In addition to these four basic questions, ask your doctor how the test is performed and what it involves. Many common tests take minutes and cause little or no pain or discomfort. More complex tests can take an hour or more, involve X-rays and probing devices, require taking a sedative or receiving a local or general anesthetic, and may produce unpleasant side effects.

Find out also where and by whom the test will be performed. Some tests are done in your doctor's office, while for others you must go to a clinic or a specialist's office, or to a hospital on an in- or outpatient basis. The person performing the test could be your doctor, a technician or aide, or a specialist.

At my last checkup, my doctor did hardly any tests. Was the doctor thorough enough?

Your doctor may have been quite thorough. More medical tests do not necessarily mean a better evaluation. Which tests to give and how often to give them are subjects of continuing debate among doctors. The cost in time and money of a given test may not be justifiable because of the test's uncertain effectiveness. Even if a test detects early signs of disease, it may not lead to any better treatment or long-term outcome than if the condition is detected after symptoms become apparent. When a test is unlikely to change the course of treatment, a doctor may avoid it, especially if it's expensive, can lead to complications, and yields a sizable number of inaccurate findings that result in unnecessary procedures and needless worry. The most beneficial checkup is generally one in which the doctor is selective about testing, focuses on your personal habits and how they affect your health, advises you about preventive steps, and helps you make changes that will improve your health.

What is a "false positive" test result?

A test result is false positive when it indicates an abnormality or a disease in someone who does not have the condition. Sometimes the testing equipment or the person administering the test may be at fault. Other times, it's the patient who causes the error by failing to follow instructions. And some patients' bodies simply register abnormal results when nothing is wrong. More often, however, a false positive result is a consequence of the limited reliability of the test itself. No test is perfect; all have certain inherent limitations.

The number of false positive results can be quite high. In some cases, less than half of those testing positive for a disease really have it. Studies show, for example, that only 30 to 43 percent of middle-aged men who have positive treadmill stress tests (p. 69) actually have coronary artery disease. When a test has such a high rate of false positives, a doctor takes a positive result simply as a sign that the patient may have the disease and makes a diagnosis through more specific tests or procedures, closer examination, or long-term monitoring.

SCREENING TESTS FOR HEALTHY ADULTS

An important part of a doctor's preventive care arsenal is an array of simple screening tests that can detect disease (or potential for it) before symptoms appear. Which tests you'll be given, when, and how often depend on your age, health, personal and family history, and your doctor's preferences.

Test	What it's for
Blood pressure test	To check for hypertension, or chronic high blood pressure. Blood pressure is the force blood exerts against arterial walls as it's pumped through the circulatory system. During each heartbeat, blood pressure varies between a high (*systolic pressure*), attained when heart contracts, and a low (*diastolic pressure*), attained when heart relaxes. Blood pressure readings are given as systolic over diastolic pressure, for example, 120/80.
Blood tests	Of the many blood tests available, the most commonly performed is the complete blood count (CBC), a series of tests that measure the number and proportion of blood components, primarily to screen for anemia (low red blood cell count). Another frequently done test measures blood levels of cholesterol.
Urinalysis	Urine provides valuable information about the health of the body as a whole and the kidneys in particular. Urinalysis is used to screen for many infections and diseases, including liver, kidney, and urinary tract disorders and diabetes.
Fecal occult blood test	To detect the presence in the stool of occult (hidden) blood, which can be a sign of a number of disorders ranging from hemorrhoids to polyps and cancer.
Electro-cardiogram (ECG or EKG)	To detect abnormal heart function by recording the electrical impulses that set off contractions of heart muscles. A resting ECG is a fairly good indicator of what has happened to the heart, but not a good predictor of future problems. An exercise ECG, or stress test, is given while the patient exercises (p.69); it is used to help diagnose chest pain, to assess heart's functional capacity, and to determine exercise tolerance.
Chest X-ray	X-rays are a form of short-wavelength electromagnetic energy. When beamed through a body onto a photographic plate, they produce images of bones and organs. Chest X-rays detect infections (mostly pneumonia), tumors and other disorders of lungs, chest cavity, and rib cage.
Pap (cervical smear) test	To detect cancerous or precancerous cells in the cervix (mouth of the uterus), often long before signs of advanced cancer become apparent. (For more on Pap tests and their accuracy, see page 251.)
Mammogram (breast X-ray)	To screen for breast cancer at an early stage, before it becomes apparent through self-examination (p.203) or a doctor's manual examination. If the mammogram is done at a facility accredited by the American College of Radiology (see Appendix), the test's accuracy rate is between 80 and 90 percent.

This chart lists the screening tests that you may be asked to take in connection with a routine physical examination. A recommended schedule for taking the tests is given in the column at right below. But there is still much controversy among medical experts about when and how often the various screening tests ought to be done. The schedule recommended by your doctor may differ significantly from this one. If a test detects a potential problem, more complex testing may be necessary (see *Diagnostic Tests,* pp. 126–127).

How it's done | **When and how often**

Inflatable cuff attached to a pressure gauge is wrapped around upper arm and inflated until blood flow stops. Listening through a stethoscope placed below cuff over brachial artery, doctor or nurse deflates cuff until sound of blood surging through arteries is heard; systolic pressure is now recorded. Cuff is further deflated until sound of blood flowing through arteries is muffled or no longer heard; diastolic pressure is now recorded.

Every 2 years if blood pressure is below 140/85. Every year if last diastolic reading was 85 to 89.

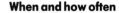

After a tourniquet has been tightened around upper arm, needle is inserted into vein at crook of elbow to draw a sample of blood into a syringe. Smaller quantities of blood may be drawn by pricking a finger tip with a needle and squeezing blood out. Sample is sent to a laboratory for analysis. Modern computerized analyzers can perform many different blood tests simultaneously.

CBC: Every 5 years before age 65; every 2 years after 65. *Cholesterol:* Every 5 years; more often if reading is above 200.

Patient is asked to urinate into a clean, dry container at home or at doctor's office. Usually a random sample is all that's required. Simple chemical analysis can be done in the doctor's office. For more complex analysis, sample is sent to a laboratory for microscopic examination or chemical testing.

Every 2 to 5 years before age 65; yearly after 65.

Doctor may take sample in the office during a rectal exam or patient may be given an applicator and sample box and asked to bring or mail in a smear to the doctor or a lab.

Yearly starting at age 50.

For a resting ECG, patient lies down, stripped to waist, while electrodes (small, flat disks) connected to a recording machine are lightly smeared with conductive gel and attached to chest, arms, and legs. With electrodes in place, recorder displays heart's electrical activity as a tracing on a screen or strip of paper. Test lasts some 15 minutes and is painless. For a stress test, the electrodes are attached to chest only.

Resting ECG: At doctor's discretion.

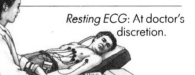

After removing jewelry, dentures, and other objects that can produce images on film, patient stands stripped to waist in front of photographic plate. Picture taking lasts only a few seconds. (For more on the risks of radiation, see page 141.)

Taken if patient smokes heavily or has signs of lung problems.

Pap test is done as part of a woman's pelvic exam (p.252). While the vagina is held open with a speculum, a spatula is used to scrape off cells from cervix. Cells are sent to a laboratory for microscopic examination. The test is not painful and usually lasts only about 5 minutes.

Three tests, a year apart, starting at age 18 at the latest; at least every 3 years thereafter.

Stripped to waist and wearing a lead apron to protect reproductive organs, patient places one breast at a time on an X-ray plate. Breast is compressed against plate (this may cause mild discomfort) and several views of it are taken. Radiation exposure is minimal; potential risks are far outweighed by potential benefits of early cancer detection.

Baseline mammogram between ages 35 and 39. Every 2 years from 40 to 50; yearly after 50.

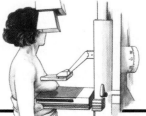

DIAGNOSTIC TESTS

To diagnose disease and monitor treatment, doctors once had to rely exclusively on their own observations and on the patient's description of symptoms. Today, sophisticated testing equipment allows doctors to view

The test and how it works	What it's for
Contrast X-ray imaging To be visible on an X-ray, blood vessels and most organs must be filled with a contrast medium—a dye or other substance that's impervious to X-rays. The contrast medium helps to outline the vessels and organs on an X-ray image.	To detect and examine a wide range of abnormalities in the organs listed at right.
Computerized tomography (CT or CAT) scanning In standard X-rays the source of the X-ray is stationary. In CT scanning the source rotates around the body part being examined. The low-dosage radiation emitted by the scanner is absorbed differently by different types of body tissue. Detectors opposite the source pick up the radiation and send signals to a computer that's programmed to sort out variations in X-ray absorption and produce cross-sectional images of the body, which are then projected onto a TV screen.	Used to explore all parts of the body. CT scans are good at detecting tumors, aneurysms, bleeding, and injuries in the brain, as well as tumors and abscesses of the abdomen; injuries of the spleen, kidney, and liver; and many different chest problems.
Magnetic resonance imaging (MRI) MRI produces cross-sectional images of the interior of the body without the use of radiation or contrast mediums. In MRI the body is exposed to a powerful magnetic field that causes the protons in the nuclei of the body's atoms to line up. Strong pulses of radio waves are used to knock the protons out of alignment. As they realign themselves, the protons emit radio waves of their own, which vary in intensity depending on the type of tissue in which they originate. A computer converts these signals into images displayed on a screen.	MRI reveals extremely subtle tissue abnormalities, such as the nerve fiber scarring associated with multiple sclerosis. It's especially useful in studying soft tissue encased in bone, such as the brain and spinal cord, but can also help diagnose diseases of the internal organs and joints.
Radionuclide scanning When introduced into the body, radioactive substances, called radionuclides, are taken up in greater quantities by some tissues than by others. The targeted tissue emits radiation that is detected by a gamma camera. The camera reacts to the radiation by emitting tiny flashes of light, which are converted to electronic signals used by a computer to produce still and moving images. The amount of radiation given off by the targeted organ depends on its cells' metabolic activity; rapidly multiplying cancer cells, for example, show up as "hot spots" on a scan.	To detect cancer and other disorders of the brain, heart, lungs, kidney, liver, and thyroid—often at an earlier stage than is possible with other imaging techniques. A state-of-the art form of radionuclide scanning, called PET scanning, is used primarily as a research tool in the study of brain and heart functions.
Ultrasound scanning In this radiation-free imaging technique, high-frequency sound waves emitted by a device called a transducer are bounced off an internal organ. The strength of the returning echoes varies depending on the type of tissue being scanned. The transducer picks up these echoes and converts them into electrical signals, which are used to build an image of the organ that can be displayed on a screen.	To view and diagnose disorders of the liver, pancreas, gallbladder, and kidneys; to monitor fetal development; to guide doctors performing prenatal screening tests (p.260). Doppler ultrasound measures blood flow in veins and arteries.
Endoscopy Endoscopy allows a doctor to view the inside of the body directly. An endoscope—a flexible tube containing fiberoptic bundles, through which light can travel—is inserted into a body cavity or surgical incision. Light beamed down one fiberoptic bundle illuminates the body part being examined. Another bundle carries the reflected image back to the instrument's eyepiece where a lens focuses and magnifies it.	To view and detect abnormalities in the body parts listed at right. Endoscopes fitted with special attachments can be used to take tissue samples for a biopsy and to perform other surgical procedures (such a removing torn cartilage from a knee joint).

the interior of the body with great precision and at little or no risk to the patient. The scanning and imaging tests described here are usually performed in a hospital radiology department and are administered and interpreted by a specialist known as a diagnostic radiologist.

How it's administered

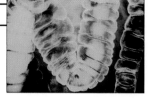

Barium X-ray of colon

The contrast medium for the gastrointestinal tract is barium (in the form of barium sulfate) given in a drink or enema. Other media are used to X-ray heart and blood vessels (angiography), uterus and Fallopian tubes (hysterosalpingography), urinary tract (urography), and gallbladder (cholecystography). The media may cause a reaction.

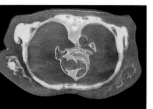

CT scan of chest

CT scanning is done in a radiologist's office or in a hospital on an in- or outpatient basis. The patient lies on a movable table that slides into the scanner's round opening. The table is positioned so that the part of the body to be examined lies within the opening. The test usually lasts from 30 minutes to an hour and is painless. Some patients experience anxiety or claustrophobia in the scanner. Contrast medium sometimes used in CT scanning may produce a reaction.

MRI scanning is done on an in- or outpatient basis. After removing all metallic objects and electronic devices, the patient lies on a movable table that slides into the scanner's hollow center. The test, which lasts about an hour, is painless; some patients may experience claustrophobia and anxiety. Pregnant women and people with pacemakers or metallic implants should not take the test.

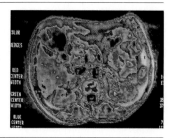

MRI scan of stomach

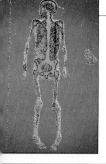

Gamma camera scan of bones

Radionuclide scanning is done on an in- or outpatient basis. Depending on the body part being examined, the radionuclide is swallowed or is injected into a vein in the arm. The patient may have to wait several hours for the radionuclide to be absorbed by the targeted tissue. During the scanning, the patient sits or lies on an examining table while the gamma camera is moved close to the body part being examined. The procedure is painless and safe (the amounts of radiation involved are minute), but is not recommended for women who are pregnant or nursing infants.

The test can be done in a doctor's office or in a hospital on an outpatient basis. The body part involved is bared and rubbed with an oil or gel to facilitate sound-wave transmission. With the patient sitting or lying down, a technologist passes the transducer over the body part. Ultrasound is inaudible and except for the pressure of the transducer on the skin, the patient feels nothing. No risks have been observed at power levels used for diagnosis.

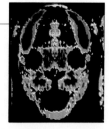

Ultrasound scan of fetus's face

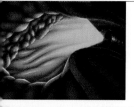

Endoscope in esophagus

Specialized endoscopes are put through the mouth to view upper gastrointestinal tract (esophagoscopy, gastroduodenoscopy), the rectum to view it and colon (colonoscopy, sigmoidoscopy), the nose to view bronchial tubes and lungs (bronchoscopy), the urethra to view it and bladder (cystoscopy), or into an abdominal (laparoscopy) or joint (arthroscopy) incision. Some are done with a sedative or local anesthetic; others with a general anesthetic. They are generally safe; some are uncomfortable.

How reliable are sidewalk tests for cholesterol and blood pressure?

Public cholesterol-screening programs in malls and supermarkets are not as reliable as testing done by a trained technician in a medical setting. One study of public testing found inaccurate results as much as 25 percent of the time, primarily because of incorrect testing techniques used by staffers with a minimum of training. Public blood-pressure screening tests, on the other hand, are relatively accurate in detecting high blood pressure.

Who should be tested for AIDS and why should they be?

When the AIDS antibody test first became available in 1985, many of those most concerned with combating the disease opposed widespread testing for the simple reason that little could be done for anyone found to be infected with the AIDS virus, known as HIV (human immuno-deficiency virus). Not only does a positive test result cause great emotional distress, it often results in job, housing, and social discrimination. Today, however, there are drugs that if administered early enough can delay the onset of full-blown AIDS and prolong the life of someone who is infected with HIV but has few or no symptoms. For this reason, most experts recommend that anyone at risk of contracting the disease be tested as soon as possible. Those at greatest risk of getting AIDS are homosexual and bisexual men and intravenous drug users. Others at high risk are hemophiliacs and anyone else who received transfusions before it became standard to test blood for HIV in March 1985.

Sex partners of anyone at risk are also at risk of getting AIDS.

Most private doctors and hospitals can test for HIV but not all guarantee confidentiality and not all give adequate counseling. To find a testing program that offers confidentiality and counseling, ask your doctor or call the AIDS hotline (1-800 342-AIDS). The best testing programs offer counseling both before and after the test. A trained adviser helps the patient understand the test and, if the result is positive, handle the emotional impact and find the best course of treatment. (See *The Facts About AIDS*, p.242.)

Do adults need to be vaccinated?

Yes they do. While many childhood vaccinations confer lifelong immunity, the vaccines for tetanus and diphtheria do not. A combined tetanus-diphtheria booster shot is recommended for all adults every 10 years. Immunity from tetanus is especially important if you garden or do yardwork. Tetanus (lockjaw) usually results from a backyard laceration and, though very rare, it can be fatal. If you suffer a severe or dirty cut before you get a booster shot, see a doctor for anti-tetanus treatment, which includes a booster.

People whose occupation, health condition, or lifestyle puts them at risk of contracting hepatitis B, or serum hepatitis, should also be immunized against it. The immunization—a three-shot procedure—is recommended for intravenous drug users, homosexual men, hemophiliacs who receive regular blood transfusions, as well as doctors, dentists, nurses, and all other health-care workers who come into contact with contaminated needles and body fluids.

I was inoculated against measles as a child. Now a friend says I should be inoculated again. Doesn't the measles vaccine give lifetime protection?

Doctors once thought that it did, but evidence now suggests that the protection wanes with time. Children should be inoculated with the combined measles-mumps-rubella (MMR) vaccine twice, at the age of 15 months and 5 years—or later if they have not received the booster shot yet (see *Childhood Immunization Schedule*, facing page).

If you were born after 1956 and were not vaccinated twice, you probably need a second shot, especially if you are at high risk for contracting the disease. High-risk groups include children and staff in day-care centers, students of all ages including college students, their teachers, and anyone in health care or other fields who comes into close contact with many people. The measles virus is airborne and highly contagious. Someone without immunity can get the disease just by being in the same room with an infected person.

If you were born before 1956, you're assumed to be immune. Most people your age and older were almost certainly exposed to the virus and had the disease or at least developed antibodies to it.

Do older or chronically ill adults need special immunizations?

Adults who are over the age of 65 or whose immunity has been impaired by a chronic condition, such as diabetes or a serious disorder of the heart, lung, liver, or kidneys, should be vaccinated against two potentially life-threatening infections. The pneu-

CHILDHOOD IMMUNIZATION SCHEDULE

Proper immunization guards your child against seven serious infectious diseases. Immunization works by tricking the body into mounting defenses against a mild form of a disease. Tiny amounts of a virus or bacteria—either killed or living but rendered harmless—are introduced into the bloodstream, causing the immune system to produce protective substances called antibodies against the same or closely related microbes. Except for the oral polio vaccine, immunizations generally involve an injection into the upper arm or buttocks. Repeated doses, called boosters, may be needed at various times to strengthen existing immunity. Although most immunizations carry little risk, always check with your doctor before having a child immunized; postpone the immunization if the child is sick.

BERT

Age	Disease	Method of immunization

TOMMY

Age	Disease		Method of immunization
2 months	✓ Diphtheria, tetanus, pertussis		Combined injection
	✓ Poliomyelitis		Oral
4 months	✓ Diphtheria, tetanus, pertussis		Combined injection
	✓ Poliomyelitis		Oral
6 months	✓ Diphtheria, tetanus, pertussis		Combined injection
15 months	✓ Measles, mumps, rubella		Combined injection
	✓ Diphtheria, tetanus, pertussis		Combined injection
	✓ Poliomyelitis		Oral
18 months	✓ Hemophilus influenzae B		Injection
4 to 6 years	✓ Diphtheria, tetanus, pertussis		Combined injection*
	✓ Poliomyelitis		Oral
5 to 21 years	Measles, mumps, rubella		Combined injection*
14 to 16 years	Diphtheria, tetanus		Combined injection*

*A single booster shot during these years.

mococcal pneumonia vaccine protects against pneumonia caused by strains of streptococcus bacteria; a single inoculation generally confers immunity for 5 to 10 years. The other recommended immunization is an annual influenza vaccination.

My company offers flu shots to its employees every fall. How effective are these shots?

Each summer a new vaccine is developed to protect against the strains of influenza virus expected to be most prevalent in the coming winter. If the mix of strains is right—and it usually is—the vaccine is about 70 to 80 percent effective in preventing influenza. Immunized people who do get the disease usually have a milder form of it.

Most communities and many companies sponsor immunization campaigns in October or November. This is the best time to get a flu shot because although the influenza season usually begins in December, people generally need 10 to 20 days to develop immunity. The shot provides protection for about a year.

Some people experience soreness around the injection site and a small number develop a slight fever, but the vaccine is considered safe for most people. It is grown in eggs, however, so if you're highly allergic to eggs, avoid flu shots.

Should a pregnant woman be vaccinated against rubella?

No, not while she's pregnant or for at least 3 months before conception. Although rubella, or German measles, is a relatively mild disease, it can cause severe damage to the developing fetus of a woman who contracts it. There's a small risk that the rubella vaccine, if administered during or shortly before pregnancy, could also harm the fetus.

Ideally, every girl should be vaccinated against rubella before she reaches adolescence. If you are a woman of childbearing age, your doctor can give you a simple blood test to find out if you have antibodies for rubella. If you lack antibodies, get vaccinated and then wait at least 3 months before conceiving.

How can I find out what shots are necessary when I travel abroad?

If you are traveling from the United States to Europe, Canada, Mexico, or the Caribbean, you don't need any vaccinations, but it's important to have received all of the standard childhood immunizations (see previous page) as well as boosters for tetanus and possibly measles. If you plan to travel anywhere else in the world, call your local city or county department of health to find out which vaccinations are required—or recommended—for the country or countries you want to visit. Local health departments receive regular updates on disease outbreaks and immunization requirements from the Federal Centers for Disease Control. You can also call the Centers for the latest and most reliable advice (see Appendix).

When asking about immunization requirements, be sure to tell the health worker all the countries on your itinerary. Many countries require a vaccination if you arrive from a country or region of a country that's infected. For example, if you stop over in a country that's infected with yellow fever but doesn't require immunization against it, you may need the vaccination anyway to enter the next country. Vaccination for yellow fever is available only at licensed health centers.

Do I have a legal right to see my personal medical files?

It depends on what state you live in. About half the states have laws that allow patients to see and obtain copies of their hospital and doctor's office records. In other states, the request may or may not be honored depending on the doctor or hospital.

As a practical matter, getting copies of your medical records can be time-consuming and may involve paying search and copying fees. In most cases, it's not worth the trouble since your doctor has a professional obligation to send your records, upon request, to another doctor who is examining or treating you. The transfer of records between doctors, however, can take time, especially if you haven't seen the first doctor in years and your records are in the inactive files. This is one reason why many patients' rights advocates recommend that all patients obtain copies of their records. This way you'd have your medical data on hand should you need to see a new doctor on short notice. Although the need to have a copy of your records is debatable, it's probably worthwhile asking for them if you are moving to another part of the country or to a foreign country; you might also want your college-bound children to have copies of their records.

Can anyone besides my doctor see my records?

As a general rule, your medical records are confidential and are seen only by your doctor and certain members of the doctor's or a hospital's staff. If a claim for payment is made with a health insurance company, the insurer can also request to see the records to verify the claim. In most

states, the company needs your authorization to do this, but the release that you sign when you first obtain the insurance is usually broad enough to cover all the claims you later make.

The law in most states requires doctors to report to state or local government agencies information on cases involving gunshot wounds, sexually transmitted diseases, and suspected child abuse.

I trust my doctor, but shouldn't I get a second opinion when making a major health decision?

If your are in doubt about a diagnosis's accuracy or a treatment's appropriateness, it is almost always a good idea to get a second opinion from a specialist (see *Medical Specialists,* p.142). Consulting with a specialist is generally recommended if your doctor diagnoses a rare or serious disease or if your doctor suggests major surgery or unusually complicated, expensive, or risky tests. Getting a second opinion is also advisable if your doctor fails to make a diagnosis after a reasonable number of visits, does not give you a satisfactory explanation for the failure of a treatment to relieve your symptoms, or attributes persistent troublesome symptoms to your "nerves" or "imagination."

Probably the most important time to get a second opinion is when your doctor advises surgery. Besides conferring with the surgeon suggested by your primary doctor, it's advisable to consult with a second qualified specialist, especially if the operation is rare, complex, potentially life-threatening, or possibly unnecessary. (Among the surgical procedures often done unnecessarily are hysterectomies, hernia repairs, coronary bypasses, and gallbladder removals as well as operations for hemorrhoids, varicose veins, and lower back pain.)

When surgery is suggested, it's often a good idea to get your second opinion from a nonsurgical specialist. If you are advised to have a heart operation, for example, you might consult with a cardiologist, who treats heart disease medically, instead of consulting with a second cardiac surgeon. Most insurance companies insist on a second opinion for nonemergency surgery—sometimes from specialists they select.

How do I go about finding a doctor for a second opinion?

The simplest way is to ask your primary doctor for a recommendation. This way you'll get someone your doctor knows and trusts. Such an arrangement also facilitates the exchange of test results and other information and saves you the trouble of finding a second doctor yourself.

If you prefer a completely independent opinion, you can find a specialist by calling a teaching hospital, a medical center, your local medical society, or your health insurance company. Look for board-certified specialists and check out their qualifications as you would those of a primary doctor (p. 119). If you find a specialist on your own, inform your primary doctor as a courtesy and have your medical records sent to the specialist. Have the second doctor's diagnosis sent to your first doctor along with any additional test results.

I'm afraid that asking for a second opinion will upset my doctor. Should I do it anyway?

By all means. A truly professional doctor is unlikely to be offended by the request. Actually a good doctor is often the first to recommend that you see a specialist if you have unusual or hard-to-diagnose symptoms. Most doctors know that they are not infallible beings and value the opinions of other doctors. They themselves often obtain second opinions, in effect, by consulting with colleagues when treating a difficult case or before recommending surgery or other radical treatment. If your doctor feels challenged by a reasonable request for a second opinion and reacts in a defensive or hostile manner, that person may be the wrong doctor for you.

What should I do if the second doctor's opinion conflicts with my primary doctor's?

When a specialist's second opinion agrees with a primary doctor's, it is reassuring and helpful to both the patient and the primary doctor. But sometimes the two opinions do conflict. When this happens, the doctors are usually able to reach a consensus, if not on the actual treatment itself, at least on a plan of action. For example, the doctors may agree to try a conservative nonsurgical treatment for heart disease for a certain period of time. If there's no improvement at the end of that period, the patient becomes a candidate for bypass surgery. If no such consensus can be reached, you may have to seek a third opinion, preferably from a nationally recognized expert on the condition you're suffering from. Before seeking a third opinion, ask the first two doctors for a clear explanation of their positions and find out exactly why they oppose each other's views. Discuss the situation with your family and friends to get their feedback. Then choose the option you feel is best.

Do doctors ever hide diagnoses from their patients?

Few doctors still subscribe to the idea that the doctor knows best and should withhold information from a patient for the patient's own good. Today, most members of the medical community adhere to the principle of informed consent. This means that before starting any treatment your doctor will obtain your consent, but only after informing you of the nature of your illness, the kind of treatment proposed, the risks and benefits of the treatment, and any alternatives to it.

To be fully informed, tell your doctor that you want to know as much as possible about your condition, even if the news is bad or uncertain. Ask direct questions. What is my prognosis? Will the proposed treatment harm me? What are the odds that it will work? What are the odds I'll get better anyway if I don't have it? If you decide against a recommended course of treatment, it's prudent to get a second opinion first.

How can I learn more about a diagnosis and its treatment?

If you have a common serious disease, the easiest way to get up-to-date information in most cases is to contact the local chapter of the national organization for that illness—for example, the American Diabetes Association, the American Heart Association, or the Arthritis Foundation (see Appendix). Most will be happy to send you pamphlets and other information. Local chapters often sponsor meetings, lectures, and support groups (check your phone book's white pages under the name of the disorder). Your doctor or a hospital may also have helpful brochures.

ALTERNATIVE MEDICINE

The term alternative medicine is applied to any approach to healing that is not grounded in standard Western medical practices. Besides the therapies described below, other common alternative medical treatments include various types of massage (p.206); manipulation therapies, which, like chiropractic, stress hydrotherapy, the use of baths or water massage or the variety of disorders (such water therapies are often Rolfing, the Alexander technique, and other posture and proper body alignment; and drinking of mineral water to treat a wide the basis of spa cures).

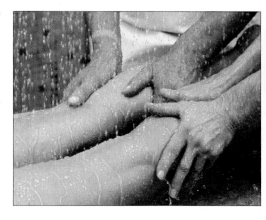

The benefits of garlic, which may even include a reduction in cancer and heart disease risk, are now being confirmed by mainstream medical researchers.

Homeopathy. This form of alternative medicine originated in Germany and was brought to the U.S. in the 19th century. Homeopathy is based on the principle that "like cures like" — the word comes from the Greek *homoios* (like) and *pathos* (suffering). A homeopathic doctor treats an illness by prescribing a small, highly diluted dose of a natural substance that in a larger, more concentrated dose would reproduce the patient's symptoms. For example, a

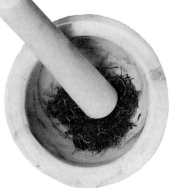

tiny amount of a laxative would be used to treat diarrhea. Homeopathic medications, called remedies, are given in the smallest dose possible and are designed to complement natural body processes. Unlike many powerful modern drugs, homeopathic remedies are not dangerous and have few or no side effects.

Other tenets of homeopathy are that the body heals itself and that people get sick in individual ways (in contrast to the traditional belief that a disease produces the same symptoms in most people).

Although some homeopaths are medical doctors who became disillusioned with the practice of conventional medicine, most mainstream physicians remain skeptical of homeopathy and point out that the success of homeopathic remedies is often due to the placebo effect.

Naturopathy. According to naturopathic doctors (N.D.'s), illness results from the accumulation of toxins in the body and can be prevented or treated by avoiding dietary, environmental, and other influences that are artificial, impure, or unnatural. Introduced in the U.S. around 1900, naturopathy is not a unified system. Rather it evolved from various 18th- and 19th-century European health practices and today encompasses different forms of steam and water therapy, massage, applications of heat and cold, herbalism, fasting, acupuncture, homeopathy, and colonic irrigation (a type of enema).

Accredited naturopathic doctors attend 4-year postgraduate colleges. They take standard medical studies during the first 2 years; then the emphasis shifts to nutrition, physical therapies, Oriental medicine, homeopathy, and behavioral counseling. Naturopathic doctors are licensed in eight states. Not all naturopaths, however, are properly accredited. Some have questionable mail-order degrees; others may engage in dubious practices, such as diagnosing illness by means of hair-shaft analysis.

Although naturopaths believe firmly in the body's ability to heal itself and stress the importance of a proper lifestyle, they will refer a patient requiring surgery or some other conventional therapy to a medical specialist. For their part, most conventional medical doctors question the effectiveness of many naturopathic practices.

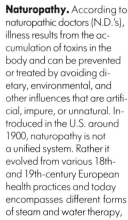

Herbalism. The use of plants to treat illness dates back to early man. Not only did modern herbalism evolve from ancient Western and Eastern practices, but many of today's conventional drugs are descendants of traditional herbal remedies. The heart drug digitalis, for example, is derived from the foxglove plant. Despite the resistance of Western doctors to folk therapies, herbalism with its natural, holistic orientation has a wide appeal. However, it is not a licensed specialty in the U.S., and some practitioners may be poorly trained.

Most herbalists dispense their own medications, usually as alcohol-based tinctures, which tend to have a bitter

Aloe vera

Different as they are, many alternative therapies share a belief in the body's ability to heal itself and in the principle of treating the whole person, physically, mentally, and spiritually. This "holistic" approach to medicine is shared to an extent by some mainstream doctors who see it as a counterbalance to the increasingly impersonal and technological practice of modern medicine. Indeed, much of the success of some alternative practitioners may be the result of the sympathetic hearing they give to patients.

Although many people are turning to alternative therapies and may benefit from them, these practices are usually not taught in medical schools and are not sanctioned by medical societies.

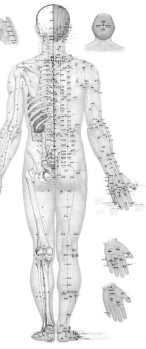

Acupuncture. This ancient Chinese practice involves inserting needles into the skin at specific points to treat disorders and relieve pain. According to Taoist theory, the Qi (pronounced "chee," also spelled Chi or Ch'i), or life force, circulates through the body along lines called meridians. Illness occurs when the meridians are blocked. Properly inserted and manipulated needles unblock the flow of Qi and restore health.

Many Western practitioners accept that acupuncture can relieve pain and other symptoms, although how and why the technique works is still being investigated. Chinese acupuncturists treat everything from eczema to menstrual problems, but in the West acupuncture is used mainly for relief of muscle and joint pain and as an anesthetic.

The needles don't hurt when inserted properly, but they sometimes produce stinging sensations. Symptoms may temporarily worsen after treatment, and some people feel lightheaded, dizzy, or drowsy; others say they feel exhilarated.

Acupuncture is licensed in over 20 states; to be accredited, most practitioners must take a 3-year course of study.

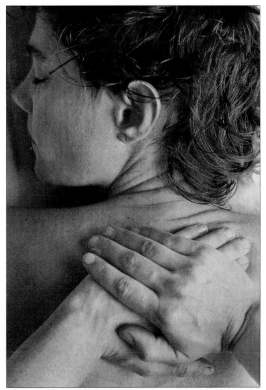

Chiropractic. Developed in 1895 by an Iowa grocer, this drugless healing method is based on the theory that misalignment of the spinal column alters the pathways of the nervous system and is a major cause of health problems. Chiropractic focuses on the manual manipulation of the spine (and sometimes other bones and joints) to relieve pain and promote health. Most practitioners also stress the importance of proper diet and exercise. Chiropractors cannot prescribe drugs or perform surgery.

Although patients sometimes claim to receive dramatic pain relief during initial sessions with a chiropractor, more often results are seen over a period of weeks or months and may come not only from manipulation but also from changes in diet, exercise, and lifestyle. While the manipulations themselves generally do not hurt, some patients feel mild, diffuse pain later on, sometimes lasting 2–3 days. This is usually considered a sign that the treatment is working.

Doctors of chiropractic (D.C.'s) must complete 2 years of undergraduate study and a 4-year course at a chiropractic college before taking national and state board exams. Every state requires chiropractors to be licensed. Nevertheless, many mainstream physicians doubt the validity of chiropractic's premises and believe that the risks of forceful joint manipulation can outweigh its benefits.

Balm of Gilead

taste. Herbal remedies may also come in the form of pills, syrups, creams, oils, gargles, and infusions (herbal teas). The effects of most herbal preparations are quite mild and certainly not strong enough to treat serious medical conditions. Like other plant products, herbal remedies can cause allergic reactions in some people; they may even be toxic if taken in the wrong combinations or in excessive amounts.

I am not really satisfied with my doctor. Should I look for a new one?

It depends on the situation and what you hope to gain by switching. If you are uncomfortable around doctors in general, switching doctors is not likely to help. If you are unhappy because you are not convinced by a diagnosis or a treatment has not been as effective as you hoped, the real solution may be to get a second opinion from a specialist.

On the other hand, if you feel your doctor doesn't spend enough time with you or isn't easily available to you, it may be better to discuss the situation with the doctor and, perhaps, reschedule your visits or calls to times when he or she is less rushed. Similarly, if you feel your doctor is not taking your complaints seriously, a discussion may reveal that the doctor has indeed examined you thoroughly and has sound medical reasons for believing your problem is not serious. Or it could lead to a closer examination or a second opinion.

However, if you really don't like a doctor's personality, find him or her uncaring, always leave the doctor's office with a negative feeling, or seriously doubt the doctor's competence, by all means look for a new one.

My doctor's behavior has become erratic recently. I suspect he may be drinking or taking drugs. What should I do?

If you observe behavior that suggests alcohol or drug abuse, senility, or some major emotional problem in a doctor, contact your state's medical licensing board. The board, which regulates a doctor's license to practice, will usually investigate the complaint and issue a report. In most cases, you won't have to testify against your doctor, but the procedure, which varies from state to state, can be slow.

You may also want to contact the local medical society, the administrator of the hospital where your doctor is on staff, and

any health maintenance organization or other health plan that your doctor belongs to.

Reporting your doctor is not an easy thing to do, but remember that you are doing his other patients—and perhaps the doctor himself—a service.

What actually constitutes malpractice, and how common are malpractice suits?

Malpractice is an error that results when a doctor (or other health-care worker) acts negligently or incompetently compared with what other "reasonable" doctors would do in the same case. A major study of hospital patients in New York state conducted in 1986 by the Harvard School of Public Health found that about 1 percent of those admitted suffered an adverse reaction as a result of negligence. Of these, more than half recovered within 30 days and 70 percent within 6 months. Only about 1 in 10 of those who suffered an adverse reaction because of negligence filed for damages. Of course, patients can suffer adverse reactions to treatment that is considered acceptable, and some of these patients also file suits.

Although malpractice awards add billions of dollars to the nation's annual health-care bill, the number of suits is quite low (about 6½ for every 100 doctors, according to the American Medical Association). Reasons for this low number include changes in the laws of some states limiting payments to patients as well as a growing tendency on the part of litigants to settle out of court in order to avoid high legal fees. Another factor is the increasing number of doctors who practice "defensive medicine," primarily by limiting the number of risky procedures they undertake.

IS THIS DOCTOR COMPETENT?

You might well worry about your chances of getting good basic medical care from a doctor who regularly exhibits any of the following patterns of behavior.

☐ Treats you without a diagnosis or treatment plan.

☐ Doesn't follow up on abnormal test results.

☐ Dismisses recurrent complaints without a good reason.

☐ Doesn't send your records to another doctor when asked to.

☐ Recommends expensive and possibly risky tests or services without a good rationale.

☐ Doesn't maintain a clean, well-ordered office.

☐ Comes to the office looking haggard or disheveled, a possible sign of personal or emotional problems.

☐ Shows obvious signs of alcohol or drug use.

☐ Misses appointments without an acceptable explanation.

☐ Doesn't return your phone calls, especially urgent ones.

☐ Harasses, intimidates, lies, or makes sexual advances.

DOES MEDICINE TREAT WOMEN FAIRLY?

Women see doctors more often than men do and are generally more involved with health care, not only their own but often that of children and aging parents as well. Yet women are more likely than men to say that doctors don't take their complaints seriously enough or that they treat them in a gruff, impersonal manner. Here are some other ways in which medicine may shortchange women.

☐ Far more tranquilizers and sleeping pills are prescribed for women than for men. Critics say pills are often quick fixes for deeper problems.

☐ Women are more likely to have unnecessary surgery. Cesarean deliveries are the most common operation in the U.S., and 1 out of 3 American women will have a hysterectomy before age 65. While many of these operations are necessary, critics think they are being performed far too frequently.

☐ Men used to be chosen much more often than women for medical research studies. Early groundbreaking studies—notably on heart attack prevention—focused only on men.

☐ Insurance companies often charge higher rates to women in their childbearing years.

If you're unhappy with your medical care, voice your complaints; if necessary, change doctors. If you're uncertain about a procedure, get a second opinion (p.130).

My doctor always keeps me waiting. What can I do about it?

Having to wait to see a doctor is frequently unavoidable. Although some doctors simply schedule patients too closely, more often the delays are caused by emergencies and other unexpected disruptions, ranging from a patient who must be admitted to the hospital to a patient who needs time to discuss a problem.

To minimize your wait, call the doctor's office before you leave home and ask how the day is progressing. You may be able to arrive an hour later rather than spend the time sitting in the waiting room. On the other hand, be sure to call ahead if you are going to be late.

It's after my doctor's office hours and I feel ill. What should I do?

If you call your doctor's office after hours, you'll almost always get a recording or an answering service that will give you a number where you can reach your doctor or another physician who is covering for him or her. If you need immediate attention, go to an emergency room, preferably at the hospital where your doctor has staff privileges. Often, a doctor on duty there will call your doctor.

I have to hold papers farther and farther away to read them. Who should I go to for an eye exam?

After the age of about 45 most people begin to lose the ability to focus on objects at close range and need reading glasses or bifocals (or special contact lenses) to read or do any kind of close work. When this happens, you can have your eyes examined by either an ophthalmologist or an optometrist. Ophthalmologists are medical doctors who specialize in the diagnosis and treatment of both vision problems and eye diseases. They not only prescribe corrective lenses but also prescribe medicines and perform eye surgery. Anyone with a serious vision or medical eye problem should always go to an ophthalmologist for treatment rather than an optometrist.

However, if you're having your eyes checked because of a normal decline in near vision, it is usually less costly and sometimes more convenient to go to an optometrist for your examination. Optometrists are trained primarily to detect vision problems and to prescribe corrective lenses. Even though they are not medical doctors, optometrists can screen for signs of eye disease, test for glaucoma (p.136), and use eye drops to dilate (enlarge) the pupils in order to get a thorough look at the inside of the eye. In some states, optometrists can even treat eye diseases and prescribe medication for them. If an optometrist does detect a serious or potentially serious condition, he or she will refer you to an ophthalmologist for further treatment.

Don't confuse an ophthalmologist or an optometrist with an optician, whose job is to fill prescriptions for eyeglasses much like a pharmacist fills prescriptions for drugs.

EXAMINING YOUR EYES

The sequence of an eye exam varies from doctor to doctor. Most ask first about your general health, specific eye problems, and activities that affect vision. The doctor will note your eyes' overall condition, check their movement, and test the pupils' reaction to light. The lids, tear ducts, and eye exteriors are examined with a *slit-lamp microscope*. This device is also used to evaluate the clarity of the cornea and lens and the condition of the iris.

To test visual acuity, or sharpness of vision, you'll be asked to read a standard eye chart (called a Snellen's chart). If you need corrective lenses, the doctor will have you look through lenses of different strengths, either in special trial glasses or in a device called a *phoropter* or *refractor*.

To examine the retina and capillaries, the doctor uses an *ophthalmoscope,* an instrument that both lights up an eye's interior and gives a magnified view of it. To get a better view, the doctor may use drops to dilate the pupils.

To test for glaucoma, the doctor uses a *tonometer,* a device with a plunger or a pressure probe, which when applied briefly to the surface of the eye measures the pressure within it (some tonometers measure eye pressure with a puff of air). Before the test, the doctor applies a drop of a quick-acting anesthetic to each eye.

Depending on your specific eye problems and risk factors, peripheral vision, depth perception, near vision, or color vision may also be tested.

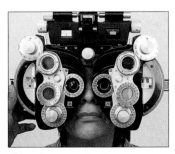

Phoropter

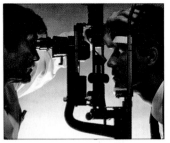

Slit-lamp microscope

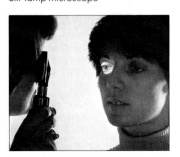

Ophthalmoscope

Tonometer

How often should I have my eyes examined?

It depends on whether or not you have a vision problem or are at risk for developing eye disease. If you wear corrective lenses already, it's a good idea to have your eyes checked every year—or any time you notice a change in your vision. If you are very myopic (nearsighted), a yearly exam is especially needed to check for retinal problems.

At around age 35, everyone should be tested for glaucoma—a sight-threatening buildup of pressure in the eyes (see *The Facts About Glaucoma,* p.398).

In the absence of a vision problem or eye disease, the American Academy of Ophthalmology recommends an eye exam every 2 to 5 years from age 35 on.

However, if you are black, diabetic, or have a family history of glaucoma, you are at high risk for glaucoma; have your eyes tested for it every year. Diabetics, who are also at risk for other eye disorders, should be especially vigilant about eye care. If you have high blood pressure or a thyroid problem, you may also need more frequent eye exams; ask the doctor treating the condition.

Have your eyes examined if you notice a decline in vision; if

your eyes hurt or are continually red and itchy; if there's a discharge from an eye; or if you find bright light bothersome or close work and reading difficult.

Do my children need regular eye exams?

An infant's eyes are examined right after birth for infection and any physical defect. From then on, the baby's pediatrician should screen for vision problems; if any arise, the pediatrician will usually recommend an ophthalmologist who specializes in treating children. If you notice that your child's eyes wander, are crossed, or are squinted excessively, an immediate eye exam is in order.

In the absence of noticeable vision problems, it's a good idea to have an ophthalmologist or optometrist examine a child's eyes around the age of 4. At this age, before the child enters school, any imbalance caused by a weakness in one eye can still be corrected fairly easily. Unless a problem develops, another exam is considered unnecessary as long as the child's eyes are checked periodically by a pediatrician.

If I give the wrong answer when my eye doctor is testing me for lenses, will I get an incorrect prescription?

Your responses to trial lenses do help the doctor to determine the prescription. But from the other side of the lens the doctor is also observing how sharply each lens brings into focus the retina in the back of the eye. The lens that gives the doctor the sharpest view of the retina is nearly always the same one that will give you the sharpest view of the world. If you give a response that is far off the mark, the doctor will know it and test again.

How often should I go to the dentist for a checkup?

If you are in good health, are not prone to tooth decay, have healthy gums and all your own teeth, and practice good oral hygiene, a dental exam once every year or two may be sufficient. But few people are so lucky (or so conscientious); most of us need to see a dentist more often. Exactly how often can only be determined by you and your dentist based on the factors listed above as well as personal habits that affect the teeth, such as

A DENTAL EXAM

If you are seeing a new dentist or revisiting one after a long absence, the examination usually begins with questions about your dental and general medical history. The dentist will ask about any chronic illnesses such as diabetes or heart disease, medications you are taking, and allergies.

After observing the overall appearance of your face and neck and feeling the temporomandibular (jaw) joint for abnormal movements, the dentist begins a complete examination of your mouth, tongue, cheeks, gums, teeth, and bite, using a mirror to check the back of the mouth and individual teeth and a metal probe to look for cavities or chips. Gums are inspected for signs of gingivitis or periodontitis. Fillings and crowns are checked for fit, jagged edges, or signs of erosion. Dentures are also checked for fit. A full set of X-rays may be taken, if previous ones do not exist or are dated. On this or a follow-up visit, the dentist or a hygienist will usually scale and clean your teeth and advise you on home oral hygiene, demonstrating the best techniques for brushing, flossing, and sometimes other procedures.

If you have a cavity, gum disease, or other problem, the dentist will explain the diagnosis, recommend a plan of treatment, and arrange for future visits.

smoking, snacking between meals, chewing sugared gum, drinking sweet or alcoholic beverages, and eating a lot of sweets. In the interest of preventive dentistry (to avoid the need for excessive restorative treatment later on), many dentists recommend a dental checkup every 6 months.

No matter what your normal checkup schedule is, see your dentist right away if you notice any of these symptoms:
☐ Gums that bleed easily or that are red, swollen, or tender.
☐ Receding gums.
☐ Pus between teeth and gums.
☐ Chronic bad breath or a persistent bad taste in your mouth.
☐ Loose teeth.
☐ A change in the way your teeth fit together when you bite.
☐ A change in the fit of partial dentures.

At what age should I take my child to have her teeth checked for the first time?

Some experts recommend a visit to a dentist as early as a child's first birthday to make sure the teeth are coming in correctly. But since the child's pediatrician usually checks this, a more practical time for a first dental appointment—either with your own dentist or with a pediatric dentist specially trained to care for children—is soon after the primary (baby) teeth have emerged, usually between ages 2 and 2½. Even at this age, children can develop dental problems, and it is important not to put off the first visit until a child has a toothache or other problem needing immediate attention. If dentistry becomes associated in a child's mind with pain, he or she may resist future trips, be upset throughout visits, and develop a lifelong aversion to dentists.

GLOSSARY OF DENTAL TERMS AND PROCEDURES

Abcess. Infection of the pulp of a tooth at the tip of the root. Treated with ROOT CANAL THERAPY.

Appliance. Fixed or removable device that is put into the mouth to reposition teeth (orthodontic appliances, or BRACES) or to replace missing teeth (prosthodontic appliances such as DENTURES and BRIDGES).

Bleaching. Procedure to remove discoloration of enamel by repeated applications of an oxidizing solution.

Bonding. Technique in which a tooth's front surface is covered with a laminate veneer (thin layers of acrylic, composite resin, or porcelain) to improve appearance.

Braces. Orthodontic APPLIANCES used to straighten or reposition teeth.

Bridge. Prosthodontic APPLIANCE used to replace missing teeth. Artificial teeth are fastened between CROWNS on adjacent natural teeth or by metal wings bonded to the adjacent teeth.

Calculus, or tartar. Calcified (hardened) PLAQUE that forms a crustlike deposit on teeth and helps inflame the gums; can lead to PERIODONTITIS. Calculus can only be removed by SCALING.

Caries. Tooth decay, caused primarily by bacteria in PLAQUE that break down food debris and create acids that erode the enamel, the dentin, and eventually the pulp of a tooth. Treated with a FILLING.

Crown, or cap. Gold or porcelain cover for top, or crown, of a tooth.

Curettage. Procedure in which a narrow spoon-shaped instrument (a curette) is used to scrape diseased tissue from lining of pockets between gum and tooth root in PERIODONTITIS; helps reattach gum to tooth.

Denture. APPLIANCE, usually removable, used to replace all or some natural teeth. Dentures have an acrylic or metal base plate with acrylic or porcelain teeth. Partial dentures are anchored to adjacent natural teeth with metal clasps or other attachments.

Filling. An inert material used to replace the decayed or damaged part of a tooth, usually amalgam (a metal alloy), gold, or, on front teeth, tooth-colored plastic.

Fluoride. Chemical added to drinking water, toothpastes, and mouthwashes that strengthens the teeth's enamel and helps prevent CARIES.

Flap surgery. Surgery in which the gums are lifted away from tooth roots

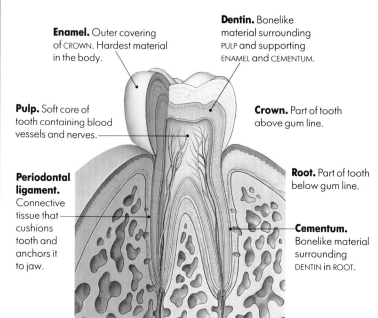

Enamel. Outer covering of CROWN. Hardest material in the body.

Dentin. Bonelike material surrounding PULP and supporting ENAMEL and CEMENTUM.

Pulp. Soft core of tooth containing blood vessels and nerves.

Crown. Part of tooth above gum line.

Periodontal ligament. Connective tissue that cushions tooth and anchors it to jaw.

Root. Part of tooth below gum line.

Cementum. Bonelike material surrounding DENTIN in ROOT.

I've never had a cavity. Do I still need regular dental checkups?

Yes. Even if you have no cavities the dentist will clean your teeth, look for oral lesions, and most important, check for periodontal disease—an inflammation or infection of the gums that can lead to loss of bone around the teeth and ultimately to loss of teeth. Periodontal disease is the most common dental disease in adults. In fact, adults lose far more teeth to periodontal disease than to tooth decay. More than half of Americans over the age of 35 are believed to have fairly advanced gum disease.

How is periodontal disease treated?

If periodontal disease is caught early when it is a relatively superficial inflammation of the gums known as *gingivitis,* a dentist can treat it by cleaning the teeth and *scaling* them to remove the *plaque* and *calculus* that causes the condition. (Words in *italics* are defined in the glossary above.)

Left untreated, gingivitis can progress to *periodontitis,* in which the inflamed gum pulls away from the teeth leaving pockets where more plaque accumulates. In its early stages, periodontitis can be treated by scaling, *root planing,* and *curettage.* To control bacterial growth, antibiotics or an antimicrobial mouthwash may also be prescribed. Once the irritants are re-to facilitate removal of CALCULUS, PLAQUE, and diseased tissue and allow reshaping of damaged bone.

Gingivectomy. Surgery in which the gums are trimmed to eliminate pockets caused by PERIODONTITIS.

Gingivitis. An early stage of PERIODONTAL DISEASE, in which a buildup of PLAQUE and CALCULUS inflames the gums. Treated by SCALING and good home hygiene.

Impaction. Failure of a tooth to erupt fully or at all through the gums. The last teeth to emerge—the upper canine, or eye, teeth and the wisdom teeth—are prone to impaction. An impacted wisdom tooth is usually extracted. Impacted eye teeth are usually repositioned with BRACES.

Implant. Replacement tooth anchored directly to the jawbone. Implants are usually attached to metal posts or a metal framework that is surgically embedded in the jawbone.

Malocclusion. Failure of upper and lower teeth to meet normally because of protruding, overcrowded, or missing teeth. Treated with orthodontic APPLIANCES (BRACES).

Periodontal disease. Inflammation and infection of the gums caused by buildup of PLAQUE and CALCULUS along gum line. GINGIVITIS and PERIODONTITIS are stages of periodontal disease.

Periodontitis. Advanced PERIODONTAL DISEASE, also called pyorrhea. At this stage, PLAQUE and CALCULUS have

Filling

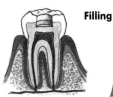
Hole drilled for filling

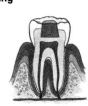
Filling in place

Root canal therapy

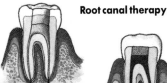
Pulp removed from pulp chamber and root canals

Tooth filled and covered with crown

Periodontal therapy

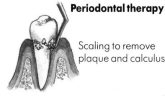
Scaling to remove plaque and calculus

Root planing to smooth root

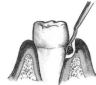
Curettage to remove diseased gum tissue

spread below the gum line, infecting and creating pockets in the gums, and eventually damaging bones around the teeth. Treatment consists of SCALING, ROOT PLANING, and CURETTAGE; advanced cases may require GINGIVECTOMY or FLAP SURGERY.

Plaque. Colorless, sticky coating on teeth consisting of saliva, food debris, and bacteria. Plaque accumulates at margins of teeth and gums; untreated, it hardens into CALCULUS. CARIES and PERIODONTAL DISEASE are caused by plaque.

Root canal therapy. Endodontic treatments used to save a tooth with an ABCESS. An opening is drilled through the crown and all the pulp is carefully removed. The root canals are cleaned, enlarged, and sterilized. The pulp chamber and root canals are packed with a rubberlike material; the tooth is then sealed either with filling material or with cement and a CROWN.

Root planing. Procedure in which surfaces of root are smoothed to promote the healing and reattachment of gums with PERIODONTITIS.

Scaling. Removal of PLAQUE and CALCULUS around the gum line to prevent or treat PERIODONTITIS. Done with a sharp instrument (a scaler) or with an ultrasonic device.

Sealant. Plastic material painted on chewing surfaces to prevent decay.

Splinting. Mechanically joining loose teeth, usually with wire or plastic, to hold them firmly in place.

moved, the gum usually heals, closing the pockets and often reattaching itself to the tooth.

In advanced periodontitis, the gums recede, pockets become very deep, bone and connective fiber suffer extensive damage, and teeth may shift or loosen. At this stage, the treatment usually recommended is surgery—either *gingivectomy* or *flap surgery*—which is performed by a gum specialist, or periodontist.

Whether periodontal disease is treated early or late, a recurrence can be prevented only by good home care and by periodic trips to the dentist for treatment. For more information on preventing gum disease, see *Caring for Your Teeth*, p. 227.

My dentist says I need gum surgery. Should I get a second opinion?

Yes. It's a good idea to get a second opinion for gum surgery, as you would for any other surgery. But first, ask your dentist about alternative treatments. Many experts believe that a nonsurgical method should be the first recourse in treating gum disease, even in some advanced cases. The treatment usually involves seeing your dentist or hygienist frequently—as often as every 3 months—for scaling, root planing, and curettage to remove plaque and calculus in the gum pockets around the teeth. To work, this course of treatment must be combined with diligent oral hygiene at home.

Fear of pain keeps me from going to the dentist. How can I overcome it?

Dental procedures are no longer the ordeal they once were. Better techniques of anesthesia have been developed. Lasers and high-speed drills are reducing the amount of time it takes to drill a tooth. If there is any pain, it is likely to be the dull ache that some procedures produce after the anesthesia wears off.

Even so, the fear of dentistry is widespread. An estimated 50 percent of Americans are afraid of going to a dentist and millions are phobic, avoiding dentists altogether or suffering from severe anxiety when they have to go. Fortunately, many dentists have become quite skilled in the use of desensitization and other techniques to calm frightened patients.

In the process of desensitization, a person overcomes a fear by becoming familiar with the very things that cause the fear. In a gentle and reassuring manner, a dentist will show the patient the instruments that are involved and give a step-by-step explanation of what is going on and what is going to happen. This promotes trust and helps the patient relax.

Learning biofeedback or practicing relaxation techniques (pp. 206–207) are other ways dental patients can help reduce their fears. Sometimes just listening to soothing music in a dentist's office is enough to calm a jittery patient.

To find a sympathetic dentist who will work with you to overcome your fears, ask your family, friends, co-workers, and doctor. And make sure you let the dentist know about your anxieties on the first visit.

How can I evaluate my dentist's work?

You can expect a good dentist to give you a thorough, unhurried examination and to stress preventive measures such as brushing, flossing, watching what you eat, and having your teeth cleaned and scaled on a regular basis. If dental work is needed, the dentist should explain the treatment plan, why you need it, how long it will take, possible complications, and how much it will cost. Although it is not always possible, the dentist should emphasize saving teeth rather than extracting them.

Realize that good dental work often takes time. It involves painstaking detail work and is as much an art as a science. Many procedures require several visits and may involve more discomfort and expenditure than you'd like. Be wary of a dentist or clinic that guarantees fast, painless, inexpensive work. But also be wary if the treatment offered seems excessive, especially if it's a radical change from what you have received from this or other dentists in the past, if it involves redoing expensive previous work, or if it is the only option offered. A good dentist lets you know your alternatives.

I'm in my mid-twenties. My dentist suggested I get braces to straighten my teeth. Am I too old for braces?

Not at all. Although wearing braces is associated with adolescence, more than a quarter of the people with braces today are over 18 years old—a trend fos-

DENTAL SPECIALISTS

Most dentists in the U.S. are general practitioners, qualified to perform all phases of dental care. They clean teeth; fill cavities; extract teeth; fit crowns, bridges, and dentures; treat gum disease; and instruct patients in good oral hygiene. A dentist is often assisted by a hygienist, a licensed professional qualified to clean, scale, and polish teeth; examine for disease; take X-rays; and teach oral hygiene. For certain problems, your dentist may refer you to one of these specialists.

Endodontist. Treats diseases of the tooth pulp, primarily through root canal therapy.

Prosthodontist. Replaces missing teeth with dentures, bridges, and crowns.

Oral and maxillofacial surgeon. Surgically treats diseases and injuries of the mouth and jaw and corrects cosmetic problems.

Pedodontist. Treats the dental problems of children from infancy to adolescence.

Periodontist. Treats diseases of the gums and bones that surround the teeth.

Orthodontist. Treats crooked, crowded, irregularly spaced, or projecting teeth, usually with orthodontic appliances (braces).

tered in part by the availability of braces that are less conspicuous than the traditional steel ones. The straightening process, performed by a specialist known as an orthodontist, usually takes about 2 years, followed by another 2 years during which the teeth become stabilized in their new positions. But because an adult's bones are denser and less flexible than a child's, it could take a little longer and might produce more discomfort. If crowding of the teeth is a problem, the orthodontist usually pulls teeth to make room for the others before putting on the braces.

Appearance is not the only reason for considering braces. Teeth that are crowded, widely spaced, badly aligned, or that bite incorrectly are more difficult to care for and may be more susceptible to decay, wear, and gum disease. They can also be responsible for tension and pain in the facial muscles and jaw.

What are the dangers of radiation from a doctor's or dentist's X-ray?

X-rays can be an important, life-saving tool (see *Screening Tests for Healthy Adults* and *Diagnostic Tests*, pp.124–127), and the risks of any single X-ray for a nonpregnant adult are usually negligible. However, your body does absorb some radiation after each X-ray (the amount varies depending on the type of X-ray) and the effect is cumulative over a lifetime. This means that the more radiation to which you are exposed, the greater your risk of injury, including cancer, damage to the reproductive cells, and for a pregnant woman, damage to her unborn child.

The general rule, which most doctors and dentists adhere to, is to avoid X-rays unless the potential benefits outweigh the potential

risks. Because children are more vulnerable to radiation than adults, it's especially important that they have as few X-rays as possible.

If your doctor advises X-rays of a body area X-rayed recently, ask if the new X-rays are likely to reveal information that will alter the diagnosis and treatment significantly. For any X-rays, ask if X-rays that are more limited in area or number will do just as well. For dental X-rays, make sure that your body is covered with a lead apron.

How should I go about finding a specialist?

Your primary physician will usually recommend that you see a specialist when a second opinion about a diagnosis or surgery is needed or if you require special care for a chronic condition. If the problem is relatively routine, the doctor generally recommends a colleague that he or she regularly works with and trusts—typically someone associated with the same hospital as the doctor. If the problem is more complex, the doctor may arrange for you to see a more prominent specialist at a teaching hospital. In either case, it's a good idea to ask your doctor why this particular specialist is being recommended. Also ask about the specialist's qualifications.

As recommended for a primary doctor (p.119), you can also check the specialist's board certification by calling the American Board of Medical Specialties (see Appendix); look up the doctor's training and other credentials in a directory of medical specialists. Ask around, too; you may be able to find a friend, neighbor, or co-worker who was treated by the specialist or you may find a nurse or other health-care worker who knows what the specialist's reputation is.

What special qualities should I look for in a surgeon?

Experience is the key quality to look for in a surgeon. Studies show that the more often a surgeon performs a particular procedure, the better the results are likely to be. Most operations require a high level of skill and dexterity and, like any other art or craft, the more frequently the person does it, the more proficient he or she usually becomes. It's proper to ask a surgeon how often he or she performs procedures similar to the one proposed for you. The doctor who performs an operation once a week or more maintains a higher level of skill—and is usually a better choice—than the doctor who does it only a few times a year. Of course, even a highly capable and competent surgeon may perform an operation infrequently because it is rare or because the surgeon's practice is in a small community where there are few cases of any particular type of surgery.

As with any other specialist, check the surgeon's board certification and other credentials. Many common procedures, such as a hernia operation, can be performed by a general surgeon but for some operations you will want a surgeon who is board certified in a special area—a cardiac surgeon, for example, to operate on the heart or a head and neck surgeon to perform surgery on the vocal cords. Also note a doctor's membership in certain voluntary medical societies. A surgeon has to meet very stringent standards to put F.A.C.S. (Fellow of the American College of Surgeons) after his or her name. And added experience and qualifications are usually required to join the national society for a specialty,

MEDICAL SPECIALISTS

A medical school graduate can become a specialist only after undergoing 3–7 years' postgraduate training as a hospital resident and then passing an exam given by a medical specialty board. Medical specialists are listed below by the body function, part, or system that they treat.

MIND

Psychiatrist. Treats emotional, behavioral, and mental disorders.

BRAIN AND NERVES

Neurologist. Treats nervous system disorders.

Neurosurgeon. Operates on the nervous system, including brain and spinal cord.

GLANDS

Endocrinologist. Treats glandular and hormonal disorders, such as diabetes.

HEART AND BLOOD

Cardiologist. Treats diseases of the heart and blood vessels.

Cardiac surgeon. Operates on the heart and blood vessels.

Hematologist. Treats blood disorders.

WHOLE BODY

Family practitioner. Provides general care for both sexes of any age; performs minor surgery; delivers babies; serves as primary physician.

Internist. Provides nonsurgical general care for adults; serves as primary physician.

Pediatrician. Provides general care for children from infancy through adolescence.

Geriatrician. Provides general care for the elderly.

General surgeon. Performs common operations on almost any part of the body.

Emergency physician. Deals with life-threatening matters, such as heart attacks, bullet wounds.

Infectious disease specialist. Treats viral, fungal, and bacterial infections.

OTHER SPECIALISTS

Anesthesiologist. Administers anesthetic; monitors patient during and right after surgery.

Oncologist. Treats cancer.

Pathologist. Tests tissue and cell samples to aid in diagnosis; performs autopsies.

Radiologist. Uses X-rays, ultrasound, and scanners to diagnose and treat disorders.

Pediatric specialist. Pediatrician who further specializes, for example, in pediatric cardiology.

HEAD AND SKIN

Allergist. Identifies and treats allergies.

Dermatologist. Treats skin disorders.

Ophthalmologist. Treats eye disorders; checks vision; prescribes corrective lenses.

Otolaryngologist (head and neck surgeon). Treats ear, nose, and throat disorders medically and surgically.

Plastic surgeon. Repairs deformed or injured body parts; performs cosmetic operations.

CHEST AND LUNG

Pulmonary disease specialist. Treats lung diseases.

Thoracic surgeon. Operates on organs of the chest (except the heart).

DIGESTIVE SYSTEM

Gastroenterologist. Treats disorders of the digestive system, including the liver, gallbladder, and pancreas.

Colon and rectal surgeon. Performs surgery on the lower intestinal tract.

UROGENITAL SYSTEM

Obstetrician-gynecologist. Treats female reproductive disorders medically and surgically; provides pregnancy care; delivers infants.

Urologist. Treats male reproductive and both sexes' urinary problems medically and surgically.

Nephrologist. Treats kidney disorders.

BONES AND MUSCLES

Rheumatologist. Treats arthritis and other diseases of the joints, bones, muscles, and tendons.

Orthopedic surgeon. Treats and operates on joints and bones.

Physical medicine specialist. Uses physical therapy to rehabilitate disabled patients.

OSTEOPATHIC MEDICINE

Doctors of osteopathy (D.O.'s), or osteopaths, are licensed physicians who use accepted medical diagnostic techniques and therapies, but stress the body's unity and ability to heal itself and emphasize bone and muscle manipulation. Like M.D.'s, osteopaths can specialize.

such as the American Society of Abdominal Surgery.

To some extent, of course, you have to rely on your own instincts and impressions. The manner in which a surgeon speaks to you and answers your questions should give you a sense of trust and confidence.

I'm undergoing surgery in a few weeks. Is it advisable to predonate blood for my own use?

Having your own blood taken and stored in advance of nonemergency surgery eliminates practically all risks associated with blood transfusions. Blood screening has reduced the odds of contracting the AIDS virus from a transfusion to a national average of 1 in 150,000; the risk of contracting hepatitis in this way has virtually been eliminated. But there is still a risk that your body may react to a transfusion by rejecting white blood cells or other substances in the transfused blood.

Blood can be stored in liquid form for as long as 6 weeks and frozen for longer periods. You can donate a unit of blood about twice a month provided you are free of any major heart or lung problems and your doctor agrees that it is all right for you to have the blood taken.

Which is better, a community hospital or a large medical center with a teaching staff?

The most common type of hospital is the community, or general, hospital, a private institution run on either a for-profit or non-profit basis. A community hospital is usually small and convenient—closer to home, family, and friends for most people—and ideally gives personalized attention to patients. If it is well staffed and has up-to-date facilities, it's likely to be fine for most ordinary medical problems and surgical procedures. Just make sure that any hospital you select is accredited by the Joint Commission on Accreditation of Health Care Organizations, which sets standards for hospitals and other health facilities.

In addition to treating patients, teaching hospitals train medical students and medical school graduates doing their postgraduate residencies; most of these hospitals are affiliated with a major medical school. A teaching hospital's full-fledged doctors, or attending physicians, are usually highly knowledgeable and experienced specialists, who teach full or part time at the affiliated school. They may also do research or have a private practice. These doctors often have access to the best technical resources and offer the latest treatments. For these reasons, a teaching hospital is often advisable if you have a condition that is unusual or difficult to diagnose or treat and needs the best care possible.

During a stay in a teaching hospital, however, you are an object of study, and can expect repeated examinations and questions from medical students, interns, and residents as well as your attending physician and specialists. Some patients find this reassuring, others find it confusing or annoying. A large medical center may also seem cold and impersonal to some patients, especially to those whose illness makes them feel weak and vulnerable.

What special qualities should I look for in a hospital for my child?

What kind of hospital care is best for a child depends on the nature of the child's illness. The pediatric unit of your community hospital is usually the best choice for a child who has a relatively routine problem that requires only a short hospital stay, such as needing an appendix removed or a hernia repaired. For a child who is seriously ill, the best choice is a special children's hospital or the pediatric unit of a large medical center. Both are equipped for long-term care and for the special needs of a child suffering from a cancer such as leukemia or for a child who needs a major operation such as heart surgery. In these cases, putting the child in a children's hospital or large medical center is usually worth the extra travel time and expense that it may entail for the parents.

Whatever type of hospital you choose, look for visiting hours that accommodate family members and young friends, a policy that allows parents to stay overnight, and a play area for the children. A play program is a nice feature, but not essential.

How can I prepare my child for an operation or extended treatment in a hospital?

First find out exactly what is going to happen, then be open and honest with your child. The more you know about your child's operation or treatment and its aftermath, the easier it will be for you to describe them honestly.

Don't gloss over the possible pain and discomfort the child may experience. Let the child know if you will be in the recovery room and if an intravenous tube will be attached to his or her arm. Also tell your child how long it will be before he or she will be able to get out of bed and be able to eat regular food.

Accept the fact that your child is going to be afraid—afraid of being separated from family and friends, afraid of being operated on, and afraid of the pain. Trying to minimize these fears and treat them as trivial is likely only to make your child angry. The fear is real; acknowledge it and try to be reassuring.

If possible, take your child to visit the hospital in advance. Many hospitals have preadmission programs in which a staff member gives children a tour and explains the unfamiliar equipment. Encourage your child to play hospital games. Testing, operating on, and bandaging dolls or stuffed toys can produce a sense of mastery over a frightening experience. Also listen carefully to what your child says to others about the upcoming operation; it can help you deal with any specific fears or misconceptions he or she has about the hospital and the procedure itself.

What information will a hospital want when I'm admitted?

The information needed varies from one hospital to another, and doctors often supply it—from their records or by asking you—when they prearrange an admission. It's a good idea to call ahead and ask if there is any special information the hospital will need. Generally, the admitting office will want to know your Social Security and insurance policy numbers and the names, addresses, and phone numbers of your employer and your next of kin (or other person to notify in an emergency). Also, your attending nurse will ask for basic medical information. This includes medications you are taking, any allergic reactions to medications you've had, a brief personal medical history covering previous hospitalizations and major illnesses, and any noteworthy family history of health problems.

Are tests required for hospital admission? Can I have them done before going into the hospital?

Tests are required, and they vary from hospital to hospital and from state to state. If you have no serious medical problems, testing is generally limited to a urinalysis and blood tests, typically a complete blood count (CBC). If you're over the age of 35, an electrocardiogram (EKG) may also be required. Some hospitals take a chest X-ray if you have not had one recently.

Nearly all hospitals have a preadmission testing program in which you can have these tests done as an outpatient, usually a few days before you are due to go in. This allows problems that could possibly affect a treatment or operation to be discovered before admission. The cost is usually covered by major hospital insurance plans.

My doctor has scheduled a biopsy for me. Does this mean I have cancer? What does the test involve?

A biopsy is the removal of small pieces of tissue or cells so that they can be examined under a microscope to diagnose an abnormality. Biopsies of the skin, breast, thyroid, and colon polyps are among the more common but almost any body part can be biopsied. A biopsy is often done to eliminate the chance that an abnormality is cancerous, but it can also be used to diagnose many conditions besides cancers. Ask your doctor why the test is being done, and bear in mind that only a small percentage of biopsies have positive results indicating the presence of cancer; most reveal benign conditions.

How a biopsy is done depends on what body part is being examined. A doctor may use a knife or a punchlike device to remove a small piece of skin, a syringe with a hollow needle to remove tissue from a breast lump, or an endoscope (p. 126) equipped with a cutting tip to remove a colon polyp. The patient receives either a local or a general anesthetic. A biopsy of an internal organ may require hospitalization; in other cases, the procedure may be done on an outpatient basis in a hospital, clinic, or doctor's office.

I have heard so much about "knife happy" surgeons. How can I be on the alert for an unnecessary operation?

It's almost always a good idea to question whether you need an operation. Did your doctor try other treatments before suggesting surgery? Have you had this condition for awhile or was the suggestion for surgery a total surprise? And before you have a nonemergency operation, consider a second opinion, preferably from a specialist who treats problems such as yours medically rather than surgically (p. 142). Ask your primary doctor, the surgeon, and the consultant giving the second opinion what the alternatives to surgery are and what is likely to happen to you if you do not have the operation. Once you have answers to these questions you'll be better prepared to decide whether surgery or an alternative treatment is the best option for you.

What questions should I ask a surgeon before an operation?

About the procedure itself, ask what are the risks involved, what the possible complications and infections are, and what kind of anesthesia will be used. You will also want to know what to expect after the operation. How will you feel when you wake up? How long will recovery take? Is there anything you will not be able to do? How long before you will be up and walking? How long will you be in the hospital? How long before you will be able to go back to work?

To find out more about a particular operation, it's useful to read patient-education literature about it and to talk to people who have had the operation.

I have been told that the anesthesiologist's role during an operation is vital. Can I find out who will be giving me anesthesia?

The anesthesiologist does play a crucial role, monitoring your vital signs and keeping you alive and well during the operation. But in nearly all hospitals today, anesthesiologists are assigned to cases on the basis of availability or by rotation. Assignments are often made the night before or the morning of the operation.

If you are concerned about receiving anesthesia, ask your surgeon whether all of the hospital's anesthesiologists are board certified. Also ask whether a nurse-anesthetist will be used and if that anesthetist's work will be overseen by a board-certified anesthesiologist. Remember that improvements in operating-room monitoring equipment and risk management have made anesthesia calamities much less frequent. Experts estimate that anesthesia causes harm about once in 200,000 operations; in 1980, the estimate was around 1 in 10,000. The risk is also a lot lower for scheduled elective surgery than it is for emergencies.

ANESTHESIA

Two types of anesthesia are used for medical purposes. A local anesthetic numbs a body part; a general anesthetic makes a patient unconscious. A sedative may be given before an anesthetic is administered to calm the patient. A muscle relaxant is sometimes used with a general anesthetic to immobilize the patient during surgery.

Type	How given	Effect
Topical	Eye drops, sprays, ointments, creams, and suppositories	Numbs skin surface to ease irritation or relieve discomfort (as from sunburn).
Simple local	Injection at site being treated	Numbs an area, as around a cut being stitched.
Nerve block	Injection near main nerve leading to treated site	Numbs a body part, such as the arm from elbow down for an operation on the hand.
Epidural block	Injection into space outside covering of spinal cord	Blocks nerve signals from lower half of body; often used to abolish pain during childbirth.
Spinal block	Injection into fluid within covering of spinal cord	Blocks nerve signals from legs and abdomen; used for appendix, prostate, and other lower body operations.
General	Gas from mask or breathing tube; or injection into vein	Patient becomes unconscious and feels no pain.

To whom should I direct complaints when I'm in the hospital?

Some hospitals have a patient representative whose job is to listen to patients' complaints and relay them to the proper authority. If you are unhappy with a hospital rule, the representative can explain its rationale.

Without such help, where you should lodge a complaint depends on what part of your care you consider inadequate. If it is nursing care, start with the head nurse for your unit, then if necessary take the matter to the director of nursing. Take concerns about a doctor or your medical care to the medical director and problems with the hospital's physical facilities or billing to the hospital administrator.

For a major complaint about the way a hospital is run, write to the administrator and to the chairman of the hospital's board of trustees. If unprofessional or seriously dangerous behavior is involved, you may also want to write to your state's department of health or other agency that regulates hospitals. If you have a serious complaint about a doctor, write to your state's board of medical examiners. If it's about a nurse, write to the board of nurse examiners.

Will my family doctor still be in charge of my care in the hospital?

Your primary doctor will often continue to be your attending physician while you're in the hospital. In this case, any specialist you see is brought in as a consultant. But if you need surgery or are critically ill, your care may be managed by a specialist throughout your hospital stay. Your primary doctor will tell you when a specialist is taking over your care. If you are not sure, ask. It's important to know which doctor is in charge and which ones are consultants. Your attending physician is the final decision-maker on your treatment and the one you should turn to if anything worries you.

You may be seen by many doctors if you go to a teaching hospital or if the doctor who admits you to the hospital has a large practice and works with associates. If you want your doctor to manage your care and perform all procedures on you, let the doctor know ahead of time and find out if it is possible.

Should I consider employing a private-duty nurse when I go into a hospital?

It depends on the kind of care you need and how good your hospital's nursing staff is. It also depends on your ability to pay. Private-duty nurses are expensive and are rarely fully covered by insurance. But having a private nurse can be a great help if you are confined to bed by traction or incapacitated by a stroke, especially if your hospital is understaffed and you do not have family members to assist you. A nurse might be affordable if hired for only a few days—after surgery, for example, when you are temporarily unable to care for yourself. If your primary need is for help rather than nursing care, consider a less costly practical nurse instead of an R.N.

The chief drawback to hiring a private nurse is not knowing what kind of experience the nurse has. You may get a marvelous nurse or you might be better off relying on a hospital's highly trained nursing staff, especially if you need specialized care. Before hiring a private nurse, ask your doctor whether he or she thinks you need one. You may be able to hire a private nurse through your hospital; if not, call a nursing agency or ask your doctor and friends for recommendations. If you use an agency, ask for a nurse with experience handling your particular type of health problem.

My wife just returned from the hospital where she found the number of different nurses who cared for her confusing. Why were there so many nurses?

The number of nurses who care for a patient during a hospital stay can indeed be confusing. In a typical large hospital the patients are attended by a nursing staff consisting of a head nurse for that floor or unit, staff nurses, licensed practical nurses, and nurse's aides. Many also have nursing assistants and student nurses. To increase this number even further, most hospitals have three 8-hour shifts daily, and weekend shifts, all staffed by different nurses. In addition, hospitals short of staff nurses often employ temporary nurses from outside agencies.

To eliminate much of this fragmented care, some hospitals now assign each patient a primary nurse, a registered nurse who, with an assistant, is responsible for the total nursing care of a small number of patients, overseeing each patient's needs from admittance through discharge. Most patients find that this continuity is comforting and improves the quality of care.

I have heard that people are often put into intensive care units unnecessarily. Is this true?

Some experts do believe that intensive care units are overused. In an ICU a patient receives more concentrated nursing care and observation, more sophisticated monitoring, and generally more intensive treatment than in an ordinary hospital room. ICU's are best used by patients who need a high level of attention for a short period of time during a serious, potentially life-threatening condition. For instance, patients recovering from complex heart or brain operations, accident or burn victims, drug overdoses, and pneumonia patients with serious complications are all candidates for ICU's.

Critics point out that the units are used not only for patients who are likely to recover but often for patients who are terminally ill, prolonging the inevitable at a cost three times that of a regular hospital room. They also note that the benefits of ICU's may not outweigh the side effects it can have on some patients. Cut off from the outside world with the lights always on, a patient can become disoriented about time and develop sleep disorders. A patient may also become fearful and anxious about being in such an environment, connected to tubes and monitors, surrounded by equipment and other gravely ill patients with a staff that is continually bustling about. If such patients can do without the close monitoring, they will often feel better in a regular hospital room and the medical outcome is usually the same. If you or a relative is faced with the possibility of going into an ICU, weigh the pro's and con's carefully with your doctor.

WHO'S WHO AT THE HOSPITAL

The array of hospital staff members presented here is likely to be found only in a large teaching hospital. But even in a small community hospital the number of staff members and their different roles may perplex a patient. Keep in mind that each hospital has its own organization and staffing system. Consequently titles and responsibilities may vary from hospital to hospital. In addition to the people listed here, who are responsible for a patient's day-to-day care, a hospital employs many others in administrative, financial, and housekeeping capacities.

GENERAL HOSPITAL

Medical staff

Attending physician. Medical doctor in charge of a patient's care. This is the doctor who orders all treatments, medications, tests, and procedures, and is usually the patient's primary physician or surgeon.

Consultant. Specialist called in by the attending physician for an opinion or to perform tests or procedures (see *Medical Specialists*, p.142).

Resident. Medical doctor training in a specialty after finishing medical school. Residency can take from 3 to 7 years. First-year residents are commonly called interns.

Senior resident. Medical doctor in the final year of specialty training. Under the attending physician's supervision, this doctor has the most responsibility for a patient's care.

Medical student. Usually a third- or fourth-year student at the school affiliated with the hospital.

Physician assistant. Health-care worker who performs some routine procedures, such as taking medical histories and blood pressure. May work for a doctor rather than hospital.

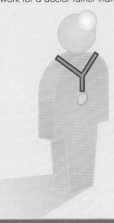

Nursing care

Head nurse. In some hospitals the registered nurse with overall responsibility for nursing on a floor, ward, or special unit, such as intensive care or emergency room.

Charge nurse. Registered nurse in charge of the floor, ward, or unit for a shift. May replace the head nurse during evening and night shifts.

Primary nurse (or team leader). In some hospitals the registered nurse in charge of a patient's nursing care; coordinates tests, procedures, and treatments.

Staff nurse (or floor nurse). Registered nurse who works with primary nurse or substitutes for primary nurse during other shifts.

Specialized nurse. Registered nurse with advanced training who specializes in one area, such as intensive care, pediatrics, anesthesia, or assisting at surgery.

Practical nurse. Usually a licensed practical nurse (L.P.N.) who gives bedside care, such as changing dressings, recording vital signs, and administering some medications. An L.P.N. can also serve as a scrub nurse in the operating room.

Private duty nurse. R.N. or L.P.N. employed by a patient; not a member of the hospital staff.

Nursing student. Student from nursing school affiliated with hospital.

Nurse's aide or orderly. Health-care worker who assists patient with bathing, eating, walking, and getting around hospital.

Ward secretary. Non-nurse at the nurses' station who keeps records and orders tests and supplies.

Others

Counselor. Hospice worker, alcohol or drug abuse counselor, minister, or other person who advises patients.

Medical social worker. Staff member who assists patient with family, financial, and work-related problems caused by illness. May coordinate post-hospital health care.

Medical technologist. Health-care specialist who conducts laboratory tests and administers some diagnostic tests and assists with others.

Therapist. Physical, occupational, recreational, speech, or other specialist who helps patient recover strength, flexibility, and skills.

Paramedic. Auxiliary medical person who responds to emergencies outside hospital and performs first-aid and other emergency procedures.

Patient representative. Administrative worker who handles patients' complaints about care, food, regulations, and other matters.

Volunteer. Unpaid assistant who may function as a nurse's aide, or may comfort and console patients or perform administrative tasks.

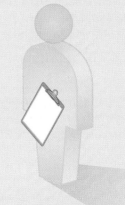

THE LANGUAGE OF MEDICAL INSURANCE

Assignment. The transfer of an insurance policy's benefits by the owner of the policy to a third party. In Medicare terms, when a doctor or health-care provider "takes assignment," he or she agrees to accept the Medicare program's payment as full payment, except for CO-INSURANCE and DEDUCTIBLES payable by the patient.

Blue Cross/Blue Shield. An independent nonprofit corporation providing insurance for hospitalization (Blue Cross) and surgical and medical costs (Blue Shield).

Claim. A request to an insurer for payment of insurance benefits.

Co-insurance. A requirement that medical costs over and above the DE-DUCTIBLE, if any, be shared by patient and insurance company. In a typical example of co-insurance, the patient pays 20 percent and the insurer 80 percent of covered medical costs after a $500 deductible.

Conversion privilege. The right granted in an insurance policy that lets an insured person change from one type of policy to another without providing evidence of insurability, such as a physical exam.

Covered expenses. Hospital, medical, and other health-care expenses that are completely or partially reimbursable under the terms of a health insurance policy.

Deductible. Amount patient must pay before insurance coverage begins.

Diagnosis-related group (DRG). A system of payment for medical services in which a hospital patient's condition is classified according to 467 diagnostic categories, each with a fixed rate of reimbursement. If the patient's care costs more than the fixed rate, the hospital absorbs the difference.

Disability income insurance. Type of insurance coverage that replaces lost income due to sickness or injury.

Exclusions. Conditions or circumstances for which benefits are not paid.

Grace period. Time that insurance protection continues after premium goes unpaid; often 31 days.

Group contract. Policy covering a group of people related by work or other affiliation.

Guaranteed renewable contract. Policy that insurer cannot cancel as long as premiums are paid.

Health maintenance organization (HMO). See question at right, below.

Hospital indemnity. Policy that pays a set sum for each day in hospital.

Limited policy. Coverage for only specified diseases or accidents.

Major medical insurance. Policy that covers all or part of the expenses of a major illness or injury after a DEDUCTIBLE has been paid.

Pre-existing condition. A physical or mental condition that existed before an insurance policy was issued.

Preferred provider organization (PPO). See question at right

Premium. Periodic payments required to keep an insurance policy in force.

Principal sum. Lump sum paid for accidental death or dismemberment.

Reasonable and customary charge. A fee that's within the usual rate charged by health-care providers in a given area for the same service. Often the basis for insurance REIMBURSEMENT.

Reimbursement. Payment by insurer to patient or health-care provider.

Supplemental health insurance (Medigap). Private health insurance policy that pays for a percentage of expenses not covered by Medicare.

I live on a small salary with no medical insurance. Can I get medical care in an emergency?

More than 35 million Americans are not covered by health insurance and have a difficult time obtaining even minimal medical care. In theory, everyone is entitled to receive treatment in the emergency room of a public hospital. But public hospitals are often understaffed and poorly funded. Many are unable to provide much beyond basic emergency care, and not every community has a public hospital. Nonprofit voluntary community hospitals often have emergency rooms and are legally bound in most states to treat an emergency case. Private for-profit hospitals must also treat emergencies, but only if they have an emergency room and not many for-profit hospitals do.

In many large cities and some rural areas, routine nonemergency medical care is available to people without medical insurance at clinics that are either free or base their fees on the patient's ability to pay.

If you are a veteran, you may be able to receive treatment at a veterans hospital. Contact your local Department of Veterans Affairs office; the eligibility requirements for treatment are complex and are subject to change.

What are the different kinds of health insurance available?

No two health plans are exactly the same. But the plans available from nongovernment insurers fall into three groups—traditional fee-for-service health insurance plans, health maintenance organizations (HMO's), and preferred provider organizations (PPO's).

THE FACTS ABOUT MEDICARE

The Federal Medicare program provides health insurance to Americans age 65 and over. Basically, anyone eligible for Social Security benefits is eligible for Medicare. (Some younger people who have a disability or chronic kidney disease also qualify.) Private insurers offer supplemental (Medigap) policies to assist with costs that are not covered.

Medicare is divided into hospital insurance (Part A) and medical insurance (Part B). Part A pays for basic and specialized hospital care, skilled nursing home care for those qualified, and some hospice and skilled home health care. For the first 60 days, Medicare pays all hospital costs after a deductible (equivalent to about 1 day's cost). For the next 30 days, the patient must make a co-payment (about 25 percent). After 90 days, benefits end until the recipient has been out of the hospital for 60 consecutive days. Then the benefits start over again. Every recipient also gets a lifetime bank of 60 days (with co-payments) that can be used to extend a hospital stay, but once used, they are no longer available.

Part B of Medicare is voluntary and covers physician's fees, outpatient treatments, therapies, tests, and some equipment, supplies, and other services. The beneficiary pays a monthly premium and must pay a certain amount (a deductible) each year before receiving benefits. Medicare then pays 80 percent of the medical service charges and the patient must make a co-payment of 20 percent—or more if the doctor's fee is higher than the Medicare schedule. Medicare sets rates for a medical service or hospital stay, based on what it considers to be reasonable for the region and for the diagnosis-related group (DRG), or diagnostic category (see facing page). Most hospitals accept these rates, but not all doctors do.

Don't confuse Medicare with Medicaid, which provides health care for lower income individuals. Each state structures the joint Federal-state Medicaid program differently.

For more information about Medicare, write to the Department of Health and Human Services (see Appendix).

There are many variations within each type. Although health insurance can be purchased by an individual, most people join a group plan offered by their employer, union, or other affiliated group. An employer may pay all or most of the premiums, but with the steep rise in insurance costs, the individual is paying a greater percentage.

☐ Traditional health insurance plans cost the most but give you the widest choice of doctors, treatments, and hospitals. They are based on fee-for-service arrangements in which you (or your doctor or hospital) submit bills to the insurance company, which pays a percentage of the total cost or the total minus a deductible (see *The Language of Health Insurance*, facing page). You often need separate policies to cover hospital expenses, surgery, and other medical costs such as doctor's office visits, outpatient treatments, dental care, and prescription drugs. Increasingly, these plans are placing restrictions on policyholders by limiting the payments for certain conditions and by requiring second opinions from insurance-company doctors for hospitalization and for costly procedures and treatments. Some plans provide a lump-sum payment for a hospitalization, which is almost always less than the actual cost to the patient.

☐ Health maintenance organizations are a form of prepaid health care. All your medical care is provided by HMO staff or contracted doctors, hospitals, and clinics for a fixed monthly fee (there is usually no deductible). The HMO provides specialists for consultations or surgery, pays hospital bills, and covers the cost of tests, outpatient treatments, and usually prescription drugs. (Dental care is normally covered by a separate HMO policy.) An HMO is more likely to pay for preventive care, such as mammograms or checkups, than a traditional plan.

HMO's generally cost less than traditional insurance plans, but they restrict your choice to doctors and specialists employed by the HMO and all treatments must first be approved by your primary doctor. Some "open" HMO's will pay a percentage of an outside doctor's fees.

☐ Preferred provider organizations are a cross between traditional health insurance and an HMO. In a PPO, the insurer generally gives you a list of doctors, hospitals, and other health-care providers who have agreed to charge a fee lower than the going rate in return for an assured number of patients. If you pick a provider from that list, the insurer usually pays the entire cost. If you go to someone else who charges more, you have to pay the difference. Before you can be hospitalized or receive a costly treatment, PPO's usually require a review and approval by their doctors. PPO's are cheaper but less flexible than traditional fee-for-payment insurance plans, costlier but more flexible than HMO's.

In addition to health-care plans sponsored by private insurance companies, government Medicare and Medicaid benefits are available to qualified recipients (see *The Facts About Medicare,* preceding page).

When I am offered a medical insurance policy, what questions should I ask?

When considering hospitalization coverage, ask these questions:
□ Does the coverage start with your first day in the hospital?
□ How much of the total cost is covered? Some companies pay 100 percent, others 80 percent.
□ How long does coverage last? Do benefits stop after a total dollar amount has been reached, or after a specified number of days?
□ What is not included? Some typical exclusions are hospital costs related to pregnancy, hospitalization for diagnostic tests, a private room, private nurses, and outpatient hospital care.
□ Are pre-existing conditions covered immediately, after a waiting period, or not at all?
□ Is specialty care, such as a stay in an intensive care unit or a coronary care unit, covered?

□ Are all hospitals and all doctors covered or only ones pre-approved by the insurer?
□ Are you guaranteed the right to renew your policy or are there conditions for which you could be denied a renewal?

If you are thinking of buying a medical insurance policy that covers doctor's fees, tests, treatments, medications, and other nonhospital medical costs, ask these questions:
□ What is the deductible? How much do you pay before the company starts paying benefits?
□ How much of your medical expenses do you have to pay? For example, the insurance company may pay 80 percent with you paying the remaining 20 percent.
□ What is the maximum amount the insurance company will pay?
□ What is not included? Does it cover home care while you are recuperating after hospitalization, physical therapy, maternity care, dental care, pre-existing conditions, pediatric care including immunizations, mental health care, or emergency care?
□ What happens if you are disabled for a period of time?
□ Are you guaranteed the right to renew the policy?
□ Can you get catastrophic coverage on this policy in the event you become totally disabled?

My husband and I are thinking of joining an HMO plan. What are the advantages and disadvantages?

The main advantage of an HMO is that it usually costs less than conventional insurance and often covers more, paying, for example, for preventive checkups and prescription medications. If the plan is large, as some are, you'll have a considerable number of doctors from which to choose your primary doctor. The doc-

tors generally receive more peer review than a private practitioner does because the HMO medical staff usually functions as a self-contained group practice and monitors itself. Because the doctors are salaried and paid the same no matter what they do, you are less likely to undergo unnecessary tests or procedures. Similarly, your primary doctor can refer you to a specialist without fear of losing you as a patient. Also, an HMO often has all medical services in a single location, making it convenient and providing more continuity of care.

The chief disadvantage of most HMO's is that they limit your choice of doctors and hospitals. If you are currently seeing a doctor who is not a member of the HMO, you'll have to switch to a new HMO doctor. At an HMO, you may not see your primary doctor at each visit; routine care may be provided by a nurse-practitioner or a physician assistant. Also you usually have to get approval from the HMO in certain situations, such as before seeing a specialist or getting treatment when traveling outside your HMO area.

Some critics believe that HMO's are good at providing routine and preventive care to basically healthy patients but are less effective in treating serious illness. However, most studies comparing HMO care with regular fee-for-service care show no difference in quality.

What should I look for in an HMO or other group plan?

When investigating an HMO or a similar plan, find out what services are—and are not—provided for in the basic monthly fee. Find out if you have to pay an additional charge (usually called a co-payment) for each office visit

Prescription

MICHAEL OTIS, M. D.

9851 Medical Center Plaza
Plainsview, CA 98476-0001

PHONE: (817) 555-4280

NAME _Joe Smith_

ADDRESS _____ DATE _3/16/92_

PHONE _____

NO MORE THAN TWO (2) PRESCRIPTIONS PER RX BLANK

℞

Erythro 500mg #40
ī PO QID   NR

REFILL 1 2 3 4 5

NO REFILL

AUTHORIZATION IS GIVEN TO:

☐ DISPENSE GENERIC BRAND UNLESS CHECKED HERE

_M Otis_____, M. D.

DEA NO. _RS 0274255_
CAL. LIC. NO. _C-62651_

04036 (REV. 12-67)

> A prescription for forty 500-milligram tablets of erythromycin, an antibiotic. One tablet is to be taken four times a day. The prescription can't be refilled.

READING A PRESCRIPTION

Hurried doctors use a Latin-based shorthand to speed the task of writing prescriptions. Here is a guide to deciphering these cryptic scribblings.

ā	before
aa	of each
ac	before meals
bid	twice a day
c̄	with
d	day
n, noct	at night
NR	do not refill
OD	once daily
pc	after meals
po	orally, by mouth
prn	as needed
qh	every hour
q2h	every two hours
qid	four times a day
rep	repeat
Rx	take, prescription
s̄	without
tid	three times a day
ut dict	as directed
i̇	one
ï	two
ïi	three
ïv	four

or medication. Ask if you can choose your primary doctor, how many doctors you can choose from, and if they are all board certified. Will you see the same doctor most times you make a scheduled visit? What happens in an emergency? Will an R.N. or physician assistant sometimes see you instead of a doctor? Can you change doctors easily if you think it's necessary? Is the doctor's office or HMO clinic convenient for you? Which hospitals does the HMO use? What kind and how many specialists are available? Is home nursing care available and does the plan offer any extra health services, such as family planning and nutrition counseling or smoking-cessation classes?

To judge the satisfaction of HMO patients with the plan, find out how many members leave each year and how much the group's membership has grown in recent years. Finally, ask about the plan's procedure for grievances and get a list of services and fees so that you can compare them with other plans.

Are there any questions I should ask my doctor about a medication he prescribes?

One way to avoid overmedication and adverse drug interactions is to become as knowledgeable as possible about all the medicines you are taking. You may even wind up reducing your drug bills

in the process. Here's a list of questions you might ask your doctor about a medication being prescribed for you:
☐ Why is the doctor prescribing the drug? What does he or she expect it to do?
☐ How much of the medication should you take and how often?
☐ When is the best time to take it—with food, before meals, or between them?
☐ What are the drug's common side effects, if any?
☐ Is there anything you should not take with it—other drugs, certain foods, alcoholic beverages? Are there any activities (such as driving, sunbathing, or exercise) that you should avoid while taking it?
☐ How long will it take the drug

to work, and how long will you have to continue taking it?
□ Can the prescription be refilled?
□ Can a generic drug or a less expensive brand-name drug be substituted for it?

If a drug causes side effects that you were not informed about or that concern you, call your doctor for advice.

What's the difference between a generic and a brand-name drug? Is it safe to substitute one for the other?

A generic drug is a medication that is sold by its general chemical name rather than by a manufacturer's trade name. Its active ingredients must be the same as those of the brand-name equivalent, and it must be approved by the Food and Drug Administration. FDA approval assures that the generic is as potent and as pure as the brand-name drug.

However, a generic drug's nonactive ingredients often differ from those in the brand-name version, and may cause the active ingredient to be absorbed at a different rate or less well. With a few drugs, mainly heart and seizure medications, which must be given in precise, closely monitored amounts, these small changes in drug levels can make a difference to some patients. (If you are concerned, ask your doctor about your situation.) But in most cases, the difference between generic and brand-name drugs is insignificant, and the two versions are essentially the same. The FDA does annual spot checks to make sure that generic and brand-name drugs are "bio-

equivalent" (that is, they function the same way in the body).

In some states a pharmacist can substitute a generic drug for the brand name if you request it; in others, your doctor must specify on the prescription that a substitution can be made. Don't automatically assume a generic is cheaper than the brand-name drug. Most generics do cost less—generally about half the amount of brand names—but studies of pharmacy pricing show that they sometimes cost more.

Should I tell my doctor that I often take aspirin or other over-the-counter medications?

Yes. Always tell your doctor about all medications that you take on a regular basis. Like prescription drugs, over-the-counter medications have side effects and may be the cause of a symptom you're experiencing. Some decongestants, for example, can cause insomnia; antihistamines can make some people dizzy or affect urination; aspirin or ibuprofen can upset your stomach.

Also, over-the-counter drugs can interact with one another or with a prescription drug. Some drugs negate another's potency; others may increase it. Some interactions can even be fatal; never mix drugs without consulting your doctor—or at least your pharmacist.

What should I look for in a pharmacy?

Because of the high cost of many prescription drugs, the first thing that most people rightly look for in a pharmacy is generally low prices. This is especially important if you take a medication regularly over a long period of time.

It usually pays to do some comparison shopping—calling several drugstores to get the best price for a particular drug. Other practical considerations are also important. Does the store accept insurance payments for prescription drugs? Does it make home deliveries (which may be crucial when you are ill)?

Many pharmacies now keep lists, often computerized, of their clients' medications. This helpful service allows the pharmacist to monitor your prescriptions. When filling a new one, for example, the pharmacist can check to make sure that the drug won't interact adversely with anything else you're taking. This serves as a double check on your doctor, who may have overlooked an interaction. More often, this is a problem when medications are prescribed by more than one doctor and you forget to tell one of them about other drugs you are taking.

Aside from filling prescriptions, how can a pharmacist help me?

A pharmacist is a trained and licensed professional, and a good one can be a very useful source of information about drugs. If you can't remember everything your doctor told you about when and how to take a medication, ask your pharmacist. Similarly, if you think that a minor symptom, such as a dry throat or constipation, is being caused by a drug, a pharmacist can usually tell you whether it is a common or known side effect. A good pharmacist can also give you advice about the effectiveness of over-the-counter medications and of home health tests.

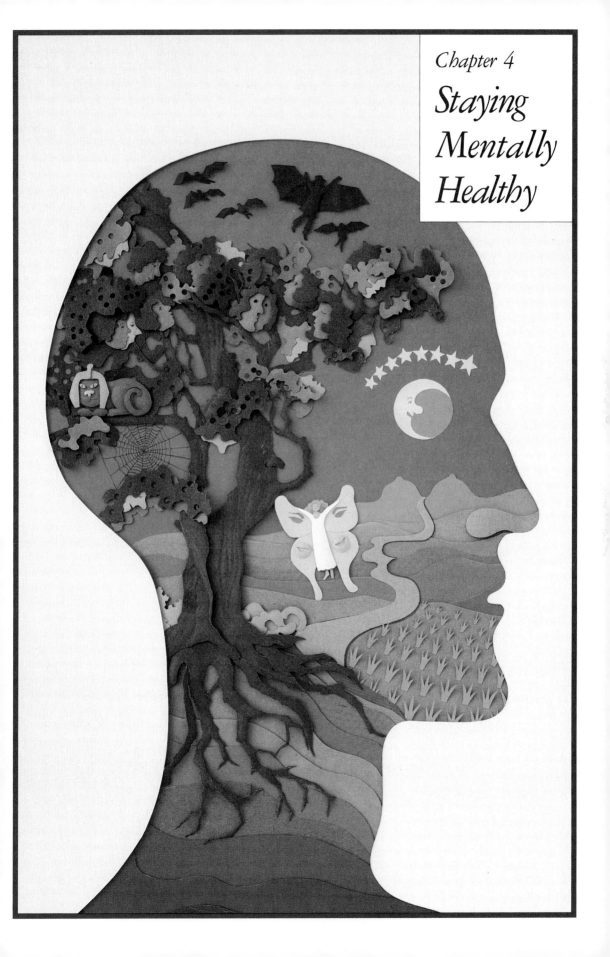

Winter Blues

Every year around the middle of December, Doug W.'s life would change. Normally good-humored and outgoing, Doug would become irritable and blue. He'd snap at family and friends, mope around, and eat voraciously. In the spring, his mood would return to normal.

One day, Doug read an article about seasonal affective disorder, or SAD—a recurrent wintertime depression apparently triggered by reduced exposure to sunlight. Recognizing his own problem, Doug contacted a clinic that specializes in treating SAD. On the basis of a detailed history and a complete physical, the doctor at the clinic confirmed that Doug had SAD.

The treatment prescribed for Doug consisted of daily exposure to a bright light source (antidepressant drugs are another treatment option). Every morning before going to work, Doug would sit in front of a light box for 45 minutes. In 3 days, his mood had improved. Delighted, he kept up the treatment until spring. This winter, instead of relying on the light box, Doug gets his sunlight from regular walks outdoors and is planning a mid-winter vacation in a sunny clime. His SAD days seem to be over.

Sober in AA

Dan M., 47, had been a problem drinker since he was 16. But he prided himself on an ability to control his drinking and go on the wagon when needed. Despite his drinking, Dan married, helped raise a daughter, and had held a good job for many years. As time passed, however, his binges became more frequent and longer lasting. He started showing up drunk at work, friends were avoiding him, and his marriage was coming apart. In desperation, he went on the wagon once again, but noticed that it was no longer so easy to stay on it. After 6 weeks without a drink and unable to stand it any more, Dan called Alcoholics Anonymous. The woman who answered told him that she was an alcoholic too, and persuaded him to come to a meeting. Eight years later, Dan still attends AA meetings regularly and has not had a relapse. He and his wife are back together, happier than ever, and his productivity at work has never been better. Looking back, Dan remembers the day he made that call as the most important of his life. It had taken him 30 years to admit that he was an alcoholic and reach out for help. But once he did, he found it.

A Fear of Dentists

As a child, Larry E. was taken to the dentist only for painful tooth extractions. By the time he was 18, he had lost several teeth and acquired a bad case of dental phobia. For the next 15 years, fear kept Larry from seeing a dentist, except for emergencies. But now he was in line for a job with a lot of client contact, and his boss gave him an ultimatum: do something about his gap-filled mouth or he would not get the job.

Determined not to lose this opportunity, Larry turned to a dental phobia clinic at a local university. During the preliminary interview, just talking about going to the dentist made Larry sweat profusely. At his first session, he learned to relax, breathe deeply, and visualize a dental exam. Next, he confronted the dental instruments themselves, first holding a dental mirror, then letting a dentist put it in his mouth. After four sessions at the clinic, Larry was able to start treatment. Thanks in part to his restored teeth, Larry's promotion came through. Today the man who once laughed with his mouth closed, greets clients with a confident open smile.

A Sound Mind in a Sound Body

What does it mean to be mentally healthy? What are positive ways of dealing with stress? How do you recognize addiction in yourself or in those you love? Is depression all in the mind? Can personality be changed? Where can you go for help in matters of the mind? Many people are reluctant to discuss or even acknowledge mental problems, yet there are few areas where basic information can be more useful. To gauge your knowledge of mental-health issues, try identifying which of the statements below are true and which are false.

1 The psychologically hardy person tends to be aggressive and cold.

_____ True   _____ False

2 Children are for the most part immune to stress disorders.

_____ True   _____ False

3 The cerebrum is the part of the brain where mind-altering drugs have their greatest effect.

_____ True   _____ False

4 Children of alcoholics are far likelier than others to become alcoholics themselves.

_____ True   _____ False

5 Drinking coffee may trigger a panic attack in some people.

_____ True   _____ False

6 Men admit to phobias more often than women do.

_____ True   _____ False

7 The vast majority of people who seek treatment for depression find relief in a matter of weeks.

_____ True   _____ False

8 A person with anorexia binges on high-calorie foods and then induces vomiting.

_____ True   _____ False

9 Dreams usually occur during the periods of deepest sleep.

_____ True   _____ False

10 Repressing emotions can sometimes cause physical illness.

_____ True   _____ False

11 A solid network of family and friends may lower disease risk and increase longevity.

_____ True   _____ False

12 Most psychotherapists use a mix of techniques from different schools of therapy.

_____ True   _____ False

Answers

For more information on any of the quiz topics turn to the pages listed next to the answers.

1. False, p.158   5. True, p.167   9. False p.178
2. False, p.158   6. False, p.168   10. True, p.183
3. False, p.160   7. True, p.170   11. True, p.185
4. True, p.162   8. False, p.177   12. True, p.192

What is mental health? Is it the same thing as being happy?

No one is happy all the time. Rather than a state of constant bliss, mental health is more like a balancing act that requires the processing and integration of constantly shifting emotions. The root meaning of *health* is wholeness. Mentally healthy people work at balancing all aspects of themselves—acknowledging and addressing the needs of their bodies, minds, and spirits. They feel generally purposeful, in control of their lives, committed to the work they do, supported by and supportive of the people around them.

Psychologists believe that the events of our lives, even the most devastating hardships, have less influence on our mental health than does the way we respond to them. Survivors of traumatic events—concentration camp prisoners, victims of terrorist kidnappings, lost polar explorers—often report triumph over pain, fear, and desolation through the conditioning of their minds. Open-minded, hopeful attitudes seem to help conquer adversity. Negative, rigid, inflexible attitudes not only decrease one's ability to cope with the inevitable stresses of life but can prevent people from fully enjoying themselves during the good times too.

A detached, defeatist outlook on life may even be harmful to health. In a study of elderly nursing home residents in Boston, Massachusetts, it was found that those who allowed every decision (what to watch on television, for example, or whether to go out to the movies with friends) to be made for them were twice as likely to get sick and die as were those who made their own choices.

What is stress and how do I recognize it?

The word *stress* is used to describe both external events and internal responses to them. Stressful life experiences range from trivial everyday hassles (a rude driver cuts you off in traffic, or the baby tips over a carton of milk) to major life-altering crises (the loss of a job, a divorce, the death of a family member). In a nationwide Louis Harris poll in 1987, 89 percent of American adults said they often operated under high levels of stress; 59 percent said they felt high levels of stress at least once a week.

Stress can be caused by any number of factors, including changes (both good and bad), personal problems, and illnesses. Listed below are some of the more common sources of stress, arranged by category:

□ Family. Death of a spouse, divorce, marital separation, death of a close family member, marital reconciliation, change in health of a family member, gaining a new family member, child leaving home, pregnancy, spouse beginning or ceasing work outside the home, problems with in-laws.

□ Personal and relationships. Death of a close friend, personal illness, sexual difficulties, change in living conditions, change in residence, outstanding personal achievement, change in sleeping habits, change in eating habits, going on vacation.

□ Work. Being fired from a job, retirement, major business readjustment, change in line of work, change in work responsibilities, change in working conditions, trouble with boss.

□ Money. Major change in financial situation, taking on a home mortgage, foreclosure on a mortgage, taking on a large loan.

Physical and psychological stress is a fact of life. What matters is the amount you face and the nature of your response. If your enjoyment of life is hampered by stress—if your relationships suffer, your sleep is disrupted, your appetite changes, your sense of physical well-being deteriorates—your body may be sending you warning signals that you are under too much stress.

What happens to the body under stress?

Certain stressful situations may set off what it known as the *fight-flight response* (see facing page). Perceiving a crisis, the brain sends out an alarm via chemical couriers called neurotransmitters. These signals from the brain trigger the production of hormones whose function is to put the body on alert and prepare it to cope with trouble. Your pulse rate accelerates, your heart pounds, your knees may shake, and your stomach may become upset.

Some of the hormones released in response to stress, especially one called epinephrine, or adrenaline, also stimulate the immune system, your body's complex mechanism for fighting off disease. While moderate levels of stress may actually hasten the healing process, high levels of stress, experienced over an extended period, deplete your supplies of stress-related hormones, slowing down the immune response and making you more vulnerable to disease.

An explosion of new research into the functioning of the immune system, much of it stimulated by the AIDS epidemic (see *The Facts About AIDS,* p. 242), is supporting long-held ideas about how emotional states can trigger physical illness. For decades, doctors have suspected that stress is a contributing factor in such conditions as ulcers, high blood

FIGHT OR FLIGHT

When confronted by acute physical or psychological stress, your brain triggers a chain reaction that prepares your body to fight the perceived threat or flee it. Though essential to survival in life-threatening situations and often useful when dealing with nonthreatening challenges, such as a job deadline, the fight-flight response is inappropriate for dealing with more routine stresses. If triggered often enough, it can lead to serious health problems. The physical reactions that make up the fight-flight response are illustrated below.

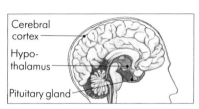

Cerebral cortex
Hypo-thalamus
Pituitary gland

The pupils of the eyes dilate.

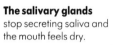

The cerebral cortex signals the hypothalamus of impending danger.

The hypothalamus releases a hormone called CRH, which activitates the pituitary gland. Nerve signals from the hypothalamus also stimulate the core of the adrenal glands to produce epinephrine (adrenaline) and norepinephrine, hormones that speed up heart and breathing rates and muscle response.

The pituitary gland, prodded by CRH, produces the hormone ACTH, which causes the adrenal gland's surface to secrete cortisol, a stimulating hormone.

The salivary glands stop secreting saliva and the mouth feels dry.

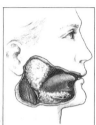

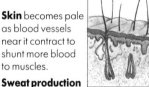

Skin becomes pale as blood vessels near it contract to shunt more blood to muscles.

Sweat production increases in order to cool a body overheated by the fight or flight.

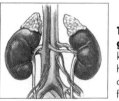

The adrenal glands atop the kidneys secrete hormones that create the fight-flight response.

Kidney function is reduced as less blood becomes available to the organs.

Heart rate increases to supply more blood to muscles.

Blood pressure rises.

Breathing rate increases to supply more oxygen to muscles.

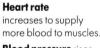

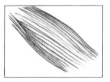

Muscle fibers contract to prepare for sudden movement.

Long-term stress can cause a variety of health problems, including head- and backache, skin rash, hypertension, cardiovascular disease, ulcers, other digestive tract disorders, impaired immune function, and sexual dysfunction.

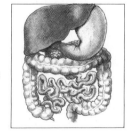

The liver increases its output of sugar and fat in order to supply more fuel to muscles.

Digestion slows or ceases. Defecation and urination are prevented by tightening muscles. (In some cases, however, diarrhea or uncontrolled urination may occur.)

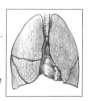

pressure, asthma, and migraine headaches. There is increasing evidence that stress makes people more susceptible to infectious diseases and may even hasten the progression of certain chronic and degenerative illnesses, such as rheumatoid arthritis.

The cardiovascular system is particularly sensitive to stress. In a study by Brigham and Women's Hospital and the Harvard Medical School in 1988, a group of cardiac patients were asked to speak publicly about personal habits they considered to be faults. As they did so, the flow of blood through their arteries was measurably reduced. Other studies show that newly widowed men face a significantly greater likelihood of developing heart disease. Along with the stress of bereavement, many of these men also suffered from loneliness and social isolation. When they remarried, their heart disease risk decreased.

It is important to remember, however, that while stress may contribute to the onset or development of illness, it is rarely the sole cause of disease.

I used to hear a lot about Type A and Type B personalities. Is it dangerous to be a Type A, and are such distinctions still valid?

There's good news for Type A's: some of the characteristics associated with forceful, ambitious personalities are now considered to be assets, not detriments, to health. While hostile, aggressive Type A behavior is certainly still a risk factor for coronary disease, physicians now make distinctions between Type A's who are angry and socially isolated and those who are able to develop supportive networks of family and friends.

Having a Type A (driven, impatient) or a Type B (easygoing) personality seems to have less of an impact on well-being and mental health than whether or not you are psychologically hardy. The psychologically hardy person has a well-developed sense of identity, feels in charge of life, and enjoys it, generally welcoming its changes as opportunities rather than threats. Such a person is also less likely to develop stress-related illnesses, such as ulcers and hypertension.

A sense of control distinguishes hardy people from those who feel victimized by stress and who overreact to minor as well as major setbacks. People who develop ulcers, for instance, don't necessarily lead more stressful lives than anyone else, but they do appear to take things more seriously and to react to their problems more negatively.

Unlike hardy individuals, who see themselves as the masters of their destinies, "pressure-sensitive" people believe that life is a matter of fate. Easily overwhelmed, they tend to be emotionally dependent; they often feel exhausted, helpless, and hopeless. They are also more likely to be depressed.

Facing life with a positive, relaxed attitude, maintaining a variety of interests, and appreciating and nurturing friendships are some of the ways anyone— Type A or Type B—can foster psychological hardiness.

How can I deal with stress effectively?

Examine your situation: what is causing the stress in your life? Concrete problems—an overbearing boss or high credit card debt—can be faced directly. Is it possible to change jobs? Or to set up a meeting with the boss to resolve your differ-

ences? Can you tighten your budget and set aside a bit more each month to apply toward reducing your credit card balance? Perhaps you could cancel all but one card and use that one only for emergency purchases.

More abstract forms of stress—long-term fears and global worries—are less easily handled. Visions of wars and famine are broadcast into our living rooms at night; troubling headlines greet us over breakfast. Our fast-paced lives pile responsibilities upon responsibilities. To be better equipped to deal with such ongoing sources of stress, it's essential to maintain a healthy mind in a healthy body. Maximize your stamina with a well-balanced diet. If you have medical problems, such as high blood pressure or elevated cholesterol levels, follow your doctor's dietary and other recommendations carefully. Regular exercise reduces tension and increases energy levels. In the past 20 years biofeedback and meditation have become recognized in the medical community as important relaxation techniques. These and other stress-reducing techniques that you can incorporate into your daily life are discussed on pages 206–207.

Are children subject to stress disorders?

Sadly, yes. Children lead stressful lives today, and often suffer the consequences both emotionally and physically. Each year since 1972 more than 1 million children have lived through their parents' divorces, and millions more watched parents fight the losing battle of an unhappy marriage. Many inner city children face risks most adults would have difficulty handling, just to get to school each day. And affluent children are subject to increasing pressures to excel, starting with admissions tests required by some *nursery* schools.

To help children deal with heightened stress levels, relaxation training could soon become a part of classroom curricula. Experts predict that teaching children to use biofeedback, meditation, and other techniques might help them ward off future stress-related diseases, such as high blood pressure.

Children most likely to remain cheerful and resilient even in the face of critical family problems, such as alcoholism or divorce, appear to be those who lead busy lives, engaging in activities in which they can proudly display their talents and forming deep, satisfying relationships with other children and healthy adults in or outside the home.

What is post-traumatic stress disorder?

After a person has been through a shocking, often life-threatening, experience, he or she may develop a number of debilitating psychological or physiological conditions that today are called post-traumatic stress disorder (PTSD). Research suggests that even one incident of overwhelming terror can alter the chemistry of the brain and trigger subsequent adrenaline surges during which victims experience anxiety attacks, mental confusion, frightening flashbacks, and other symptoms of PTSD (see box at right).

Most Americans have become aware of this problem through the suffering of veterans who were traumatized in combat. But post-traumatic stress has also been observed in the survivors of disasters, such as earthquakes or fires; in people who have suffered major accidents; and in victims of violent assaults. The condition is apt to be most ex-

TRAUMA AND ITS AFTERMATH

For many Vietnam veterans, the war is not over; the battles have simply moved from the jungle outside into their minds. According to the Department of Veterans Affairs, 12 to 15 percent of all Americans who served in Vietnam suffer from post-traumatic stress disorder (PTSD). Those who saw heavy combat are by far the most likely to experience the anxiety, recurrent nightmares, uncontrollable rages, emotional numbing, and sudden flashbacks that characterize the condition. In some cases, the symptoms disappear spontaneously within months; in others, a chronic, debilitating disease chips away at its victim's ability to hold down a job or take part in family life.

Vietnam veterans appear to suffer from PTSD in greater numbers than veterans of earlier wars, in part due to the controversial nature of the war itself and the soldiers' uncelebrated homecomings. Also, the men who fought in Vietnam were particularly young—their average age was 19, compared with age 26 for soldiers in World War II.

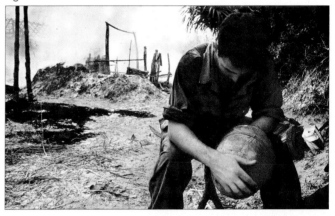

treme and last longest when the threat to life or safety was overwhelming and when all sense of personal control was lost.

Whether an individual develops PTSD seems to depend, at least partially, on the strength of the support he or she receives from loved ones. Rape victims who were criticized or felt rejected by their spouses or partners were more likely to develop PTSD than those who felt supported. People whose responses to a traumatic event are very defensive, especially if they deny the significance of the trauma or don't

share the experience with others, may also be at greater risk.

Pharmaceutical researchers are working to develop drugs that will reduce PTSD symptoms. If drug therapy can help PTSD sufferers to sleep better or to feel less anxious, psychologists say, psychotherapy for such emotional problems as numbness and guilt can become even more effective. Cognitive behavioral therapy (p. 193), in which the patient repeatedly relives the traumatic event, has proven useful in relieving PTSD symptoms in rape victims.

ADDICTION AND RECOVERY

Mood-altering drugs affect the brain in ways still not fully understood; why some of these drugs become addictive is an even more complicated matter. The language itself is confusing, with the term *addiction* being supplanted, at least among professionals, by the term *dependence.* Physical dependence on a drug, such as heroin, is characterized by *tolerance* to it—that is, the user has to take ever larger doses in order to achieve the same "high"—and *withdrawal symptoms* experienced when the drug is denied.

A drug such as marijuana may not produce a true physical dependence, but rather psychological dependence, in which the user has a compulsive emotional need for the drug. However, since both types of dependence have a biochemical basis in the brain, the distinction between the two terms is blurring.

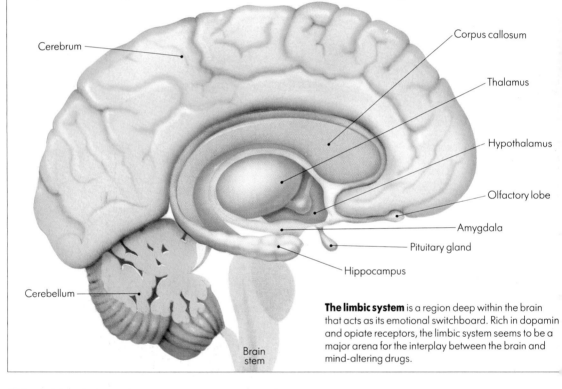

Cerebrum

Corpus callosum

Thalamus

Hypothalamus

Olfactory lobe

Amygdala

Pituitary gland

Hippocampus

Cerebellum

Brain stem

The limbic system is a region deep within the brain that acts as its emotional switchboard. Rich in dopamin and opiate receptors, the limbic system seems to be a major arena for the interplay between the brain and mind-altering drugs.

Why is it that some people who take drugs become addicted while others don't? Is there really such a thing as an addictive personality?

Although human beings have used mood-altering drugs since their earliest history, no one yet fully understands why one person can take these substances casually while someone else will become dependent on them.

Ongoing scientific research is revealing how psychoactive drugs interfere with the workings of the brain (see above). But biochemical descriptions alone only partially explain the process by which an individual develops a dependency on drugs. The same is true of personality and environment. The concept of an addictive personality is a controversial and not terribly useful one. It suggests, on the one hand, that "weak-willed" people are to blame for their drug problems, and on the other, that they are not responsible for their behavior. While the tendency to abuse drugs may be encouraged by psychological traits such as low self-esteem and by certain environmental factors, such as poverty, family upheavals, and social and peer pressures, it remains a fact that people from all walks of life and of vastly different psychological makeups become habitual drug users.

Three overlapping factors appear to affect anyone's reaction to intoxicants: the nature of the drug, the nature of the user, and the setting in which drug use takes place. The kind of drug—

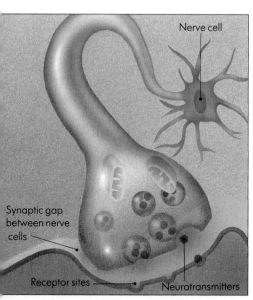

Nerve cell

Synaptic gap
between nerve
cells

Receptor sites — Neurotransmitters

Drugs that influence mood do so because they alter electrochemical activity in the brain. Essential to that activity are electrochemical "messengers" called neurotransmitters that carry signals from one nerve cell to specific receptor sites on nearby nerve cells. A stimulant like cocaine binds to receptor sites for the neurotransmitter dopamine, preventing its reabsorption into nerve cells. The resulting increase of dopamine levels in the brain produces the euphoria characteristic of a cocaine high.

Heroin and other opiates imitate the action of natural pain-killing neurotransmitters called endorphins. When heroin is available to the brain, endorphin production is suppressed. If drug use suddenly stops, the brain is left without a buffer against pain; the result is withdrawal.

Depressants like alcohol and Valium may enhance the action of the inhibitory neurotransmitter GABA; alcohol seems to affect several other neurotransmitters as well.

Whether the drug is nicotine, alcohol, or heroin, breaking a drug dependence can be a difficult, sometimes painful process. The first step is recognition that a problem exists, followed by detoxification, either abrupt or gradual, depending on the drug and the user. Withdrawal symptoms also vary with each drug, as well as in kind and severity. Withdrawal from heroin, for example, which should take place only under expert medical supervision, can cause sneezing, cramps, chills, tremors, vomiting, seizures, coma, and sometimes death. Rehabilitation measures for the recovering addict include psychotherapy to deal with the underlying psychological and behavioral problems that may have led to the dependence, personal counseling, and membership in support groups (see *The Facts About 12-Step Programs,* p.164).

The vicious spiral of drug abuse and its cost to individuals, their families, and society at large have heightened scientific interest in finding medical treatments to facilitate withdrawal from drugs, or even to eliminate the desire for them. Antabuse and methadone were the first drugs used to treat alcoholics and heroin addicts. More recently new antidepressant, anticonvulsant, and antianxiety drugs have been yielding promising results in animal trials. Although such drugs may one day help win the battle against drug addiction, today relapses remain common among recovering addicts, and it may take several attempts before someone can permanently break a drug dependence.

---

its physically and psychologically addictive chemical properties—interacts with an individual's biological and temperamental makeup and with his or her background and environment to determine whether that person will become an addict. The availability of a drug and whether its use is condoned or condemned in a particular social setting play a critical role in determining how widely the drug will be used and what its use will mean to those who take it and to those around them.

I'm finding it almost impossible to quit smoking? Why is it so hard?

Most smokers try their first cigarettes when they are teenagers, and habits formed early in life are usually hard to break. Over the years, long-term smokers develop automatic connections between lighting up and virtually every activity of their daily lives. The morning coffee break cigarette means it's time to get going; the cigarette after dinner

signals time to relax. Cigarettes provide energy as well as relaxation to smokers when levels of nicotine, a highly addictive substance, ebb and flow in the bloodstream. Although most smokers don't actually feel intoxicated when they smoke, they will recall feeling flushed and dizzy when they first started smoking, and will likely experience withdrawal symptoms when they try to stop.

Because nicotine is both physically and psychologically addictive, giving up cigarettes is quite

IF YOU DRINK

☐ Know why you are drinking. A sociable drink with friends is a pleasurable experience; drinking to dispel feelings of depression or to fall asleep can easily set up a dependency.

☐ Before you drink, eat some high-protein, high-fat food, such as meat or cheese. Avoid anything salty that would make you thirsty.

☐ Learn approximately how much you can drink without becoming intoxicated. Then stay within your limit, rather than trying to keep up with friends.

☐ Control the time you take to finish a drink. (Try to sip it slowly.)

☐ Dilute your drink with plenty of ice and noncarbonated mixers.

☐ If you're having a second drink, have a glass of juice or water first, and continue snacking.

☐ Of course, never drive after you have been drinking.

☐ If you take medication *of any kind,* even an over-the-counter drug, be sure you know how it interacts with alcohol.

a challenge for many people. But the hazards of smoking—from greatly increased risks of developing lung cancer, cardiovascular disease, and emphysema to the embarrassments of being a smoker in a society that increasingly disdains the habit—motivate most smokers to give it a try. For suggestions on how to quit smoking, see page 201.

How does alcoholism happen?

Alcoholism is a progressive disease; it begins when social drinking gradually builds up to heavy drinking (six or seven drinks per day) or to alcoholic binges. Once the central nervous system develops a tolerance to alcohol, the result is a physical dependence. The drinker gets cranky and uncomfortable when alcohol is not available. As the disease progresses, an alcoholic loses interest in other activities, eats poorly, loses control over the drinking, and becomes obsessed with it. The condition perpetuates itself as the alcoholic feels depressed about his drinking, feels isolated

and remorseful, and attempts to drown all these unbearable emotions in yet another drink. It may only be after many years of hard drinking that the effects of alcoholism become obvious, and that psychological, social, and physical degeneration can no longer be denied.

My husband and I argue a lot about his drinking. He says it's no problem. I'm afraid he he may be becoming an alcoholic. How can I tell who's right?

In most people, the development of alcoholism is insidiously gradual, hard to trace and easy to ignore. Alcoholism affects one of every four families in this country, and while families react to drinking problems in different ways, here are some of the common signs that a problem does exist.

☐ Do you and your children find yourselves tiptoeing around your husband when he's been drinking? Most families of alcoholics live in a constant state of insecurity; family members never know whether this will be a

pleasant day or whether the alcoholic will make life miserable for everyone by drinking.

☐ Do tension levels in your home rise when your husband starts to drink? Are you afraid to talk about or to criticize his drinking habits?

☐ Does your husband miss work frequently after evenings of heavy drinking?

☐ Has he been involved in traffic violations or fights when he drinks?

☐ Does he begin to drink in the morning, try to hide his drinking, feel guilty about drinking bouts, and make promises to quit?

☐ Has he tried to stop drinking and been unable to?

The very fact that you and your husband argue frequently about his drinking habits may in itself be a sign that he is becoming an alcoholic.

Drinking problems seem to run in my family. Can alcoholism be inherited?

There's strong evidence that a *tendency* can be inherited. Studies of twins and adopted children have shown that heredity can play a more critical role than environment in the development of alcoholism. Children of alcoholics tend to tolerate greater amounts of alcohol when they begin drinking and are apt to start drinking at a younger age. Later their reactions change—more sensitive to alcohol than others, they tend to get sicker after being intoxicated. Such children stand four to six times the risk of developing alcoholism than others do.

Much scientific research is being devoted to identifying a genetic basis for alcoholism. In one study, a receptor gene for dopamine, a neurotransmitter (p. 161) that plays a part in pleasure-seeking behavior, was located in the brains of 77 percent of alcoholics, compared with only 28 percent of nonalcoholics, during autopsies. Exactly what role the gene may play in the development of alcoholism is unclear. By activating the release of dopamine, it could affect the degree of pleasure felt when an individual drinks alcohol, and may lead to a craving for more alcohol to release more dopamine.

However, no single biological explanation for the development of alcoholism is entirely satisfactory. Social and cultural factors can lead people to abuse alcohol whether or not they are genetically predisposed to the disease. And the way families pass on a tendency toward alcoholism may not be entirely biological but may also stem from familial relationships, as well as from the way alcohol is used and drunkenness is regarded in the home.

My close friends are telling me that I am becoming codependent. What does that mean?

The term *codependency* is widely used these days to describe the unhealthy dynamics and mutual dependence between an addict and those closest to him or her. Anyone whose life is deeply affected by involvement with an addict is said to be at risk. According to some interpretations, it's possible to be codependent not only with an alcoholic or a drug abuser, but also with a compulsive gambler, an overeater, or anyone with a problem that's viewed as an addiction.

In such relationships it's the codependent who throws away the addict's pills, pretends not to notice the slurred speech, and hides their mutual nightmare from friends and family. Collusion is the motor of a codependency. Lies are told, facts are hidden, evidence is covered up for the family member with the "problem." Codependents may believe they are helping the addict by holding things together, but what they're actually doing is preventing the addict from seeking help.

Many people have found the concept of codependency useful as a way to think about their responses to a loved one with an addiction problem and to cope with what is often an impossible situation. But blaming the family or intimates of an addict for "enabling" the addiction can have detrimental consequences and is not supported by scientific research. For more information on dealing with an addiction problem in your family, contact your local chapter of Al-Anon, the family group associated with Alcoholics Anonymous (see Appendix).

ALCOHOL AND YOUR HEALTH

Statistics indicate that taking an occasional drink is not injurious to health, as was once thought, and may even be helpful. People who sometimes have a drink or two in the evening tend to live longer than strict teetotalers. However, excessive alcohol consumption still takes a high toll in disease and unnecessary deaths in the United States.

In the short term, frequent heavy drinking leads to

☐ Loss of judgment and emotional control.
☐ Loss of motor coordination; slower reflexes.
☐ Increased risk of car and other accidents.
☐ Insomnia.
☐ Headaches and nausea "the morning after."

☐ Risk of a dangerous reaction if alcohol is taken with certain other drugs, including common over-the-counter medications, such as aspirin and antihistamines.
☐ Damage to unborn children (p.261).

The long-term price of alcohol abuse is higher and includes

☐ Irreversible, sometimes fatal, liver disease (cirrhosis).
☐ Deterioration of memory and general mental functioning.
☐ Malnutrition.
☐ Impairment of the immune system.
☐ Greater than normal risk of cancers of the mouth, larynx, esophagus, liver, breast, thyroid, and the digestive tract.

☐ Increase in the cancer risks posed by smoking.
☐ A higher incidence of gastrointestinal problems, pancreatitis, and phlebitis.
☐ Temporary or permanent visual impairment.
☐ Dramatic rise of heart attack and stroke risk, in part because alcohol raises blood pressure and blood levels of triglycerides, which contribute to clogging of the arteries.

THE FACTS ABOUT 12-STEP PROGRAMS

What are they? The 12 steps are a set of guidelines for self-help groups that form to address a wide range of issues, from battles with alcohol and other drugs, to crippling phobias or even the suffering faced by the parents of murder victims. From 1980 to 1990 the number of self-help groups in this country quadrupled. In 1990 more than 15 million Americans were attending some 500,000 meetings each week. Alcoholics Anonymous, the first and still the largest of the 12-step programs, has an estimated membership of 1.73 million people around the world, about half of whom live in the United States. People who cannot afford the considerable expense of professional psychiatry and those who wish to supplement psychotherapy by meeting with others who are staring down the same demons find 12-step groups to be invaluable vehicles for self-improvement.

How do 12-step programs work? Based on the precepts of Alcoholics Anonymous, the original self-help group founded in 1935, 12-step programs operate on the assumption that people with a common problem can cure themselves by helping each other. The central principles are honesty, tolerance, and faith in a "higher power," as defined by the individual member.

Groups meet regularly, usually twice a week, in church basements, members' living rooms, and hospital conference rooms. The members share their experiences and help motivate each other to "work the steps" first devised by Bill Wilson, an alcoholic who was one of the founders of Alcoholics Anonymous. A member takes the first step by ad-

mitting that he has lost control to his compulsion. With each other's encouragement, members progress step by step—from introspection to compassion, from resolving past problems to facing the future with good cheer. Familiar slogans such as "One Day at a Time," "Live and Let Live," or "Let Go and Let God" are reminders of the programs' blueprints for living.

What are the drawbacks? Twelve-step programs have been criticized for their emphasis on spirituality. It has been suggested that people who might otherwise benefit from the mutual support offered by such programs are turned off by talk of a higher power. Ironically, other critics claim that 12-step programs are usurping the place of religious organizations and contributing to the rise of atheistic humanism by allowing members to define a higher power in their own way.

Within the AA program there is also controversy over appropriate criteria for membership. Some old-line members see AA as a haven for alcoholics only and believe that alcoholics with drug problems should join such spinoff groups as Narcotics Anonymous or Cocaine Users Anonymous.

Some addiction experts question the proliferation of spinoff groups for such diverse problems as compulsive shopping, overeating, even excessive consumption of cola drinks. As often happens in our culture, a good idea may be taken too far. But for the millions of people who have been or are being helped by the various 12-step programs, what counts most is that the programs work for them.

I've heard that alcohol affects men and women differently. Is this true?

Research suggests that a woman feels the effects of a drink more quickly than a man of the same size. When men drink, much of the alcohol they consume is digested in the stomach, broken down by an enzyme that prevents it from ever reaching the bloodstream. Women appear to have much less of this enzyme; when they drink, more alcohol flows through the stomach wall directly into the bloodstream and from there to the brain, making women feel and act more intoxicated sooner than men.

Does recovery from alcoholism mean giving up alcohol completely?

While some people with drinking problems (especially younger ones who do not yet have a full-blown dependence) report that they are able to control the problem while continuing to drink socially, most of the evidence suggests that total abstinence is the safest bet for anyone struggling with a severe dependence.

The recovery process can take several forms, including stopping cold turkey on one's own (see *Addiction and Recovery,* pp.160–161). Many alcoholics, however, find the support of a program like Alcoholics Anonymous an invaluable aid in getting through the first days and months of recovery. (See *The Facts About 12-Step Programs,* facing page.)

What, if any, are the long-term effects of smoking marijuana?

To date, most studies of chronic heavy marijuana use have failed to produce clear evidence of physical or psychological damage. However, possible connections between long-term, heavy marijuana use and chromosomal damage, birth defects, impairment of the immune system response, lower levels of the hormone testosterone in males, and menstrual irregularities in females are suspected and are still being studied.

In the short term, there is evidence that memory loss and anxiety reactions occur in some users. Schizophrenics and people who are clinically depressed may experience a worsening of their symptoms. Because marijuana smoke is inhaled very deeply and held in the lungs for several seconds, smoking four marijuana cigarettes per week is potentially as damaging to respiratory capacity and as carcinogenic as smoking a pack of cigarettes every day. Driving under the influence of marijuana is also a hazard, since intoxication can impair judgment, slow reaction time, and impair visual tracking (the ability to follow moving objects accurately).

Although there is no clinical evidence that smoking marijuana leads inevitably to addiction to other drugs, statistics show that many abusers of heroin, cocaine, and psychedelic drugs smoked marijuana before they became addicted to hard drugs.

DRUGS ON THE JOB

The estimated cost to the U.S. economy of on-the-job drug abuse exceeds $60 billion per year. Many large companies now routinely screen job applicants for drug use and have instituted random drug tests for employees with safety-related jobs. This testing—usually by urinalysis—is very controversial. Employees may see it as an invasion of their privacy; and experts acknowledge that the tests are not foolproof (the poppy seeds on a morning bagel, for example, can show up as heroin).

Computer performance tests of hand-eye coordination and reflexes may one day replace drug tests in judging employee fitness to handle safety-related jobs. Still experimental, these tests promise a practical, on-the-spot measure of impairment.

Meanwhile, the best corporate drug policies refer employees suspected of drug abuse to an Employee Assistance Program (EAP) for a confidential evaluation and, if necessary, referral to a treatment program. Seeing colleagues getting help instead of losing their jobs may encourage other employees to seek help.

I've heard that crack is more dangerous than cocaine. Is that true?

Yes, it is. Cocaine in any form is dangerous and potentially lethal. It constricts the blood vessels, reducing the flow of blood to the heart, and can cause severe cardiac inflammation and arrhythmia. But the risks are considerably higher when cocaine is taken in the form of crack.

Sold on the streets in pellets and flakes, crack is a cheap, potent, and highly addictive form of cocaine. Because it's heated and smoked, crack reaches the brain faster than sniffed cocaine does. Crack provides a very brief ecstatic rush and, in about 20 minutes, a deep letdown.

All forms of cocaine artificially boost energy and self-confidence, but since the effects of crack are so fleeting, these feelings quickly subside. To maintain their high, users must smoke crack again and again.

Emotionally, crack addiction can paralyze the user, eradicating even the most basic human instincts, such as the desire of parents to protect their children. More than the victims of other forms of drug abuse, mothers of crack babies seem to lack interest in their children, often neglecting them or abandoning them to the care of others. Women who use crack during pregnancy expose their unborn children to the risk of deformities and other birth defects. Once they are born, crack babies are subject to ongoing behavioral and developmental problems.

If there is any good news in this area, it's that recent surveys indicate that the use of crack and other forms of cocaine is declining, at least among middle-class youngsters and probably across a broader spectrum of American society.

STREET DRUGS

The term *drug abuse* refers to any use of a drug that harms the user physically, psychologically, economically, legally, or socially. The abuse may entail using an illegal substance (heroin, cocaine) or misusing a drug obtainable legally (alcohol, nicotine, glue) or only through a doctor's prescription (analgesics, amphetamines, barbiturates, steroids; see also *The Facts About Steroids*, p.86). Ironically, alcohol and nicotine, the drugs with perhaps the most detrimental effects on the nation's health and productivity, are not only legal, but their use is widely promoted.

Drug	Effects	Long-term hazards
Amphetamines Street names: *meth, crank, ice, bennies, speed, uppers.* Taken orally, sniffed, injected, or smoked.	Hyperactivity, quickened pulse, restlessness, insomnia, sense of self-confidence and excitement followed by depression.	Weight loss, tolerance, dependence, paranoia, nervous exhaustion, palpitations, violent behavior.
Barbiturates Street names: *bluebirds, downers, goofballs, blues, reds, yellow jackets, nembies.* Taken orally or injected.	Slowed heart rate and breathing, slurred speech, unsteady gait, confusion, lethargy, limited attention span.	Tolerance, dependence, risk of fatal overdose (especially if taken with alcohol). Serious infections (such as hepatitis and AIDS) from shared needles if injected.
Cocaine Street names: *blow, coke, free base, lady, nose candy, snow, toot, crack.* Sniffed, smoked, or injected.	Faster pulse, appetite loss, euphoria and self-confidence followed by agitation, anxiety, depression.	Dependence, damage to nasal passages from repeated sniffing; risk of seizures and cardiac arrest from overdose, serious infections from shared needles if injected.
Heroin Street names: *dope, horse, junk, smack, scag, H, hombre.* Sniffed, smoked, or injected.	Euphoria, lethargy, slurred speech, mood swings, shallow breathing, loss of self-control.	Tolerance, dependence, malnutrition, risk of AIDS or hepatitis from shared needles, fatal overdose.
Inhalants Airplane glue, rubber cement, cleaning fluid.	Giddiness, euphoria, confusion, flushed face.	Risk of brain, liver, or kidney damage or of death from heart failure or asphyxia.
LSD Street names: *acid, haze.* Taken orally or smoked with tobacco or marijuana.	Sensory distortions, muscle rigidity, hallucinations, paranoia, panic, unpredictable or violent behavior.	Tolerance, recurrence of effects without use of drug, risk of suicide or fatal accident, long-term psychological damage.
Marijuana Street names: *dope, grass, pot, tea, weed.* Smoked or ingested with food or as a tea.	Euphoria, giddiness, mood swings, dry mouth, hunger, loss of coordination and sense of time.	Large doses may cause panic, confusion, and paranoia. Long-term use may damage lungs and reduce fertility.

I think my son is abusing drugs. How do I talk to him about it?

Promptly, and as calmly as you can. Few parents sit down to talk about drugs until a family member is suspected of using them. Then a child may be grounded or ordered to just say no, without being given ammunition to help him resist peer pressure and without an informed explanation of the dangers of taking drugs.

The best way to help your child make sensible decisions about alcohol and drug use is to set a good example and to make sure he knows the *facts* about drugs—their short-term effects and long-term hazards (see *Street Drugs,* facing page). Make sure you understand how alcohol and drugs can interfere with your child's physical and emotional development so that you can explain these things to him. To learn more about the dangers of drug abuse, write the National Clearinghouse for Alcohol and Drug Information (see Appendix).

Successful school antidrug programs intervene early to provide teenagers with plenty of information and to encourage them to discuss the issues, resist peer pressure, and form their own conclusions about drug use.

Parents who hope to help their teenagers avoid drug problems can't be hypocrites. Examine your own use of alcohol, nicotine, and prescription drugs and be prepared to honestly discuss your personal attitudes about legal and illegal drugs. If your own experience with alcohol or drugs will shed any light on the issues, you may want to share that experience with your child.

Encourage your son's interest in healthy alternative activities and help him think of face-saving ways to turn down peers who offer him drinks or drugs.

I know someone who had a terrible time withdrawing from Valium. Is this drug still widely prescribed?

Prescriptions for Valium are way down nationwide. In the 1960's benzodiazepines (a family of drugs that includes Valium, Dalmane, and Librium) were regarded as wonder drugs and were widely prescribed to help people, especially women, relax during the day and sleep through the night. But in the mid-1970's severe withdrawal symptoms were reported, even in people who were taking relatively small therapeutic doses on doctor's orders. Symptoms such as anxiety, depression, nausea, and convulsive seizures could last for weeks if withdrawal was not accomplished gradually.

While Valium prescriptions are down, new tranquilizers are taking its place. Halcion, a short-term sedative that offers the promise of a good night's sleep without drowsiness in the morning, accounts for nearly half of the 20 million prescriptions written for sleeping pills annually. But reports of Halcion-based delirium and short-term amnesia are making some physicians think twice about prescribing it.

In general, pills are not a good long-term solution for insomnia, which often responds to safer nondrug treatments (see p. 208).

I occasionally become very agitated for no apparent reason. What could be causing this?

You may be having a panic attack—an intense burst of anxiety accompanied by such physical symptoms as heart palpitations or chest pains, dizziness, numbness of the hands or feet, sweating, trembling, or a choking sensation. Fear and a sense of unreality may be overwhelming. Sometimes flashes of bright light may alternate with a clouding of vision. If the attack occurs in public, the victim may feel an urgent need to rush home. Panic attacks usually begin suddenly and unpredictably; when attacks recur, the condition is called a panic disorder.

Some people suffer panic attacks for a brief and limited period, and then their problems mysteriously vanish. Others with long-term panic disorders may develop agoraphobia (literally meaning "fear of the marketplace"). Afraid to go out because a panic attack might overwhelm them, these people eventually become housebound.

The causes of panic attacks are not yet fully understood. There is increasing evidence that an individual's patterns of thinking—the catastrophic messages that the victim of panic attacks sends himself—are directly related to the problem.

Connections between panic attacks and mitral valve prolapse, a generally benign abnormality of the heart, indicate that the attacks may also have a biological basis. High blood levels of adrenaline and other fight-flight hormones (p. 157) have been observed both in people with mitral valve prolapse and in people with panic disorder. An increase in the flow of such hormones could set off an attack.

Improper functioning of the autonomic nervous system, which regulates the body's blood supply, heart rate, and other involuntary functions, might also cause the fainting spells, dizziness, heart palpitations, and feelings of anxiety characteristic of this condition.

And according to some experts, caffeine consumption is a possible trigger of panic attacks.

Can my panic attacks be treated?

No sure cure exists, since no one knows exactly what causes panic attacks, but several treatments are being used successfully. The most effective psychological treatment combines techniques of cognitive and behavioral therapies (p. 193) that focus on the patient's physical sensations and on his or her catastrophic interpretations of these sensations. Panic attacks are also treated with antianxiety or antidepressant drugs or with certain MAO inhibitors (p. 171).

People prone to panic attacks are urged to eliminate coffee, tea, and other caffeinated beverages from their diets. Regular exercise provides a healthy outlet for anxiety and can help soothe tensions. You might also try some of the relaxation techniques described on pages 206–207.

I live in a neighborhood with a high crime rate, and I'm growing more and more afraid of going out. How can I cope with my fears?

Some fears are realistic. If the streets in your neighborhood are not safe at night, it makes sense to take precautions. When a friend or cab driver drops you off at your home, have him wait to see that you're safely inside. If you must walk home alone, walk briskly and purposefully. Hold your keys ready so you won't have to fumble for them at the door. Wear a whistle around your neck so you can summon help when you need it. If your beloved old neighborhood has become particularly dangerous, you may want to consider moving; holding on to pleasant dreams of the past won't lower the crime rate.

On the other hand, if your neighbors don't seem to worry as much as you do, you may be suffering from the early stages of agoraphobia, or fear of public places. Agoraphobics particularly fear being caught in crowded places from which there is no easy exit, such as department stores, buses, or busy city streets. In its advanced stages, this disease keeps people captives in their own homes, where depression can exacerbate the original problem.

When does a fear become a phobia?

Only in the movies or on Saturday morning TV are you likely to encounter heroes and superheroes who have no fears. The rest of us are reasonably prudent when it comes to climbing ladders, swimming out over our heads, or wading through deep grass where snakes could be lurking. Such rational fears protect us from getting hurt.

Many of us also harbor irrational fears—fears of crossing bridges, encountering large dogs, or visiting the dentist. What distinguishes these common fears from phobias is their intensity and the degree to which avoiding the feared object or situation interferes with daily life. A fear of frogs, for instance, does not present much of a problem to a city dweller unless it prevents him from ever visiting friends in the country. A fear of tunnels is not a problem if a driver merely feels ill at ease while driving through one and eager to reach the light at the end; but if he maps out elaborate strategies for avoiding tunnels, circuitous routes that add miles to the journey, the fear has become a phobia. Some phobias are so intense and all-encompassing that they dominate a person's life.

What are the most common phobias?

Among the most common phobias are fear of public speaking, fear of heights (acrophobia), fear of snakes (ophidiophobia) and dogs (cynophobia), fear of enclosed spaces (claustrophobia), fear of thunder (brontophobia) and lightning (astraphobia), fear of darkness (nyctophobia), and fear of flying (aerophobia). People with these phobias usually realize how disproportionate their worries are but feel helpless to prevent the overwhelming anxiety provoked by the feared objects or situations. Phobias affect about 12.5 percent of the population at some point in their lives. Women admit to phobias more often than men do.

Phobias can be divided into two groups: simple phobias, which involve single objects or situations (cats, elevators, thunder), and complex phobias, which are usually accompanied by intense panic attacks and often combine more than one simple phobia. Complex phobias are generally much more disabling; agoraphobics, for instance, may fear not only leaving the house but also heights, enclosed spaces, and germ contamination. Agoraphobia is the most common phobia for which people seek psychiatric treatment.

Are there any effective treatments for phobias?

Yes, although they're not always needed. Many people suffering from mild, simple phobias never seek treatment. Some conquer their own fears over time; others don't, but manage to work around their fears. People who do seek treatment find that simple phobias are often easily cured.

The most common treatment is to expose the phobic person to the object or situation he fears by gradual degrees. Usually a therapist (or, in the case of a child, a parent) helps ease the phobic into the situation. The first step in overcoming a fear of flying, for example, is gradual acclimation in an airplane that remains on the runway. Only after weeks of preparation do the patients actually fasten their seat belts for takeoff. People with complex phobias—especially agoraphobics—can also benefit from exposure therapy, usually with the help of both a spouse or friend and a therapist. Antianxiety or antidepressant drugs may be used in conjunction with therapy to reduce the severity and frequency of panic attacks associated with phobias.

What's the difference between being depressed, anxious, or just plain blue?

Every normal person feels sad at times. There are life events— marital problems, the loss of a job, the death of a loved one— that will temporarily depress anyone. Psychiatrists draw the line between the blues and more serious forms of depression when a person's gloomy feelings predominate for weeks instead of days, are intense, and are associated with sleep and eating disturbances. Clinical depression often begins when those low, lethargic feelings we all experience from time to time simply will not go away.

Depression is quite common; about 8.3 percent of Americans will suffer a depressive disorder at some point in their lives. It is a highly treatable illness, but unfortunately it is also among the most misunderstood by the average layman. Most of us will say we are depressed on a day when we feel down in the dumps or just grumpy, and this casual

use of the word only adds to popular misconceptions.

Casual references to anxiety muddy the waters too. Any teen-ager who's a little nervous or fidgety before a Saturday night date will say she's anxious. But true anxiety, as it is observed in about two-thirds of clinically depressed people, is a state of inner distress in which dread, fear, and foreboding dominate one's thoughts; its physical symptoms include heart palpitations, sweating, rapid pulse, and stomach upset.

What are the signs of depression?

Feeling sad (blue, hopeless, gloomy) all or most of the time for more than 2 weeks is the most common symptom of depression. These feelings of sadness may be pervasive, not tied to a specific event. Many people lose motivation or their interest in things they normally enjoy; nothing seems to matter, nothing means anything. Some may have suicidal thoughts.

Restlessness, difficulty concentrating, sleep problems, and a decrease in sexual desire are also common complaints. About 70 percent of depressed people lose their appetite, while a minority feel hungrier and eat more, especially at night.

Other physical symptoms of depression include head, neck, and back pain, a tightness in the throat, blurred vision, nausea, muscle cramps, painful urination, indigestion, and constipation.

Depressed people are often put through a series of diagnostic workups in search of a medical explanation for their symptoms. Too often, physicians don't suspect that their patients' physical complaints could be symptoms of depression. In one recent study, doctors failed to

recognize severe depression in half the patients they saw who suffered from it.

My brother has been down in the dumps lately, but his wife says it's all in his imagination. Is she right?

No. Many people believe that depression is a sign of personal weakness, a condition that can and should be willed away. But anyone who thinks that depression isn't real is wrong and grossly underestimates the suffering caused by this illness.

Signs that depression has a physical component abound. PET scans (p.126) and electroencephalographic recordings of brain waves (EEG's) vary from normal in some depressed patients. Scientists are exploring connections between depression and thyroid abnormalities, coronary artery disease, and head injuries. But the most compelling evidence that much depression is based in a biochemical imbalance is the fact that drug treatment affords relief in a majority of cases.

Severe depression that responds to treatment with antidepressant drugs is thought to be caused by a reduction in the levels of certain excitatory neurotransmitters—chemical messengers that alter mood by stimulating brain cell activity (p.171). Even when depression has a primarily psychological basis (childhood traumas such as incest are at the root of some cases) it can be as real a physical condition as diabetes or heart disease, and just as debilitating. If ignored and left untreated, depression can deepen; thoughts of suicide may turn into attempts. And even if one episode subsides without treatment, the condition cannot be counted as cured. At least 50 percent of depressed people experience recurrences. Unfortunately, the stigma attached to depression prevents many people from seeking the help they need.

My father suffered from depression for many years. Does that mean that I am at risk too?

A genetic vulnerability appears to exist, at least in some forms of depression. Manic depression (p. 172) shows the most likelihood of being genetically based. If you are genetically susceptible, ordinary setbacks and normal periods of grief—illness, a financial or even a midlife crisis—could trigger a serious depression.

But even if depression runs in your family, you may never develop the disease. Continuing research suggests that personal, social, and biochemical factors combine in a complicated interaction to determine whether an individual will become depressed.

What should I do if I get depressed?

If your depression continues unabated for 2 to 4 weeks, talk to your family doctor and get an evaluation from a counselor, a psychologist, or a psychiatrist. Depression is a highly treatable disease; at least 80 percent of those who seek treatment get significant relief in a matter of weeks from drug therapy (p. 171), psychotherapy, or a combination of the two. Many people who are mildly depressed will improve quickly with only short-term, goal-oriented counseling (p. 193). Such time-limited therapy works best for temporary depressions triggered by specific events; instead of delving into childhood experiences, treatment focuses on the present.

Vigorous exercise can sometimes ease a mild, short-term case of the blues. But jogging will not cure a major depression. Unfortunately, some people turn to alcohol, marijuana, cocaine, or even cigarettes to relieve their depression. While drug use can mask depression temporarily, in the long run alcohol and other drugs seriously exacerbate the problem. Depressed smokers not only damage their health but have a harder time giving up cigarettes than other smokers do.

Support groups can help sufferers feel that they're not the only ones on earth who experience such terribly dark periods. But for most people who suffer from major depression, psychotherapeutic help is an important key to recovery.

A friend of mine is often depressed. What can I do to help?

Lend a sympathetic ear. Studies show that a caring listener can often lighten the burden of a mildly depressed person as much as drug treatment or psychotherapy can. Whatever you do, don't tell your friend that her problem is in her head. Urging her to "snap out of it" may only make your friend, whose self-esteem is already low, feel even worse.

If her feelings of depression persist, you can encourage her to see a psychotherapist by stressing that she's suffering from a common condition for which effective relief is available.

Is it true that women are more likely to become depressed than men?

Yes, it is. Statistics show that women are twice as likely as men to suffer from every kind of depression (except manic depression). Men are more likely to experience other mental disorders, including alcoholism, drug abuse, and behavioral problems in childhood and adolescence.

It is possible that men actually do get depressed as much as women but are diagnosed less often. Women tend to seek medical care, including psychological counseling, more frequently than men do, and they tend to be more open with their emotions, more expressive about their sorrows and disappointments. A man could be just as depressed as a woman but might act less depressed and thus escape attention. On the other hand, because women are generally in closer touch with their emotions, they may feel losses more deeply, especially losses in relationships, and so be more vulnerable to depression. The more passive, less assertive attitudes many women have been taught to assume may also be a factor.

Is depression more likely to occur in the winter months?

Seasonal affective disorder (SAD) afflicts some 6 percent of Americans during the cold, dark months; another 14 percent suffer from milder cases of the blues as the days shorten and temperatures fall. Reluctant to face the bleak winter days, people with SAD sleep an average of 2 extra hours each night and hate to get up in the morning. They eat more (especially sweets and starchy foods), often lose interest in sex, and go about their daily routines feeling bored and discontented.

Although most SAD sufferers live in climates with long, icy winters and suffer winter depressions, a few are adversely affected by the summer. Cases of people who grow despondent in summer and elated as the weather gets colder have been recorded since the 1800's. Symptoms of

A GUIDE TO PSYCHOTHERAPEUTIC DRUGS

The drugs used to treat mental disorders can be very effective in relieving symptoms. Like other drugs, psychotherapeutics produce different effects in different people and entail a risk of adverse reactions or unwanted interactions with other drugs and certain foods; antianxiety drugs can also cause dependence. Never use or mix psychotherapeutic drugs without medical supervision.

Drug Class	Common Drugs*	Risks
Antianxiety drugs, or minor tranquilizers, help alleviate feelings of nervousness and tension. BENZODIAZEPINES reduce agitation and promote drowsiness and relaxation; they are also used to treat insomnia. BETA BLOCKERS reduce shaking, sweating, and palpitations.	1. BENZODIAZEPINES: *chlordiazepoxide* (Librium), *diazepam* (Valium), *oxazepam* (Serax) 2. BETA BLOCKERS: *propranolol* (Inderal)	Dizziness, daytime drowsiness, and forgetfulness. Regular use may result in dependence. Withdrawal symptoms may follow abrupt cessation. Fatigue, cold hands and feet, breathing difficulties, slowed heartbeat.
Antidepressants are usually prescribed for serious depression, but are also effective for treating some anxiety and eating disorders. Both TRICYCLICS and MAOI's raise levels of the neurotransmitters serotonin and norepinephrine, chemicals that stimulate brain cell activity. *Fluoxetine* (Prozac), one of a new generation of antidepressants, affects only serotonin levels. Because it appears to have fewer side effects, *fluoxetine* is now the most widely prescribed antidepressant in the U.S.	1. TRICYCLICS: *amitriptyline* (Elavil), *imipramine* (Tofranil) 2. MONOAMINE OXIDASE INHIBITORS (MAOI's): *isocarboxazid* (Marplan), *phenelzine* (Nardil) 3. *Fluoxetine* (Prozac)	Dry mouth, blurry vision, dizziness, drowsiness, constipation, difficult urination. Overdose can cause seizures, coma, and death. Can cause dangerous increase in blood pressure when taken with certain drugs or foods rich in tyramine (such as pickles, beer, red wine, cheese). Overdose may result in seizures and death. Headache, nausea, insomnia, nervousness, weight loss. Severe adverse reactions, including suicidal impulses, have been reported; long-term risks are unknown.
Antimanic drugs may reduce the intensity and frequency of the mood swings of manic-depressive illness, probably by reducing levels of the neurotransmitter norepinephrine.	*Lithium* (Eskalith, Lithane)	Overdose can cause blurred vision, twitching, tremors, electrolyte disturbances, vomiting, and diarrhea. Blood levels of *lithium* must be monitored carefully.
Antipsychotic drugs (also called major tranquilizers or neuroleptics) help suppress grossly abnormal behavior in psychotic patients. One effect of these drugs is to block the action of the neurotransmitter dopamine.	1. PHENOTHIAZINES: *chlorpromazine* (Thorazine), *thioridazine* (Mellaril) 2. BUTYROPHENONES: *haloperidol* (Haldol)	All antipsychotics require careful management and dosage monitoring. Can cause drowsiness, involuntary movements of face and limbs, dry mouth, dizziness, blurred vision, and difficult urination.

*Drug families are in SMALL CAPITALS, generic names are *italicized*, brand names are Capitalized.

SAD have also been observed in desert regions when searing summer heat keeps residents indoors. After long-term confinement in their homes, both desert dwellers and northern natives may develop signs of cabin fever: restlessness, a short fuse, and a tendency to drink too much alcohol. In the worst cases, people hallucinate and turn violent.

What causes SAD, and is there a treatment for it?

Although the causes of SAD remain unclear, the latest research is focusing on melatonin, a hormone produced in the pineal gland deep within the brain. Melatonin helps set the body's biological clock and also influences sleep patterns. Its production appears to decrease as a person is exposed to more sunlight.

One promising treatment is phototherapy, in which people suffering from sunshine deprivation are exposed to high-intensity, broad-spectrum sources of light. When exposed to incandescent light that is 10 to 15 times brighter than room light—approximating the light of a spring sunrise—from as little as 30 minutes to as long as 6 hours per day, many SAD sufferers notice significant improvement in mood and energy levels after only a few days. Such quick results (without side effects) compare favorably with those of antidepressant drugs, which generally take several weeks to work.

Is there anything I can do on my own to shake the winter blues?

If it's only a mild slump, you can take a cue from SAD research. Simply turning on more lights in the house or office should brighten your mood. Move a desk or the kitchen table closer

to a window to catch all the light a winter day has to offer. Wear bright colors to cheer yourself and those around you. Bring fresh flowers into your home whenever possible. Get outdoors as often as you can. Take up cross-country skiing (p. 98) or jogging (for tips on exercising safely in the cold, see page 110). If all else fails, and you can afford it, plan a winter vacation to a tropical island.

For people who get SAD when the temperature starts climbing, turning up the air conditioner and taking long cold showers seem to help lift spirits.

FACT OR FALLACY ?

Depression is a common symptom of menopause

Fallacy. New research is shaking long-held beliefs that women are at increased risk for depression during menopause. A menopausal woman is no more likely to be depressed than are women at other stages of life, according to several studies. The same holds true for women who've had a hysterectomy. Recent British and French research finds the likelihood of depression after a hysterectomy to be no greater than for other major surgical procedures. However, women who undergo a mastectomy appear to be at much higher risk of depression than had been previously realized. But this psychological distress is often relieved after reconstructive surgery is performed.

I've read that several great artists have been manic depressives. Is there a link between creativity and this disorder?

There is no clearly demonstrated link between creativity and manic depression. Many artistic people—including Vincent Van Gogh, Ernest Hemingway, and Edgar Allan Poe— are thought to have suffered from it, but so have people in other walks of life. Manic depression is a mental illness in which a severely depressed state is punctuated by hyperactive, elated episodes. During manic periods, a person feels greatly heightened self-esteem, uncritical self-confidence, grandiosity, and bursts of energy. Such episodes are characterized by spending sprees, sexual escapades, and the start of ambitious projects. When talented manic depressives go through a manic period, their creative outbursts are particularly productive. Manic episodes do not last as long as the depressive parts of the cycle; they generally begin and end abruptly, typically lasting from a few days to a few weeks.

Manic depression, or bipolar disorder, as it's technically called, is rare: While about 20 percent of women and 10 percent of men will experience the more common, or unipolar, form of depression (p. 169) at some point in their lives, only about 1 percent of the population will suffer a bipolar disorder. Unlike unipolar depression, manic depression is equally common among men and women. It is more likely to run in families and is more apt to recur if not treated. Lithium salts have proven highly effective in controlling manic depressive mood swings, but have no effect on unipolar depression (see *A Guide to Psychotherapeutic Drugs*, p. 171).

Is shock therapy still used to treat depression?

Highly criticized in the 1950's and 1960's, shock therapy—or, more accurately, electroconvulsive therapy (ECT)—has recently reestablished credibility with mental health professionals. The treatment consists of applying electric current to the patient's temples for a fraction of a second. The patient loses consciousness, has a convulsion similar to an epileptic seizure, and then falls into a comalike sleep for a few seconds. More than 30,000 patients each year—primarily the victims of severe depression—undergo new, improved forms of ECT without fear of physical harm or significant memory loss.

Much has changed since the days of Olivia De Havilland's horrifying portrayal of the experience in *The Snake Pit,* or of Ken Kesey's indictment of its misuse in *One Flew Over the Cuckoo's Nest.* Patients are thoroughly anesthetized and given muscle relaxants before treatment to prevent the jerky movements that once caused bones to break. Oxygen is administered during treatment to prevent brain damage, and new techniques dramatically reduce the risk of memory loss. In unilateral ECT, for instance, electrodes are attached not one on each temple but one on the right temple and one on the top right half of the head to avoid transmitting current through the brain's left hemisphere, where verbal memory centers. Brief-pulse therapy uses the lowest effective electrical current; voltage ascends rapidly to a high point, is maintained momentarily, and then drops precipitously before the cycle is repeated again.

Curiously, doctors still aren't sure how shock therapy works.

The prevailing theory holds that electrically induced seizures produce changes in brain chemistry. While some critics still maintain that even improved methods can result in memory loss, the National Institutes of Health gave the treatment its approval in 1985, after a blue-ribbon panel concluded that shock therapy is "demonstrably effective for a narrow range of severe psychiatric disorders, including depression, mania, and schizophrenia."

There have been lots of headlines lately about teen suicides. Is suicide in any way "catching"?

Suicide is not contagious in the literal sense. However, if a friend's or classmate's suicide brings the possibility of self-destruction closer to home, makes it seem more like a reasonable solution, then another's suicide could precipitate suicidal thoughts in the mind of a teenager who is already looking for a way out of a tough situation.

For the past 20 years or so, the dramatic rise in the rate of teenage suicide has paralleled the rise in the divorce rate, and many experts are drawing conclusions about the damaging effects of divorce, particularly on adolescent males. Sons of absent fathers have a hard time controlling their impulses, studies show, and an inability to control angry impulses is a hallmark of male suicidal behavior. Research also shows a statistically significant incidence of separation and divorce among parents of teenagers who attempt and commit suicide. (Four to five times more male adolescents actually *commit* suicide than female adolescents do; however, four to five times more females than males *attempt* to take their lives.)

Parents who are separated or divorced cannot change this basic fact, but they should always keep in mind the importance of remaining close to their children, whether living with them or not, and of carefully maintaining open channels of communication with their teenagers.

Families in which both parents work significantly more than 40 hours a week may create a dangerous environment too. Sons (both nursery school age and adolescents) are more likely than daughters to show adjustment problems in homes where both parents work. The overwhelming bulk of evidence indicates that the absence, whether physical or emotional, of supportive, caring adults can put a child's well-being in jeopardy.

My 16-year-old son has suddenly become uncommunicative, and his grades have dropped in school. I'm pretty sure he's not doing drugs. Should I be alarmed?

You should take the situation seriously and talk to your son. Years ago psychiatrists saw adolescence as a time of such colossal emotional upheaval that unpredictable behavior tantamount to mental illness was deemed to be typical of the American teenager. No longer. Now the experts believe that while most children's passages from childhood to adulthood are occasionally stormy, teenagers are generally no more miserable than the rest of the population. Your son's sudden withdrawal and the deterioration of his schoolwork could well be warning signs of a condition more serious than ordinary adolescent moodiness and rebelliousness.

When a child suddenly becomes quiet and withdrawn, forsaking activities that normally interest him, he may be exhibiting symptoms of depression. As early as age 8, depressed children act pessimistic, lose interest in play, and don't want to talk about what's bothering them. By age 12, a depressed child may have physical symptoms such as sleeping problems, loss of appetite, and stomachaches. A depressed 17-year-old may have nightmares and thoughts of suicide as well.

The risk of depression increases with age; 17-year-olds are four times more likely to be depressed than 8- to 12-year-olds, according to one study, which concludes that early recognition and treatment of depression can prevent a melancholy 8-year-old child from becoming a suicidal teenager.

How can I tell if someone is in danger of committing suicide? What can I do to help?

The person most likely to commit suicide sees himself in an unbearable and hopeless predicament. Death seems preferable to continuing to live under such circumstances. Lacking self-esteem, the potential suicide sees no way out of his crisis; he feels not only hopeless, but helpless as well. Alcoholics, drug abusers, the terminally ill, and the chronically depressed make up a high-risk group for suicide.

Someone contemplating suicide may or may not give clues to his intentions. Here are some of the signs to watch out for:
☐ Social withdrawal. The person becomes increasingly withdrawn, socially isolated, often after suffering a major trauma or life stress, such as financial reverses, divorce, the death of a loved one, or chronic illness.
☐ Talk of suicide or death. Con-

trary to popular belief, people who say they want to take their own lives may actually do so. Repeated threats or the revelation of specific plans should be taken as a signal that someone is seriously contemplating suicide.
☐ The giving away of treasured possessions.
☐ The return of a cheerful or calm demeanor. Once a person has decided to commit suicide, he may feel a sense of relief at having finally reached a resolution for his problems. The risk of suicide is greater when a person seems to be recovering from a deep depression.

If you suspect that a friend or relative is in danger of committing suicide, here are some steps you can take to help:
☐ Listen. A potentially suicidal person needs an empathetic ear. Don't criticize, argue, disapprove, or offer too-easy answers. Just be there to help share the burden.
☐ Talk about it. Talking about suicide won't put the idea into a person's mind; it's already there. Help him focus on alternative ways to resolve his problems. Encourage him to talk to a clergyman, mental health professional, or to use the suicide prevention hotline, listed in many local phone books.
☐ Don't leave the person alone. If you feel there is a crisis and you can't handle it yourself, take him to a psychiatrist or physician or to the emergency room of the nearest hospital.

Is grieving a form of depression?

Grief is an unavoidable human emotion, a natural response to life experience and not always a symptom of depressive illness. In reaction to a major loss, such as the death of a beloved spouse, it is a normal and essen-

tial process through which the bereaved mourns the loss and survives it.

Studies have shown that grieving generally progresses through three stages. At first, the bereaved is preoccupied with the person who has died, with his image and memory. Denial very often characterizes this stage. The grieving person tries to hold on to the loved one by holding conversations with him, wearing an article of clothing he used to wear, or developing a taste for food he especially enjoyed. Newly bereaved people often lose things absent-mindedly and then search desperately for them, rejoicing when the seemingly meaningless objects are found; the search is a way to act out hopes that the lost loved one might somehow appear again. While some of this behavior may seem quite bizarre to other people, it is a natural part of the grieving process.

In the second stage, the pain of loss becomes more pronounced as the bereaved works it through and begins to accept the fact that the loved one's absence is permanent. Anger, feelings of despair and emptiness, thoughts that life is really not worth living predominate. Grief colors every experience. It may be felt more strongly at certain times—when a memory overwhelms or a visit to a place enjoyed with the deceased brings on a wave of sadness—but it is always there. "Her absence is like the sky, spread over everything" is how author C. S. Lewis described the pain he felt after the death of his wife.

In the third and final stage of the mourning process, the bereaved returns to normal functioning and behavior. Friendships, often ignored during the second stage, become important again. The constant pall of grief begins to lift, but the pain can return unexpectedly—when the phone rings and a widow hears a salesman ask for her husband, for instance. Anniversaries and holidays will also rekindle the pain of loss, especially during the first year.

When my father died, my mother showed few signs of emotion. Is this normal or even healthy?

A stoic response to death, especially to the death of someone so close as a husband, may not be a good sign. Your mother may not be dealing with her loss, may be denying that your father is gone, and her unresolved grief may present problems later on. If you can get her to talk about your father, perhaps her memories will bring tears and allow her to give in to the natural process of grieving.

Suppressed emotion is only one possible sign that the mourning process may not be proceeding normally. Hysterical grieving—prolonged screaming, fainting, and the development of psychosomatic symptoms—can also be an abnormal reaction to loss. Overreaction and underreaction must be judged, however, in terms of the bereaved's personal and cultural background; what seems an extreme expression of grief in one culture may be normal in another.

Other danger signs include hyperactivity that doesn't leave time for acknowledging the loss; fury at doctors or a hospital that overshadows the loss; and self-destructive behavior (giving away treasured belongings or signing contracts for bad business deals). Unrealistically memorializing the person who has died—either as a faultless saint or as a total villain—is also a sign that grief is unresolved.

HELP FOR A GRIEVING FRIEND

☐ Just by showing up, you let a grieving friend know that you are available for support and solace. The mourner is often in a state of shock and may not remember the words you say but will be comforted by an embrace, a hand to hold, an empathetic ear.

☐ The simplest words—"I'm sorry"—are often the best. Avoid empty cliches—"It's better this way" or "Life goes on"—which seem to deny the bereaved's pain.

☐ The weeks after the funeral, when the initial numbness wears off, can be even more trying than the funeral itself. This is when friends who don't forget are invaluable. Send notes, letters, flowers.

☐ Set up a time to visit; bring old photographs, postcards, or letters to help savor pleasant memories of the deceased. Bringing food, offering to take the children out for a while, or coming up with some other specific plan to help is better than just saying you're available if needed.

☐ See that your friend is not alone on holidays and anniversaries at first.

☐ Perhaps the greatest gift you can offer is to simply sit with a friend and listen while she sobs out her anger and grief or reminisces about the loved one. You will help the bereaved to work through her grief with your act of friendship.

How long does grief usually last?

Research shows that four out of five people emerge from the most acute stages of mourning after about 3 months. Most bereaved people benefit by returning to work or other normal activities in 3 to 6 weeks after a loved one dies, even though their loss will continue to be felt in many ways. And depending on the nature and intimacy of the relationship, the period of intense bereavement varies. Widows and widowers, for instance, remain at increased risk of death for the first year following the death of their spouses. Parents often take many years to recover from the loss of a child. The survivors of murder victims or suicides similarly suffer extended periods of bereavement.

What's the difference between neurosis and psychosis?

In psychoanalytic terms, the words *psychosis* and *neurosis* are used to differentiate the more serious from the less grave types of mental disorders. A psychosis is a major organic or psychological impairment that causes a person to feel, think, or act in seriously deviant ways. Psychosis implies that an individual is out of touch with reality, that his thoughts and actions are so disturbed that he can't cope with the demands of daily life. Psychoses require intensive treatment and sometimes hospitalization.

The most common psychotic disorder is major depression with psychotic features, such as hallucinations and paranoid delusions. Advances in drug therapy now enable many people formerly hospitalized with this disorder to lead symptom-free lives between episodes. Other types of psychoses are schizophrenia (see below) and paranoia. The latter is a persistent delusion usually involving a dangerous personal threat.

Neurosis is an umbrella term for nonpsychotic personality disorders that has fallen out of favor with diagnosticians. Disorders once called neuroses are usually now labeled under more specific categories, such as phobias, anxiety and panic disorders, obsessive-compulsive disorders, and hypochondriasis. People with neuroses generally continue to function in society, although not always at full capacity.

I've heard of drug-induced psychosis. Can drugs really cause a psychosis?

Yes. Heavy long-term use of some drugs, especially amphetamines, can result in psychotic episodes resembling schizophrenia. In one study, which followed drug abusers for 6 years, 55 percent of the chronic stimulant users developed schizophrenic psychoses. Even single doses of PCP, a powerful hallucinogen, can bring on a psychotic episode in which users become disoriented, extremely impulsive, antisocial, and violent.

How common is schizophrenia?

Schizophrenia afflicts more than 2.5 million Americans and costs society at least $20 billion each year. About 1 out of every 100 people will be diagnosed as schizophrenic at some point in their lives. Although the disease can begin at any time, it usually first appears during late adolescence or early adulthood, affecting males and females equally. Perhaps the most feared form of mental illness, schizophrenia, with its hallucinations, delusions,

and separation from reality, is what most people think of when they try to imagine insanity.

No one knows exactly what causes schizophrenia. While drugs can control its symptoms, no cure exists. Enlargement of brain ventricles and excessive sensitivity to the neurotransmitter dopamine have been observed in some studies of schizophrenics. While heredity appears to be a factor in some cases, it does not ensure the development of the disease. An external factor— a viral infection, an obstetrical complication, a traumatic event, or a prolonged period of stress— is needed to trigger the onset of schizophrenia.

Our son is schizophrenic, and his behavior is seriously disrupting our home life. Would it be better to put him in an institution for the sake of the rest of the family?

Schizophrenia causes tremendous suffering, not only to the people afflicted with the disease but to those who love them. Treatment with antipsychotic drugs allows many schizophrenics to function outside a hospital setting much of the time. But the success of this alternative hinges on two conditions: that the schizophrenic will consistently take the drugs, and that the family can provide a sheltered living situation.

Many families cannot withstand the burdens. It's not easy to live with someone who does not bathe; who sits in one place for hours, staring into space and wringing his hands; who hears voices; who screams, curses, and accuses; who may be prone to violent outbursts. A schizophrenic, particularly one who does not always take prescribed medication, may do all

these things. Even if they wanted to and could make the allowances necessary to live with this person, most families can not prevent a schizophrenic from periodically roaming off to destinations unknown. When the problems overshadow the benefits of providing a sheltered setting, placement in a hospital (or day hospital or group home) is a reasonable solution.

Temporary hospitalization during acute episodes is often necessary to provide the family with some relief from the burden of care. Longer-term hospitalization is required for schizophrenics who don't respond to outpatient treatment and consistently refuse to take antipsychotic drugs.

Choosing among the variety of private and public hospitals that exist can seem a formidable task; however, what matters most is the competence of the treating physician. The best way to find expert psychiatric care is to ask every doctor you trust and any other families of schizophrenics you may know. Inquire also about local organizations set up to help schizophrenics and their families.

If the schizophrenic will not agree to voluntary admission, commitment may be necessary. Commitment laws vary from state to state but usually require a petition from an adult relative and an examination of the patient by one or two physicians.

I have a colleague who is obsessively neat and always seems to be washing his hands. Is there a name for this behavior?

He may be suffering from an obsessive-compulsive disorder, a condition that affects up to 5 million Americans. Once in a while most people have fleeting urges to check that the stove has been turned off or that the front door is locked. When you were a child, you probably lined up toy soldiers quite neatly and became furious if anyone interfered with their order. Imagine such feelings vastly magnified and constantly felt, and you will have an idea of what obsessive-compulsive disorder (OCD) is like. OCD sufferers may constantly wash their hands or pull their hair or disinfect their houses. An obsessive-compulsive may stop his car every few blocks to convince himself he has not run over anyone. Or he may feel compelled to leave work repeatedly to make perfectly sure that he has not left a cigarette burning in a wastebasket at home.

Psychotherapy has not been very successful in treating OCD. Although in the past the condition has been linked to childhood conflicts or emotional traumas, such as overly rigid toilet training, the evidence is mounting for a physiological cause. CAT scans have shown physical aberrations in the brains of people with OCD. Treatments with clomipramine and fluoxetine, antidepressants that increase levels of serotonin production in the brain, have helped, offering hope that the repetitive behavior of OCD might be controlled by neurochemical adjustments.

My young niece, an aspiring ballerina, has put herself on a radical weight-loss plan. Is it possible that she's becoming anorexic?

The profession your niece has chosen puts her at higher risk for developing an eating disorder such as anorexia nervosa. Her age and sex do too. Almost all the victims of anorexia are female, and most of them begin to exhibit eating problems during early adolescence. (From 5 to 10 percent of adolescent females suffer from eating disorders, including anorexia nervosa and bulimia.) Whether your niece is actually developing anorexia depends in part on her body image. A ballerina is necessarily concerned with her weight and with the way she looks, an occupational hazard that may predispose your niece to excessive dieting. Does she often talk about herself as being fat even when she is far from overweight? Are her eating habits extremely restrictive—does she limit herself to fewer than 900 calories per day? Does she exercise constantly? Has her weight dropped considerably below the normal range for her bone structure and height? So many young women in our society are preoccupied with thinness that it is difficult to know when such obsession becomes pathological. Talk to your niece about your concerns. If she is not receptive, talk to her parents. If they are worried too, they should get her to agree to see a doctor, preferably one who specializes in eating disorders.

How does anorexia differ from bulimia?

Anorexics compulsively starve themselves and are usually extremely thin. In the worst cases, anorexics lose more than 25 percent of their body weight and require hospitalization to keep them from literally starving themselves to death. Bulimics, in contrast, binge on high-calorie food and purge themselves afterwards, usually by vomiting or taking laxatives. They may be thin, fat, or of normal weight.

Bulimics feel guilty about their food binges and try to keep them secret, making their condition hard to detect. Some signs of bulimia include erosion of tooth enamel from stomach acids that remain in the mouth after vomiting, abrasions on fingers and knuckles from forced vomiting, chronic diarrhea, and dehydration. In severe cases, bulimics may suffer rupture of the esophagus and stomach, kidney failure, and electrolyte imbalances that can lead to heart failure.

Both anorexics and bulimics tend to be young women in their teens or twenties, but they can be older. The distinction between the two conditions is sometimes clouded by the fact that half of all anorexics binge and purge when they are at very low weight, and bulimics may alternate periods of binging with periods of strict dieting.

Anorexics and bulimics alike see themselves as fat even when they are extremely underweight. In their relentless pursuit of thinness, they may exercise so much that they stop having menstrual periods. Their blood pressure and pulse rate will be low, and they may develop an irregular heartbeat. Gastrointestinal problems are also common.

Although the incidence of anorexia has doubled over the past 20 years, it's still a rare condition, affecting less than 1 percent of U.S. teenage girls. Bulimia is far more common, affecting from 4 to 10 percent of female high school and college students.

I have a friend who seems to be a hypochondriac. How can I tell when he's really sick?

Hypochondriasis is a chronic fear of illness and injury. The hypochondriac is so afraid of getting sick that he becomes obsessed with bodily sensations, magnifying them until they feel like aches and pains. Hypochondriacs may in fact have more sensitive nervous systems than most people do, and normal aches and pains may feel more ominous to them. The symptoms hypochondriacs describe are often bizarre and usually don't follow any pattern recognizable as ordinary illness. Because the hypochondriac visits doctors frequently, however, he usually has a good grasp of medical terminology and can sound very expert on the subject of illness.

Anxiety and depression often underlie the hypochondriac's preoccupation with physical pain; he hides his emotional difficulties behind his medical complaints. Like most people, hypochondriacs will develop the symptoms of real diseases sooner or later. It is very difficult—even for doctors and psychiatrists—to distinguish a genuine disease from one presumed to be imagined. As a friend, you shouldn't even try to diagnose. The best help you can give is a referral to a reputable doctor.

The number of hypochondriacs in our society may be on the rise. Since the 1930's the average number of doctor visits Americans make has doubled, to five per year, even though we are no sicker than our ancestors were; 60 percent of our visits to the doctor's office reveal no serious medical condition. We now seek medical care for the common cold, minor backaches, general fatigue—symptoms that went untreated a generation ago.

I am having a lot of trouble sleeping these days. What could be causing my insomnia?

Just about everyone has trouble falling or staying asleep at one time or another. Noisy neighbors or other minor disturbances disrupt sleep. So do major life transitions such as moving to a new town or starting a new job. Older people typically take longer to fall asleep and tend to wake up more often during the night. Half of all men and women over 50 suffer from insomnia, at least occasionally. People on shift work who must change shifts (from day to night or evening) can throw off their biological rhythms, triggering sleep difficulties.

Snoring disturbs the sleep of about 60 million Americans nightly, both the snorers themselves and those who sleep near them. See page 209 for tips on how to stop snoring.

Another cause of insomnia is sleep apnea, a condition usually accompanied by loud snoring, in which the sufferer stops breathing briefly and has to gasp for air up to several hundred times each night. It can be caused by obstructions of the breathing passages (often by enlarged tonsils or adenoids) or by a disorder in the central nervous system that interferes with normal breathing. Although in extreme cases sleep apnea can bring on a stroke or heart attack, the most common result is daytime drowsiness. About 90 percent of those who suffer from sleep apnea are overweight middle-aged men. Treatments for apnea include weight reduction, medication, and in rare cases, surgery.

According to sleep researchers, however, more than half of all insomnia stems from psychological causes, usually anxiety or depression; fears and worries kept at bay during the day return to haunt people at night. Alcohol and drug abuse also interfere with natural sleep cycles.

For several effective ways of dealing with occasional sleep disturbances without the use of sleeping pills, see page 208. If your sleeplessness persists, consult your doctor.

What is the function of dreams?

Freud called dreams the "royal road" to the unconscious and used them to decipher his patients' hidden wishes. Although their function and meaning remains a matter of dispute, we do know that most dreams occur during the light stages of REM sleep, so called for the rapid eye movements triggered by a hyperactive nervous system. While the body rejuvenates itself during states of deeper slumber, the mind seems to go through a process during REM sleep in which information crucial to survival that has been acquired during the waking hours is committed to memory. Thus the contents of dreams often bear a close resemblance to events of the day, but distorted or couched in symbols.

Are nightmares a sign of psychological problems?

Not necessarily. New research shows that people have frightening dreams more often than they think they do (on average, once every 2 weeks) and that the frequency of a person's bad dreams bears no relationship to waking levels of anxiety. Younger people are more apt to have troubled dreams, and frequency tapers off with age. From the age of 8 into their late twenties, people report 10 times as many nightmares as they do in their middle years. Children younger than age 8 are most prone to "night terrors," distinct entities from nightmares, which cause panic so vivid that the dreamer wakes up in the middle of the night screaming.

Also distinct from the occasional bad dream, and more troublesome, are chronic nightmares. These dreams are often lifelike and detailed, with richly observed colors, sounds, pains, tastes, and smells. Dreamers may become someone else in their nightmares or even another species. They have dreams within dreams, and once awake, it often takes them a long time to shake off the dream. In extreme cases, it can take the dreamer 30 minutes or more to figure out whether he is asleep or awake.

The latest theories pinpoint a personality type most likely to have chronic nightmares. So-called thin-boundaried people are unusually open, introspective, and vulnerable. Often artistic and imaginative, they don't quickly dispense with negative emotions as most people do but allow fears and angers to expand and become more intensely felt. In some cases, their fluid emotional states resemble schizophrenia. A significant number of people who suffer from chronic nightmares show some symptoms of schizophrenia or have a family history of mental disorders, especially schizophrenia. They don't necessarily need psychotherapy. But if nightmares are often so vivid that the dreamer wakes in terror and is afraid to go back to sleep, or if fear of nightmares keeps a person from falling asleep, therapy can help.

Post-traumatic nightmares are quite different from chronic nightmares. They tend to occur during the first stages of the sleep cycle (most nightmares occur during REM sleep in the early hours of the morning), and the content of these dreams directly reflects a disturbing experience. The trauma is reenacted in realistic detail and, as the event recedes in memory, the experience gradually weaves itself into less upsetting dreams. The dreams are part of working through the trauma emotionally; therapy is often effective in causing such nightmares to subside.

DREAMWORK

Dreams, it's been said, can provide intuitive solutions to practical problems; they may also help you work through emotional ones. The "meanings" of dreams are usually encoded in symbols and metaphor (there are often puns and jokes, too). Some of the more common dream images are illustrated below.

Most people dream every night, but many don't remember their dreams. Drinking alcohol or taking drugs, especially sleeping pills, impedes dreaming. To increase your recall, try suggesting to yourself "Tonight I will dream" before you go to sleep. Keep pad and pencil by your bed to write down whatever you can remember upon awakening. While deciphering dreams may or may not help you solve problems, the exercise can be fun as well as enlightening.

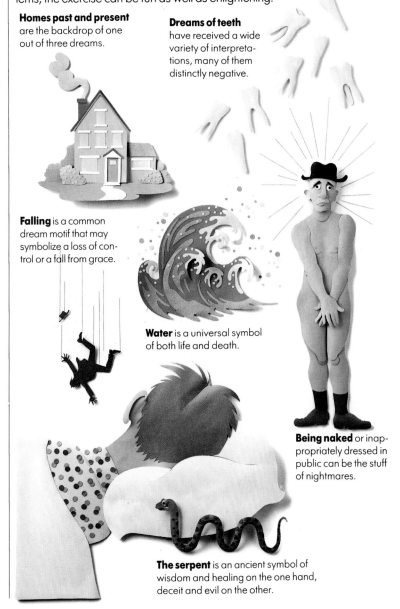

Homes past and present are the backdrop of one out of three dreams.

Dreams of teeth have received a wide variety of interpretations, many of them distinctly negative.

Falling is a common dream motif that may symbolize a loss of control or a fall from grace.

Water is a universal symbol of both life and death.

Being naked or inappropriately dressed in public can be the stuff of nightmares.

The serpent is an ancient symbol of wisdom and healing on the one hand, deceit and evil on the other.

I tend to lash out at people a lot. Can a hot temper be controlled?

As natural as it may feel, a hair-trigger temper isn't something you're born with, like red hair or freckles. It's a habit you've learned, and it can be broken.

Your body reacts to anger-provoking stimuli—a ball thrown through a window or an irritating remark—by releasing epinephrine, norepinephrine, and other hormones. It's the dynamic interplay among these hormones that fuels all our emotions, from fear to excitement, from joy to anger. As hormones flood your system, you feel intensely, but their release does not determine your *reactions* to emotions. You do, depending on the circumstances of the moment and on the habits you have developed for processing feelings. One man will react to a ball thrown through his living-room window by charging out of his house and grabbing the first child he sees by the scruff of his neck. Another will look out the window, see boys playing ball, and fondly recall his own days on the sandlot. Then he'll go out and talk calmly to the boys about paying for the broken glass.

No matter how hot your temper is, you can learn how to respond constructively and appropriately to anger.

☐ Think about your reaction. Count to 10 before you open your mouth, to give yourself time to cool off.

☐ Try putting yourself in the place of the person who's making you angry. Maybe he's having a horrible day or is in pain or has personal problems you know nothing about.

☐ Develop your sense of humor; it's impossible to laugh and scowl at the same time.

☐ Before a crisis erupts, work at reducing your general level of tension. Take up yoga; learn self-hypnosis or another relaxation technique (pp. 206–207).

☐ Try just taking a few deep breaths the next time you feel your temper flaring.

FACT OR FALLACY ?

It's always healthy to vent your anger

Fallacy. People who express their anger don't necessarily feel better. To be cathartic, anger must be expressed appropriately—to the right person, at the appropriate time, and in a constructive way. People who are always furious can build up a pattern of behavior that keeps their blood pressure high and their hearts pounding. Family counselors report that most couples who yell at each other feel more, rather than less, angry afterwards. Also, experts now believe that ulcers, migraine headaches, and other conditions once believed to be the symptoms of repressed anger and agitation, can have multiple causes, including an individual's genetic makeup, habits, and environment.

Jealousy has cost me several important relationships. How can I control this terrible emotion?

There are essentially two kinds of jealousy. The first, usually romantic in nature, is addressed to a person about other people

and has to do with fear of love's loss. The second type, more properly called envy, relates to possessions; what others have detracts from the envious person's happiness. Because both jealousy and envy can be such destructive emotions, they are well worth purging, or at least tempering.

To help dilute the intensity of a dependence that makes you jealous, develop friendships and interests outside your primary relationship. Think about what you have, not what you don't have, when envy haunts you. Television commercials notwithstanding, no one has it all; everyone has problems, and you probably wouldn't want to exchange your life for someone else's if you were to live it in every detail, good and bad. If chronic envy or jealousy is eroding your relationships, talk to a counselor or therapist, who is trained to help you identify any deep-seated sources for your insecurities.

Is competitiveness a healthy trait?

Competitiveness certainly came in handy in primitive times when survival went *only* to the fittest. Today it continues to serve a purpose when it brings out people's best efforts and drives them to fulfill potential. But when a comparative attitude clouds all other points of view, it fosters unhealthy competition. We Americans are prone to excessive comparisons; watching television, we can gauge our progress against the lifestyles of movie stars and millionaires and come up short. In the business world, some people are so driven by their competitive instincts that they resort to unethical practices. Measuring well-being by the numbers and in terms of other people, we sometimes forget that there are other, more rational ways of measuring things. We forget that we are not all the same and that we don't necessarily want the same things. When a young scientist resents the success of a former classmate, even though that classmate is a lawyer and has done well in a field completely unrelated to science, his competitive instincts no longer serve his best interests. Competitiveness is a healthy trait only when it is balanced by generosity and a sense of proportion.

They say that women are more comfortable talking about their emotions than men. Is this a good thing?

Women and men experience very similar feelings but differ dramatically when it comes to showing them. In one study, participants were asked to write descriptions of themselves. Although men and women revealed about the same amount of information, the women's revelations were of a much more intimate nature. Researchers conclude that, despite the revolutionary social changes of recent decades, women still express their feelings more naturally.

There are two exceptions: anger and sexual arousal. In scientific experiments, when men were presented with situations meant to make them angry, they got angry; women said they felt disappointed, hurt, or sad. When men and women listened to tapes of an erotic story, almost half the women claimed that they were not sexually aroused; all of the men reported being aroused.

Social expectations are still strong enough, apparently, to make some men suppress such emotions as sadness and compassion, which are considered "unmanly," while some women suppress anger and sexuality.

That both sexes are limited in emotional self-expression by rigid ideas of what's appropriate for men and women is unfortunate. Men can be damaged by losing touch with their emotions; women can suffer too, if they personalize life's difficulties. Men tend to view the world concretely and more readily attribute failures to external factors, while women are apt to see things in terms of relationships and tend to blame themselves when things go wrong, a characteristic that can lead to depression. Such disparate viewpoints often make it hard for men and women to communicate with each other.

My husband tends to keep things to himself, and I feel left out. How can I get him to open up more?

Your husband has been brought up in a culture where boys are still raised differently from girls. Recent studies show that parents ask their 18-month-old daughters how they're feeling much more often than they ask 18-month-old sons. Mothers talk about feelings with 2-year-old girls more than they do with 2-year-old boys. When parents tell stories to their preschoolers, they tend to use more emotional emphasis with girls—except when the emotion concerned is anger. Parents urge little boys to control their feelings and reward little girls for expressions of emotional closeness.

Assuming he wants to change, it will take time and effort for your husband to do so. Try drawing him out. Ask him how he's feeling more often. Wait for him to respond, and show him that you're interested and appreciative when he does express his emotions. You might want to pay attention to how you're raising your children, too, so that you don't inadvertently pass on outmoded stereotypes to them.

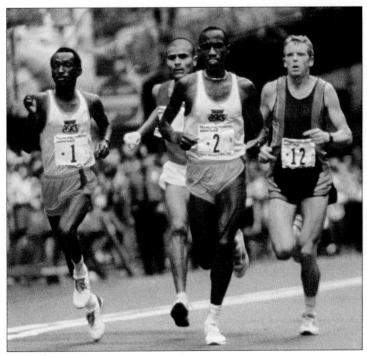

Competitiveness, if properly channeled, can fuel winning efforts.

I grew up in a very strict household, feeling guilty about many things. Now that I'm an adult, how can I overcome this pervading sense of guilt?

Most people live with a certain amount of guilt; a little is not necessarily a bad thing because it helps us to distinguish right from wrong, to use our conscience and compassion.

Pervasive guilt is another matter altogether. If you constantly feel ashamed of yourself, unsatisfied with your accomplishments, unworthy of what happiness you have achieved, your experience of life is marred. Try to distinguish between healthy guilt (which focuses on distinct problems you can do something about) and unhealthy guilt (a constant sense of responsibility for everything, including circumstances beyond your control). Pay attention only to the former.

The typical victim of unhealthy guilt is an overcommitted, perfectionistic, apparently selfless person who grants herself little time or pleasure but still manages to feel guilty about having any sort of a life at all. Perhaps because their roles have changed dramatically within the last generation, women (particularly working mothers of young children) are more likely to suffer from guilt than men. If this describes your predicament, try drawing up two lists—one with all the things you could change (spend more time reading to the baby or taking her to the park, for example) and the other with those things you really can't change. Work on the items in the first list; don't worry about the second. Removing the responsibility for carrying the whole world on your shoulders will help alleviate the dull ache of constant guilt.

Can guilt be used positively?

Guilt is an emotional compass; it points us in the right moral direction. Pangs of guilt help us correct our behavior when we are at risk of hurting ourselves or others. Like many things, guilt is good in moderation. A reasonable dose of guilt motivates us to make changes; when we correct our mistakes, we still those internal recriminations. People who always feel guilty take too much blame on themselves and should learn to distinguish between what they can and can't control.

People who almost never experience guilt are sociopaths, capable of committing all sorts of crimes with little remorse. Without guilt, Freud said, there would be no counterforce to the pleasure principle. Humans would be no different from animals, and society would plunge into chaos.

We're a black family living in a largely white area. How can I instill ethnic pride in my children while encouraging them to partake fully of our society?

Nurture your children's self-esteem so that they can take pride and pleasure in the ways that they are different, as well as in the ways that they are the same as others around them. Love and affection, open communication, and a sense of spiritual values are the basis for any family's contentment.

Family reunions and get-togethers with black friends will help your children develop ethnic pride. Make African American art, music, and literature a natural part of your family's cultural life. Read African fables to a toddler at bedtime. Allow a grade-schooler to choose among dolls of different complexions, and seek out games with multiracial themes. Help a teenager decorate his room with a Caribbean motif. Celebrate the birthdays of black American heroes—not only Martin Luther King, Jr., but Harriet Tubman, Marcus Garvey, and Sojourner Truth, for example. Keep a close eye on what your child is absorbing about blacks from the media. When your children encounter racism, talk about these experiences. Make sure they know that something is wrong with racist attitudes, not with them. Finally, the best way to ensure your child's ethnic identity is to be proud of your own. Setting an example is the most effective way to educate a child about almost any subject.

I seem to put myself down a lot. What causes low self-esteem? What can I do to build myself up?

We are all constantly talking to ourselves, sending private messages about who we are and how likely we are to get what we want and need. Frequently these messages are negative, and the accumulation of self-inflicted insults eventually lowers self-esteem. Here are a few typical examples: "I'm a loser." "I can't do anything right." "I always say the wrong thing."

Certain ways of thinking characterize negative messages. Globalizing—seeing things as black or white with no room for gray areas—makes it hard to regard yourself as anything but perfect or perfectly awful. The key words *always* and *never* reflect the belief that you are fated to repeat the same mistakes over and over. We all know people who can listen to a litany of compliments and nevertheless fixate on one less-than-glowing comment. They sift through praise searching for criticism. Many of us discount successes and highlight failures; when we achieve something, it's no big deal, but when we fail to achieve, we punish ourselves.

If this scenario sounds familiar, try revising your internal dialogue. The first step is to listen to yourself. The next time you're feeling low, ask yourself what you're thinking. What was the last thought you had about yourself? Get a notebook and write down these thoughts, along with your feelings about them and some information about the situation that triggered them. Identify words like *all, nothing, always,* or *never* and edit them out. Think through what's really true about you in the situation. If you made a mistake on a report at work, is that what you "always" do, or are you actually pretty competent? Revise your message to yourself by writing it out in your notebook. Then practice sending yourself more realistic and positive signals by being conscious of—and consciously altering—your interior monologues.

To build up your self-esteem, you must not only revise your thinking, but also act on the positive new messages you are sending yourself. If you are living in an oppressive environment, try to find ways to alter it or leave it. Set realistic goals and credit yourself for small changes.

I often let people walk all over me and then feel angry about it when it's too late. How can I learn to assert myself more effectively?

Standing up for your rights promptly prevents the buildup of hostility. It also saves you from holding on to your anger and

ASSERTING YOURSELF

Classes in assertiveness training are being given all over the country today. Their aim is not, as is often supposed, to make people more aggressive but to defuse anger before it builds up and to enhance communication between people who live and work together. Here are some of their basic strategies:

☐ Experiment with simple assertions first. Choose a waiter who's just served you a cold bowl of soup before confronting your mother about the way she's been belittling you since you were 3 years old.

☐ Focus on nonverbal cues. Make eye contact. Stand straight and tall, with your head high. Don't smile nervously or giggle when you're telling someone you are angry. Don't whisper or scream; speak in a well-modulated voice.

☐ Make sure that your timing is opportune, and choose a quiet, private place to talk.

☐ Don't spend so much time fretting over which words to use that you delay speaking up. Expressing your needs, even if imperfectly, is better than saying nothing at all.

☐ Remember to listen to what the other person is saying. Don't focus so much on what you're getting off your chest that you miss the apology you got all fired up to elicit in the first place.

turning it against yourself. Nevertheless, it's seldom too late to own up to your feelings and to assert yourself appropriately. If a troublesome situation has gone on for a long time, you can start by saying something such as, "I've been concerned about this for quite some time and…" or "I've been meaning to talk to you about…"

Asserting yourself means taking responsibility for your own feelings. Center your comments on how the situation makes *you* feel. "I'm angry…" or "It really upsets me…"—not "You drive me crazy when…" or "You always take advantage of…" Then offer a constructive suggestion for how you would like to see the situation improved.

Happily, you don't have to go through a major personality change to start becoming assertive. Changing your daily behavior—standing up for yourself in specific situations—will eventually strengthen your attitudes. Being assertive gets easier each time you try.

Can holding in emotions cause physical illness?

Evidence exists that people who stifle their feelings may be more vulnerable to certain illnesses. According to several British and U.S. studies of patients with breast, skin, and other cancers, emotionally repressed people are more likely to develop cancer than people who express themselves.

However, the exact mechanism by which biological and psychological factors may interact to cause disease is still unclear. It's important to remember that most physical illness stems from physical causes and is rarely, if ever, solely emotional in origin.

It's also true that nobody is doomed to an emotionally arid existence. If you are suppressing long-buried feelings, psychotherapy can help you ventilate them. You can also help yourself. Learn to respond appropriately to anger and frustration when you're feeling them and you may prevent the buildup of acute stress, which can lead to physical and emotional breakdown. Practice a relaxation technique (pp. 206–207) and exercise regularly. Seek out the emotional support you need. Foster your friendships and family relationships so that people are there for you to turn to in times of trouble.

Is there anything to the theory that humor and positive thinking can cure disease?

"A merry heart doeth like good medicine." Long before scientists began to explore the relationship between humor, positive thinking, and health, the Bible reported their healing effects. Today, we know more specifically how laughter helps people breathe easier, massages the heart and other vital organs, and how it may increase the release of disease-fighting cells in the immune system. Like exercise, laughter quickens the pulse and stimulates the cardiovascular system. In experiments, students who watched funny movies were found to have an increased flow of infection-fighting proteins in their saliva.

A positive outlook also guards against illness and may even increase longevity. Optimistic World War II veterans followed for 35 years after the war ended developed fewer health problems—including hypertension, diabetes, and back trouble—and lived longer than their pessimistic counterparts. Scientists now connect pessimism not only with depression but consider it a risk factor for disease, just like high blood pressure or smoking. Pessimists are more likely to develop physical illnesses when stressed and take longer to recover after surgery.

Children are naturally cheerful, and psychologists speculate that their emotional buoyancy may be part of our species' survival mechanism, that optimism helps protect the young from disease until they can reach puberty and reproduce. Optimism may also have helped to preserve the species in prehistoric times. Although realism saved cave men and women from being gobbled up by tigers, without an optimistic sense of adventure, they would never have ventured away from the cave in the first place.

I'm incapable of getting anywhere on time. What can I do to change?

People who are chronically late may be expressing unconscious hostility. By making others wait, you are covertly telling them that your time is more valuable than theirs. If this describes your emotional state, think about why you're angry and work on expressing anger in a more direct, positive way. Not only does your chronic tardiness cause you to miss appointments and disappoint or anger others, but being late all the time probably makes you a nervous wreck.

First, recognize that everyone has bad habits and that while it may not be easy, habits can be changed. The first step should be a small one. Perhaps you might sit down at a time when you can relax and jot down the experiences of a typical day. Analyze your schedule. Are you trying to accomplish too much? Are there any activities you can drop? Ways to streamline? Pockets of time wasted that could be recovered?

CHANGING HABITS

Bad habits detract from your enjoyment of life and may lead to health problems. Attack an unwanted behavior or trait on four fronts: physical, emotional, cognitive, and situational.

☐ Learn how to relax. When you're tempted by, say, a bag of potato chips, sit down, close your eyes, and do the relaxation exercises described on pages 206–207. Take a few deep breaths; keep in mind that the urge will pass.

☐ Recharge yourself emotionally, using meditation or another form of mental relaxation. Reward yourself for small victories over your bad habit. When in doubt, smile. People who try to find something funny in their dilemmas feel better sooner than those who have a good cry.

☐ Adapt the techniques of cognitive therapy (p.193) for your own use. List, then analyze, the reasons you want to quit drinking, for instance, and the reasons you don't. Get a clear view of what drinking means to you, and reinvent yourself as an ex-drinker.

☐ Situational triggers— places, people, or events— may elicit unwanted behavior. If watching TV is your cue to snack, take a walk or read a book instead, or try doing exercises while you watch. If those tactics fail, at least substitute a healthful snack for that calorie-rich dish of ice cream.

Develop a habit of promptness one day at a time. Make your first goal a fairly easy one. If you're a morning person, try getting to work on time or a little early. If the afternoon is an easier part of the day, make a commitment to pick the baby up at day care on time every day for a week. Be realistic about accomplishing your goal and reward yourself for achieving it.

Seek out support. Find another friend who's also late all the time and make a bet. Whichever one of you can be on time for aerobics class 3 days running treats the other to a salad after the third workout. Soon you'll start to notice the benefits of being on time. You will feel more relaxed, friends and family will appreciate your efforts to respect their time, and your smoother-running life will become its own reward.

My 15-year-old daughter has always been shy and shows no signs of coming out of her shell. Is there anything I can to do to help her?

Shyness is a common childhood experience, and teenage girls in particular are apt to be shy. The importance of being popular at this age and the budding of sexuality can escalate insecurities.

You can help your daughter cope with this difficult stage by encouraging her to learn and practice social skills. Give her dancing lessons for her birthday. Help her learn to play the guitar or the piano. Since looking her best will bolster her confidence, make sure she is well groomed and dresses stylishly.

Breaking free of shyness is not accomplished overnight, so don't try to force her to become the life of the party before she is ready.

Respect her natural inclinations and support small, step-by-step changes. Perhaps going off to college or taking a summer job will nurture her independence.

I've always enjoyed being by myself. Is having many friends a necessary component of mental health?

People do need people. A time and place for solitude exists in all of our lives, and a quiet walk in the woods or a meditative afternoon on a deserted beach can be delightful, but too much isolation is not good for your mental and physical health. The true loner, the hermit who habitually prefers his own company to that of others, is a rare individual.

A solid network of family and friends can help you deal with stress and make it less likely that you will suffer from depression, anxiety, and other mental health problems. (A rewarding social life has also been found to increase longevity and lower the risk for developing cancer, heart disease, and other major illnesses.)

On scales of psychological satisfaction, friendships measure lower than stable marriages as a source of happiness but rate higher than work or leisure pursuits for most people. Friendships are usually strongest in youth, from adolescence until marriage, and again in old

---

IF YOU ARE SHY

Shyness is an almost universal experience. In a national survey conducted at Stanford University, 80 percent of those interviewed reported being shy at some point in their lives. Over 40 percent said they were presently shy and only about 7 percent had never experienced feelings of shyness.

Most shyness is a learned response to specific situations that are viewed as threatening. Shy people generally feel uneasy with strangers, authority figures, or members of the opposite sex. The experience ranges from mild discomfort in unfamiliar settings to intense, panic-like fear of any social interaction.

In recent years, workshops and clinics have sprung up to help people overcome what can be a disabling emotional handicap. They are proving that, contrary to popular belief, even chronic wallflowers can blossom into social butterflies when they understand what makes them shy and take small, slow steps to change their behavior. Here are some of the social exercises that are taught in these workshops:

☐ Instead of focusing on the impression you think you are making, focus on the other person. Put yourself in that person's shoes; empathize with his or her feelings.

☐ Start saying hello to every person you normally see.

☐ Begin to strike up simple conversations with strangers in nonthreatening public places, such as doctors' waiting rooms, libraries, banks, and lines at the supermarket or the movies.

☐ Don't expect an instant metamorphosis.

☐ If you think someone deserves a compliment, offer one, and allow yourself to enjoy the compliments you receive.

age, when retirement and bereavement can decrease other social attachments. The fact that women usually manage to make better psychological adjustments than men after divorce or the death of a spouse is due at least in part to the broader social networks they develop.

Exactly how friendships guard mental (and physical) health is not completely clear. Some psychologists surmise that friends act as buffers, protecting us from stress, and when they make us feel loved and appreciated, nurture one of our most vital assets, self-esteem.

I live alone in a big city and am sometimes lonely. Would it be a good idea to get a pet?

If you're willing to accept the responsibilities involved, a pet makes an excellent companion. Dogs are notoriously uncritical fans of their owners. Cats are a bit harder to please but are easing out dogs as America's favorite pet. Naturally independent, they require less attention than dogs do. Tropical birds and fish also make fine pets.

The sort of creature you invite to share your home will depend on your personality. But feline or canine, fish or fowl, any pet is good for your health. In one study, pet owners proved five times less likely to die a year after suffering a heart attack than did petless people. Stroking your cat—or even watching goldfish swim in a tank—has been shown to lower blood pressure. Like human friends, pets bring you out of yourself by connecting with you and relying on you. You can talk to them, and though they seldom talk back, they make excellent confidantes. Most pets are never in a bad mood and seldom criticize what you're watching on television.

Making friends is easy for me, but committing to a love relationship isn't. Should I be worried?

You are not unique; commitment isn't always easy. People run all the possible unhappy endings through their minds, question their own feelings, and doubt that those feelings are shared. Many wind up choosing the safety of independence over the risks of rejection. And then, in solitude, they yearn for connection.

The qualities that attract us to lovers are not all that different from the qualities that draw us to friends. People tend to like people who are similar to them, who have compatible interests and attitudes. One salient distinction between friendship and romance (in addition to passion) however, has to do with commitment.

With romantic love, the emotional stakes are considerably higher. Except in times of crisis, friends don't expect to head your list of priorities; lovers do. To get closer to someone, you must open up and trust that person enough to reveal things about yourself—your values, experiences, expectations, your triumphs and failures, joys and sorrows. Shy people, and people who have been burned before, are particularly reluctant to do this.

Worrying about difficulties with commitment won't help, but working at your problems with intimacy will. Anxious and afraid that trust will be betrayed, many people set up conscious or unconscious barriers to commitment. These must be taken down slowly and gingerly, sometimes with the help of professional counseling. But the struggle is worthwhile; the alternative is to deny your very human need for love and understanding.

I've just begun dating again after a divorce and am uncomfortable with the whole process. Any suggestions?

Once you've been on the sidelines for a while, this mysterious mating dance called dating can be petrifying. Men wonder whether

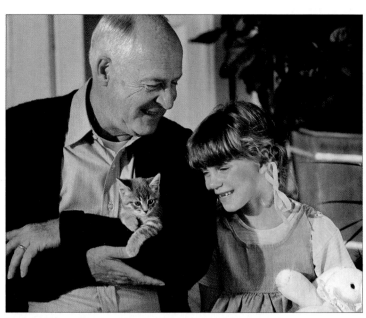

The health benefits of owning pets have been well documented.

they should still take full responsibility—for making the phone call to set up the date, for deciding where to go and what to do, for making the first move sexually. Women don't know whether they must wait for a man to make all the traditional moves. Should they still sit by the phone, willing it to ring? Social attitudes are changing; it's now permissible for a woman to ask a man out on a date and for a man to accept. Sex-role reversals can be liberating, but sometimes these switches only make matters more confusing.

Whether you're male or female, fear of rejection is the central issue in post-divorce dating. No matter how much you think you're over your ex, you may find the slightest hint of disapproval brings the pain rushing back.

If you look for rejection, you will find it. Don't set yourself up by being apologetic and self-effacing. Instead, pamper yourself before you go out on a date. Dress to look your best; visualize yourself as gorgeous, fascinating, self-assured. While you're out, assume your date is attracted to you. If you still get dumped, don't personalize the rejection; the reason behind it may have little or nothing to do with you. Some dating disasters are unavoidable. Have faith in yourself, maintain your sense of humor, keep trying, and the odds for success will be in your favor.

I've always been nervous and shy with the opposite sex. How can I overcome this?

If everybody were a raving extrovert, the world would be a rather noisy place, wouldn't it? Many people—male and female—find a quiet, modest, refined personality refreshing. Gregarious sorts are always pleased to meet good listeners. Others, as socially inhibited as you are, will bask in the presence of a kindred spirit. When you're feeling nervous and shy, you may imagine that everyone is analyzing you with special attention to all your shortcomings. The truth is, most people are thinking about themselves, how uncomfortable they're feeling, and what kind of impression they're making on *you*.

Don't try to overcome your shyness with alcohol or drugs. Chemical courage will only add to your problems. And don't worry about presenting a polished image; relax and be yourself. What's different about you is often the quality that makes you most endearing.

How do I tell the difference between love and sexual attraction?

It's not easy. A strong sexual attraction is dizzying and can feel, at least at first, just like falling in love. Physical closeness seems to spill over into emotional intimacy, and the desire to be together is strong.

Sexual attraction plays a crucial role in the initial stages of romantic involvement, but other qualities, such as honesty, reliability, emotional stability, become more important when a real, multidimensional relationship develops. If you're in love, you'll enjoy each other's company when you're not in each other's arms. You become best friends. Trust develops. You tell each other your life stories and begin to include each other in the present chapters of those tales. Passion continues to play a vital part in the most successful love affairs, no matter how many wedding anniversaries have passed. But mutual care and concern become more important, enduring signs of love.

FACT OR FALLACY?

Being married is good for your health

Fact. Married people generally live longer than single people do. In a 1987 study of populations in 16 industrially developed countries conducted at Princeton University, the average death rates for unmarried men were found to be twice as high as those for married men and one and a half times higher for unmarried as for married women. Divorced people, especially men, had the highest death rates. The researchers who conducted the study said that two factors might account for these statistics. Healthier people could be more likely to marry; and sharing the stresses of life with a partner may increase longevity by making those stresses easier to bear. One final note: The benefits of marriage appear to apply more strictly to men than to women. Married men have been found to have fewer mental illnesses, fewer physical complaints, and to be generally happier than unmarried men. Married women, however, have higher rates of depression than married men or than single women have; one possible explanation is that single women are more likely than single men to maintain supportive networks of family and friends.

Can someone be addicted to sex?

People claim to be addicted to everything from shopping malls to hot fudge sundaes. There are 12-step groups, based on the principles of Alcoholics Anonymous (see *The Facts About 12-Step Programs,* p.164), not just for alcoholics and drug addicts, but for their families, for neurotics, overeaters, gamblers, and those who say that sex enslaves them.

Certainly some people behave compulsively when it comes to sex, and 12-step groups are of great help to many people. But whether sexual activity is literally habit-forming is another matter. Certain celebrities, blaming their behavior on sex addiction, appear to be letting themselves off the hook. Most people who have sex want to have it again, but people deprived of sex do not have physical withdrawal symptoms, as addicts do. The issue is often one of responsible control.

I've recently developed a strong attachment to someone of the same sex, and for the first time in my life, I'm confused about my feelings. Could I be bisexual?

You are confused about a confusing and inadequately studied subject. In his famous studies of sexual mores in the 1940's and 1950's, psychologist Alfred Kinsey found that 37 percent of men and 13 percent of women had direct homosexual experience at some time in their adult lives. Fifty percent of the men Kinsey studied had been sexually attracted to other men, whether or not they had acted on it. Kinsey found that 18 percent of white men in his study had equal amounts of homosexual and heterosexual experience for at least 3 years between the ages of 16 and 55. Between 4 and 11 percent of unmarried women had homosexual experiences as frequently as heterosexual experiences between the ages of 20 and 35. Bisexual orientation, Kinsey proved, is far from rare.

Your attachment to a member of the same sex doesn't necessarily mean that you are bisexual or homosexual. Among other things, the Kinsey Reports supplied evidence that sexual orientation is a matter of degree, and that sexual behavior varies widely across a spectrum, from exclusively heterosexual to exclusively homosexual.

Although research is scanty in this area, there is evidence that bisexuality is a true sexual orientation that can exist in one of three ways: 1) transitionally, as Freud suggested, 2) historically, as a particular experience in the sexual history of a basically homosexual or heterosexual person, or 3) sequentially, as an ongoing situation in which relationships with both sexes alternate.

Because bisexuality is generally regarded as rare, if not mythical, most bisexuals discover their orientation relatively late in life, usually not until they are in their twenties or thirties. If you are disturbed about the ambivalence of your feelings, you might benefit by discussing them with a psychotherapist.

Between work and family, I no longer seem to have time for my friends. What role should friendship play in adult life?

Friends are often the closest social attachments, not only for singles but for married people too—particularly married women whose spouses are not natural confidantes. No spouse should be expected to fulfill all your needs for intimacy. Friends help married people maintain an identity outside the confines of coupledom, and this independence will bolster a good marriage. Psychologists note a high correlation between loneliness and depression, so solid friendships help keep you emotionally healthy.

Make time for your friends, no matter how busy your life has become. Be there in a crisis; when a good friend needs you, do everything you can to help. Arrange get-togethers just as you would book business meetings or the children's dental appointments. Even if it's just a half-hour for coffee, maintain and enjoy regular contact with treasured friends. If you can't find time to write letters, send greeting cards or postcards to friends who live far away. You can also make telephone calls to their answering machines during the day even though you know they'll be at work. A 1-minute electronic visit costs only pennies and will be a pleasant surprise for your friend.

What are the qualities of a good friend?

Friends care about you. At work they make the day pass more smoothly, by helping and advising you as well as by making the workplace more fun. Neighbors can also be good friends, feeding the cat while you're on vacation, lending a cup of sugar, sharing a beer while admiring your newly mowed lawn. The parents of your children's friends can become your friends too, since you have major interests in common. Swapping babysitting or chauffering services are among the many practical ways you can help each other.

But the best friends are usually

long-term ones, linked to you by a common past. The friends you've known the longest provide perspective on life's changes; your shared history can be buoying in times of transition and stress. These lasting connections don't rely on geography or circumstance for glue. Years can pass and oceans can divide, but one phone call can erase time and distance.

Of course, even the dearest, oldest friends can be estranged when tumultuous changes— marriages, births, divorces— create tension. Good friends feel free to tell you what they *really* think. Such heartfelt honesty can hurt feelings and stir up controversy, even as it proves a friend cares. Although they can't always be objective, true friends will stand by you, offering their opinions but ultimately supporting, with all their strength, your right to be yourself.

___

I've been accused of being abrasive at work, but my male colleagues are rewarded for the same behavior. How can I reconcile my natural competitiveness with my boss's expectations of "feminine" work habits?

This is a two-sided problem involving your behavior and his. Women in positions of authority are still a novelty for many in the business world, and even today some men perceive ambitious women as tough and pushy. Unfair or not, it's realistic to recognize that women are still often judged by different standards than men are.

The best policy is one of honesty coupled with tact. Be assertive, not hostile. Go after your goals calmly and straightforwardly. Camouflaging your career goals with soft speech and softer outfits won't work. You must carefully balance your image. Take your boss's (and your co-workers') feelings into consideration; respond sensitively and respectfully to others' needs, but don't sacrifice your legitimate ambitions to them. When you must criticize others, do so in a constructive, nonjudgmental way. Do all you can to let your boss know you are a talented team player.

If you are following this scenario, you are not, in fact, too abrasive. If your boss continues to treat you differently from your male colleagues, calmly point out the discrepancy to him. Then, if he can't change, you may want to consider changing your job situation.

___

I have a hard time taking criticism. How can I use it more constructively?

You will have a hard time taking criticism if you let it affect your self-esteem. It's easier said than done, but try not to take every criticism to heart. Remember, you're the final arbiter of your own success. Criticism is easiest to take when it's expressed privately in a respectful, nonparental way. When you're read the riot act in public, made to feel like a naughty child or a useless fool, it's harder to concentrate on the value of the advice. But you can do it.

The way to use criticism constructively is to weed out any emotional reactions you may feel about the incident and the criticizer and, like an editor or a shopper, identify and isolate those elements that might be of value to you in learning more about yourself and advancing your own future. Concentrate on the rewards you'll reap by changing. Then develop reasonable goals, define what steps are needed to achieve them, and take that first step.

___

My boss is always putting women down or making unwanted advances, and it's affecting my ability to work with him. How should I handle this?

Sexual harassment in the workplace is illegal today. The regional office of the Equal Employment Opportunity Commission can evaluate your situation and advise you, and your state bar association can refer you to an attorney experienced in labor law. However, unless your boss's behavior is totally disruptive or dangerous, suing him should be your last resort.

In your best interests, try to handle the situation intelligently and prudently. When put-downs or come-ons are hurtful, respond immediately in a dignified, nonaggressive way. Don't answer insults with insults; your goal is not to humiliate the boss or to engage him in ideological debate. Find out whether he is capable of learning and changing. Take him aside and calmly explain that women have been judged more on appearance than ability for too long. Keep your sense of humor. Don't stomp all over the boss's ego. If you publicly criticize his sexist behavior, he may get back at you— consciously or unconsciously— by withholding a promotion.

Some old-fashioned men still regard flirtation as a form of flattery, and it would take a monumental effort to raise their consciousness. In such cases it may be better policy to ignore stupid remarks and to concentrate on career goals that will gradually move you out of the sexist's domain.

I was promoted recently and instead of rejoicing, became depressed. Is there such as thing as fear of success?

In the late 1960's psychologist Matina Horner conducted a study of people's reactions to professional achievement. When told the story of Anne, a medical school student at the top of her class, 62 percent of Horner's female subjects expressed conflict over Anne's success, while only 9 percent of the male subjects reacted negatively to the story of a man's success. What the women associated with success were social rejection, doubts about their normality, and denial that the success was real.

Times and sex roles have changed, and these kinds of tests no longer have such a female bias. Fears that success will bring rejection, conflict, overwork, or stress seem to grip as many contemporary men as women.

Fear of success, sometimes rooted in guilt over surpassing the achievements of one's parents, is by no means uncommon. Such feelings may drive people to self-defeating behavior that sabotages their own best efforts.

A related problem for some successful people is an "impostor" complex: capable achievers doubt their abilities and believe that they have become successful only by fooling everybody around them. Seemingly poised and confident, they are tormented by a fear of being found out.

Sometimes, just recognizing that many other people are grappling with these same problems is enough to overcome them. Try exploring your own feelings about your new position with your spouse or a close friend. If your fears become debilitating, however, you should seek help from a professional counselor.

IF YOU ARE FIRED

Losing your job, like divorce or a death in the family, is one of life's most stressful events. No matter why it happened—company cutbacks, layoffs after a merger, differences with your boss—you can't help feeling shocked and betrayed. Your livelihood and your self-esteem have suddenly been pulled out from under you. If you don't deal realistically with the situation, your health can suffer too. Here are some guidelines for coping:

☐ Vent your feelings among sympathetic family and friends who will let you safely explore all your emotions. This is a major, sometimes unforeseen change in your life, and you'll need time to come to terms with your sense of loss, your anger, and your fears about the future. If your bitterness persists, consider some professional counseling.

☐ Take stock of yourself. Analyze what happened. Were you in any way at fault? What can you learn about yourself from this experience? Did you *like* that job, or might boredom have affected your performance? Think about what you really *want* to do. A firing can be a great opportunity to make changes in your professional life that you may have been afraid to try before.

☐ If the services of an outplacement firm are included in your severance package, take advantage of the counseling to help you reevaluate your aptitudes and to explore other types of work that might be more fulfilling for you. Otherwise, consider hiring an outplacement firm with a strong counseling service yourself. Such companies don't find you a job; they help you to evaluate your own potential and to develop an effective job-hunting strategy appropriate for your field.

☐ Keep up your health routines. It's easy to slip into bad habits when you are upset—eating or drinking too much, slacking off on your exercise regimen—but it is during emotional turmoil that you need your health disciplines most. This kind of stress affects the immune system and makes you more susceptible to viruses, headaches, and high blood pressure. Practicing your own preventive medicine is your best defense.

☐ Make the job search your full-time work. If you have use of an office through an outplacement firm, go to it every day. Or set up an office at home and keep regular 9-to-5 hours. Work as hard selling yourself as you would on your ideal job.

I've been passed over for a job I really wanted. How can I use this failure constructively?

Don't label yourself a failure because you lost out on one promotion; the only people who never fail are those who never take chances. Pessimists see failure as defeat; optimists see it as an opportunity to learn and try again. Try to separate your emotional reaction to losing out from the reality of what occurred. If you analyze what went wrong, the incident could yield some valuable lessons: how to present yourself better, how to develop an argument, how to use the right timing to ask for and get what you want. The sooner you put your loss into perspective, the better you'll feel.

☐ Be objective. If you lost the job because you lack a certificate or don't have a particular skill, use this experience as an impetus to get the training you need to advance.

☐ If your credentials are impeccable, how do you get along with others at work? Success in business depends not only on competence but on politics, strategy, and human relations skills.

☐ If you're not advancing fast enough, reconsider your line of work. It's possible that you're not well suited to the field you've chosen. Changing careers may be the best way to get ahead.

Taken constructively, failure is a great reality check. Stumbling helps you to distinguish your true goals, to separate them from daydreams and fantasies. Only when you know what you really want can you dedicate yourself thoroughly to success.

My fear of public speaking is beginning to affect my career. What can I do about it?

Almost everyone hates to speak in public. In one recent poll, public speaking surpassed flying, loneliness, and even *death* as the experience people feared most. With that in mind, here are some commonsense tips for relatively painless public speaking.

☐ Practice in front of friends first. Ask them to tell you when you're coming across effectively and when you're not.

☐ Videotape (or audiotape) yourself to get an audience's view of you. Take notes on your strengths and weaknesses and use them to make changes in your presentation.

☐ If your speech is well organized and focused, you'll be less nervous. Keep it short and simple; don't try to fit everything you know into one speech. People will only absorb one or two main points anyway. Telegraph your main ideas with spoken "headlines" and flesh them out with one or two specific examples.

☐ The first few moments on stage are usually the scariest. Clear your throat *before* you get to the podium. Take a few deep breaths to relax while you're being introduced. When you rise to speak, smile, thank your introducer, and then wait. Don't begin to speak until you have the audience's attention.

☐ Establish eye contact with three friendly-looking faces— one toward the back of the room, one to your left, and one to your right. As you divide your glances among these people, your eyes sweep the room and you give the impression of speaking personally to everyone assembled. Focusing on individuals also helps make the audience seem less amorphous and less threatening.

☐ Use your hands to help control anxiety. Moving slightly and making gestures help manage the adrenaline your system is pumping. Keep your hands waist high. Fold them lightly, don't tighten into fists. If there's a podium, rest your hands flat on it; don't grip the podium as if it were your sole source of support.

☐ If you begin your speech with a joke, be sure it's actually funny. One of the fastest ways to alienate an audience is with a joke that falls flat. It's safer to start with an intriguing rhetorical question to arouse curiosity.

☐ Consider your tone of voice. Clipped, staccato speech patterns can make you sound tense or authoritarian. If you end a sentence on an "up" note, you will seem to be asking for agreement; lower your voice to appear more sure of yourself. A voice that's resonant, rich, and relaxed will go a long way toward improving your presentation and make you feel more comfortable giving it. Concentrate on using your voice effectively and you may forget how nervous you were in the first place.

I put in long hours at a demanding job and still bring problems home. How can I strike a better balance between work and family?

It is easy to fall into a workaholic routine today. During the inflationary decade of the 1980's, the percentage of Americans who spent more than 49 hours a week working rose from 18 to 24 percent. In the early 1990's, belt-tightening companies made increasing demands on fewer employees. More people today are moonlighting, too, holding two or three jobs because salaries aren't keeping pace with inflation. And technological advancements—fax machines, car phones, laptop computers, paging devices—are speeding up the pace of work and making it easier to blend distinctions between work and home.

To strike a better balance between work and family, be clear about your priorities. If you treasure family weekends, for example, you may have to concede a promotion to someone willing to work Saturdays. Work hard when you're on the job, but organize your tasks so that you cut down on overtime, then concentrate on your family when you get home. For ideas on how to make the most of limited family time, see pages 283–284.

Although many companies still frown on employees who are less than driven, others are recognizing the need for employees to balance work and family. Exhausted working parents are starting to ask for more time at home. A growing number of businesses are responding to the needs of families by offering flexible work options—part-time hours, job-sharing, even sabbaticals for long-term employees.

If you decide to approach your boss about such alternative working arrangements, research your company first. How many people have negotiated flex time before you? Will you still be eligible for promotions and fringe benefits? Decide which parts of your job you wish to keep doing and come up with reasonable ways for the rest of the work to get done. Is there someone in the company who would want to job-share with you?

If the boss denies your request, you may wish to consider other employment or self-employment. More than 6 million Americans currently work for themselves and make their own hours (although this doesn't always mean that they work less). In the future, as the labor market shrinks and the economy undergoes further restructuring, more companies may offer flexible job options as a way of attracting and keeping the valuable employees they need.

I think I could benefit from therapy. What qualities should I look for in a therapist?

The kind of therapist who'll serve you best depends in part on what kind of help you're looking for. Some therapists specialize in particular areas—marital counseling or habit control through behavior modification,

for instance. You may want short-term intervention to work on a stressful situation in your present life. Psychoanalysts usually take a longer-term approach and work on major personality changes. You'll want to consider this more intensive, more expensive sort of treatment if you suspect that you suffer from a chronic problem like pervasive depression, low self-esteem, or ongoing difficulties in relationships.

Often, the best way to find a good therapist is to ask friends for referrals. Many therapists won't treat two relatives or very close friends (for reasons of confidentiality) but most will be happy to confer and recommend colleagues. Comparison shopping for therapy is difficult because it usually happens at a time when you're under emotional stress, but it's important to make a clear and rational choice. Don't just fall into a relationship with anyone who's hung out a shingle. Check credentials; most states have some kind of licensing procedure. But even more important than a therapist's training and degrees are the trust and rapport you feel, the sense that you (and your problems) are being understood by an intelligent, empathetic human being.

I just can't imagine spilling all my problems to a perfect stranger. What actually happens in a therapy session?

There are many schools of psychotherapy, and most therapists will tell you which they most espouse. Freudians are famous for steering their patients to couches and never giving much feedback. The Freudian depicted in cartoons restricts his remarks during sessions to one question, "Can you say more about that?",

and one response, "Mm-hm." Strict Freudians are rather rare, however. Most therapists blend the wisdom of various schools to come up with their own eclectic approach. Most people in therapy expect interaction, a give and take with someone who talks and responds, offering understanding and new insights into problems. A good therapist does maintain a certain level of neutrality. He won't chit-chat about his family life. You're paying for the session, after all, and you're not there to listen to his problems. By maintaining some distance, the therapist also makes it easier for you to disclose personal information. He is not there to judge you or to compare his outlook with yours. His task is to help you see more clearly into your own emotions, behavior, and assumptions.

Can religious counseling take the place of psychotherapy?

Religious counseling can provide a good alternative to psychotherapy, especially for deeply religious people. Most major religions share a common view of reality in which the ups and downs of daily life are seen in the context of a greater moral purpose. Seeing the changes you go through as part of your progress on a spiritual path contributes to a healthy sense of proportion and promotes emotionally stable, well-adapted behavior.

Many churchgoers feel more comfortable discussing their problems with religious counselors, whose role as advisers and helpers is centuries old. Some members of the clergy are also trained therapists. Others may not be as well equipped to handle serious psychological problems, but may be able to refer you to professional help.

TYPES OF PSYCHOTHERAPY

There are dozens of different methods of psychotherapy. Each involves a fairly specific approach to assessing and treating personal problems and disorders, and each has its supporters and detractors. Some of the better-known methods, and their philosophy and course of treatment, are listed below. All of these therapies are usually used to treat individuals on a one-on-one basis. But they can also be used to treat patients in groups (p. 195) or as a family or couple.

Therapy	Basic approach	Course of treatment
Behavior	Focuses on modifying or neutralizing unwanted aspects of a patient's behavior and encouraging desirable aspects.	Most frequently employed as short-term therapy to resolve specific difficulties, such as phobias.
Cognitive	Emphasizes the influence of a patient's thoughts on his feelings and behavior.	Generally used to relieve depression and specific difficulties, such as oversensitivity to criticism; one to three sessions a week.
Gestalt	Analyzes responses to present-day experiences rather than ones in the past; dreams and conflicts are reenacted.	Long-term analysis, usually with one or more sessions a week.
Humanist/ existential client-centered	Focuses on individual's subjective experience and ability to make choices and take responsibility for own self. Emphasizes potential for growth.	Time frame varies with therapist's orientation or school; usually one to five sessions weekly.
Hypnosis	Therapist uses hypnosis to suggest behavioral change or to delve into past experiences, often as a supplement to traditional therapy.	May be used to combat smoking, phobias, and psychosomatic illness. Time frame varies with type of basic therapy.
Psychoanalysis	Intensive analysis of patient's past with emphasis on early experiences, free association, and interpretation of dreams.	Used to treat well-established personality problems, usually with three sessions a week over a period of 3 to 5 years or more.
Psychoanalytically oriented	Uses psychoanalytic theory but therapist takes a more active role and may use different techniques.	Offers either short-term assistance during a crisis or long-term analysis of a year or more; one to three sessions a week.

Can a therapist prescribe drugs?

Only a physician or a psychiatrist, who is also an M.D., can write drug prescriptions. A psychologist or other trained counselor, however, can work in conjunction with a psychiatrist or other physician if drugs are a necessary part of treatment. A patient may continue to see a nonprescribing practitioner for regular weekly talk therapy and visit the prescribing physician periodically for monitoring and adjustment of medication. Some states are considering new licensing procedures that would allow practicing psychotherapists who are not M.D.'s to do some prescribing on their own.

I've just started seeing a therapist and I'm very embarrassed about it. Why is there such a stigma attached to mental health issues?

Perhaps because emotional wounds can't literally be seen, many people take psychological pain less seriously than physical pain. They question whether emotional illnesses actually exist and tend to blame the victims for their own suffering. Tragically, this stigma prevents some people, who feel alone and ashamed of their problems, from seeking the help they need. Some men, in particular, think it a sign of weakness to disclose emotional problems. Aware of this hesitation, some clinics are setting up men-only therapy groups where issues of inadequacy and self-worth can be addressed in a safe setting.

According to the National Institute of Mental Health (NIMH), mental illness is just as common an everyday condition as high blood pressure. At some point in their lives, one-third of all Americans will face a mental or drug-related problem.

In a major NIMH study, more than 15 percent of the 18,500 people surveyed said they had had an emotional problem during the previous month. Only one in five, however, said they had sought help for their mental health problems.

How can I tell if therapy is working? How do I know if a therapist is not right for me?

A patient's frustration with the course of therapy is not always the sign of a genuine impasse. Could you be delaying progress by refusing to confront important issues? Are your expectations too high? Do you expect change to come too easily?

Of course, it's possible that this therapist is the wrong person to help you. He or she may be extremely talented, but if the therapist is not temperamentally suited to work with someone like you, the therapy won't progress. The daughter of an overbearing mother, for instance, may need a flexible, accepting therapist. A man who suffers from high anxiety will want someone who is calm and relaxed. All sorts of things enter into the match between therapist and patient, even such seemingly minor matters as whether you like her sense of humor or the way she has decorated her office.

Therapy often rolls along at a glacial pace, and frustrating periods—when it seems you're going over the same material again and again—are inevitable. However, if you are not experiencing relief of any symptoms after 6 months to a year of regular sessions, you may reasonably question where, and at what pace, your therapy is going. Let your therapist know you are frustrated. His response will help you decide whether you're in the right place. A good therapist will be honest and straightforward with you; direct, but not arrogant or hostile; able to convince you that he understands your experience, at least most of the time. Some patients tend to deify doctors. Therapists are not omniscient gods, but human beings with their own foibles; however, you have the right to expect them to be well-trained and helpful human beings.

I want to end my relationship with my therapist. How do I go about it?

☐ First, tell him or her directly and clearly that you wish to end the relationship. Be willing to consider and discuss whether you are truly dissatisfied or whether you are temporarily angry at the therapist for bringing up uncomfortable issues.
☐ Consider getting a second opinion on the course of treatment your therapist has recommended. If your therapist objects to this, there really is a problem.
☐ Most therapists will ask you to continue with your appointments for a time, often about a month, so that you can thoroughly examine the problem and allow time to process the end of the relationship, if that is to happen. However, if you feel extremely uncomfortable with the therapist, if you feel intimidated or humiliated, there is no need to continue your sessions.
☐ If a psychotherapist makes sexual advances, leave immediately. There is no therapeutic excuse for such behavior, and you may be helping others by reporting such abuse to the proper authorities (p. 134).

Our 16-year-old son has agreed to see a therapist. Other than paying the bills, what is our role and what rights do we have as parents?

When a child is in therapy, parents may have a natural desire to communicate their concerns to the therapist and to receive feedback from him or her about their child's progress. These are important questions that need to be discussed with your son's therapist up front. Some therapists encourage family sessions on a regular basis. Those affiliated with a hospital or a mental health center may suggest separate family therapy with another therapist on the staff, or they may refer you to a parents' group. But you can insist that a way—agreeable to all concerned—be worked out for you to express your concerns about your child and to get a response.

Although this may sound needlessly complicated, there are good reasons for such formal procedures. A therapist is ethically and legally bound to keep confidential anything a patient says in a therapy session. Without that assurance, your son will not feel free to talk about what is on his mind and there will be no healing. Also, a good therapist will not talk to you behind your son's back. To be effective, the therapist must win your son's trust. Talking to you without your son's being present would be a betrayal of that trust.

This doesn't mean that you have no rights. If you are disturbed about something your son has done, you should be able to arrange a meeting with the therapist and your son together to talk about it. And if you feel, after a year or more, that your son is not making progress, or if you are uncomfortable with things the therapist appears to be encouraging your son to do, you can ask a second therapist to make an evaluation. Such a person will talk individually to you, your son, and your son's therapist, and then make recommendations. If your son's therapist objects to this, you then have grounds for taking him or her off the case.

We think that our teenage daughter might benefit from therapy, but she refuses to go and accuses us of thinking she is crazy. How can we get help for her?

This is a frustrating situation that many parents face. A resistant patient is not likely to benefit very much from therapy. Sometimes, however, youngsters who begin therapy reluctantly come in time to trust the therapist and appreciate the process.

One approach that you might try is to take the whole family to a family therapist. You can tell your daughter that you feel unable to communicate effectively within the family, and you need her help in solving your problem. This takes the onus of craziness off your daughter and shows her that *you* are willing to get help when you can't cope.

If she finds the family therapy helpful, she may be encouraged to go a step further and see a therapist on her own. If not, you will at least have learned ways to deal with her problems more effectively within the family.

Aside from drugs and therapy, what other techniques are available for treating emotional problems?

Biofeedback and other relaxation techniques (pp. 206–207) can help anxious people cope with stress. Behavior modification is often used to help overcome phobias and control habits. Caring and supportive family and friends will provide sustenance through emotional crises. Relationships with people, pets, and even plants help draw individuals out of themselves and into a larger involvement with life, a healing connection. A basic philosophy of life, whether religious or secular, puts problems in perspective and provides a structure for incorporating changes.

Are there any advantages to group therapy over individual therapy? Are self-help groups effective?

Group therapy allows people to see how they are viewed and accepted by peers. In groups, people may re-create family constellations and reexperience childhood interactions from an adult perspective. Groups awaken empathy. By listening to others' stories, people learn more about their own problems and how to cope with them. Hearing the pain others endure, people better understand their own suffering and learn to put it in perspective. Group therapy is particularly helpful for those who have problems with interpersonal relationships, and it often works well in conjunction with individual therapy. (Group sessions are less expensive than individual work and can be successfully substituted for it in some cases.)

The healing power of talking with others who have "been there" explains the proliferation of self-help groups. There are self-help groups that address the problems of cancer patients, people with phobias, bereaved parents, victims of rape and incest, single parents, and a variety of other issues (see *The Facts*

About 12-Step Programs, p.164). Most experts recommend that self-help groups be used as a complement to, not a substitute for, psychotherapy, at least during times of acute crisis. But after completing therapy, many people continue to participate in self-help groups to continue dealing with their problems.

I sometimes feel that I'm not living up to my potential. Are there techniques for developing creativity?

Researchers have found that creative people performing at the peak of their ability experience something called flow. Painters merge consciousness into the canvas. Writers engage in dialogue with the characters in their stories. By studying how artists, scientists, and other creative people work, psychologists have been able to identify the characteristics of situations that encourage creative flow.

Challenge and skills must be well matched. If a task is too difficult, anxieties arise. If it's too easy, boredom sets in.

Developing skills primes the pump for flow. An exhilarating sense of control is part of the flow experience and hard work is the only route to such mastery. Intuition also flourishes best the more a person knows about a given subject. Flashes of brilliance don't just come out of the blue, scientists say, but occur when a solid base of knowledge allows the brain to access the right chunk of information at the right time.

One interesting sidelight of flow research shows that while people think they'd rather spend time relaxing than spend time working, the average person is much more likely to experience flow at work.

I am reasonably content with my life, but something—joy, a sense of fun or adventure— seems to be missing. What can I do to relish life more?

One thing you can do, psychologists suggest, is to make pleasure a priority; too many people tend to postpone it, bogging themselves down in the routines of daily life. People who equate success with happiness, for instance, often lose sight of the end in their pursuit of the means.

Make a list of your favorite activities. Then do the things you like, and do them often. Take credit for making yourself happy. People get the most joy out of life not only when things go well but when they feel they've helped things go that way.

Happy people look on the bright side, view other people more positively, and recall events more favorably. A well-developed sense of self-esteem nurtures joy. The resolution of inner conflicts clears the way for happy feelings.

Researchers report that life satisfaction is generally highest among individuals whose work breaks down into short-term goals that can be accomplished in the company of others, enjoyably and without too much difficulty. Happy people also seem to be better organized; they make and keep plans, are punctual and efficient.

Although poverty can obviously make life miserable, wealth doesn't necessarily make people happy. Seventy to 80 percent of Americans (a much higher percentage than anywhere else in the world) consider themselves happy, but money isn't at the root of their joy. From 1946 to 1978, when real income rose dramatically, Americans reported no increase in happiness.

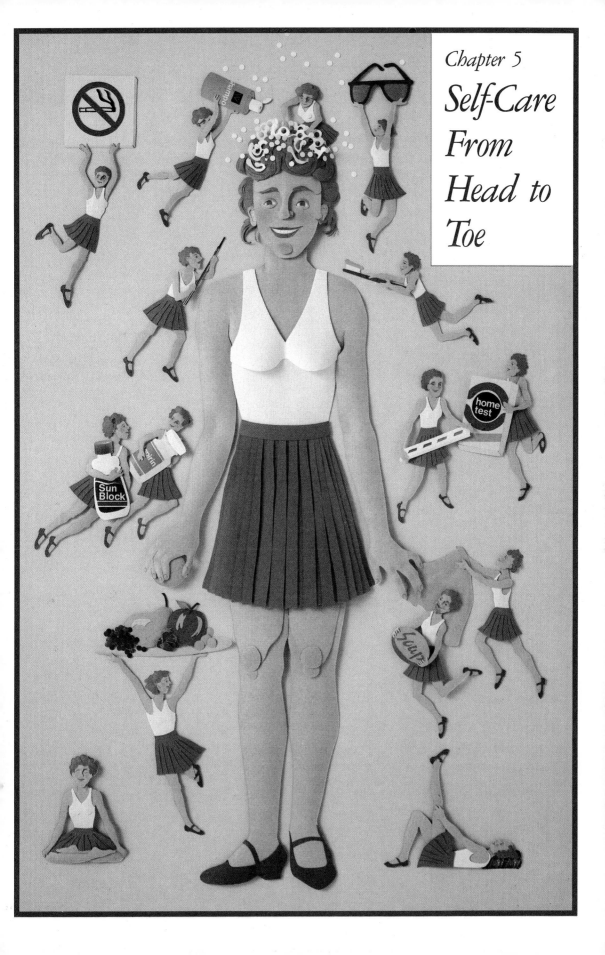

Turning Over a New Leaf

J ohn G.'s heart attack came as no surprise to his colleagues. A hard-driving achiever in his late fifties, John was quick to anger when frustrated. And in the months before his heart attack, he had known plenty of frustration as several projects under his direction either went sour or failed to take off with the smooth precision he always demanded. On top of that, John's blood pressure was dangerously high; he also favored fatty foods and had the paunch to prove it.

While John was still in the hospital recovering from his heart attack, his doctor persuaded him to sign up for the hospital's stress-reduction program. Every week for 8 weeks after his re-lease, John attended a group workshop, where he learned progressive muscle relaxation, controlled breathing, and other stress-relieving techniques. He soon learned to pinpoint sources of stress both at home and at work and to use relaxation techniques to control his body's stress response and reduce demands on his heart.

Now back at work, John has become adept at dealing with situations that trigger frustration. Instead of getting angry, he calms himself by using controlled breathing. He practices muscle relaxation at home and has taken up yoga. John's temper, his wife reports, is under better control, and he's even stopped grousing about their new low-fat, heart-healthy diet.

Vigilance Rewarded

 S carcely ill a day in her life, Diana B., 42, still made a point of seeing her doctor regularly, having a mammo-gram every 2 years, and doing a breast self-exam at the same time every month. While examining her breasts one day, Diana noticed an unfamiliar lump in the left one. After the first wave of panic had passed, Diana felt the breast once again. The lump was small—no bigger than a pea—but it was definitely there. Diana immediately went to see her gynecolo-gist. An ultrasound scan ruled out the possibility that the lump was a benign cyst; a mammo-gram confirmed the presence of a possibly cancerous lesion in the breast.

The following week, Diana underwent a biopsy, in which the lesion was removed and examined. Although the growth was malignant, a subsequent lymph node biopsy indicated that the disease hadn't spread. After 6 weeks of radiation therapy, Diana's prognosis is excellent. Following her doctor's advice, she has a yearly mammogram and continues to perform the monthly breast self-exams that saved her life.

Self-Care for an Aching Back

T en-hour work days were not unusual for Sandy T., a 42-year-old lawyer. These long, strenuous hours, most of them spent hunched over her desk, eventually took their toll on Sandy's back. Increasingly frequent attacks of lower back pain cut into her productivity, made her miserable and moody, and even led her to give up her weekend tennis. One day, a coworker who had noticed Sandy grimace in pain gave her a copy of a magazine article on ways to relieve a bad back. At home that night, Sandy read the article and decided to try the series of exercises recommended for strengthening the lower back and abdominal muscles. The routine, which took no more than 10 minutes each morning, soon proved beneficial. Sandy also bought a back support cushion for her desk chair and began taking short walks around the office every 40 minutes to relieve stress on her back. Two months later, Sandy was back in action at the office and on the tennis court.

TEST YOUR HEALTH I.Q.

How Good Is Your Day-to-Day Self-Care?

Whether it's brushing your teeth regularly to prevent decay or reaching for an aspirin to relieve a headache, most of our daily health-care activities are almost automatic. Other preventive steps, such as examining your body for signs of disease, are often overlooked. How valid are your personal theories about day-to-day health care? Start to find out by selecting the phrase or phrases that most accurately complete each statement below.

1 If you quit smoking today, your risk of developing heart disease and lung cancer drops to that of a nonsmoker in _____ years.

- **A.** 2–4
- **B.** 5–9
- **C.** 10–15
- **D.** 15–20

2 Acetaminophen, ibuprofen, and aspirin are all effective pain relievers. As a side benefit, aspirin also _____ .

- **A.** neutralizes acidic urine
- **B.** thins the blood
- **C.** strengthens fingernails

3 Your best defense against the common cold is _____ .

- **A.** avoiding chills and drafts
- **B.** washing your hands often
- **C.** taking high doses of vitamin C
- **D.** getting a flu shot every year

4 To relieve occasional mild constipation, it's best to _____ .

- **A.** take mineral oil
- **B.** increase the fiber in your diet
- **C.** drink more fluids
- **D.** step up your exercise

5 A sunscreen with a sun-protection factor (SPF) of 15 _____ .

- **A.** protects against intense sunshine for 15 minutes
- **B.** offers 15 times the protection of plain sun oil
- **C.** lets you stay in the sun 15 times longer than with no sunscreen

6 To avoid back problems, you should sleep _____ .

- **A.** on your side in a fetal position
- **B.** on your back
- **C.** on your stomach
- **D.** with a pillow under your knees

7 When buying sunglasses, most people should _____ .

- **A.** get a prescription from a doctor
- **B.** favor green or gray lenses
- **C.** select the darkest lenses
- **D.** look for a "special purpose" label

8 Eating _____ neutralizes mouth acids, which helps to limit plaque buildup and tooth decay.

- **A.** apples
- **B.** peanuts
- **C.** cheddar cheese
- **D.** yogurt
- **E.** potatoes

9 You can minimize the effects of jet lag by _____ .

- **A.** getting lots of exposure to sunlight
- **B.** drinking plenty of water or other nonalcoholic beverages
- **C.** arriving in the morning
- **D.** making stopovers on long flights

Answers

For more information on any of the quiz topics turn to the pages listed next to the answers.

1. C, p.200	4. B,C,D, p.216	7. B, p.220
2. B, p.205	5. C, p.219	8. C, p.228
3. B, p.209	6. A,B, p.219	9. A,B,D, p.232

I've heard a lot of talk about "preventive medicine." What do people mean by it?

As the term implies, preventive medicine focuses as much on what keeps you from getting sick or injured in the first place as on how to treat medical problems.

A generation ago medical students were taught very little about the impact of nutrition, exercise, and lifestyle on health. Today, the cumulative impact of hundreds of scientific studies on the causes of disease have changed that. First, the irrefutable connection between smoking and cancer was established. The role of saturated fat in building up plaque in the arteries became clearer (see *The Facts About Atherosclerosis*, p. 329). The benefit of aerobic exercise was documented.

The new preventive approach to health care calls for periodic "wellness" checkups with your primary care physician (pp. 122–124) in addition to visits you make because of illness. During the checkup, you are tested for potential health problems and you and your doctor discuss what you can do to protect yourself and lower your health risks. In effect, you become a partner with your doctor in managing your health and assume greater responsibility for your own well-being.

Although preventive medicine for adults is still relatively new in the United States, its effectiveness can already be seen in such statistics as fewer lung cancer deaths in men under 45 and reduced rates of stroke.

What steps can I take on my own to live a longer, healthier life?

First, change your dangerous habits for healthy ones. If you smoke, stop. If you drink, do so moderately (see *If You Drink*, p. 162). Don't take drugs except under a physician's care. Avoid risky sexual practices (p. 243). Fasten your seatbelt when you get in a car. Wear goggles when you play sports or use tools that can injure your eyes. Wear a helmet when you ride a bicycle or a motorcycle. Don't keep a loaded gun in the house.

Then work at staying healthy. If you don't exercise very much, choose one or more physical activities that you can enjoy on a regular basis and start doing them at least three times a week (pp. 66–67). If you are too heavy, find out what your target weight is (pp. 68–69) and pick a program that will get you there. Educate yourself about nutrition. If your diet misses the mark, make changes.

Finally, pay attention to your body so that you will notice changes if and when they occur (p. 211). Learn to recognize the symptoms of common diseases. Call your doctor when you notice a condition that is more than a transient and routine complaint.

Is there such a thing as a safe cigarette?

No. Theoretically "safe" cigarettes billed as "low tar" and "low nicotine" can do great damage to your health. Even if manu-

IF YOU QUIT SMOKING TODAY

You'll feel better, smell better, sleep better, and breathe easier. You'll cough less and have fewer headaches, stomachaches, and respiratory infections. The level of oxygen-depleting carbon monoxide in your blood will decline right away, and your stamina will increase. You'll feel less guilty and, of course, you'll have more money in your pocket.

In addition to these immediate payoffs, quitting smoking now—no matter what your age or how long you've been smoking—will give you a number of long-term benefits:
☐ Your heart disease risk starts declining within a year. After 10 to 15 years of not smoking, your chances of having a heart attack will be the same as those of the general population.

☐ Your risk of developing lung cancer also begins to decrease within a year. After 2 years of not smoking, your likelihood of getting lung cancer will decline by almost a third. And after 10 to 15 years, your lung cancer risk will be almost normal.
☐ Your risk of all health problems related to smoking will decline steadily for 15 years. Then your risk of dying will return nearly to that of someone who has never smoked.
☐ If you're pregnant and quit before the fourth month, your baby will likely have a higher birth weight than a smoking mother's infant. If you stay off cigarettes, your risk of having a low-birth-weight baby in your next pregnancy will be the same as that of a nonsmoker.

A QUIT-SMOKING DIARY

More than 90 percent of the 43 million Americans who have stopped smoking in recent decades did it on their own. Most quit cold turkey and most did not succeed on the first attempt. It takes the typical smoker 4 to 10 tries to kick the habit for good.

An effective aid for the smoker trying to break his or her addiction is the quit-smoking diary illustrated here. Maintaining a daily record of your smoking habits, cigarette by cigarette, allows you to analyze when and why you light up. Just by keeping track, you may wind up reducing the number of cigarettes that you smoke without thinking. Studying several days' worth of diary entries can help you identify and change the behavior or activities that trigger smoking.

Time/Trigger/Thoughts and feelings

7:30 a.m./Morning coffee
This cigarette gets me going.

8 a.m./Driving to work
Helped pass the time when traffic slowed to a halt; kept me from feeling irritable.

9 a.m./Accepting a phone call
Seemed to be an automatic response; I was smoking before I even realized what I was doing.

10 a.m./Coffee break
Coffee just doesn't taste right without a cigarette. It's the cigarette that makes the break refreshing.

10:30 a.m./Writing up proposal for new training program
Cigarettes helped me to concentrate. Before I knew it I had smoked four.

1:30 p.m./After-lunch coffee
Cigarette tasted good and seemed to relax me before getting back to work. I had two.

4 p.m./Discussion with colleague after the budget meeting
He offered me a cigarette and I took it without thinking. It seemed to give us something to share while we reviewed the meeting.

5:15 p.m./Driving home
Smoking seems to calm me down in traffic.

Time/Trigger/Thoughts and feelings

6:30 p.m./Drink before dinner
Drinks and cigarettes go together. I'm not sure I would want a drink without a cigarette, but the combination is refreshing after a long day.

7:30 p.m./After-dinner coffee
The most relaxing cigarette of the day. I actually had two before I even noticed.

10 p.m./Editing work proposal
Working for two hours at my desk I smoked five cigarettes. (I know by the butts I count in the ashtray.) It was so habitual, I didn't think as I lit up each one. I seem to do this almost unconsciously when I am concentrating hard.

Helpful programs

If you have trouble giving up smoking on your own, professional counseling and group support can help. Quit-smoking programs employ a variety of techniques, from behavior modification to acupuncture and hypnosis, to help smokers break the tobacco habit, either gradually or cold turkey. These organizations offer effective and inexpensive programs nationwide (see Appendix for addresses and phone numbers):
The American Lung Association (Freedom from Smoking Clinics)
The American Cancer Society (Fresh Start)
The General Conference of Seventh-Day Adventists (Breathe Free Plan to Stop Smoking)

Nicotine gum

Smokers trying to quit may experience withdrawal symptoms such as headaches, fatigue, drowsiness, and difficulty concentrating. To help relieve these symptoms, your doctor may prescribe nicotine chewing gum. Because acidic beverages such as coffee, tea, and fruit juices interfere with nicotine absorption from the gum, don't drink them before or while you chew. Use nicotine gum only under a doctor's supervision.

facturers *could* screen out all tar and nicotine (they cannot), there are other toxic gases in cigarettes that disturb the healthy balance of the respiratory system and, in turn, each of the other systems dependent upon it. Smoking introduces carbon monoxide into the blood, which takes over a significant share of the red blood cells that are ordinarily used to transport oxygen throughout the body. The resulting oxygen depletion, if it becomes severe enough, can stress the heart sufficiently to bring on a heart attack.

Even allegedly "safe" cigarettes contain some tar and nicotine, and these materials in any concentration cause sticky resins to be deposited in fragile lung tissue, promote arterial plaque, raise heart rate and blood pressure, interfere with fetal development during pregnancy, depress the body's immune function, and produce carcinogenic changes in cells.

To compensate for the reduced tar and nicotine in these cigarettes, smokers tend to consume more per day, making "safe" cigarettes as dangerous as conventional cigarettes.

I've cut down my smoking from a pack to two or three cigarettes a day. Have I cut my risk of developing heart disease and lung cancer proportionately?

Any *significant* reduction in the number of cigarettes smoked per day will improve your overall health picture (see *If You Quit Smoking Today,* p.200), but not proportionately. A smoker who can keep his cigarette consumption down to three a day still has a much higher risk of developing serious diseases than a nonsmoker. In one epidemio-

logical study, for example, a man who smoked more than 40 cigarettes a day had a risk of dying of lung cancer that was 23 times greater than that of a nonsmoker, while a man who smoked fewer than nine cigarettes a day still had nearly four times the risk of the nonsmoker. Similar findings exist for people who continue to light up cigarettes, but have stopped inhaling.

And, as the U.S. surgeon general has pointed out, smoking is an addiction. If you simply cut down the number of cigarettes you smoke rather than giving them up altogether, you are much more likely to resume heavy cigarette smoking whenever you feel under stress.

My teenage son has recently begun chewing tobacco. Is this any less harmful than smoking?

Chewing tobacco and snuff are two types of "smokeless" tobacco; both can create serious health problems. Held directly in the mouth, often for hours, chewing tobacco can cause tooth decay, gum disease, and pre-cancerous white lesions on the inside of the mouth called leukoplakia. Snuff, which is inhaled through the nose, irritates the nasal lining. In time, the use of smokeless tobacco may lead to full-blown cancers of the mouth and throat (or of the nose if snuff is used) and to nicotine-related atherosclerosis, or narrowing of the arteries.

Because smokeless tobacco puts higher and more sustained concentrations of nicotine into the system, dependency on this form of tobacco tends to be harder to break. Sad to report, of the estimated 10 million American users of smokeless tobacco, more than half begin the habit by the time they are 13 years old.

Is smoking a pipe or a cigar safer than smoking cigarettes?

Since most pipe and cigar smokers don't inhale, they avoid the high risk of lung cancer and emphysema that cigarette smokers incur. However, smoking a pipe or a cigar is not a risk-free activity. Either form of tobacco use can lead to cancer of the lips, tongue, and esophagus. And like cigarette smoking, pipe and cigar smoking can accelerate the development of atherosclerosis (p.328), which so often results in a heart attack or stroke.

How often should I perform a breast self-examination?

Starting at approximately age 20, a woman should examine her breasts once a month, and continue the practice throughout her life. Premenopausal women should pick a time 2 or 3 days after their period ends when their breasts are least likely to be tender, swollen, or lumpy. Postmenopausal women can chose a date that's easy to remember, like the first day of the month or the first Monday in the month. If in the course of the exam (see facing page) you detect a new lump, a nipple discharge, or a significant change in the shape or appearance of your breasts, see your doctor right away.

Is there such a thing as a "benign" lump in the breast, or should I just assume that any lump that I find will probably be malignant?

Nearly 90 percent of the lumps women find in their breasts are no cause for concern. Most are caused by fibrocystic disease, a common condition in which small

THE BREAST SELF-EXAM

The process takes only a few minutes once a month, and the benefits may be lifesaving. In the beginning, practice examining your breasts every day until you are comfortable with the procedure. As you become more familiar with the normal feel of your breasts, you will become more sensitive to changes that you should mention to your doctor.

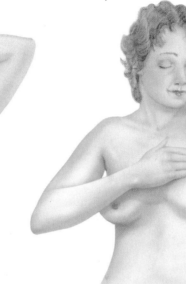

1. Stand directly in front of a mirror, your arms by your side, and study both breasts for anything unusual: puckering, dimpling, scaling. Then, clasping your hands behind your head, look for changes in the shape or contour of each breast. Keep checking as you turn from side to side.

2. In the shower, raise your left arm. Using the middle fingers of your right hand, firmly explore your left breast in a circular pattern from the outside inward. Feel for lumps or thickened tissue. Then raise your right arm and examine your right breast with your left hand.

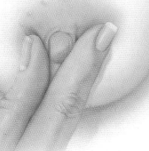

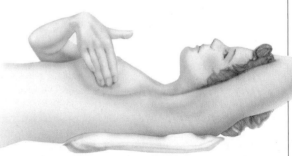

3. With your left arm raised, gently squeeze the nipple of your left breast with your right hand. You are looking for a discharge. Repeat the process on the right breast with the right arm raised and the left hand squeezing.

4. Lying down with a pillow under your left shoulder and your left arm raised, explore your left breast, pressing firmly with the pads of the middle fingers of your right hand. Reverse the procedure for the right breast. Feel the entire breast area for lumps from the armpit to the top of the collarbone.

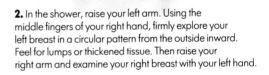

COMMON CANCERS: ASSESSING YOUR RISK

Some cancer risk factors, such as smoking and sun exposure, are controllable; others, like age and gender, aren't. Having a risk factor for a cancer does not mean that you'll get it, but it is prudent for you—and your doctor—to be on the lookout for symptoms (see *The Body's Warning Signals,* p.211) and to eliminate controllable risks. Regular checkups (p.122), self-examination of the breasts (p.203) and skin (pp.371–372), and fecal occult blood tests, Pap smears, and mammograms (pp.124–125) are important early detection measures, which could prevent some 150,000 cancer deaths a year, according to the American Cancer Society. (The figures below are 1991 estimates.)

Type	Yearly toll	Risk factors*
Breast	175,000 new cases 44,800 deaths	Family history of breast cancer; obesity, late childbearing, and childlessness.
Bladder	50,200 new cases 9,500 deaths	Smoking (nearly half of cases); bladder cancer is more common in men than in women.
Cervical	13,000 new cases 4,500 deaths	First intercourse at an early age, multiple sexual partners, smoking, history of genital herpes.
Colorectal	157,500 new cases 60,500 deaths	Being over 50 with colon polyps or ulcerative colitis; a family history of these disorders or of colon cancer; a high-fat, low-fiber diet.
Leukemia	28,000 new cases 18,100 deaths	Exposure to radiation, benzene, and other chemicals.
Lung	161,000 new cases 143,000 deaths	Smoking (83 percent of cases); exposure to asbestos, radiation, and secondhand tobacco smoke.
Lymphoma	44,600 new cases 20,300 deaths	Being over 50; no other known risk factors.
Oral	30,800 new cases 8,800 deaths	Smoking, chewing tobacco, and heavy alcohol use.
Pancreatic	28,200 new cases 25,200 deaths	Smoking, high-fat diet.
Prostate	122,000 new cases 32,000 deaths	Risk increases with age; more than 80 percent of cases occur after 65.
Skin	600,000 new cases 8,500 deaths	Fair skin, severe sunburn in childhood, frequent sun exposure, and family history of skin cancer.
Uterine	46,000 new cases 5,500 deaths	Being postmenopausal with a history of infertility, ovulation failure, or abnormal bleeding; also obesity, hypertension, diabetes.

Hormone replacement therapy has been linked with an increased risk of breast, uterine, and other cancers in women. For more on this subject, see page 377.

fluid-filled sacs, or cysts, form in response to hormonal changes just before menstruation each month and disappear soon after. Although they may feel like tumors, such cysts are quite normal and benign in origin. Fibrocystic disease may come and go throughout a woman's fertile years, or it may become increasingly noticeable as a woman ages.

Less common but also noncancerous are breast growths called fibroadenomas, which are firmer and typically larger than cysts. Their genesis may be related to fat consumption in the diet. Unfortunately, a biopsy is the only definitive way to identify a fibroadenoma. If the lump is found to be benign, it may be left alone or, if it causes discomfort, it can be removed surgically in a doctor's office under local anesthesia.

How common is testicular cancer? How often should a man examine himself, and how is the exam done?

For men between the ages of 15 and 34, particularly those who have an undescended or partially descended testicle, testicular cancer is one of the most common types of cancer.

Early signs include a slight enlargement of one of the testes, and a change in its consistency. There may be no pain, although a dull ache in the abdomen or groin is common.

Men under 35 should examine their testes regularly once a month, a procedure that takes no more than 3 minutes. After a warm bath or shower, when the skin around the scrotum is most relaxed, roll each testicle gently in both hands. If you find any hard nodules, see your doctor. The lump may be benign, but only a doctor can determine that.

Treatment of testicular cancer depends on the stage of the disease. A localized tumor usually requires surgical removal of the testicle. If the malignancy has spread to nearby areas, a follow-up treatment of chemotherapy and radiation is prescribed. Cure rates are high: 95 to 97 percent of men treated early survive, and even in cases where some spread has taken place, 85 percent respond positively to aggressive further treatment.

How effective are breast and testicular self-exams in lowering the risk of cancer death?

There is still not enough evidence from scientific studies to make a definitive judgment on the value of these tests. The vast majority of lumps that patients find themselves are benign and perhaps result in unnecessary biopsies. On the other hand, patients *have* found cancerous tumors by self-examination and have sought medical attention early enough to be treated successfully. While a self-examination can't take the place of a physician's checkup, it is important for people to become conscious of their own bodies and to note changes that should be discussed with a doctor.

Is it really possible to lower one's risk of having a heart attack?

We all start out with certain genetic factors that determine how likely we are to develop heart problems as we age, but research makes it clear that a significant part of the risk is in our own hands.

Doctors consider high blood pressure, cigarette smoking, and high blood cholesterol to be the three most important contributors to heart disease.

There are a number of things you can do yourself to lower your blood pressure (see next question). You can quit smoking on your own or through a program (see *A Quit-Smoking Diary*, p. 201). Restricting the cholesterol and the cholesterol-producing fat in your diet and exercising regularly will help lower your blood cholesterol level.

FACT OR FALLACY ?

Women are not as prone to heart attack as men

Fallacy. For decades, it was believed that heart disease was primarily a man's problem. Research was generally restricted to male subjects. Recent studies, however, paint a different picture. Although men under 60 do have a significantly higher risk of heart attacks than women of comparable age, the gap narrows as women enter menopause. By age 60 the two sexes are at the same risk for heart attacks, but women are more likely to die from them. Scientists believe that the hormone estrogen, which is produced naturally until a woman reaches menopause, may protect younger women from cardiovascular disease. A woman can improve her heart disease risk after menopause by following the same diet and exercise programs recommended for men. Her doctor may also advise estrogen replacement therapy.

What can I do on my own to lower my blood pressure?

Once your doctor has determined that you have hypertension, there are several things you can do to help yourself. If you smoke, stop (p. 201). If you're overweight, just losing 10 to 20 pounds will often significantly lower your blood pressure. An aerobic exercise program, if practiced regularly for at least 20 minutes three times a week (see *The Facts About Aerobics*, p. 71), will also help bring blood pressure down. (Avoid heavy weight training and isometric exercises, which can increase blood pressure).

Limit the amount of salt in your diet. Reduce your alcohol consumption to at most two drinks a day or eliminate alcohol from your diet completely.

If stress contributes to your hypertension, learning a relaxation technique (see *Learning to Relax*, pp. 206–207) and practicing it regularly may help keep your blood pressure within bounds.

If your doctor has prescribed antihypertension medication for you, don't forget to take it.

I've heard that an aspirin a day can lower the risk of heart attack. Does that mean everyone should take a daily aspirin?

Along with reducing pain, lowering fever, and relieving inflammation, aspirin also blocks certain clotting factors in the blood. For this reason many physicians recommend that patients with a high risk of heart attack and stroke take one aspirin tablet (325 milligrams) daily or every other day as a form of preventive medicine.

At least two major studies have indicated that at this low

Continued on page 208

LEARNING TO RELAX

Relaxation techniques are designed to help you relieve muscle tension, achieve mental calm, and relax. They're also effective in reducing blood pressure and alleviating anxiety symptoms. Learning to relax is an active process in which you retrain mind and body to release tension and not overreact to stress. Pick a technique such as progressive relaxation, meditation, or yoga (p.103) and practice it regularly, 2 or 3 times a day. Begin each session with controlled breathing; take a few minutes afterward to enjoy your relaxation. In time you'll be able to relax at will and achieve control over your responses to stress.

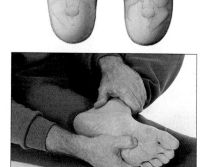

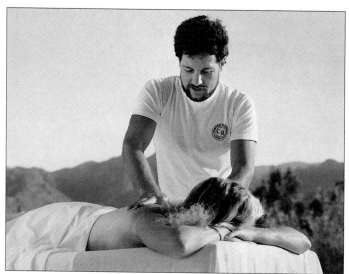

Massage, the systematic manipulation of skin and muscles, is an ancient form of therapy and a very effective relaxer. In Western, or Swedish, massage, the masseur uses hands and fingers to rub, knead, squeeze, and pound the client's body. Shiatsu is a Japanese style of massage based on the same principles as acupuncture (p.133). The Shiatsu practitioner uses the tips of his thumbs and fingers, as well as knees, elbows, and feet, to apply pressure to specific points along the body. Sports massage combines elements of the two schools. Although massage is most beneficial when administered by an experienced professional, it's a good technique to learn with a partner. Schools of massage therapy offer workshops, or you can learn the basics from a manual or video tape. Even without a partner, you can teach yourself strokes that will help relieve an aching neck, back, or shoulder.

Foot massage is very relaxing and easy to practice on yourself. The Asian technique called reflexology is based on the theory that different areas of the feet govern different parts of the body (top) and that massaging the proper area will relieve symptoms in the corresponding part. Thumb-walking (above) is a basic reflexology technique in which you press the tip of the thumb against the sole of the foot and creep forward by bending and unbending the thumb.

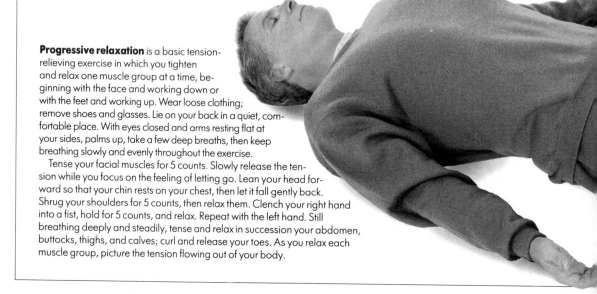

Progressive relaxation is a basic tension-relieving exercise in which you tighten and relax one muscle group at a time, beginning with the face and working down or with the feet and working up. Wear loose clothing; remove shoes and glasses. Lie on your back in a quiet, comfortable place. With eyes closed and arms resting flat at your sides, palms up, take a few deep breaths, then keep breathing slowly and evenly throughout the exercise.

Tense your facial muscles for 5 counts. Slowly release the tension while you focus on the feeling of letting go. Lean your head forward so that your chin rests on your chest, then let it fall gently back. Shrug your shoulders for 5 counts, then relax them. Clench your right hand into a fist, hold for 5 counts, and relax. Repeat with the left hand. Still breathing deeply and steadily, tense and relax in succession your abdomen, buttocks, thighs, and calves; curl and release your toes. As you relax each muscle group, picture the tension flowing out of your body.

Meditation is the practice of concentrating on an object, word, or idea to clear the mind, relax the body, and achieve a state of heightened awareness and enlightenment. Meditation has been a feature of many religions, but it can also serve as a practical, calming therapy. To try a simple form of meditating, find a quiet place and a comfortable sitting position that keeps your back straight, either on the floor or in a chair. Close your eyes and concentrate on an image (a flame or flower) or on a sound or word (known as a mantra) that will help clear your head of any extraneous thoughts. Breathe deeply and rhythmically, focusing attention on the chosen object or sound for 20 minutes.

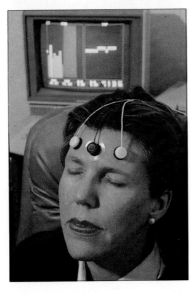

Visualization, or imaging, is a related technique in which you use your imagination to reduce anxiety and achieve a state of deep relaxation. Find a comfortable position either lying down or seated in a quiet place. Close your eyes and begin breathing deeply and evenly. At first, focus your mind's eye on an object or a color, and use your chosen image to banish other thoughts from your head. As you gain experience, focus on more complex images. Picture yourself relaxing in a pleasant, calming locale, such as along the shore of a tropical island. Imagine the sights, colors, and smells of your island paradise in as much detail as possible. Prolong your mental holiday for 10 to 15 minutes.

Biofeedback is an aid to relaxation that helps you to recognize and eventually control your responses to stress. A biofeedback machine—either a sophisticated lab device or a simpler home model—monitors blood pressure, heart rate, perspiration, temperature, muscle tension, or brain waves and alerts the patient to changes by means of a sound, light flash, or fluctuating needle. Guided by this feedback, the patient applies relaxation techniques to bring about changes in the readings. With practice, many people learn to exercise such control even without a machine.

Biofeedback has been used successfully to treat migraines, hypertension, chronic pain, anxiety, and depression. For more information about biofeedback applications and clinics, contact the Association for Applied Psychophysiology and Biofeedback (see Appendix).

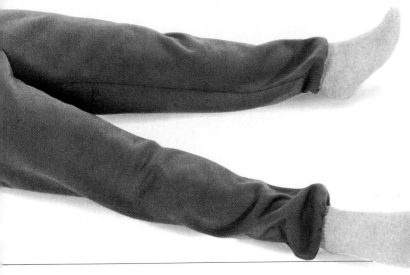

CONTROLLED BREATHING

An emphasis on deep, rhythmic breathing from the diaphragm is a feature of many relaxation techniques. In addition to helping you relax, controlled breathing has been shown to lower heart rate and to prevent or relieve anxiety symptoms. Often recommended for patients with bronchitis and other chronic chest diseases, controlled breathing is also effective in helping women to relax and relieve pain during labor and childbirth (p.262).

To practice controlled breathing, place one hand on your chest and the other on your diaphragm, just below the breast bone. Breathe in deeply through your nose or mouth. Slowly exhale through your mouth, letting your abdomen relax as you do so. The hand on your diaphragm should rise as you inhale and descend as you exhale. If you are breathing properly, the hand on your chest should hardly move.

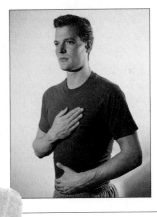

dosage aspirin can actually reduce by half the risk of heart attack in healthy, middle-aged men as well as lower the risk of a second stroke or a second heart attack by 25 to 50 percent. A more recent study shows that women, too, may benefit from aspirin therapy.

Another study of aspirin's blood-thinning properties involved patients with a heartbeat irregularity called atrial fibrillation that afflicts more than a million Americans. Test results suggest that daily doses of a single aspirin tablet (or another blood-thinning drug called warfarin) reduce stroke risk in both men and women patients by 80 percent.

Good as it sounds, aspirin is not entirely safe, and the decision to undertake aspirin therapy should be made with your doctor. Although aspirin is an over-the-counter drug, it should not be taken by people who are anemic, who have peptic ulcers, or who bleed easily from other causes. Aspirin can also be hazardous to pregnant and nursing women, asthma sufferers, and individuals with stomach problems.

Incidently, neither acetaminophen (Tylenol, for example) nor ibuprofen (Nuprin) is a viable aspirin substitute in this case. Both are comparable painkillers, but don't thin the blood.

I'm often tired even though I get 8 hours of sleep every night. What could be causing this?

Although 7½ to 8 hours is widely thought to be the optimum length for a good night's sleep, adult sleep needs vary considerably, and you may be one of the almost 50 percent of the population who need more. To determine your own requirements, sleep researchers suggest that you try going to bed an hour or even 90

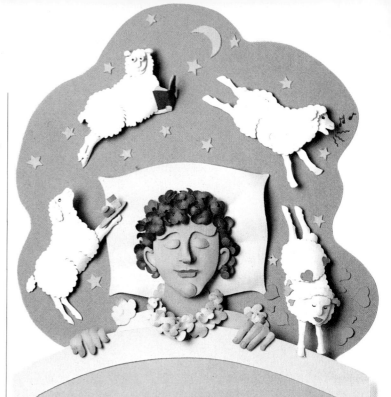

FALLING ASLEEP

If you have serious, debilitating insomnia, ask your doctor to refer you to a sleep clinic. You might, however, first try a few lifestyle changes. Give up alcohol, smoking, and caffeine—three primary causes of sleeplessness—and step up your daytime exercise regimen. (Evening workouts may give you a second wind and keep you awake.) For an occasional bout of insomnia, there are simple, time-proven remedies that may help.

☐ Drink a glass of warm milk with honey at bedtime. Both contain small quantities of the amino acid L-tryptophan, which is believed to have sleep-inducing qualities. (Meat and lettuce also have L-tryptophan, if you crave a bedtime snack.) Stay away from tea and hot chocolate, soothing as they sound. They contain caffeine, and will keep you awake.

☐ Avoid loud music, big meals, heated arguments, and exciting television shows that might overstimulate you at night. Make the countdown to bed a relaxing routine that keeps your mind off the day's problems. Take a warm bath. Listen to soothing music. Read a good book that isn't related to your job (reading or thinking about work may set your mind racing with ideas or worries).

☐ Save your bedroom for bedroom activities: sex and sleep. Entering it should not make you think of the bills you haven't paid or the notes you need to write the next day. Making love, incidentally, is considered by many sleep researchers to be the best natural sedative of all.

☐ Once in bed, try the relaxation and imaging techniques described on pages 206–207 to take your mind off worrisome thoughts. The old saw about counting sheep to get to sleep is a kind of imaging technique, and unless you happen to be a shepherd, it's an effective one.

minutes earlier for at least 10 days. Keep a diary. Note how refreshed you feel during the day and how your ability to carry out difficult tasks compares with the way you felt and performed before the experiment. You may be surprised to find that a few extra z-z-z's are all you need to perk up your energy and spirits.

If extra sleep does not relieve your tiredness, you may have a sleep disorder that is undermining the *quality* rather than the *quantity* of your sleep. Or your fatigue may be a secondary symptom of some other disease—a viral infection, thyroid disease, or depression, for example. Depression is the most common cause of chronic tiredness. To get at the source of your fatigue, see your doctor.

Are over-the-counter sleep aids effective? Are they habit-forming?

Most nonprescription sleep drugs rely on antihistamines, which have sedative side effects, to make you drowsy. They work for some people, but about one in four users experiences unpleasant side effects such as dry mouth, dizziness, urinary retention, constipation, nausea, blurred vision, or increased heart rate. And another smaller percent get no sleep benefit at all.

OTC sleep aids are less powerful than their prescription counterparts, so they are less addictive. However, they can in time become habit-forming. To be safe, never take them for more than two nights in a row.

Is it better to sleep without a pillow?

If you sleep on your back you will put less strain on your neck by doing without a plump foam pillow under your head. Switch to a

soft fiber- or down-filled pillow, or don't use a pillow at all, presuming you can still get a good night's sleep without it. If you sleep on your stomach, which is not good for your back, and you find it impossible to change, put a pillow under your waist to lift and straighten your back. Or try sleeping on your side, with one or both knees drawn up and pillows in front of you to support upper shoulder and knee.

I'm told I snore. How can I prevent this?

Snoring is usually caused by a stuffy nose that makes you breathe through your mouth while you sleep. The rattling noise of a snore is created by an obstruction in the throat that vibrates like the reed of a wind instrument as you breathe.

The obstruction can be the soft palate or enlarged adenoids, but it's usually just lax throat muscles. In chronic snorers this condition is associated with overweight, but other causes of an overly relaxed throat are a deviated septum, a sinus or other respiratory problem, smoking, or drinking too much alcohol.

Since most people snore while sleeping on their backs, a simple remedy is to sew a "snore ball" into the back of the snorer's night clothes. (It will be just uncomfortable enough to make the sleeper turn over without waking.) Or prop the head end of the bed an inch or two higher than the foot. This way, your nose will drain more easily and you'll breathe better without snoring.

How important is bed rest when I have a bad cold or the flu?

Bed rest does nothing to alter the course of the common cold, a viral infection that usually takes

about a week to clear up. But a day at home can make you feel better and perhaps prevent the cold from developing into a more serious secondary bacterial infection, such as bronchitis or strep throat. If you are feeling miserable, you won't accomplish very much at work anyway.

Influenza, or flu, is a more severe type of viral infection than a cold. Its symptoms include chills, fever, headache, muscle ache, and severe fatigue accompanied by a cough, chest pains, a sore throat, and a runny nose. Several days of bed rest are almost mandatory to get your strength back. For the elderly and those with lung or heart disease, a bout of influenza cannot be treated lightly: it often leads to serious secondary infections such as bronchitis or pneumonia.

Is there any way to avoid catching a cold?

Your best defense against colds is to wash your hands often. You catch a cold when you come in contact with cold viruses. Just turning a door knob or picking up a telephone recently touched by someone with a cold may be enough to infect your system, particularly if you rub your eyes or your nose right afterwards. Eyes and nose, not the mouth, are frequently the routes for self-infection with cold viruses. In fact, you're more likely to catch a cold by shaking hands with someone than by kissing him or her.

Lacking the immunity that adults build up over time, children are the most common cold carriers (preschoolers average 6 to 10 per year). Teach your children to wash their hands often with soap and water. Children and adults should sneeze and blow noses into tissues rather than handkerchiefs, and discard used ones promptly in a wastebasket.

FACT OR FALLACY ?

Chicken soup is an effective cold medicine

Fact. Chicken soup was already a well-established home remedy for the common cold when Jewish philosopher and physician Maimonides prescribed it for an Egyptian caliph nearly 800 years ago. In 1978 a Florida physician tested the effects of what has come to be known as "Jewish penicillin." He found that chicken soup did open clogged nasal passages and let the patient breathe more easily. These respiratory effects were short-lived, and could probably be duplicated by other steaming hot beverages. However, there may be another benefit to chicken soup. It is usually bestowed with love, and that alone may make the sufferer feel better.

Chills, drafts, and wet feet cause colds

Fallacy. In the 1950s researchers in both England and the United States set out to test this old bit of folklore about colds. On both sides of the Atlantic scores of volunteers walked about with wet feet, sat in drafts, and endured chilling temperatures without proper clothing. No correlation whatsoever was found between the incidence of colds and the misery of the volunteers.

How effective are the many cold remedies sold over the counter?

Commercial cold remedies can't cure or shorten the duration of a cold (usually 7 to 10 days), but some of them can relieve a cold's more irritating effects. In reports prepared over the last 20 years by panels of experts for the U.S. Food and Drug Administration, 115 active ingredients commonly used to treat six different cold symptoms were reviewed.

The panels endorsed analgesics for reducing aches and fever, antihistamines for relieving sneezing and runny nose, nasal decongestants for clearing sinus passages, antitussives for suppressing cold-related coughs, and the expectorant guaifenesin for loosening coughs. Anticholinergics, sometimes included in cold remedies to relieve watery eyes and nose, were found to have no proven cold-relief value.

The experts also looked into the effectiveness and safety of "multisymptom" cold remedies. Although the FDA has recommended combination products with as many as four different ingredients, the panels emphasized the need to take only the ingredients necessary to treat the symptoms being experienced at each stage of a cold and not to load the body with superfluous and inappropriate chemicals.

Most doctors endorse the panels' advice: stick with safe, proven cold-relief ingredients and take each only as needed. And remember that generics (p. 152) are often cheaper and just as effective as brand-name products.

Can antibiotics cure colds or flu?

Antibiotics such as penicillin, tetracycline, and erythromycin are specifically designed to attack certain disease-causing bacteria. They have no effect at all on the hundreds of different viruses that cause colds, flu, and other upper respiratory infections.

The reasons have to do with the distinctly different nature of bacteria and viruses. Bacteria are living microorganisms that are equipped to survive and reproduce on their own, given the right environment. Antibiotics destroy bacteria by interrupting their life cycle. Viruses (which can be one-hundredth the size of bacteria) are far more primitive in structure. They survive only by invading a human target cell and reproducing within it. For a drug to destroy a virus, it either must destroy the entire host cell, a cure more costly than the disease in the case of colds, or prevent the virus from invading the host cell, a procedure that is theoretically possible but still not practicable.

It should be noted, however, that a prescription drug has been developed for treating Type A influenza, one of the three main types of influenza. Called amantadine, the drug works in a way that is not yet precisely understood. It appears to either block the Type A flu virus from attaching to healthy cells or inhibit the virus from reproducing within cells it has penetrated.

Amantadine not only helps prevent infection with the flu virus, but if taken early in a bout of flu, it can also shorten the duration of the infection.

Does vitamin C really help prevent colds?

In 1970 Linus Pauling, one of the nation's most distinguished chemists, published a book called *Vitamin C and the Common Cold*. In it he made a case for taking daily supplements (1,000 to 2,000 milligrams) of ascorbic acid (vitamin C) to prevent colds and even higher doses (4,000 to 10,000 milligrams) to combat existing colds. He cited a variety of studies to support his claims.

Pauling's ideas were eagerly seized upon by millions of American cold sufferers, with the result that sales of vitamin C soared. The medical establishment, however, has never been able to duplicate the results of Pauling's vitamin C studies and remains, for the most part, steadfast in its opposition to his theory.

Despite serious questioning of Pauling's studies, the controversy surrounding vitamin C continues to be very much alive. More recent evidence suggests that there may be some truth to Pauling's claims that vitamin C stimulates the body's immune response, but the effect is not strong enough to warrant the vitamin's use in preventing or treating colds.

Medical researchers also warn that taking large doses of vitamin C over extended periods can adversely alter the balance of acid in the body, interfere with the action of other medications, foster the development of kidney stones, and have an undesired laxative effect.

When, if ever, does a cold become serious enough to warrant a call to the doctor?

Complications arising from a common cold are rare, but when they do occur you should see your doctor promptly. Such complications are usually caused by bacteria that get trapped in or invade a blocked passageway, where they multiply into a full-blown secondary bacterial infection.

Staphylococcus bacteria, for example, can infect the lungs to produce a form of pneumonia that is particularly severe in in-

---

THE BODY'S WARNING SIGNALS

Recognizing a symptom that merits a call to your doctor is critical to your good health. Although such symptoms often turn out to be caused by minor problems, they sometimes indicate a serious disease requiring prompt action. Here's a basic list of danger signs. The first seven are the American Cancer Society's warning signs of cancer. Unexplained weight loss, persistent fever, and recurrent vomiting can also signal the presence of cancer.

1. Unusual bleeding or discharge. In women, vaginal bleeding between periods, during pregnancy, or after menopause; bleeding or discharge from the nipples. In both sexes, rectal bleeding or blood found in feces (they will look black and tarry), urine (it may range from pink to brown), vomit, phlegm, or sputum.

2. Any marked change in bowel or bladder habits.

3. A sore that doesn't heal in about 3 weeks.

4. A change in the size or appearance of a mole, freckle, or skin blemish.

5. A lump, swelling or, thickening in a woman's breast or, in either sex, elsewhere in the body.

6. Nagging hoarseness or coughing; a worsening smoker's cough.

7. Chronic indigestion or difficulty in swallowing.

8. A sudden, unexplained drop in weight.

9. Recurrent vomiting.

10. Unexplained chronic pain; new or severe pain in the head, chest, or abdomen.

11. Chronic fever or sweats.

12. Unexplained light-headedness or fainting spells.

13. Blurred vision; seeing halos around lights.

14. Severe, unexplained shortness of breath.

15. Bluish lips, eyelids, or nail beds.

16. Chronic ankle swelling.

17. Excessive thirst.

18. Unusual weakness or fatigue.

19. Yellowing of the skin or the whites of the eyes.

20. In men, frequent, difficult, or painful urination or a discharge from the penis.

---

fants and the elderly. Pneumococcus bacteria cause another serious type of pneumonia. Streptococcus bacteria can trigger pneumonia, middle ear infections, and painful, sometimes deadly, strep throat.

A persistent fever (above 102°F in adults, 103°F in children) is usually the first sign of a secondary infection, but swollen glands, breathing and swallowing difficulties, chest pains, a skin rash, a cough that produces yellow, pink, or rust-colored mucus, neck stiffness, earaches, thick white or yellow spots at the back of the throat, or any other symptoms that are not commonly associated with a cold should prompt a phone call and perhaps a visit to the doctor's office.

Even in the absence of such symptoms, you should consult your doctor if a cold lasts more than 2 weeks, or if you find yourself becoming increasingly sicker instead of better. While it is not probable, your "cold" may not be a cold at all, but some other disease that in its early stages mimics a cold.

How can I best protect myself against the flu?

The same practices that reduce susceptibility to colds (p.209) apply in general to cutting down your chances of getting the flu: wash your hands frequently (anything touched by someone with the flu will likely carry the virus), try not to rub your eyes and nose (they are the primary entry points for cold and flu viruses), and avoid direct contact with infected people when you can.

However, if the flu is epidemic, and you are not lucky enough to be immune to the particular strain causing this year's outbreak, you may become infected anyway. If you are otherwise healthy, the infection will put you to bed for a few days and slow you down for several more but generally will have no serious or lasting consequences.

There are people, however, for whom flu poses a significant risk of complications: everyone over 65, anyone with a blood disease or who suffers from chronic heart, lung, kidney, metabolic, respiratory, or immune disorders. If you are in a high-risk group, you should receive an annual flu shot (p.129). If for some

reason you miss getting vaccinated in the fall, you may want to ask your doctor about taking the prescription drug amantadine in case of a flu outbreak.

Should I avoid driving when I have the flu?

Whenever you are down with an infection, coping with fever, or otherwise feeling miserable, your reactions will be slowed to some degree and your judgment will be impaired. Add to this the sedative effects of any drugs— over-the-counter or prescription—that you may be taking to treat flu symptoms and your risk of being involved in an auto accident rises significantly.

By the same token, avoid operating any sort of dangerous machinery at home or at work when you have the flu or are otherwise not feeling up to par.

Is it true that keeping a humidifier in the house can help prevent colds and coughs?

A humidifier will make heated indoor air more comfortable to breathe, especially when you have a cold. As to whether a humidifier can actually prevent colds and coughs, the scientific research is inconclusive, and the Association of Home Appliance Manufacturers makes no health claims for the humidifiers made by its member companies. (Skeptics point out that people who live in desert areas without humidifying the air are no more cold prone than anyone else.) In addition, the devices do pose a certain health risk. Unless they are properly cleaned and maintained, humidifiers can disperse harmful mineral particles into the air and serve as a breeding ground for fungi and other disease-causing organisms.

Which thermometer is more accurate, the new digital type or the old mercury thermometer?

Both kinds of thermometers are about 98 percent accurate. The chief difference between them is that the more expensive digital is easier to use. It may buzz when it has a reading, and it spells out the temperature clearly on a lead crystal display screen. A mercury thermometer must be shaken down to a base reading level before each use. Once you have inserted it in the patient, you have to wait for the mercury inside to warm and climb to its proper level on the calibrated scale—about 3 minutes. To read a mercury thermometer, you need good light and an agile wrist.

An electronic digital thermometer costs three times what a standard glass mercury thermometer does and needs a new battery every 2 years. A mercury thermometer won't run down, but it may shatter if dropped.

Whichever thermometer you pick, the oral version is preferred for most situations. Place the bulb end of the thermometer under the patient's tongue with the mouth closed around it. To get an accurate reading, don't take a temperature immediately after the patient has eaten, taken a drink, or soaked in a tub.

For young children, use a rectal thermometer. Putting an oral thermometer in the armpit (normal readings are about 1°F lower) or using a flexible temperature indicator strip across a child's forehead gives a less precise reading.

What medicines help lower fever?

Both aspirin and acetaminophen are effective in lowering fever associated with colds and flu in adults. For children with fever,

HOME MEDICAL TESTS

Kits sold at pharmacies enable you to perform a variety of important medical tests. Designed to be used under a doctor's supervision, most do-it-yourself tests involve the use of a dipstick or a test pad coated with bands of chemicals. When exposed to certain substances in urine or blood, the chemicals change color in characteristic ways. If performed correctly, many home medical tests are no less reliable than lab tests. Read instructions carefully — and remember that self-diagnosis is not a substitute for a doctor's diagnosis and treatment.

Test	Purpose	How it works
Blood glucose	To monitor glucose levels in diabetics	*Reagent strip:* Glucose in a drop of blood causes a chemically treated test strip to change color. The strip is then compared with a color chart. *Electronic meter:* Strip is inserted into a device that analyzes blood and displays glucose reading digitally.
Occult blood	To detect occult (hidden) blood in feces, a sign of possible colon cancer	A stool sample is brought into contact with tissues, pads, or slides that change color in the presence of blood. Take specimens from three consecutive bowel movements; follow diet and other instructions carefully. See a doctor promptly if test results are positive.
Urinary tract infection	To detect urinary tract infections and early signs of bladder or kidney diseases	*Nitrite test:* A dipstick changes color in the presence of bacteria-produced nitrite in a urine sample. *Leukocytes test:* The dipstick changes color if there is an excessive amount of bacteria-fighting white blood cells, or leukocytes, in the urine.
Ovulation prediction	To pinpoint the time a woman is most likely to conceive	A chemically treated strip is dipped in a urine specimen every day for a week midway in the menstrual cycle. A characteristic color change indicates an increase in the level of a hormone that triggers ovulation, usually within 24 to 36 hours. (This test should not be used for contraceptive purposes.)
Pregnancy	To determine whether a woman is pregnant	Many different types of home pregnancy tests are available, but all are based on the same principle—chemicals mixed with drops of urine change color or form a characteristic deposit in the presence of HCG, a hormone found in urine only during pregnancy.

acetaminophen is the medicine of choice. Aspirin has been known to increase the risk of Reye's syndrome, a relatively rare but serious disease that children under 15 can contract in the wake of a viral infection.

Do colds really cause cold sores?

Cold sores and fever blisters are misnomers. These small, itchy, sometimes painful skin eruptions that appear around the edges of the lips are not caused by colds or fevers per se, although colds and fever do trigger them. Rather, they're symptoms of infection with the herpes simplex type 1 virus. This virus infects most people early in life and can remain dormant for years at a time until it's reactivated by any number of physiological or psychological stresses, such as a bad sunburn, menstruation, or anxiety. Often, the trigger remains unknown.

An attack of herpes simplex typically begins with tingling and itching around the mouth followed by the appearance of one or more blisters. Several days later fluid in the blisters oozes out and a crusted scab forms. As the fluid contains live virus, it's easy to spread the infection to other sites on the body or to someone else. Wash your hands often and avoid kissing during an outbreak. Keep fingers that have touched the blisters away from your eyes: a herpes simplex infection of the eye can be severe and lead to corneal damage and permanent vision impairment. Cold sore outbreaks usually last about a week to 10 days.

When you feel an attack coming on, rest and avoid alcoholic drinks. Over-the-counter antibiotic ointments can reduce skin cracking and the possibility of an opportunistic bacterial infection. For a particularly uncomfortable outbreak, your doctor may prescribe acyclovir ointment (Zovirax), an antiviral drug that usually clears up the sores quickly. (Although it has been approved by the U.S. Food and Drug Administration for the treatment of genital and other herpes infections, the use of acyclovir for cold sores is still being tested.)

What is the difference between a cough suppressant and an expectorant?

Cough suppressants, or antitussives, are intended to relieve and suppress dry, irritating nonproductive coughs. Expectorants, on the other hand, are formulated to liquefy and loosen the sticky secretions produced by the mucous membrane so that they can be coughed up and expelled from the lungs.

Antitussives come in lozenges and liquids. Over-the-counter preparations typically contain dextromethorphan, a synthetic narcotic that is generally considered safe and somewhat effective in its ability to suppress the urge to cough. Stronger preparations, often required for more persistent and painful coughs, contain codeine, an opium derivative available only in prescription form. So long as the cough remains dry, an antitussive may have value, but suppressing a cough for a period of several days can cause an unhealthy

buildup of mucus in the lungs. Consequently, an antitussive should be used only briefly and according to package directions.

Expectorants are not regarded as particularly effective by the U.S. Food and Drug Administration unless they contain an ingredient called guaifenesin. However, no adverse effects have been associated with their use. The FDA is specifically opposed to cough medications that claim to be both a suppressant and an expectorant. Doctors agree that it is irrational to mix medications that have diametrically opposed purposes.

How effective are throat lozenges?

Throat lozenges, troches, and cough drops are all variants of medicated candy. Most of them contain tiny amounts of a topical anesthetic, which is released as you suck on them. The soothing effects begin almost immediately and often last for up to 30 minutes. But like all medications, they should not be taken more often than recommended on the package or for extended periods of time. If throat pain persists or becomes more severe, it's time to see a doctor.

I got over the flu several weeks ago, but I am still coughing. What could this mean?

Most healthy people recover from the flu and are essentially back to normal within 2 weeks. But the elderly and people with an underlying heart or respiratory problem can develop a secondary infection, often associated with the bronchial tubes, sinus cavities, or lungs. A persistent cough, particularly one that is accompanied by a low-grade fever, may be symptomatic of

such an infection, and should be investigated by a doctor. Similarly, if you experience earaches, shortness of breath, or chest pains in the wake of influenza, consult your doctor.

Does heartburn have anything to do with the heart?

Heartburn is simply a popular name for acid indigestion and has nothing to do with the heart except that you may feel a burning sensation in the chest area.

Heartburn is generally caused by a reflux, or backflow, of stomach acid into the esophagus, the connecting tube between the mouth and the stomach. Under normal circumstances, the sphincter muscle, or valve, between the esophagus and the stomach stays closed except when you are swallowing. Stress or emotional upset can trigger heartburn by affecting the nerves that control the sphincter muscle. Other factors that can cause the sphincter muscle to malfunction are obesity, pregnancy, smoking, an unhealthy diet, an excess of intestinal gas, or a hiatal hernia, a condition in which part of the stomach bulges through the diaphragm into the chest.

I recently had chest pains so severe that I thought I was having a heart attack. Luckily, it was indigestion. How can I tell the difference next time?

Most people who experience severe chest pains assume they're having a heart attack. Without evaluation by a doctor it can be difficult to distinguish between that dire possibility and a host of other far less serious conditions affecting the chest wall, abdomen, and gallbladder.

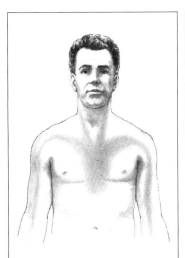

A heart attack feels as if a heavy weight had been dropped inside you. The dull, crushing pain usually starts in the center of the chest and spreads upward into the neck and jaw or into either or both arms; it may be accompanied by nausea, vomiting, and a strong sense of impending doom.

If there is a single generalization that can be made, it's that a heart attack typically involves severe, crushing chest pain that often radiates from the center of the chest to the jaw, neck, and arms.

By contrast, a pain that is more burning and irritating than crushing, that gets worse when you bend over or lie down, or that develops soon after eating, is more likely to be from a hiatal hernia or indigestion. If a chest pain is localized and the region is tender to the touch, you probably have a pulled muscle or some other sort of injury to the rib cage. If a pain is accompanied by coughing and spitting up blood, or shortness of breath, you may have pneumonia or another serious lung condition.

Prompt attention is crucial in treating heart attacks and serious lung conditions. Call for help immediately if you have doubts about the cause of any chest pain.

I know someone who pops antacids like candy. How effective are they? Can taking too many be harmful?

Over-the-counter antacids, which neutralize excess gastric acids, are helpful in relieving heartburn and sour stomach, as well as the pain of peptic ulcers (p. 216).

Although there are scores of antacids on the market, all contain one or more of four active ingredients: sodium bicarbonate, calcium carbonate, magnesium salts, and aluminum salts. None of these products should be taken indiscriminately.

Bicarb is rapid acting but offers only short-term relief. It may cause abdominal discomfort, belching, and other side effects, especially with prolonged use. Because bicarb contains sodium, it's not recommended for people with heart disease, high blood pressure, or kidney problems.

Calcium carbonate is also fast acting, but with prolonged use may cause constipation and acid rebound (a condition in which stomach acid levels rise even higher after the antacid is absorbed). When taken by people on a bland, high-milk diet, calcium carbonate can cause blood levels of calcium to rise excessively.

Magnesium and aluminum antacids are slower acting, longer lasting, and usually safe if used in moderation. However, magnesium antacids can cause diarrhea; aluminum-based ones, constipation.

In addition to taking antacids, there are other self-help remedies for heartburn:

☐ Avoid caffeine, alcohol, aspirin, fatty or highly acidic foods, and any food that you identify as contributing to your problem.
☐ Don't wear tight clothing, particularly around the waist.
☐ To keep stomach acids flowing in the right direction while you sleep, elevate the head of your bed on 4- to 6-inch blocks.
☐ Don't lie down after eating.
☐ If stress triggers heartburn, try to relax, especially at mealtimes.

Persistent abdominal pain, even if relieved temporarily by antacids, should be evaluated by a doctor within 2 weeks.

Is it harmful to lie down right after eating?

It may not be exactly harmful, but it can cause uncomfortable heartburn. Try to stay upright for at least 2 to 3 hours after meals. Better yet, schedule a modest walk right after a big meal. And avoid eating within 2 hours of your bedtime.

I have a tendency to belch a lot. Is there anything I can take to relieve this problem?

Belching is a form of relief, a way of getting rid of excess air that gets trapped in your stomach when you eat or drink too fast. (Some people develop an unconscious habit of swallowing gulps of air when they talk.) The expelled air rises through the throat, passes the vocal cords, and makes a sound. In some parts of the world, that sound is considered a sign of contentment; in the West, however, it gets a mixed review, depending on the situation and the company.

There is no medication that has proven effective in controlling this problem. If you want to curtail belching, try eating more slowly and chewing your food more carefully so that you take in less air as you eat. If belching becomes a persistent problem for you, consult your doctor. Excessive belching can be a symptom of hiatal hernia or chronic indigestion. (For ways to curtail flatulence, see p. 33.)

How can you tell the pain of an ulcer from ordinary indigestion?

Peptic ulcers are open sores that form in the lining of the upper gastrointestinal tract—the esophagus, stomach, and duodenum (the first part of the small intestine). If ulcers are left untreated, they may cause internal bleeding or a perforation of the tract wall that can lead to serious infection. (For more on the causes and treatment of peptic ulcers, see pages 345–346).

Distinguishing between ulcers and ordinary indigestion is often a matter of recognizing a consistent pattern of symptoms over a period of weeks. To begin with, ulcers are not a transient occurrence. Like the occasional stomachache, they may produce a gnawing, aching, or burning sensation in the abdomen just above the navel, but the pain is likely to recur several times a day, every day, for weeks at a time. Sometimes the pain comes when the stomach is empty and eases or stops altogether after you eat or drink something. In other cases, the pain starts immediately after eating.

If the ulcerative condition is advanced, the pain may become quite severe and be accompanied by blood in the stool, extreme weakness, fainting, and unusual thirst, all of which are symptoms of internal bleeding.

If you suspect you have ulcers, you may be able to treat them with antacids, but make sure to see your doctor for an evaluation.

Is persistent mild diarrhea a sign of a serious problem?

If it occurs infrequently and for short periods of time, diarrhea is generally not a cause for concern. Indeed, it is often part of

---

THE FACTS ABOUT REGULARITY

What's "normal." The normal frequency of bowel movements varies from person to person, depending on diet, fluid intake, physical activity, medications, and genes. Three a day is normal for some people; once every 3 days for others. Going a day or two beyond your usual pattern is not generally a cause for concern. However, if constipation lasts for more than a few days or if it is accompanied by sudden unexplained weight loss, abdominal pain and bloating, or very hard or bloody stools, consult your doctor.

The most effective remedy for occasional mild constipation is to increase the amount of fiber in your diet. Eat more vegetables, fruits, and whole-grain breads and cereals. Drink more fluids and step up your exercise. And when you feel the urge to defecate, give yourself time to do so; ignoring your bowel needs is a common cause of constipation.

Laxatives are drugs designed to produce a soft, easy-to-pass stool. Excessive use may cause diarrhea; prolonged use may cause the bowels to become dependent. Stimulant laxatives (bisacodyl, senna), lubricants (mineral oil), and saline laxatives (magnesium sulfate, sodium phosphate) may cause adverse effects. If you must use a laxative, take a bulk fiber laxative (psyllium), and stop using it as soon as regularity is restored.

---

the digestive system's effort to rid itself of an irritant or an infectious agent. Such mild cases of diarrhea are best left untreated for the first few hours; then, if necessary, try an over-the-counter antidiarrheal medication and avoid high-fiber foods for the next few days.

But diarrhea that persists can cause dehydration, especially in infants and the elderly; it can also be a signal of serious intestinal disturbances. As a general rule, if adult diarrhea continues beyond 4 days, or is associated with other physical problems such as black or bloody stools, severe abdominal pain, or signs of dehydration, seek medical attention. Diarrhea causes damage much sooner in infants and very young children because of their small size and tendency to become dehydrated. Consult

your pediatrician if an infant has had more than three watery stools in 24 hours or if a child has had diarrhea longer than 2 days.

How effective are over-the-counter hemorrhoid medications?

A variety of remedies can soothe the affected area while normal healing is taking place, but their role in "curing" hemorrhoids is very limited.

Similar to varicose veins on the legs, hemorrhoids are swollen and distended veins either inside the rectum or surrounding the anal opening. The best and most natural remedies are those that increase blood flow in the veins and decrease pressure on the rectum. Starting an exercise program (or simply walking around more during the day), eating more fiber, straining less during bowel movements, and taking hot baths can often clear up a mild problem and prevent its recurrence.

Among helpful over-the-counter products are rectal wipes and ointments containing zinc oxide, which soothe the irritated area. Hemorrhoid remedies that promise to anesthetize the pain (their names often end in "-caine") may in fact lead to even more irritation after repeated use.

If self-treatment doesn't bring relief, see your doctor. For hemorrhoids located inside the rectum, "banding" may be suggested. In an office procedure that requires no anesthesia, each of the swollen—and essentially superfluous—veins is tied off with a tiny rubber band and left to wither away. Alternatives include injecting the hemorrhoids with a scar-inducing chemical (sclerotherapy) or burning them with electric current.

Unlike internal hemorrhoids, external hemorrhoids are too pain-sensitive to be removed by banding or sclerotherapy. They can be excised surgically in a procedure that requires a hospital stay and general or epidural anesthesia. Or in a simpler procedure performed in a doctor's office with a local anesthetic, external hemorrhoids can be burned with infrared heat, lasers, or electricity.

Are all over-the-counter painkillers equally good for all kinds of headaches, or should I pick and choose according to symptoms?

It may be hard to believe, but there are only three active chemical ingredients—aspirin, acetaminophen, and ibuprofen—in all of the many headache medications that line the shelves of supermarkets and drugstores. All three of these painkillers are equally effective.

Aspirin has been around the longest, is the best known, and costs the least (only a few pennies a tablet if you buy a generic product). But aspirin should not be taken by people with bleeding disorders or ulcers because it thins the blood slightly and can irritate the stomach. Aspirin is also not recommended for children with a fever or for anyone anticipating surgery or major dental work within 5 days.

"Enteric-coated" aspirin, which dissolves in the intestines rather than in the stomach, is useful for people who take aspirin frequently and experience stomach discomfort. Buffered aspirin tablets contain an "acid-neutralizer," whose value is questioned by many medical authorities. (The U.S. Food and Drug

---

TYPES OF HEADACHES

Tension headaches are the most common type of headache. Pain is caused by a tightening of the muscles of the neck, face, or scalp, usually triggered by emotional stress (worry, anxiety, depression) or physical stress (sitting in a stuffy room or working too long in the same position). The pain often feels like a band of dull, steady pressure around the head. Most tension headaches respond to aspirin or other over-the-counter analgesics, but some can last all day, and recur frequently. These may require evaluation at a headache clinic, where a variety of treatments are available: hypnosis, behavior modification, acupuncture, and drug therapy. Prevention for most people lies in avoiding—or changing—the stressful life situations that trigger headaches.

Vascular headaches are caused by changes in the diameter of blood vessels that supply the brain and scalp. The most common type of vascular headache is the *migraine headache*—sharp, throbbing pain often on one side of the head and often associated with nausea. Migraines affect more women than men and tend to run in families. For more on migraines, see page 356.

Cluster headaches affect more men than women, do not seem to run in families, and are rare. Characterized by a piercing pain in one eye or on one side of the face, cluster headaches may occur a few times a day for weeks or months, and then disappear. They often start in the middle of the night, waking the sufferer up. Though painful, cluster headaches are not signs of a more serious problem and they do respond to drug therapy.

Other common headaches are caused by excessive caffeine or alcohol consumption; certain foods, food additives, and drugs; and in some cases, even orgasm. Most headaches are not a sign of a serious underlying problem. However, if a headache is accompanied by visual loss, vomiting, confusion or loss of memory, numbness in some part of the body, lack of coordination and slurred speech, or high fever and a stiff neck, seek medical attention right away.

RELIEF FOR AN ACHING BACK

The best defense against back trouble is to get in shape and learn how to use your body properly. It's especially important to stretch back muscles and strengthen abdominal muscles, which do most of the work of supporting the back. The exercises shown here, as well as *curl-ups, buttock squeezes,* and *side tucks* (p.88), are all good for your back.

Proper posture is also important. When standing or walking, contract your abdominal muscles and tuck your buttocks under slightly. Keep your shoulders back (but not in an exaggerated arch) and your torso loose. If you must stand for a long time, raise one foot to take some weight off your lower

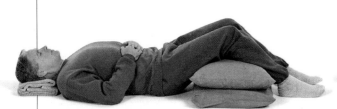

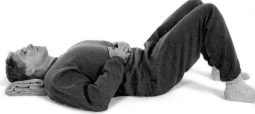

To relieve a back spasm, lie on your back on the floor (or on a very firm mattress), with a small pillow under your head and two large pillows under your knees. Keep your spine pressed against the floor. Rest in this position for at least 20 minutes. Do not attempt any exercises until the pain has fully abated.

Pelvic tilts. Lie on your back on the floor, with your knees bent and a small pillow under your head. Place your hands on your abdomen. Press the small of your back against the floor by tightening your buttocks and pulling in your stomac You should feel your pelvis tilting up. Hold for a slow count of 5. Release and repeat 5 times.

Administration, however, has found that buffered aspirin is absorbed faster than regular aspirin.) Some analgesics (Anacin, for example) contain aspirin and caffeine, a combination that may give some people greater relief from the pain of tension headaches than aspirin alone.

Acetaminophen does everything aspirin does except reduce inflammation. It's a good substitute headache remedy for people who can't take aspirin, and it's the over-the-counter analgesic recommended for reducing fever in children. However, long-term use of acetaminophen has been found to cause liver and possibly kidney disease in some people.

Ibuprofen, which fights pain, fever, and inflammation, is no better than aspirin or acetaminophen in treating headaches, and generally costs more. Ibuprofen should not be taken during pregnancy. Prolonged use can cause kidney damage.

Besides taking a pain-killer, is there anything else I can do to relieve a tension headache?

Often the best way to treat an occasional tension headache is to lie down in a darkened room with a cool cloth over your forehead. Massaging tight neck muscles or taking a hot shower may also provide some relief.

If tension headaches are a regular part of your life, then you need to address the source of the tension and resolve it in some way. If practiced regularly, the relaxation techniques described on pages 206–207 can be very beneficial.

How can I best protect myself from the sun's harmful effects?

Ultraviolet radiation from the sun is the main cause of skin cancer, a major cause of premature wrink-

ling, and a contributor to cataracts and other eye problems. Recognition of the sun's harmful effects has come just as changes in the earth's ozone layer have made ultraviolet rays even more potent. Although fair-skinned people are most at risk, dramatic increases in skin cancer cases since the 1960's have convinced doctors that it's foolish for anyone to pursue a tan.

If you're out in the sun a lot, protect your eyes with sunglasses (p.220) and keep yourself covered up. Wear a broad-brimmed hat, long pants rather than shorts, and a long-sleeved shirt. (Ultraviolet rays can penetrate many loosely woven fabrics.) Remember that sunlight reflected off sand, water, and snow can also burn the skin. Stay out of the summer sun when it's most intense, between 10 A.M. and 2 P.M.

Use sunscreen regularly, and for long stints outside, protect nose, lips, and cheeks with a

back. Wear comfortable shoes; avoid high heels. Use straight-backed chairs and a firm mattress. Try not to sleep on your stomach. If you can't sleep on your back, try lying on one side in the fetal position.

When lifting a heavy load, let your legs, not your back, do the real work. Get close to the object to be lifted, spread your feet apart, and slowly bend your knees. Lift by pushing up from your knees while keeping your back straight. Don't bend at the waist. Most minor back problems respond to bedrest, moderate applications of ice or heat, and aspirin or other mild analgesics. For more information on the causes and treatment of chronic back pain, see page 357.

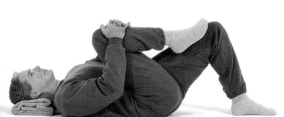

Knee hugs. Lie on your back on the floor, with your knees bent and a small pillow under your head. Grasp one of your knees with both hands and draw it gently toward your chest. Hold this position for a count of 10, then release the knee, and repeat the same procedure with your other knee. Repeat 10 times for each knee.

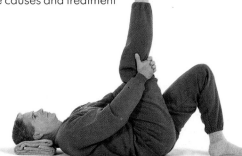

Hamstring stretches. Lie on your back, as for *knee hugs*. Grasp one knee with both hands and draw it gently toward your chest. Straighten the leg and pull it toward your head without bouncing. Bend knee; return foot to floor. Slide leg down, relax, then bend knee again. Repeat with other leg. Repeat 5 times for each leg.

blocking agent. These two sun protection products are the key to preventing skin damage.

Sunscreens don't block ultraviolet rays; rather, they slow them down, allowing you to stay in the sun longer without burning. The degree of protection provided is indicated by the product's SPF (sun-protection factor) number. If you ordinarily can stay in the sun for 10 minutes before starting to redden, using a sunscreen with an SPF of 15 lets you spend 2½ hours (15 x 10 minutes = 150 minutes) in the sun without burning. Some people are sensitive to an ingredient used in many of the early sunscreens, para-aminobenzoic acid (PABA), but there are many formulas now that don't contain PABA. Sunscreen comes in lotion, cream, or lip salve form; some versions are waterproof. Whether you are very fair or dark-complexioned, always apply an SPF 15 or higher sun-

screen to exposed parts of your body when you go out into the sun for any length of time— winter or summer. Apply it 30 minutes before going out, and reapply it every 2 hours (sweat can remove sunscreen) and after swimming. Use sunscreen on babies 6 months or older; keep younger infants in the shade.

Blocking agents, which do stop ultraviolet rays, are the white or brightly colored creams you see lifeguards wearing on the nose and in stripes under the eyes. If reapplied frequently, blocks do a nearly perfect job of protecting sensitive skin areas from sun damage.

Are tanning salons safer than direct exposure to the sun? What about tanning pills?

Dermatologists take a dim view of tanning parlors. The ultraviolet rays of an indoor sun lamp are

actually more intense than the sun's rays. You can become overexposed in a matter of minutes instead of hours. And that overexposure exacts a cumulative price: rough, wrinkled skin and, in time, a heightened risk of skin cancer. The eyes also are at greater risk in a tanning salon. If you go to one, you need to wear goggles, not just sunglasses, and never look directly into one of the lamps.

Tanning pills provide pigment to cells just below the surface of the skin (as well as throughout your body). Taking the pills for a certain number of days causes enough pigmentation to build up to produce a noticeable color (more orange than tan); to maintain the color, you must keep taking a minimum dosage of the pills.

Beta-carotene and canthaxanthin, the main ingredients in tanning pills, are not approved by the U.S. Food and Drug Administration for tanning purposes, although both chemicals are approved for use as food dyes. (Tanning pill dosage of these chemicals is 20 to 30 times the amount ingested in a normal diet.) Some people get dry, itchy skin from taking tanning pills; others may experience nausea, cramps, and diarrhea. Doctors are also concerned that the pills may cause liver damage and retinal problems.

If looking tanned is terribly important to you, the safest route is to use either a chemical tanning product containing dihydroxyacetone (DHA) that you rub on your skin or a bronzing gel that simply paints on color.

Is it really important to wear sunglasses in the summer? What type of sunglasses should I look for?

It's very important to protect your eyes from too much sun in both winter and summer. Over time, exposure to the sun's visible light and ultraviolet rays can damage the lens, the retina, and the cornea of the eye, and may cause cataracts.

Unless there are special circumstances (you need prescription glasses, you've had cataract surgery, you're taking tetracycline or other drugs that make you more sensitive to sunlight, your job or sport keeps you in the sun all day), you needn't buy expensive sunglasses from an optometrist. Safe, effective, and inexpensive sunglasses are available at drugstores and department stores. Here's what to look for:

□ Rating label. The American National Standard Institute (ANSI) sets consumer standards for sunglasses. Glasses with an ANSI "general purpose" label are suitable for most normal outdoor activities. They block from 60 to 95 percent of visible light (the

bright sunlight that makes you squint), 95 percent of UVB, or ultraviolet B, rays (the rays that cause your skin to burn and that are most harmful to your eyes), and 60 percent of the less intense UVA, or ultraviolet A, rays. Glasses with an ANSI "special purpose" label are designed for very bright environments like beaches or ski slopes. They may block as much as 97 percent of visible light (depending on how dark they are), 99 percent of UVB, and 60 percent of UVA. The ANSI "cosmetic" label goes on sunglasses that are intended more for show than for protection. They block less than 60 percent of visible light, 70 percent of UVB, and 20 percent of UVA. Although sunglass labeling is voluntary, it's a good idea to look for ANSI-rated glasses that block as much UV radiation as possible and at least 75 percent of visible light.

□ Darkness. The ability of a lens to block ultraviolet rays is not a function of its darkness (it's a special chemical coating that does the job). However, for sunglasses to stop 70 percent or more of visible light, the lenses must be quite dark.

To judge if sunglasses are dark enough, put a pair on and look in a mirror; you should barely be able to see your eyes. On the other hand, glasses that are too dark can reduce your vision excessively and cause accidents. Try to test glasses outdoors in bright light before buying them.

□ Color. Both drivers and pedestrians need to distinguish between red and green traffic lights. Gray and green lenses transmit colors most faithfully for most people. Blue and purple distort the most. Brown and amber are in the middle.

□ Optical characteristics. Check lenses for distortion of shapes and lines: With the glasses on,

look at a vertical line and then rotate your head from side to side. Does the line bend or ripple? If so, don't buy the glasses.

□ Lens types. Glass lenses are heavier but less likely to get scratched than plastic. Polarized lenses have a filter that cuts glare. Mirrored lenses cut glare, too, but scratch easily. Gradient lenses that are dark at the top and lighter at the bottom allow a driver to read numbers on the dashboard more clearly. Phototropic lenses, which turn darker in the sun and lighter in the shade, don't work well behind glass and should not be used for driving.

□ Fit. Look for glasses that fit snugly and comfortably. Lenses should be large enough to give protection and shafts narrow enough not to block side vision (wraparound lenses are best).

How effective is Retin-A in eliminating wrinkles?

Tretinoin, marketed under the trade name Retin-A, is a derivative of vitamin A that was developed as a treatment for severe acne. When word got out that Retin-A could also reverse the wrinkling effects of sun exposure, people rushed to dermatologists for Retin-A prescriptions, even though the U.S. Food and Drug Administration had not (and still hasn't) approved Retin-A for the removal of wrinkles. (Once a drug has been approved for one use, doctors are allowed to prescribe it for other things.)

Clinical studies seem to confirm some of the positive effects attributed to Retin-A. On some patients, fine lines do soften, dark spots lighten, and the skin takes on a rosy glow (the last effect is due partly to irritation).

Some users of Retin-A, particularly those who blush easily, have experienced severe skin irritation. Because this problem is often the result of misapplication, doctors should instruct their patients carefully on how to use the product.

The wrinkle-removing effects of Retin-A last only as long as you continue to use it. To maintain good results, you must commit yourself to an expensive lifetime regimen. No one yet knows what the effects of such long-term usage may be.

Caution. Retin-A makes the skin more sensitive to the sun's ultraviolet rays and significantly increases your risk of burning. If you use it, make sure you apply a sunscreen with a minimum SPF 15 rating anytime you go out into the sun.

Which is the better skin saver, aloe vera or vitamin E?

There is no firm evidence that vitamin E—whether taken internally or applied topically—is beneficial in the treatment of any common skin problem. In fact, doctors have reported cases in which patients who squeezed the liquid contents of a vitamin E capsule onto their skin broke out in rashes. The manufacturer of a deodorant containing vitamin E had to withdraw the product from the market for the very same reason.

Folklore and legend attribute almost miraculous powers to the liquid extract of the aloe vera plant, but hard scientific evidence does not seem to support such claims. The juice of the plant is 99.5 percent water, with the 0.5 percent balance containing about 20 amino acids and carbohydrates, none of which has any demonstrated ability to produce the remarkable curative results ascribed to the plant. Aloe is a good but not miraculous skin moisturizer, however, and it can be soothing on minor burns.

Are there any specific types of cosmetics I should avoid?

For most people, the answer is no. However, certain cosmetics contain substances (usually perfumes) that can produce skin irritation in some people.

Such allergic reactions to cosmetics are very rare. When they occur, they are usually caused by hair dyes, nail polish, eye makeup, and lipstick. These and other cosmetic products are now available in hypoallergenic versions, which are less likely to trigger allergic reactions.

If you know yourself to be somewhat sensitive, try a patch test before you use a new cosmetic. Apply some of the product to a small area of skin and cover it with an adhesive bandage. After 2 days examine the area for signs of irritation. If there are none, the product is probably safe for you to use according to the directions on the package.

My teenage son is very self-conscious about his acne. What causes acne and what's the best treatment for it?

Acne breaks out when oil produced by the sebaceous glands around hair follicles in the skin plugs up pores. Trapped bacteria multiply and the pores become inflamed and infected, resulting in the characteristic pimples, blackheads, whiteheads, and in serious cases, cysts that are symptoms of acne. Hormones are thought to play a role in causing acne, as are genetics (the condition tends to run in families). Acne afflicts teenage boys in particular, but many teenage girls suffer from it too.

There is no cure for acne, but treatments can improve the condition. Since all are slow acting,

youngsters must be prepared to follow a regimen for months before seeing any benefit.

To prevent the buildup and spread of bacteria, your son should wash his face gently with a mild soap twice a day and avoid touching his face as much as possible. Shampooing often will prevent oily hair from aggravating the condition. Diet doesn't seem to play a role in acne breakouts, as doctors once thought; so giving up chocolate or french fries won't really prevent or shorten an acne attack.

Many over-the-counter acne medications are simply a waste of money; greasy or oily ones can even aggravate the problem. However, for mild cases of acne, topical medications containing benzoyl peroxide can help dry the skin, kill off some of the bacteria, and promote healing.

Topical antibiotic creams, which a doctor must prescribe, can also be effective in treating mild cases of acne. If the problem is a persistent one, long-term therapy with oral antibiotics such as tetracycline can be beneficial. In such cases, however, the patient has to be careful in the sun and always use sunscreen, since tetracycline makes the user particularly sensitive to the sun's ultraviolet rays.

For severe acne, drugs derived from vitamin A, such as tretinoin (Retin-A) and isotretinoin (Accutane), are often effective. Because these drugs can have serious side effects, they must be used under a doctor's close supervision. Accutane, one of the strongest vitamin A derivatives used to treat acne, can cause serious birth defects if used by pregnant women.

Mild cases of acne usually clear up on their own by the time a youngster passes his teens. More serious cases should be evaluated and, if necessary, treated by a doctor.

Are warts a sign of poor personal hygiene?

Warts are minor local infections caused by the papilloma virus. No one knows why some people get warts and others don't, but personal hygiene plays no role. Warts are mildly contagious, particularly where no immunity to the virus exists, which is why children and adolescents are most likely to develop them.

Left alone, warts will disappear on their own within 2 years or less, which may be how some of the superstitious remedies got started. If you picked up a frog one day and your wart fell off the next day, you too might assume that the frog did the trick. Other old cures, such as rubbing a wart with earwax or dandelion juice, are no more effective than handling a frog.

Common warts are easy to remove. You can paint and repaint the growth with an over-the-counter acid compound; this burns off successive layers until the wart is gone. Other methods—freezing with liquid nitrogen or surgical removal—entail a visit to a doctor.

Plantar warts, which grow on the bottom of feet, and genital warts both require professional medical attention. Women with recurrent genital warts should undergo frequent Pap tests (p. 124) since a link has been found between genital warts and cervical cancer.

Is blow-drying bad for hair? What about permanents and dyes?

A blow dryer will not damage your hair as long as you keep the nozzle moving and don't train it too long on any one spot. A properly functioning dryer heats air to no more than 185°F—a temperature well below the

FACT OR FALLACY?

There's still no hope for the balding

Fallacy. It is true that none of the creams, lotions, vitamins, massagers, and other products that are widely advertised as baldness remedies work. They have no effect on the number of hairs that grow on the head, their thickness, or the rate of natural thinning. These are mainly hereditary factors. However, one new drug, minoxidil, has shown some promise in treating thinning hair. Developed as a treatment for high blood pressure, it was found to stimulate hair growth when applied topically. Early studies show good results for 39 percent of the test subjects. To keep the new hair growing, however, you must continue the applications. A prescription drug, minoxidil appears to be safe for long-term use, but it's most effective in people with the least amount of baldness. Hair transplants are another option for the balding. Tiny plugs of hairy scalp are removed from areas of thick growth and grafted onto bald areas. The transplants continue to produce hair in the new position. And looking to the future, British scientists have stimulated hair growth in a test tube; they expect some day to duplicate the feat on human scalps.

300°F it takes to damage hair.

Excessive shampooing, bleaching, dyeing, streaking, too vigorous brushing, straightening, and teasing the hair, as well as swimming in chlorine-treated water or exposing the hair to salt water and sunshine on a regular basis, are all hard on hair.

Conditioners, usually applied immediately after shampooing, offer a measure of protection against all these abuses. Cream rinses add surfactants (substances that act on the surface) that recoat hair and neutralize static electric charges so that hair is more manageable and combs out with less pulling and snarling. Protein conditioners contain other surfactants that lubricate and add luster and body to damaged hair.

What is the best way to get rid of a persistent case of dandruff?

Your scalp, like other parts of your body, is constantly renewing itself; in the process dead skin flakes off producing dandruff. For most people, ordinary hair brushing plus regular washing with a mild shampoo is enough to remove the oily flakes and keep hair and scalp free of unsightly accumulations of dandruff. But in a minority of cases—probably because of hormonal activity—the condition becomes extreme and earns the name of seborrheic dermatitis, an adult form of cradle cap.

For a moderate case of dandruff, avoid scratching and irritating your scalp and try an over-the-counter antidandruff shampoo. Products containing selenium sulfide, sulferon, tar, or zinc pyrithione in low, nonprescription concentrations are often effective, especially if you alternate them periodically.

You can't expect dandruff to

go away for good, but it should come under control after a few weeks of home treatment. If it doesn't, consult a dermatologist. If your condition really is dandruff, you may be given a prescription for a stronger anti-dandruff shampoo. If it turns out to be psoriasis, ringworm, or some form of allergy, other treatments will be prescribed.

What are hangnails?

A hangnail is a crack or split in the skin along the sides of a nail. It can develop from excessive skin dryness, from a nervous habit of picking or biting the skin or nail, from some minor injury, or even from inexpert manicuring. Hangnails are unattractive at best and often irritating as well.

The problem can be greatly reduced if you protect your hands from excessive dryness. Use emollient creams several times a day if you are prone to dry skin, especially following a plunge in hot, soapy water, or after gardening, which can be very desiccating. Better yet, wear cotton-lined rubber gloves for tasks that put your skin at risk. And if a hangnail does develop, resist picking or pulling at it, which can injure the live skin attached. Rather, use a sharp pair of manicure scissors to neatly trim the damaged skin.

Can biting your fingernails damage them permanently? What's the best way to break this habit?

Nail biting is more than just an unattractive habit. It can disfigure the nail, injure the finger, and cause skin infections. And because the hand is involved in so many things we do, it can also become an effective vehicle for spreading disease from the

nail biter to others and vice versa. Nail biting is a frequent but usually transient childhood habit—a handy means of dispelling tension and anxiety when youngsters need it. But if you are still biting your nails and want to stop, it will probably take more than willpower to succeed. The habit often has become so ingrained that the biter remains unaware of it.

Some nail biters have gotten good results by painting their nails with a nonprescription liquid that tastes bitter enough to catch their attention. Wrapping bits of tape around the fingers is another way to stop the habit, as is keeping idle hands busy: try knitting, whittling, doodling, or some other activity for those occasions when the desire to nail bite is strongest. Hypnosis aimed at modifying nail-biting behavior can also be helpful.

However, if the habit is an important personal device for relieving tension, you may need to explore and resolve underlying issues with a professional therapist before the nail biting can be stopped permanently.

What causes styes and how are they treated?

A stye is a small abscess that forms on the leading edge of the eyelid, usually at the base of an eyelash; it is caused by an infection with staphylococcus or some other bacteria. As the infection progresses, the lid becomes red and inflamed, and a small pimple develops. Shortly after the stye comes to a head—usually in a matter of hours or days—it discharges pus. Once this happens, the pain and irritation diminish and the abscess clears up.

A stye is likely to hurt as it is growing, but it doesn't require a doctor's treatment or antibiotic ointments unless the condi-

tion persists or recurs often. To help bring a stye to a head, hold warm compresses on the area for 15 minutes at a time, 3 or 4 times a day. Try not to rub the stye; if you do, you may spread the infection to the other eye.

My eyes are frequently red and irritated. Can eyedrops help and are they safe?

Eye irritation has many causes, from environmental pollutants such as dust and smoke, to colds and allergies. Severe cases, especially when accompanied by a discharge, may be a sign of conjunctivitis, an infection that should be treated by your doctor, not with over-the-counter eyedrops. If you have a mild eye irritation, eyedrops will "get the red out," as the ads promise, but the relief is only temporary and it's not without risk.

Many over-the-counter eyedrops contain decongestants, which reduce the appearance of inflammation by shrinking blood vessels in the eye. These drops may trigger allergic reactions in some people and should be used only with the approval of an eye doctor by anyone who wears contact lenses or has glaucoma.

Excessive use of decongestant eyedrops can also cause a rebound effect—the eyes become so accustomed to the constrictor in the eyedrops that they redden automatically as the medicine wears off. Don't use eyedrops casually or for more than 2 weeks at a time. If irritation persists, try to identify the source and either remove it or protect your eyes from it. Wear watertight goggles when you swim in a chlorinated pool, for example.

Another problem with eyedrops is that they can help spread infection. New drops come from manufacturers in sterile containers, but once you break the seal, you open the way to contamination. Squeeze bottles are the safest dispensers, as long as you don't touch the nozzles; eyecups are the worst. Eyedroppers are acceptable if the applicator end is *never* set down on a surface. Be sure to wash your hands carefully before and after you roll back your eyelid to apply the medication, and don't touch any part of the eye with the applicator. Don't share eyedrops with anyone.

Is eye makeup bad for the eyes?

Two problems are commonly associated with eye makeup. Like other cosmetics, some types of eye makeup cause allergic reactions (including eye irritation) in a small number of women. And an open container of eye makeup is an excellent medium for the growth of disease organisms. Among teenagers, who are prone to sharing makeup, it's quite common for a case of infectious conjunctivitis to be introduced and spread far and wide in a matter of hours.

In general, however, eye makeup is safe to use as long as it is applied in moderation to relatively insensitive parts of the outer eye, is removed carefully with gentle washing at the end of the day, and—most important—is free of infectious organisms. To lessen the risk of spreading infection, discard mascara after 4 to 6 months. To keep bits of mascara from flaking into your eyes and irritating them, don't use too much or apply it too close to the eyelid's edge.

If you wear contact lenses, choose eye cosmetics labeled "hypoallergenic" or "safe for use with contact lenses," and be extra careful when applying them. You don't want microscopic bits of mascara to get under the lenses.

Why do my eyes sometimes get dry?

Dry eye—the gritty, burning, sometimes itchy, or painful sensation that often occurs in one eye only—is a sign that the tear gland connected to the eye is not producing sufficient fluid to keep your cornea healthy. The other eye may respond by watering copiously as it tries, fruitlessly, to compensate.

Dry eye can have several causes, including pollution and old age. It can also be the symptom of an underlying health problem such as rheumatoid arthritis. If left untreated, dry eye can lead to blurred vision and other serious eye problems.

If you experience dry eye longer than a few days, see your doctor. The usual treatment is artificial tears, mild over-the-counter eyedrops that more or less duplicate the chemical composition of real tears. As with other kinds of eyedrops, it's important to keep the drops and the applicator scrupulously clean. And if you wear contact lenses, be sure to use a product described as suitable for your kind of lens.

Are there any health or safety reasons for choosing eyeglasses over contact lenses?

The design of contact lenses has come so far in recent years (see box at right) that many of the concerns people once had about wearing them are no longer valid. However, contacts don't correct all vision problems, and they are still not suitable for everyone.

Many ophthalmologists believe that contact lenses should not

CARING FOR YOUR EYES

☐ Read and do close work in a good light: shine a 100-watt incandescent bulb or a 20-watt fluorescent over your shoulder onto the book or work area to avoid glare and shadows.

☐ When using a computer, reading, or doing close work, remember to rest your eyes every 30 minutes or so by looking at distant objects.

☐ Keep your computer and television screens sharply focused when you are viewing them.

☐ Wear safety goggles whenever you use caustic chemicals, do carpentry, work under the car hood, or run power tools.

☐ Wear shatterproof sports goggles during active sports, particularly in games like squash and racquetball.

☐ Wear watertight swim goggles in chlorine pools or in any water of doubtful cleanliness.

☐ Don't look directly at the sun, especially during eclipses; the darkened sun can cause severe and permanent damage. Similarly, avoid staring at any bright or glaring lights.

☐ Don't rub your eye to remove a foreign object. Try blinking and irrigating it with running water, or see your doctor.

be prescribed for people who are clumsy with their hands—and this includes most children—because of the risk of eye injury during lens insertion and removal. If you are highly allergic, your eyes may have difficulty accepting contact lenses.

Even seasoned contact lens wearers go back to ordinary glasses for comfort in certain situations. Dry airplane cabins (or dry climates in general) can make contacts feel gritty. It also may be unpleasant to wear contacts when your eyes are watery from a cold or, conversely, when you've taken a decongestant, which dries out your eyes by reducing tear flow.

For some women, pregnancy, birth control pills, and menstruation make contact lenses temporarily intolerable. And people who live and/or work in an environment containing high levels of dust, chemical pollutants, and other airborne irritants may not be able to wear contacts because particles that get trapped under their lenses cause discomfort and may scratch the cornea.

I can't seem to get used to my bifocals. Any suggestions?

Bifocals are a convenient substitute for carrying two pairs of glasses. They are particularly useful for people who wear glasses for long-distance vision and then develop, usually in middle age, additional problems with close-range vision.

Conventional bifocals are made with two distinctly separate lenses per eye, the upper one ground to correct for distance vision, the lower, often smaller one for close-up sight. The trick to wearing them successfully is to get accustomed to looking through the appropriate portion of the glasses for each task. Mid-

CONTACT LENS BASICS

Today's contact lenses offer more comfort, more convenience, and even more fun (you can change your eye color with tinted lenses) for people whose eyes, vision, and health can tolerate them. Have your eye doctor help you pick the type of lens that is best for you—hard, rigid gas-permeable, or soft.

Hard lenses. These are the original contact lenses, and they still offer the best vision correction for people with astigmatism and irregular corneas. They're less expensive than other types of contacts, more durable, and easier to clean. However, it takes 2 weeks or more to get your eyes used to wearing hard lenses.

Rigid gas-permeable lenses. With openings that allow oxygen to get through to the cornea, this type of contact lens offers the sharp vision of hard lenses, with some of the comfort of soft lenses. Rigid lenses need custom fitting and cost more, but last longer and are easier to clean than soft lenses.

Soft lenses. Easier to fit and more comfortable at first than other lenses, soft lenses don't provide the same sharpness of vision as hard or rigid lenses. Soft lenses begin to dry out as soon as they are inserted and consequently require eyedrops. And because they soak up tear proteins, mucus, and microorganisms, which can irritate the eye, soft lenses require complicated cleaning and disinfecting. Extended-wear soft lenses, which you keep in your eyes continuously (most eye specialists would limit you to 7 days), cut down on cleansing chores, but may cause irritation. Disposable lenses (wear them a week and throw them away) free you from maintenance.

---

range vision—the kind involved in descending a flight of stairs or stepping off a curb—is sometimes blurry because it literally "falls between the cracks" of the lenses. If you are just starting out with bifocals, begin wearing them indoors during relatively sedentary activities. And practice going up and down stairs at home until you feel confident enough to move with ease in public places.

In seamless bifocals one lens blends into the other without a line between the two. Some people find these glasses more attractive, but many have difficulty getting used to them. Seamless bifocals are also more expensive than the standard version.

Is it all right to purchase reading glasses off the rack at a drugstore?

If you notice any change in your vision, have your eyes checked by an optometrist or ophthalmologist. If you are simply farsighted (you have difficulty reading small print or doing other close work), or if you already wear contact lenses and just need additional magnification for reading, nonprescription eyeglasses may be just fine. Sold in pharmacies and dime stores, the glasses are available in a variety of magnification strengths and frame styles. To select a pair, you try on frames until you find one that feels comfortable, and then test different lenses on the lines of a display chart or on other small-size type. When you can read the small print, you have found your "prescription."

However, if you have astigmatism, a form of visual distortion caused by irregularities in the cornea, or if the refractive errors are different in each of your eyes, you'll need lenses ground to your own prescription.

FACT OR FALLACY?

Wearing the wrong glasses can worsen your vision

Fallacy. Eyeglasses can't diminish your vision or damage your eyes. Lenses that are too strong or otherwise unsatisfactory, however, can interfere with your daily life and may cause you to have an accident. If you think your glasses are wrong for you, have them checked by an eye specialist.

Going without your glasses doesn't hurt your eyes either. Even reading in dim light won't ruin eyesight. It might bring on a headache, but it won't make you "go blind," as your parents may have warned.

Although wearing the wrong glasses won't worsen vision, there are cases in which wearing the right glasses can actually cure a vision defect. Eyeglasses are usually part of the treatment for childhood strabismus (crossed eyes) or amblyopia (lazy eye).

I've always been told not to stick anything in my ears. Yet my ears generate a lot of wax. Must I go to a doctor to get my ears cleaned?

Earwax is a natural protective substance produced in the ear canal. Because it usually dries up and washes away with showering and shampooing at just about the rate that it is produced, wax buildup is not a serious problem for most people. However, if wax does build up in your ears, try using a liquid softening agent (drugstores carry several nonprescription products for this purpose). A few drops used as directed over several days usually take care of the problem.

Ear specialists continue to urge that you not put "anything smaller than your elbow" in your ear; this includes poking at earwax with cotton swabs, a practice that may wind up driving wax deeper into the ears.

If home efforts fail to reduce wax buildup, see your doctor. He or she may use a spoon-shaped instrument called a curette to remove the wax manually, or the doctor may irrigate the ears and suction the wax out.

I want to have my ears pierced. Who should I go to? What precautions should I take?

Ear piercing is not a complicated procedure. Any reputable jeweler who offers the service and uses sterilized instruments in a sanitary setting should do a satisfactory job. In most cases it takes just a few minutes to apply a topical anesthetic, locate a site for the hole, and pierce the lobe.

Most infections from pierced ears—and they are almost epidemic among the young—result either from failure to keep the

earlobe clean during the healing phase, from an allergic reaction to the metal alloys used in some earring posts, or from pushing the back piece on a post earring too close to the earlobe and pinching it. Fortunately, most infections are minor and easily treated at home.

Symptoms of infection include a swollen, overly sensitive, reddened lobe and a yellowish discharge. When these occur, remove the earring immediately, wash the area and apply hot compresses several times a day. Allow the wound to heal in the open air. If the condition persists for a week or more, see your doctor; you may need an oral antibiotic. Don't return the earring to the pierced hole until the infection is entirely gone.

If you suspect an allergic reaction, confine your choice of earring posts to pure gold or stainless steel. Oxidizing silver can irritate skin; don't use silver posts for at least 6 months after piercing.

I'm prone to nosebleeds. Why is this and what's the best way to treat them?

The fragile capillaries of the lining and septum of the nose lie near the surface and can easily rupture and bleed. An injury to the nose, a spell of vigorous nose blowing, a cold or other viral infection, or sometimes just being at a very high altitude can bring on such ruptures. If you live in a very dry climate, or produce less nasal mucus than average, the inside of your nose may be prone to cracking and bleeding.

To stop a nosebleed, sit upright with the fingers of one hand pinching the soft lower part of the nostrils; hold a bowl in the other hand to catch the flow. Keep the nose in this "finger tourniquet" for 5 to 10 minutes,

CARING FOR YOUR TEETH

Good dental hygiene takes only minutes a day, but pays off in healthy teeth and gums for a lifetime. Here are the basics of mouth care:

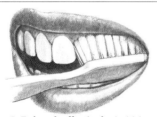

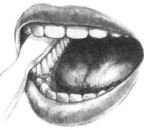

1. To brush effectively, hold the brush against the outside surface of the teeth at a 45° angle so that the bristles point toward the gum line. Move the brush side to side, using a light scrubbing motion.

☐ Select a fluoridated toothpaste or gel that has the American Dental Association's seal of acceptance.

☐ Choose a brush with soft, end-rounded bristles in a size that's comfortable for your mouth and capable of reaching every tooth. Replace your brush every 3 or 4 months. A manual brush is generally no better or worse than a power brush; what counts is how well you use either.

2. Using the same short back-and-forth stroke, brush the biting and inner surfaces of the back teeth. You'll find it easier to brush the back teeth if you close your mouth slightly.

☐ Brush teeth at least twice a day, after meals. Brush after every meal if your gums are prone to gingivitis (p.139).

☐ Floss, using the waxed or unwaxed variety, once a day after brushing for routine plaque control. Rinse well after flossing.

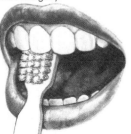

3. To clean the inside surfaces of the front teeth, hold the tip of the brush vertically at the gum line and use short up-and-down strokes.

☐ Brush your tongue for fresh breath and cleaner taste.

☐ Don't use your teeth to tear, pull, turn, or open objects.

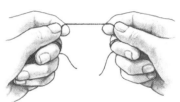

1. Proper flossing requires a bit of practice. Break off an 18-inch length of dental floss and wind most of it around each of your middle fingers. Hold 1 or 2 inches of floss taut between your thumbs and forefingers as shown above.

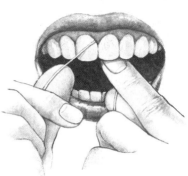

2. Using a gentle sawing motion, slide the taut floss between two teeth until it touches the gum line. Curve the floss into a C-shape around one tooth and gently slide it into the space between tooth and gum. Draw the floss away from the gum, scraping the side of the tooth as you do so. As you proceed, wind the floss from one middle finger to the other to gain a clean piece of floss. Rinse your mouth well after flossing.

---

then release slowly to see if the bleeding has stopped. Resume if necessary. A cold compress or an ice pack placed on the bridge of the nose may also help. Only if the bleeding keeps up for 20 minutes or more, or if it's associated with a trauma to some other part of the head, should you seek medical attention.

Incidentally, the old practice of having the nosebleeder lie down is *not* recommended: it maintains a higher-pressure blood flow and diverts the leaking blood into the throat and stomach.

If nosebleeds become a recurring problem, and they are not clearly associated with any of the circumstances described above, check with your doctor. It's rare, but multiple nosebleeds can be a symptom of an underlying blood-clotting problem.

Can a toothpaste or mouthwash prevent gingivitis?

Fluoridated toothpastes and mouthwashes help fight cavities, but there is still no scientific evidence that any toothpaste removes plaque or tartar below the gum line, where periodontal diseases such as gingivitis begin (see *Glossary of Dental Terms and Procedures,* pp. 138–139). However, brushing your teeth thoroughly—3 to 5 minutes—at least twice a day does reduce plaque, and you may brush better with a toothpaste you like.

Most over-the-counter mouthwashes simply mask bad breath. When buying a mouthwash, check the label to make sure it has been approved by the American Dental Association's Council on Dental Therapeutics as a legitimate preventive agent against the growth of plaque above the gum line.

Dental researchers are investigating more effective ways of treating all stages of gum disease, and it's probably only a matter of time before toothpastes and mouthwashes will be reformulated as the important plaque and tartar fighters they now claim to be. Meanwhile, a toothbrush and dental floss—used correctly and regularly—remain your best weapons against periodontal disease.

Are some foods worse than others in promoting tooth decay?

A diet high in sugar creates the best environment for the bacteria responsible for the buildup of plaque in your mouth and the development of tooth decay. Sticky, slow-dissolving sweets that adhere to teeth, such as hard candy, caramels, honey, brownies, icing, and raisins, are the worst culprits.

Your teeth's only natural defense against plaque-caused decay is saliva. By far the best dental rinse, saliva washes over teeth, diluting and neutralizing the destructive acid in plaque that eats through tooth enamel.

How much you salivate depends on your genes, on your health and diet, and on medications you may be taking. (Salivation virtually stops when you are asleep; so eating bedtime snacks is an invitation to decay.)

While some foods promote decay, others seem to guard against it. Potatoes, whole grains, pasta, bread, nuts, raw vegetables, and cocoa apparently stimulate the production of saliva in your mouth. Cheddar cheese, eaten at the end of a meal, does even more. It has been found to neutralize mouth acids, creating an oral environment that is less conducive to plaque buildup and tooth decay.

FACT OR FALLACY ?

Cloves can relieve toothache

Fact. The dried buds of the clove tree have been used by folk doctors to treat toothache since ancient times. Contained within the aromatic oils of the clove bud are substances that act as a local anesthetic and antiseptic.

Most toothaches are caused by a cavity or an infection, conditions that a dentist should treat. But while you wait for an appointment, try this old remedy. Saturate a tiny wad of surgical cotton with oil of clove (sold over the counter at many pharmacies) and put it on the aching tooth for a few minutes until the pain subsides.

What causes bad breath?

The most common cause of bad breath is probably insufficient cleaning of teeth or dentures. Without proper oral hygiene, food particles become lodged between teeth and along the gum lines and decay, forming plaque and emiting a foul odor in the process. Better brushing and flossing will take care of transient problems; a thorough workup in the dentist's chair may be needed if the plaque is extensive and the gingivitis is advanced.

Smoking is a second major offender. The residue of tobacco tars in the mouth combine with the tainted air being expelled from the smoker's lungs to leave a stale smell. Bad breath can also be an early sign of a mouth infection or ulcer, or the side effect of a sore throat. Use an antiseptic mouthwash until the condition heals.

Eating onions or garlic is another common cause of bad breath. Although teeth brushing may help, some of the pungency will remain in the blood, and thus in the lungs and mouth, for up to 24 hours. Stick with other garlic and onion lovers, and no one is likely to complain.

If bad breath is new to you and not due to the common causes listed here, consult your doctor. In rare instances, bad breath is a symptom of stomach and lung infections, strep throat, or certain kinds of cancer.

How serious is it if I occasionally miss taking a prescribed drug?

It depends on the particular drug and your condition. For example, if you forget to take your blood pressure medication every once in a while, your blood pressure probably won't be affected. However, a diabetic who misses one dose of insulin risks going into shock; a woman who skips one contraceptive pill can become pregnant.

When you are taking medications, it's also important to take them on schedule. If a prescription calls for your taking a pill at mealtimes, for example, the drug probably causes irritation in an empty stomach. On the other hand, a pill that is prescribed for 2 hours after meals probably does not work very well when it has to compete with a full stomach.

If you do miss taking your medication at a given hour on a given day, don't decide on your own to double dose later without checking with your doctor first. With some medications, you can safely take a missed dose as soon as you remember, but with others you could be risking a very high concentration of the drug in your system, which might be more hazardous than having skipped the earlier dose.

What's a good way to remind myself to take my pills at the right time?

Plastic dispensers with separate snap-lidded compartments for each day of the week are one inexpensive and effective way to keep track of your daily doses. Fill them with an entire week's supply once a week, preferably in conjunction with some other routine activity such as Sunday breakfast. Then make a habit of checking yourself at least once a day to see if you have emptied the correct compartment.

You can also develop your own reminder systems. Use an alarm watch, for example, or if you are a person of regular habits, try coupling pill taking with another activity. A simple example: You must take a teaspoon of a liquid medicine twice a day. Keep the bottle and a spoon beside the bathroom basin so you will see it when you brush your teeth. Each morning after your first dose, place the bottle on the right-hand side of the sink; at night after your second dose, put it on the left side. You'll always know at a glance where you stand.

STOCKING YOUR HOME MEDICINE CABINET

Every household needs medical supplies to treat minor accidents and illnesses. The best place to store medicines is in a small cabinet or closet in a room other than the bathroom, where heat and humidity cause drugs to deteriorate and lose potency. If you have children at home, keep medicines locked up and out of their reach. Certain drugs must be stored in the refrigerator; check labels. Clean out your medicine cabinet periodically, discarding aspirin that smells vinegary, medicines past their expiration date, prescription drugs from a past illness, and any medicines without a label. Flush old medicines down the toilet. The following items will handle most medical problems in the home.

FIRST-AID EQUIPMENT

- ☐ Assorted small adhesive bandages
- ☐ Individually wrapped sterile gauze pads
- ☐ Roll of sterile gauze bandage
- ☐ Roll of adhesive tape
- ☐ Triangular bandage and large safety pins (for a sling)
- ☐ Cotton swabs and balls
- ☐ Measuring spoons
- ☐ Heating pad or hot-water bottle
- ☐ Ice pack
- ☐ First-aid manual

- ☐ Small blunt-tipped scissors
- ☐ Tweezers and a packet of sewing needles (to remove splinters)
- ☐ Thermometers (oral for adults, rectal for infants)

MEDICINES

- ☐ Antacid
- ☐ Antibiotic ointment or antiseptic for cuts
- ☐ Antidiarrheal medication
- ☐ Antihistamine
- ☐ Anti-itching lotion or spray (or baking soda)
- ☐ Aspirin or acetaminophen
- ☐ Burn ointment
- ☐ Children's acetaminophen (if needed)

- ☐ Cough syrup with expectorant
- ☐ Decongestant
- ☐ Foot powder
- ☐ Mild laxative
- ☐ Powdered activated charcoal (to absorb poison)
- ☐ Syrup of ipecac (to induce vomiting)
- ☐ Rubbing alcohol (70 percent solution)

Can taking too many aspirins cause harm?

Taking too much of any medication can have adverse effects, and this applies even to aspirin, which is no less powerful for being an over-the-counter drug. The standard dose of aspirin for the relief of pain and fever is two regular tablets (650 milligrams total) every 3 to 4 hours. In certain circumstances, such as a case of severe inflammation, a patient may safely take 16 or more tablets in a single day, but should do so only under a doctor's supervision.

If taken in excess over several days, aspirin can interfere with blood clotting, trigger internal bleeding, and cause stomach irritation as well as such neurological side effects as ringing in the ears. And because aspirin is something of a superdrug, it can mask symptoms that ought to be examined without delay by a doctor. (For a discussion of the role of aspirin in the treatment of heart disease, see page 205.)

A friend of mine takes megadoses of vitamins. Is this necessary? Can it be dangerous?

Megadoses of vitamins and minerals are doses in excess of the National Academy of Sciences' Recommended Dietary Allowances (RDA's), the widely accepted standards by which a healthy diet is measured. Unless you are being treated by a physician for a specific disorder that calls for exceptional quantities of a particular vitamin or mineral, there is no medical reason to take megadoses. Self-treatment with vitamin megadoses not only does no good, but can be quite harmful. Toxic quantities of certain vitamins and minerals may accumulate in the body faster

GUARDING AGAINST HEALTH FRAUD

Every year, Americans spend at least $10 billion on products promising anything from quick weight loss to a cure for cancer or AIDS. At best, these remedies are unproven and useless; at worst, they cause real harm or divert people from seeking sound medical advice.

Health charlatans prey on people's insecurities about their appearance, on the desperation of the terminally ill, and on the very human hope that a miracle *can* indeed happen. Arthritis sufferers, for example, spend some $3 billion a year for copper bracelets, snake venom treatments, and other false cures.

Diet is another fertile field for the quack. Beware of "miracle" diets, fat-dissolving ointments or wraps, electrical muscle toners, or other weight-loss schemes that sound too good to be true.

Learn how to decipher ads for health products. Phrases like "gets the poison out of your body" or "balances your chemistry" are just come-ons. Be wary, too, of simple treatments for complex diseases such as cancer or AIDS. Consult your doctor before experimenting with new health treatments or products. Report health frauds to the U.S. Food and Drug Administration, your state attorney general's office, or the National Council Against Health Fraud (see Appendix).

than it is able to process and eliminate them. In some instances, the results can be very serious, ranging from nerve damage and numbness to kidney stones and liver disease.

I often see ads for vitamins that are supposed to relieve stress or bolster the immune system. Do these vitamins really work?

So-called "stress vitamins" are high-potency formulations that generally combine vitamins C, E, and B complex. Advertised as miracle-working supplements for people who live high-tension lives, they actually have little or no value in relieving the effects of emotional stress. Vitamin megadoses may be recommended for patients who have undergone a *physical* trauma such as a major surgical procedure, a serious infection, or a bad burn, which can deplete the body's store of essential vitamins.

Vitamin C tablets have gained a reputation as immune system stimulants, credited by some with raising resistance to everything from the common cold to cancer. Once again, no significant correlation has ever been found between taking large supplements of vitamin C and resisting colds or cancer. On the other hand, according to studies by the American Cancer Society, people who eat a substantial amount of foods rich in vitamin C—citrus fruits, celery, green peppers, and tomatoes, for example— show a lower incidence of cancers of the stomach and esophagus. This suggests two things: that vitamin C may have some influence on the immune system after all, and that supplements may not be necessary as long as you eat sufficient quantities of foods rich in Vitamin C.

HEALTH MAINTENANCE ON THE ROAD

Nobody wants to seem to be a hypochondriac while traveling, but getting sick far from home where you may not understand the language or recognize the names of familiar medications is a daunting prospect. You'll fare better (and feel less vulnerable) if you go prepared.

□ If you're taking medication, bring enough to last the entire trip plus 3 days.

□ Pack an antibiotic (ask your doctor), analgesic, decongestant, diarrhea medicine, mild laxative, antacid, sunscreen, anti-itch ointment, antiseptic, and adhesive bandages.

□ Call the CDC International Travelers' Hotline or the IAMAT (see Appendix) for the immunization requirements of countries you plan to visit (p. 130).

□ If you use a pacemaker, have it checked before you go (p.331). Take with you a basic dossier of information about the make and model of the equipment. Bring a letter from your doctor (with his telephone number) about your need for a pacemaker. Airport security devices are activated by pacemakers but don't interfere with a pacemaker's workings.

□ Carry medications with you rather than packing them (luggage may be lost) and keep them in their original bottles (customs officials may assume unlabeled drugs are illegal).

□ If you suffer from asthma or emphysema, ask your doctor to contact the airlines for you about carrying standby oxygen.

□ Take a spare pair of prescription eyeglasses and an extra copy of the prescription.

□ If you have diabetes and take insulin daily, ask your doctor how to adjust your food and drug intake during flights across several time zones and how to synchronize your system to the new time once you reach your destination. Take along a supply of appropriate snacks for the trip; that way, if meals are delayed you can still keep your blood sugar at its proper level.

How can I avoid traveler's diarrhea?

Most cases of traveler's diarrhea are caused by local bacteria invading your intestinal system. You build up immunity to many bacteria in your part of the world, but you may be susceptible to strange bacteria elsewhere.

If followed carefully, these measures should keep you well wherever you travel:

□Avoid local tap water. Stick to bottled drinks like beer, soda, or mineral water, and don't use ice in them (it's made from local tap water). Use bottled water to brush your teeth.

□Eat only fruits and vegetables that you peel yourself; avoid salads and sliced fruit.

□Pass up dairy products. There is no way you can tell whether milk or fresh cheeses have been pasteurized or not.

□Don't eat raw shellfish or meats cooked "rare."

□Never buy snacks or other food from street vendors.

What causes jet lag and are there ways to lessen its effects?

In response to cues from the rising and setting sun, a complex internal clock within our bodies synchronizes body functions and rhythms—heartbeat, temperature, mental acuity, the release of hormones, the desire to eat and sleep, for example—to time of day. The approximately 24-hour cycle of each of these body mechanisms is known as its circadian rhythm.

When you travel rapidly across several time zones—overnight from New York to Paris, where the sun rises 6 hours earlier, for example—your body is thrown into a state of circadian confusion. It wants to stay on New York time, but circumstances demand that you wake, sleep, work, and eat on Paris time. The result for most people is "jet lag," a combination of symptoms that include fatigue, sleeplessness, a sluggish body, and general disorientation.

Jet lag generally dissipates over a few days, as body clocks gradually shift to the light cycle of the new locality. The readjustment rate averages about a day for each time zone crossed, with eastward shifts somewhat more difficult to overcome than westward ones.

To minimize the effects of jet lag, take the following steps:
☐ If you're heading east, try going to sleep earlier for a few days before the trip; go to sleep later if you're traveling westward.
☐ During the flight, drink plenty of water and other nonalcoholic beverages, avoid alcoholic drinks, and eat lightly.
☐ Try to break up a long flight with a stopover.
☐ If at all possible, plan your trip so that you arrive at your destination in the early evening and then try to get to bed early.
☐ You can speed up the readjustment process by spending several hours outdoors in sunlight each of the first few days of your stay.

I am frequently carsick. Is there anything I can do to prevent this?

Carsickness and its nautical equivalent, seasickness, usually indicate that your brain is getting conflicting signals from several sensory centers simultaneously: your eyes are reading one kind of movement, the balance sensors in your ears are interpreting something else, and the motion sensors in your skin, muscles, and joints are reporting yet another kind of movement.

Scientists are still not sure how the connections work, but your overloaded brain in effect short-circuits, triggering nausea and vomiting. The most likely candidates for carsickness are children from 2 years old to 12.

The simplest way to combat mild carsickness is to eat sensibly before and during the trip, avoid alcoholic beverages, stop reading while the car is moving, and keep your eyes focused outside the car windows, on the horizon. For many people sitting in the front seat of the car, where the ride is smoother and visibility is better, is helpful.

If these recommendations don't work, try one of the over-the-counter motion-sickness pills sold at your pharmacy. For intractable cases of carsickness a prescription drug, scopolamine, may be effective. Administered via a transdermal patch placed behind the ear shortly before setting out on a car trip, scopolamine slowly releases a drug that blocks carsickness symptoms in the central nervous system where they begin.

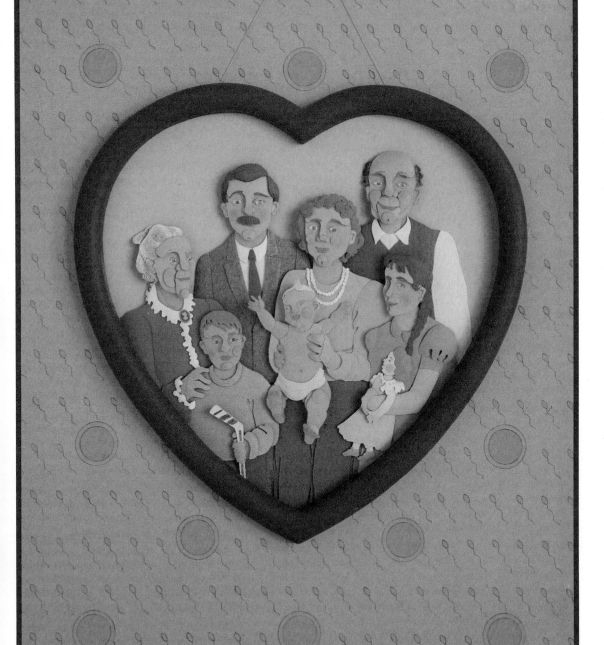

Taking Time to Recharge

With three young children and two full-time jobs, Tom and Diane M., both in their mid thirties, were beginning to feel like business partners rather than lovers. Their lives seemed to revolve exclusively around work, child care, and juggling schedules and responsibilities. By the end of a typical day, both were too tired even to engage in relaxing conversation, much less to make love.

As the distance between the couple increased, so did the number and intensity of their quarrels. Eventually, Tom and Diane came to realize that their marriage was in jeopardy; frightened into action, they made an appointment with a marriage counselor.

The first thing the counselor suggested was that the couple review their schedules for the past year or so. The results were eye-opening. Tom and Diane had not spent significant time alone with each other in months. Their lovemaking had been even less frequent than either of them had cared to admit.

The therapist's "prescription" was a simple one. Every week, Tom and Diane were to go out on a real date—no family or friends allowed, no talk of work, finances, or the children. The couple were definitely encouraged to touch one another, but sex was not necessarily part of the agenda.

Two days later, over a quiet dinner away from home, Tom and Diane began to relax and focus on each other's needs and attractions as they had not done in quite a while. Not surprisingly, lovemaking was very much on the agenda that night.

Tom and Diane's weekly date is now a much-anticipated part of their schedule. They're also doing more of the things they used to do together when they were first married—hiking, bicycling, and other outdoor activities, which they now enjoy sharing with their children. Instead of allowing themselves to drift apart, Tom and Diane are communicating better and enjoying each other more than they ever did.

A Struggle to Conceive

Christina S. gave birth to her first child by cesarean section at age 32. Since her labor had been long and difficult, Christina and her husband, Jay, decided to wait awhile before having another baby. Two years later Christina become pregnant but soon miscarried. After a year of trying to conceive again, a worried and frustrated Christina consulted her gynecologist.

The doctor reviewed Christina's history and ordered a sperm count for Jay, the results of which were normal. The next step was a complete fertility workup on Christina. A basal body-temperature chart suggested that she was ovulating, and a postcoital test showed that her cervical mucus and her husband's sperm were compatible. The cause of Christina's problem finally showed up on a hysterosalpingo-gram (a contrast X-ray of the uterus and fallopian tubes). The fingerlike projections at the ends of the tubes had enlarged and grown together, keeping them from catching the eggs released by the ovaries and conveying them to the uterus.

The gynecologist referred Christina to a surgeon, who confirmed the diagnosis after viewing Christina's fallopian tubes through a laparoscope, a fiber-optic tube that is inserted into the pelvic cavity through an abdominal incision. Using microsurgical techniques, the surgeon was able to separate and turn back the ends of the tubes, freeing the fingerlike projections.

Although the operation was a success, the surgeon advised Christina to wait a month and a half, or until she had her first normal period, before trying to become pregnant. When the time came, Christina used an ovulation prediction kit to determine when she'd be most likely to conceive. The kit was accurate, and today Christina and Jay are the grateful parents of a second happy, healthy baby.

All in the Family

Few areas in life give rise to as much anxiety and misinformation as do sexuality and human relationships. The goal of this chapter is to shed light on a wide range of sexual and family matters—from rekindling marital passion to assessing methods of birth control, from problems of the urogenital tract to talking to your children about sex. Nurturing loving relationships requires patience, communication, and knowledge. See how knowledgeable you are by taking this True/False quiz.

1 There is a direct relationship between frequency of lovemaking and the success and happiness of a marriage.

_____ True   _____ False

2 New scientific findings are confirming the effectiveness of traditional aphrodisiacs, such as ginseng.

_____ True   _____ False

3 Being physically fit can increase your enjoyment of sex.

_____ True   _____ False

4 Fewer than 25 percent of married people have extramarital affairs.

_____ True   _____ False

5 The AIDS virus can't be transmitted through casual kissing.

_____ True   _____ False

6 A vasectomy makes a man immediately sterile.

_____ True   _____ False

7 A sudden increase in sexual activity can cause urinary tract infections in women.

_____ True   _____ False

8 Women over 30 have a much higher risk of having a problem pregnancy or an unhealthy baby than younger mothers do.

_____ True   _____ False

9 The average woman should try to gain no more than 20 pounds in the course of her pregnancy.

_____ True   _____ False

10 A newborn's Apgar score is an important predictor of the child's future health and intelligence.

_____ True   _____ False

11 Tonsils serve no useful purpose and should be routinely removed in early childhood.

_____ True   _____ False

12 Sex education should start before a child reaches puberty.

_____ True   _____ False

Answers
For more information on any of the quiz topics turn to the pages listed next to the answers.

1. False, p.236	5. True, p.243	9. False, p.261
2. False, p.237	6. False, p.247	10. False, p.265
3. True, p.238	7. True, p.248	11. False, p.272
4. False, p.241	8. False, p.258	12. True, p.277

After 25 years of living together, my wife and I seldom have sex even though we love each other. Is this normal?

There's really no normal frequency of sex. Although the average seems to be about twice a week, couples in one survey said they make love from 0 to 20 (or more) times a week. It's also common for the frequency of intercourse to vary at different stages of a relationship. A couple may make love often early in their relationship, then once or twice a month when they're busy with careers and children, then perhaps more often again in middle age. A Canadian survey of 365 people, most under 40 and married for an average of 11 years, showed that a third went without sex for long periods; half of this third had stretches of abstinence lasting 8 weeks or more.

The fact that you and your wife seldom make love is not necessarily a cause for concern if you have talked about it and are content with the arrangement. If you aren't, discuss the matter with your doctor or a qualified counselor or therapist.

How can I tell normal from abnormal in sex?

What a culture considers normal sexual activity depends on complex social and historical factors. Because sexual behavior includes a wide range of activities and so strongly influences how we think of ourselves, each of us must make personal judgments about what is appropriate. When evaluating a situation, ask yourself whether it is physically or emotionally harmful to you or others and whether you and your partner are participating of your own free will. Activities such as rape, incest, and sadomasochism clearly

do not meet these criteria. And in the age of AIDS, neither does unsafe sex (p. 243).

Feelings of coercion, degradation, and physical or emotional pain are not generally considered normal, even in nonsexual situations. If you associate such negative feelings with lovemaking, discuss them with your spouse and possibly with your doctor or a therapist.

On the other hand, experimenting with new activities is normal and healthy as long as both you and your spouse feel physically, emotionally, and morally comfortable with them.

What causes lack of interest in sex? What can be done about it?

Temporary lulls in sexual interest are to be expected in almost any relationship. More worrisome, however, is a persistent lack of desire (loss of libido) in general or for a certain person. Technically known as inhibited, or hypoactive, sexual desire, this is a common sexual problem, whose causes may be psychological, physical, or both.

Psychological factors—stress, depression, grief, anxiety, anger, guilt, fear, confusion, marital discord, boredom, and concerns with self-image and body image—are the most common cause of loss of desire. Marital counseling and sex therapy are often helpful, but the condition may not respond to therapy as rapidly as other sexual problems, because the underlying issues are often more complex.

Physical factors include hormonal imbalances, illnesses, and the use or abuse of drugs. Some experts believe that low levels of the male hormone testosterone (secreted by both men and women) may decrease libido, although the connection has not

been proven. It is known, however, that stress lowers testosterone levels in men and women, and that people under stress report lowered desire. Thyroid problems, pituitary tumors, diabetes, and depression may also decrease libido, sometimes even before the underlying condition is diagnosed.

Certain prescription medications, including some tranquilizers and antidepressants (p. 171), oral contraceptives, and antihypertensive drugs, can cause loss of desire as a side effect. In addition to creating many other problems, alcohol, barbiturates, marijuana, heroin, and morphine can also depress sexual desire and inhibit performance.

Keep in mind that there is no standard for assessing sexual desire. If the problem arises in your relationship, try to discuss the subject openly, admitting your frustrations, fears, desires, and concerns. If necessary, consult an expert for help with healing the underlying causes.

Can certain vitamins or minerals make a man more potent?

Although a good diet is essential for sexual function, there is no single nutrient that will make men more potent. Unfortunately, some vitamins and minerals, including zinc, the B vitamins, and vitamin K, have been promoted as potency-enhancers, and enough people have believed these questionable claims to keep the business alive.

If you think your diet, or another physical factor, is detrimental to your sex life, see your doctor. Impotence (p. 238) has many possible medical causes, and a thorough physical examination (including an evaluation of your eating habits) should pinpoint any problems.

Are there any real aphrodisiacs?

Substances thought to stimulate sexual desire and enhance performance are called aphrodisiacs, after Aphrodite, the ancient Greek goddess of love. Although love potions have been touted for centuries, there is no evidence that any of them work. And some, such as Spanish fly (cantharides), a powder made from ground beetles, are outright dangerous and potentially fatal.

Although foods rich in zinc (such as oysters) do contribute to the development of reproductive organs in children, there is no evidence that eating zinc-rich foods or taking zinc supplements improves sexual performance in adults. In fact, taking too much zinc can interfere with iron absorption and cause other health problems.

Alcohol is often used to reduce shyness and inhibition, which makes it easier for some people to relax and respond to a sexual encounter. But mixing alcohol and sex should be done judiciously, especially among those who lack experience in either area. Even small amounts of alcohol can impair judgment, diminish physical coordination, and decrease testosterone production. Alcohol can also impair the parts of the brain that regulate the release of sex-related hormones. Large doses can make a man temporarily impotent. In women, heavy drinking is linked to difficulties in becoming aroused and achieving orgasm.

Drugs with reputed aphrodisiac powers, such as marijuana, cocaine, amphetamines, heroin, some hallucinogens, and amyl nitrate, actually reduce sexual capability and enjoyment—and can have grave health consequences.

My husband often reaches orgasm too quickly for me. Is this common?

Premature ejaculation is a common male sexual problem. But reaching orgasm "too quickly" means different things to different people. Experts define premature ejaculation variously as ejaculation before penetration, from 30 seconds to several minutes after penetration, or before the woman has an orgasm. A general rule followed by many sex therapists is that a man ejaculates prematurely if he can't delay his orgasm long enough to satisfy his spouse most of the time or if he usually reaches an orgasm before he chooses to.

The condition is frequently caused by anxiety about performing adequately. Other causes may include a man's early interpretation of sex as something dirty, to be gotten over with as quickly as possible, or early sexual experiences in which speed was of the essence, such as secretive masturbation, sex in the back seat of a car, or sex with prostitutes. Some men are brought up to feel that women find sex unpleasant and therefore hurry for their wife's sake.

What can my husband and I do to prolong his lovemaking?

As with most sexual difficulties, the place to start looking for a solution is in frank and caring

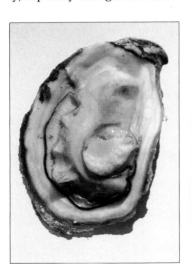
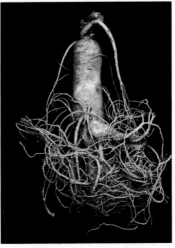
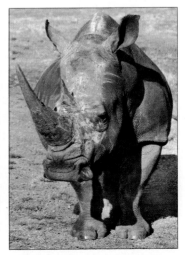

Power to enhance lovemaking has been attributed to zinc-rich oysters, the Oriental root herb ginseng, and the horn of the endangered East African rhinoceros. In the age-old quest for better sex, people have ascribed aphrodisiac properties to some other surprising substances, including honey, ginger, sea cucumbers, strychnine, alcohol, cocaine and other street drugs, and the notorious Spanish fly. All of them are equally ineffective and some are potentially fatal.

IMPROVING YOUR SEX LIFE

That happy couples have the best sex has been confirmed by many studies. Having a trusting, loving relationship does more to enhance lovemaking than any exercise, technique, or therapy yet invented. However, there are things every couple can do to promote a better sex life:

Stay in shape. Just being physically fit tends to improve your enjoyment of sex. If you're out of shape, especially in the stomach, hip, and thigh areas, which are used during lovemaking, consider a firming and toning program (pp.88–89).

Try Kegel exercises. Developed by a gynecologist to help women with bladder control after childbirth, this regimen strengthens the pubococcygeal (PC) muscles, helping many women to reach orgasm more easily and giving many men better control over ejaculation. To locate the PC muscles, try to stop the flow during urination (it is the PC muscles you'll be using). If you can't, or can't do it completely, practice contracting those muscles throughout the day. For the most benefit, women should work up to 20 contractions (holding each for 1 to 3 seconds) three times a day; men should do 10 to 15 contractions (holding each for 3 seconds) twice a day, working up to 60 to 70 contractions in each session. Both men and women who do these exercises report more intense orgasms.

Practice touching. Often recommended by sex therapists, hour-long sessions of touch therapy focus on the pleasures of intimate touching without the pressure to perform in intercourse. Partners take turns caressing or massaging each other; the receiving partner tells where to stroke and how it feels.

Make time for sex. Busy couples, particularly after they have children, have trouble fitting lovemaking into their lives. Make dates to spend time alone together; this may or may not lead to intercourse, but it will allow intimacy.

Respect your partner's problems. Depression and stress can cause a decline in sexual interest. A trauma like losing a job can affect your partner's self-esteem so badly that sex is no longer a pleasure. Discuss difficult situations and seek counseling if necessary. Be supportive during a partner's distress.

Resolve conflicts outside the bedroom. Marital discord is the most common reason for avoiding sex. Don't use your bedroom as a battleground; resolve disagreements elsewhere, either by yourselves or with the help of a marital counselor.

Experiment. To avoid getting into a stale routine in bed, try new words, positions, places, and times to stimulate each other in different ways. And remember that not every sexual encounter has to include intercourse to bring both of you satisfaction.

conversation. You may just need to assure your husband that you do enjoy sex with him and that longer foreplay and intercourse would give you even greater pleasure. Sometimes a man may need to learn the physical sensations that signal orgasm in order to develop more control. Slowing the rhythm of intercourse, changing positions, or pausing altogether until control is regained may be all that's needed.

If necessary, consult your doctor or a sex therapist about learning techniques designed to help a man delay his orgasm and develop greater control. One technique that therapists recommend involves a stop-start approach. The man masturbates, stops before ejaculating, then starts again, repeating the cycle for increasingly longer periods. After a few weeks, he can try the same thing with his partner, having her stimulate him, then stop, then start again, until he is able to delay his orgasm for as long as they both want.

Another technique that therapists have also found successful involves squeezing the penis to control the urge to ejaculate. Just before the man thinks he is about to ejaculate, either partner squeezes the head of the penis between the thumb and two fingers. The technique can be repeated as often as it is needed during intercourse.

A couple should also remember that one partner's orgasm need not signal the end of lovemaking. An affectionate and playful relationship will inspire more than enough methods of expression to keep you both satisfied.

Should I worry about occasional impotence?

Erectile dysfunction, commonly called impotence, is a man's inability to achieve or maintain an erection. Its causes are often psychological, although many cases are the result of a physical disorder and some are caused by both physical and psychological factors. Impotence is a common problem, affecting some 10 million American men. Many more experience occasional impotence due to stress, fatigue, drinking too much alcohol, or other passing problems. Episodes of impotence tend to increase as a man ages.

An occasional "failure to perform" is natural and should not be a cause for concern. In fact, worrying about it can aggravate the problem. Instead of worrying, a man with erectile difficulties should not hesitate to see his doctor and explore the many treatment options available today.

How is impotence treated?

A man who experiences impotence regularly (that is, who is unable to have an erection at least 25 percent of the time) should be evaluated by his doctor for a possible physical disorder. Some diseases, such as diabetes and arteriosclerosis, can inhibit erection. So can neurological and glandular disorders, spinal-cord injury, surgery, drug or alcohol abuse, and certain medications, such as some antihypertensive and psychoactive drugs. If the cause is not readily apparent, a doctor may use a Doppler ultrasound device (p. 126) to evaluate blood circulation to the penis.

Whatever the underlying problem, most cases of physically based impotence are treatable. Not all hypertension medications, for example, cause impotence in all men; if you are having problems with your medication, ask your doctor about switching to another type. Treating a drug or alcohol problem often leads naturally to the recovery of potency.

Other conditions are treated by improving blood circulation to the penis, either by vascular surgery or by the injection of drugs known as vasodilators.

Thousands of men with erectile dysfunction have been helped by penile implants, either semi-rigid plastic rods or inflatable devices that are filled with fluid from a surgically implanted internal reservoir. Also effective is a nonsurgical vacuum device that fits over the penis. The vacuum draws blood into the penis to produce an erection.

Psychological causes of impotence can be transitory (fatigue, stress, or boredom) or longer-lasting and more deeply rooted, such as fear, performance anxiety, anger, depression, dissatisfaction with the relationship, guilt or confusion about sex, and loss of self-esteem (a possible result, for example, of being fired). Often, a self-perpetuating cycle is set up: Impotence makes a man anxious about sex, which inhibits his ability, which makes him more anxious, and so on.

Sometimes simply acknowledging the problem and talking it over with an understanding spouse will cure temporary impotence. When more complex psychological factors are involved, a couple may need the help of a therapist to define and correct the problem.

Is it unusual for a woman to reach orgasm only by being manually stimulated?

Not at all. Studies suggest that at least half of all women need direct stimulation of the clitoral area in order to achieve orgasm. Such stimulation can be done during intercourse as well as before and after, and some positions, such as having the woman on top, may make touching easi-

er to do. It's a good idea to discuss this with your partner, to share your feelings with him and find out how he feels about it. It may also be helpful to show him what feels good by guiding his hand during lovemaking.

Sometimes I find that intercourse is painful. What could cause this?

Many women experience occasional pain during intercourse. Among the common causes are tenderness in the pelvic area around the time of ovulation and insufficient lubrication because of brief foreplay or because the woman is going through menopause. Another possible cause is a vaginal infection. If you suspect that you have an infection, see your doctor for treatment.

If a woman experiences pain every time she has intercourse, the problem could be endometriosis (p. 252) or, less commonly, vaginismus, the involuntary tensing of muscles in the outer third of the vagina. Mild vaginismus is often experienced as an uncomfortable, burning sensation upon penetration. It has also been compared to the reaction of flinching when an injured part of the body is touched. In severe cases of vaginismus, the involuntary contractions of the vaginal muscles prevent not only penetration but tampon use or a pelvic exam. The noted sex research team of William Masters and Virginia Johnson found that most women with this condition have normal sexual desire, can be aroused, and can experience orgasm. Vaginismus can be treated successfully and quickly by a patient and knowledgeable doctor. However, when the problem has an underlying psychological cause, such as a rigid upbringing or childhood sexual abuse, psychotherapy may be necessary.

What really happens in sex therapy?

Many people have misconceptions about sex therapy. It does not mean having sex in front of your therapist, with your therapist, or with a surrogate. Sex therapy generally involves the evaluation and treatment of sexual problems that have nonphysical causes. It is also used when a physical condition cannot be corrected and a couple needs guidance in reorienting their sexual activity. Sex therapy is not the same as marital counseling, which deals with a wider range of marriage and family issues.

Besides psychologists, sex therapists include clergy, social workers, educators, doctors, and nurses. The best qualified usually have had training in psychotherapy and are certified by the American Association of Sex Educators, Counselors and Therapists. They should be in some way associated with a physician or a hospital so that they can refer clients for medical treatment.

Sex therapists treat couples and individuals—the latter for problems with sexual inhibitions or concerns about sexual identity. It's usually recommended that a couple enter therapy together, even if one partner "doesn't believe in it" or thinks "it's not my fault."

To evaluate the problem and develop a course of treatment, a therapist will ask you and your partner to talk about yourselves individually and as a couple. The discussions may include your childhood, your relationship with your parents, your diet, your job, and other aspects of your life beyond the strictly sexual. Based on the talks, the therapist will suggest exercises for you to do on your own to help you relax and to promote intimacy. Quite often these focus on touch or massage and, at least initially, exclude intercourse. Treatment may last from a few weeks to several years, although most couples report improvement within a few months.

Sometimes people are embarrassed to seek sex therapy, thinking it means they have a bad marriage, an awful sex life, or are personally inept or undesirable. But a sexual problem is simply that—a problem for which there's usually a solution.

How do I go about finding a sex therapist?

Before seeing a sex therapist or counselor, it's a good idea for both partners to have medical checkups to rule out any physical causes for the problems that concern them. If there are no physical problems, you can find a reputable sex therapist by either asking your doctor for a recommendation or contacting the American Association of Sex Educators, Counselors and Therapists (see Appendix) for a free state-by-state listing of certified therapists. Don't be shy about contacting several therapists before making a choice. It's vital to have a therapist whom you trust and feel comfortable with.

Individual practitioners set their own fees, which are usually comparable to those for other types of psychotherapy. As with other therapies, the costs may be covered in whole or in part by medical insurance.

Is there any reason not to have sex during a woman's menstrual period?

As long as both partners are healthy, and in the absence of religious prohibitions, there's no reason to avoid sex at this time. Certain religious groups, such as Muslims and Orthodox Jews, forbid sexual intercourse between husbands and their menstruating wives. Such restrictions are rooted in ancient traditions. They also have the effect of increasing a couple's chance of conceiving a child (the most fertile time in a woman's cycle is soon after her period ends, which is when Muslim and Jewish codes allow sexual relations to resume).

Some couples prefer not to have sex during the woman's period; they may not want to deal with the inconvenience, the woman may not feel sexy, or the man may not be aroused by her at that time. Other couples don't mind the menstrual fluid, or use a diaphragm to hold it back; their enjoyment of sex may even be enhanced by the fact that a menstruating woman is less likely to become pregnant (this does *not* mean that birth control isn't necessary during menstruation). Some women feel more aroused during their periods; others say that orgasm helps relieve cramping and discomfort. In general, the decision to have sex or not during the woman's period is almost always a matter of personal preference and seldom creates problems for couples. **Caution.** A woman carrying the AIDS virus is more likely to transmit it when she's menstruating and, if uninfected, she is at greater risk of contracting it from an HIV-positive partner.

Does the fact that a married man or woman masturbates indicate an inadequate sexual relationship?

Masturbation was considered an unnatural act by many authorities until well into this century, and many religious groups still have a strong prohibition against it. But the early Kinsey studies in the

1940's and 1950's (and many surveys since) revealed that most men and women masturbate at some point. Many start to experiment in early adolescence before sexual activity with another person is permissible or possible. Others start later, after they are sexually experienced.

Even though they may not consider masturbation unnatural, many people have a lingering belief that a happily married person shouldn't need to masturbate if he or she has a truly satisfying sexual relationship in the marriage. But masturbation appears to be common even among happily married people. They may be fully satisfied with both the quality and quantity of sex they have with their spouses, and simply masturbate as another way to add sexual feelings and experiences to their lives. Some couples derive pleasure from mutual masturbation. Of course, if the chief reason one member of a couple masturbates is because he or she is unhappy with some aspects of their lovemaking, the couple might be well advised to discuss the problem and, perhaps, seek counseling or therapy for it.

Psychologists who study sex say that masturbation is a way for people, married or not, to learn their own patterns of arousal and to discover what gives them the most pleasure.

Does being attracted to someone other than your spouse mean that something is wrong with your marriage?

Not necessarily. It's normal and healthy for people in established relationships to have fantasies and dreams about celebrities, characters from books or movies, strangers, slight acquaintances, former partners—even

close friends. It's also normal for married people to have close friendships and work relationships with people of the opposite sex. These relationships may or may not be accompanied by occasional sexual thoughts by either or both parties.

Such fantasies are usually not wishful thinking, but rather a harmless way of experiencing something different and forbidden. For example, a woman may daydream about having sex with her husband's best friend or with the carpenter working next door, without having the slightest intention of fulfilling this wish. Whether you tell your spouse about your fantasies is up to you; many people choose to keep them to themselves, but some couples find that sharing fantasies about others can be a way to affirm their trust in the relationship.

However, a persistent attraction to someone other than your spouse and a growing desire to act on your sexual urges may be signs that something in your relationship needs attention.

Does an affair always signal the end of a marriage?

It is estimated that 40 to 50 percent of husbands and 35 to 40 percent of wives have sex outside their marriage at some time. Yet adultery is the stated reason for less than 2 percent of all divorces in the United States. Even though adultery is no doubt a factor in many divorces filed for "incompatibility" or "mental cruelty," it would seem that most marriages affected by adultery survive. A brief affair or a single incident usually affects a marriage less than an ongoing relationship, which may involve more than simple lust. Still, the impact of any extramarital affair can be

devastating. Both men and women report being shaken to the core by the loss of trust in their spouse. Occasionally, an affair strengthens a marriage by providing a catalyst for confronting issues and working toward change, but there are usually far less disruptive ways of initiating improvement in a relationship.

Recent research indicates that an affair can have a profound negative effect on children, even if it's hidden from them. Children seem to sense that something is going on and may feel anxious, frightened, or rejected, or become convinced that they have done something wrong.

The reasons for having an affair are as many and varied as human beings themselves; they include lust, boredom, curiosity, anger, revenge, sexual frustration, loneliness, intoxication resulting in loss of inhibition, a need to prove one's attractiveness or self-worth, concerns about aging, and confusion about sexual orientation.

Whatever the reasons for an affair, psychotherapy, sex therapy, marital counseling, or marriage and family therapy can be very helpful to a couple or a family dealing with its consequences. Although talking to friends or relatives can be comforting, they probably won't be able to help you uncover the issues that led to the problem. Because they are likely to see only your side, they won't be much help in correcting the situation. A trained therapist, on the other hand, can help both partners express their feelings about the affair and other issues in the marriage, and work toward deciding how, or whether, to continue the relationship. The American Association of Marriage and Family Therapists (see Appendix) can provide a list of qualified therapists in your area.

THE FACTS ABOUT AIDS

What is it? AIDS (*Acquired Immune Deficiency Syndrome*) is a breakdown of the immune system resulting from infection with the human immunodeficiency virus (HIV). Once AIDS is diagnosed, it is considered fatal. The first cases of AIDS were detected in 1981 in the United States; since then the disease has been reported and tracked worldwide.

Who gets it? AIDS has struck men, women, and children of all ages, races, and sexual orientations. In Africa, where the disease is now widespread, most AIDS patients are heterosexual, with men and women affected equally. In the United States, the disease first broke out among homosexual and bisexual men, who still account for 60 percent of U.S. AIDS patients. The second-largest group consists of intravenous drug users, who spread the infection first among themselves by sharing needles, then among their sexual partners through unprotected intercourse. About one-third of the babies born to HIV-infected mothers also become infected. Transfusions of contaminated blood products in the early 1980's were responsible for some AIDS cases. This route of infection was virtually cut off in 1985 when new blood-screening techniques were put into practice.

How is it spread? HIV is spread mainly through contact with infected body fluids, such as semen and blood. The most common methods of transmission are sexual intercourse with an infected person and the sharing of needles and syringes among intravenous drug users. The "safer sex" practices outlined on the facing page will reduce the risk of getting HIV from sexual contact, but they won't completely eliminate it.

Misconceptions. You can't get AIDS by touching, hugging, or sharing living quarters with an infected person. Nor can your child contract AIDS from an infected classmate in routine school or playground activities. You certainly can't get AIDS by *donating* blood (sterile disposable needles are used), and the current odds for getting HIV from a blood transfusion are less than 1 in 150,000.

How does HIV infection affect a patient? HIV attacks T4-lymphocytes, a type of white blood cell that defends the body from a host of disease-causing organisms and cancers. As the T4-lymphocytes are destroyed, more and more infections or cancers are able to overwhelm the immune system. Having an HIV infection, however, is not the same as having AIDS. People who test HIV-positive usually experience no symptoms for several years, sometimes for as long as 10 years, possibly longer. Symptoms begin to develop gradually and may include swollen glands, fatigue, a whitish coating on the tongue, fevers, and, in women, chronic vaginal yeast infections and repeated bouts of pelvic inflammatory disease (p.250). In its most severe form, HIV infection makes an individual susceptible to some serious disorders that are rare in people with sound immune systems; these include Kaposi's sarcoma (a cancer), lymphoma of the brain, pneumocystis pneumonia, and vision-threatening cytomegalovirus infection of the eye.

How is AIDS diagnosed? A blood test, developed in 1985, can detect the presence of HIV antibodies—substances formed by the immune system to fight off the infection; more sophisticated tests confirm HIV infection. Because it can take weeks or months for antibodies to form, a person who has engaged in high-risk behavior and tests negative should be retested 6 months later. (For more on HIV testing and counseling, see p.128.) The diagnosis of AIDS is based on positive HIV test results together with a T4-lymphocyte count below 200 per cubic millimeter of blood (about 1,000 is considered normal).

How is it treated? There's still no cure for AIDS, but the sooner HIV infection is detected and treatment begun, the more effective that treatment is likely to be. Antiviral drugs such as AZT have prolonged the asymptomatic period for some HIV-infected persons and improved the quality of life for AIDS patients. Preventive treatments are available for pneumocystis pneumonia and other AIDS-related disorders.

What is "safe sex"? Are you ever 100 percent protected against AIDS?

According to the U.S. Public Health Service, the best protection against AIDS is to abstain from sexual relations or to have a long-term mutually monogamous relationship with an uninfected person (that is, the relationship predates 1977, you are both absolutely sure that neither of you is infected, and you both have sex only with each other). Deciding if someone is infected, however, is not easy. The AIDS virus (HIV) can live in the human body 10 years, and possibly longer, before symptoms become apparent (an infected person, however, may test positive for HIV antibodies as early as 6 weeks after infection). That's why many public-health officials consider abstinence and long-term exclusive monogamy with an uninfected partner to be the only totally safe sex practices.

Other practices, referred to as safer sex, can reduce your HIV risk but do not eliminate it. Avoid casual sex and sex with multiple partners, and be sure to take the following precautions:

☐ Limit your sexual activities to those that do not involve the exchange or passage of semen and other body fluids between you and your partner. Cuddling, massaging, body rubbing, kissing your partner's skin, and mutual masturbation fall into this category.

☐ If you engage in vaginal or anal intercourse, the two activities associated with the highest risk of HIV transmission, use a latex condom with a spermicide (see right).

☐ If you practice oral sex, use a condom without a spermicide.

Passionate open-mouth kissing poses a theoretical, but low, risk of HIV transmission; casual (mouth-to-skin) kissing is generally considered safe.

USING A CONDOM CORRECTLY

A condom's effectiveness in preventing pregnancy or lowering the risk of transmitting a disease depends on proper use. Condoms come in individual packets, rolled and ready to use, and are sold without prescription at any drugstore. Buy only latex condoms with a semen reservoir at the tip. (Lambskin condoms are less effective in preventing disease transmission.) Store condoms in a cool, dry place. Before using one, examine it for brittleness, stickiness, or deterioration.

Use condoms with a water-based spermicide containing 5 percent nonoxynol-9. (Some condoms come with a spermicide already applied; it's a good idea to add more.) Petroleum-based lubricants, such as petroleum jelly, mineral oil, or cold cream, weaken latex; use water-based lubricants.

Place a condom on the penis once it is fully erect but *before* penetration or oral sex. Squeeze the reservoir at the condom's tip to remove air. Still squeezing the tip, unroll the condom over the penis. If the condom tears or does not fully unroll, discard it and open a new one. After ejaculation but before the erection is lost, withdraw, holding the bottom of the condom securely to prevent semen spillage. If lovemaking continues, use a new condom.

These guidelines apply to HIV. Other sexually transmitted diseases (STD's) may be passed on differently (you can catch herpes, for example, from casual kissing). For more information see *The Facts About AIDS*, facing page, and *Sexually Transmitted Diseases*, p. 244.

What is "date rape"?

Like all rapes, date rape (also called acquaintance or nonstranger rape) is sexual intercourse with an unwilling partner through the threat or use of force or violence. The distinction in this case is that the people involved know each other.

Most rapes are committed by people known to their victims. The rapist might be someone the victim just met (on a date or at a party, for example), someone she knows slightly (such as a neighbor or co-worker), or a close friend, relative, or spouse. Acquaintance rapes are less likely to be accompanied by physical violence than nonacquaintance rapes—and it's thought that they are less likely to be reported. Many women who are raped feel that the rape was their fault, and if they were raped by someone they know, they may believe that "it wasn't really rape."

What should a woman do if she is threatened with rape?

Law-enforcement officers and other experts advise that when a woman is faced with the threat of rape her chief goal should be to survive. This may mean trying to run away, screaming to attract attention, reasoning with the rapist, fighting, or submitting (especially if the assailant is armed).

A rape should always be reported to the police, if only to help prevent an attack on someone

SEXUALLY TRANSMITTED DISEASES

A sexually transmitted disease (STD) is an infection passed on primarily, but not exclusively, by sexual contact. Genital herpes, hepatitis B, and AIDS are caused by viruses for which there are no cures. Herpes outbreaks, however, can be controlled with antiviral drugs, and hepatitis B (formerly called serum hepatitis) can be prevented before exposure with a vaccine. Most STD's are caused by bacteria or by other microorganisms known as chlamydiae and can usually be treated with antibiotics.

People with many sexual partners are at highest risk of contracting an STD. Practicing safer sex (p.243) will reduce your risk. If you think you have been exposed to an STD, avoid any sexual contact until after you see a doctor for a diagnosis, receive any necessary treatment, and take a test showing that you are not infected. Your sexual partner(s) should also be tested and, if necessary, treated.

Disease	Symptoms	Treatment	Possible outcome if untreated
AIDS	*See* The Facts About AIDS, *p.242, for information about this disease.*		
Chlamydial infection	Often symptomless. Mild burning when urinating; discharge from penis or vagina. Vaginal bleeding. Infections in genital area.	Antibiotics.	*Men:* Sterility. *Women:* Pelvic inflammatory disease, infertility. Pneumonia and serious eye infection in infants born to infected mothers.
Crab lice	Itching; visible infestation of pubic and other hair.	Pesticide shampoo or ointment.	Progressive infestation.
Genital herpes	Recurring eruptions of painful blisters and sores around genitals or mouth. Possible fever, headache, swollen glands, malaise.	Antiviral tablets.	*Women:* Risk of cervical cancer, miscarriage, or premature delivery. Active sores can seriously infect newborn.
Gonorrhea	Often symptomless. Painful urination; discharge from penis or vagina. Abnormal uterine bleeding.	Antibiotics (but some strains have become resistant to antibiotics).	Arthritis, heart disease, brain infection, sterility. *Men:* Blockage of urethra. *Women:* Pelvic inflammatory disease. Serious eye infection in newborn.
Hepatitis B	*See* The Facts About Hepatitis, *p.349, for information about this disease.*		
Nonspecific urethritis	Abnormal urethral or vaginal discharge; painful, difficult urination; pelvic pain. May be symptomless.	Antibiotics.	*Women:* Pelvic inflammatory disease, inflamed cervix. *Men:* Cystitis, inflamed testes or prostate, urethral narrowing.
Syphilis	*First stage:* Chancre (sore) on genitals or other sex-contact area that heals in a few weeks. *Second stage:* Rashes, fever, malaise, swollen glands, hair loss; then no symptoms, often for years.	Antibiotics.	*Third stage:* Brain and nerve damage causing blindness, paralysis, insanity; heart and blood vessel damage; death. Infected newborn may be malformed or stillborn.
Trichomoniasis	May be symptomless. *Women:* Inflamed genitals; vaginal discharge. *Men:* Inflamed glans or urethra.	Antibiotics.	No serious complications.
Venereal warts	Flat or cauliflower-shaped warts in genital area or on mouth.	Laser, chemical, or electrical burning; freezing; surgery.	Warts may spread. Linked to abnormal Pap smears, cervical cancer, and genital tumors.

else. Don't bathe or shower if you think you may want to prosecute—you'll wash away evidence. Even if you do not have any serious injuries, you need prompt medical attention; it's suggested that you go straight to the police or, if necessary, a hospital emergency room. If possible, have a friend, relative, or rape-crisis counselor go with you. The police may question you in detail about the rape; provide as much information as possible. In the past some women have felt intimidated by police questioning, although rape-crisis counselors say this seldom happens now.

Medical care should include a pelvic exam (with collection of semen), examination and treatment of any injuries, treatment with antibiotics for sexually transmitted diseases, and possibly treatment to prevent pregnancy. A 6-week follow-up visit is often recommended.

How should a woman handle the emotional aftereffects of rape?

The emotional impact of rape can persist for a long time. The victim may have feelings of fear, anger, depression, anxiety, and guilt for weeks, months, even years. She may dread being alone or having sex. She may begin abusing alcohol or drugs, develop compulsive behaviors (such as frequent washing or checking door locks), or become agoraphobic (fearful of going out in public). She even may suffer post-traumatic stress disorder (p.159) and have flashbacks of the attack during normal sex.

It's important for the victim to deal with her feelings about the rape and to talk about them with people she is close to and trusts—her spouse, family, and friends. Therapy, counseling, and support groups—both for the victim and for her partner or family—can also do a lot to help a woman work out her feelings and rebuild her wounded confidence, self-reliance, and self-esteem. Prosecution of a rapist can be a long, exhausting process, making support essential.

What are the health risks of abortion? How far into a pregnancy is it safe to have one?

Abortion is the deliberate ending of a pregnancy before term. The earlier in a pregnancy that a woman has an abortion, the safer it is for her.

Most first-trimester abortions are done by vacuum aspiration: the woman is given either a local or a general anesthetic, her cervix is dilated, and a tube is inserted through the cervix into the uterus. A suction machine attached to the outer end of the tube draws tissue from the uterus into a vacuum bottle. The physician then examines the uterus to make sure that none of the fetal and placental tissue has been left behind. The procedure is over in about 5 minutes. There may be some pain and cramping during it, and cramping and bleeding afterward. If performed by a professional in a hospital, doctor's office, or clinic, a first-trimester abortion has a low risk of failure or complications, such as infection or excessive bleeding. The woman usually goes home within a few hours, and recovery is quick (sexual relations can be resumed after 2 or 3 weeks).

Second-trimester abortions are generally more complicated and riskier, and may involve an overnight hospital stay. The most common method, called dilation and evacuation (D and E), is similar to vacuum aspiration, except that the dilation process, which involves a series of small rods of graduated size or a device known as an osmotic dilator, can take several hours. Once the cervix is sufficiently dilated, a suction machine is used to empty the contents of the uterus. For later second-trimester abortions, a saline solution or a labor-inducing hormone (prostaglandin) is injected into the uterus to induce contractions and a miscarriage. The contractions are painful and may last several hours. The fetus is expelled within 8 to 24 hours. Side effects may include cramping, nausea, diarrhea, and uterine bleeding.

The health risks and potential for complications increase with the length of pregnancy. Third-trimester abortions are usually performed only when the mother's life is in danger.

After an abortion, some women (and their partners) may feel sadness and a sense of loss.

I want to take the pill. Should I be concerned about its side effects?

The pill is a highly effective contraceptive, but it can cause a variety of side effects. The combined pill contains synthetic forms of the female hormones estrogen and progesterone; its side effects may range from relatively simple problems such as nausea, vomiting, weight changes, and tender breasts to much more serious conditions, including the formation of blood clots that can threaten the heart, brain, and lungs. The pill also increases the risk of heart attack and stroke in women over 35 who smoke or have high blood pressure.

The minipill, which contains only synthetic progesterone, produces milder side effects, such as irregular periods and bleeding. It is somewhat less

PREVENTING PREGNANCY

A risk-free, 100 percent effective contraceptive doesn't exist. But your doctor can help you match your personal needs with a suitable contraceptive and check that you know how to use it properly. In addition to preventing pregnancy, a latex condom provides good STD protection, especially when used with a spermicide (p.243). Other barrier methods (diaphragm, cervical cap) and sperm-killing methods (spermicides, sponge) offer only limited disease protection. Hormonal contraceptives (the pill, implants), the IUD, and natural methods do not provide STD protection.

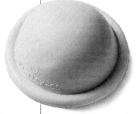

Diaphragm. A soft rubber cup stretched over a flexible frame blocks entrance to the uterus; must be used with spermicide. Requires fitting and training to use. Can be inserted up to 6 hr. before intercourse, but spermicide must be reapplied (with the diaphragm in place) within an hour before intercourse or repeated intercourse. Must be worn 6 to 8 hr. after last intercourse (but no longer than 24 hr.). *Failure rate: 6–18 percent.**

Spermicide. Chemicals in a cream, jelly, foam, or suppository create a sperm-killing barrier in the vagina. Easy to obtain and use. Effective 10 min. after application for up to 1 hr. Must be reapplied before repeated intercourse. *Failure rate: 3–21 percent.*

Contraceptive sponge. A wet polyurethane sponge is inserted in vagina, where it releases spermicide. Requires no prescription. Effective for 24 hr. Must be worn for 6 hr. after last intercourse (up to 30 hr. total). Not for use during period. *Failure rate: 6–28 percent; highest for women who have borne a child.*

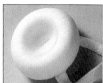

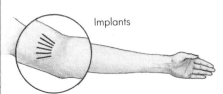
Implants

Implants. Soft capsules inserted under the skin of a woman's arm slowly release the hormone levonorgestrel, which makes the woman infertile. Effective for 5 yr. Can be removed to allow conception. Implants have fewer side effects than other hormonal contraceptives. *Failure rate: 0.04 percent.*

Condom. A thin sheath, usually latex, covers erect penis to contain the ejaculate. Easy to obtain and use (p.243). But putting it on before penetration can interrupt lovemaking. Also can reduce penile sensation or break or slip off. *Failure rate: 2–12 percent.*

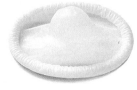

Intrauterine device (IUD). A small plastic device wrapped in copper or containing the hormone progesterone is inserted in the uterus and prevents fertile eggs from implanting. Convenient but increases risk of ectopic pregnancy, miscarriage, and pelvic inflammatory disease. May be expelled or perforate uterus. *Failure rate: 0.8–3 percent for copper-wrapped; 2–3 percent for hormone type.*

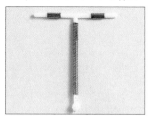

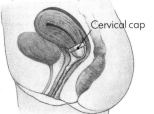
Cervical cap

Cervical cap. A small, firm rubber cap fits over cervix; must be used with spermicide. Needs careful fitting and training to use. Can be worn 48 hr. No need to reapply spermicide for repeated intercourse. Must stay in 8 to 12 hr. after intercourse. *Failure rate: 6–18 percent.*

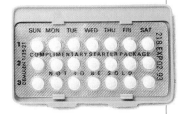

Oral contraceptives. Synthetic hormones progesterone and estrogen (in combined pill) or progesterone alone (in minipill) prevent conception. Most effective nonsurgical method. But requires prescription, must be taken regularly, and may have side effects (p.245). *Failure rate: 0.1–3 percent for combined pill; 0.5–3 percent for minipill.*

Natural family planning. A couple avoids intercourse during the woman's fertile period, calculated by calendar, by observing changes in her temperature or cervical mucus, or by a combination of these methods. Acceptable to religions that prohibit pills or devices. Requires motivation and precise record keeping. *Failure rate: 1–20 percent.*

*A contraceptive's failure rate depends on several factors, among them the user's motivation to prevent pregnancy and his or her knowledge of proper contraceptive use. The failure rate is lowest when a method is used correctly and consistently over a period of time. The higher failure rates listed on this page, however, are more typical.

effective as a contraceptive than the combined pill, but its failure rate is still lower than that of barrier types of contraceptives.

Overall, the side effects of taking the pill must be balanced against its convenience and benefits. Besides its proven effectiveness, the combined pill reduces the amount of bleeding and pain during periods and may have a protective effect against various conditions, including cancer of the ovaries, benign breast disease, pelvic inflammatory disease, and rheumatoid arthritis. Over the years hormones in the pill have been modified to reduce side effects and to produce a range of doses so that a woman can take the smallest dose that is effective for her.

Can sterilization be reversed?

Until recent years, a man's vasectomy was irreversible. But developments in microsurgery have increased the success rate of vasectomy reversals. Today about half of attempted reversals are successful, and the couple is able to achieve a pregnancy. The procedure is technically difficult and must be done by a trained microsurgical specialist; it is also expensive and not universally available. A man considering a vasectomy should always assume that it will make him sterile for the rest of his life.

A woman should also consider a tubal ligation permanent, although reversal is possible if the tubes were constricted or clamped rather than cut or cauterized. About 70 to 75 percent of women who undergo surgical reversal of sterilization are later able to become pregnant normally. But they have 10 times the normal risk of having a life-threatening ectopic, or tubal, pregnancy (p. 262).

STERILIZATION

Both female and male sterilization are simple procedures performed with local anesthesia. Women must go to a clinic or hospital, but men need only visit their doctor's office. Performed correctly, both operations are virtually 100 percent effective—immediately for women and after a few months for men.

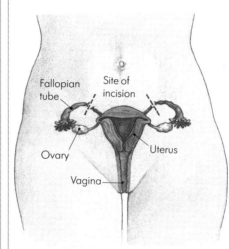

A woman is most often sterilized in an operation involving two small incisions in the abdomen. The fallopian tubes are cut and tied, clamped, or cauterized (burned) to prevent sperm from reaching an egg. The procedure is the single most common form of birth control worldwide. Among women who use birth control in the United States, some 28 percent have elected to be sterilized.

Male sterilization, or vasectomy, involves cutting and sealing the two sperm-carrying tubes—the vas deferentia—in the scrotum. The procedure does not make a man sterile immediately. Sperm present in the tubes must be either expelled (20 or more ejaculations) or allowed to die over time (3–4 months). Until then the man or his partner must use another form of birth control.

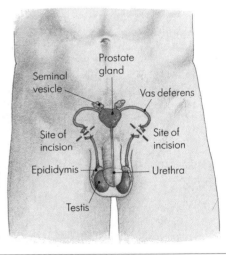

If I get a vasectomy will it affect my sex life?

No. A vasectomy has no effect on desire, arousability, performance, or any other aspect of a man's sexuality except his fertility. Postoperative soreness causes most men to avoid sexual intercourse for a few weeks. But after that, they should not experience any difference in feeling or performance or even notice a difference in the volume of semen ejaculated. Sperm cells make up only a very tiny percentage of semen. Most of this fluid is produced by the prostate and seminal vesicles, and their functioning is not affected by a vasectomy.

A lot of men I know have prostate trouble. What is the prostate?

The prostate is a gland lying under the bladder and in front of the rectum in men. It is about the size and shape of a chestnut and surrounds and feeds into the urethra as it descends from the bladder. The prostate produces the milky part of semen, which makes up 95 percent of semen's total volume (the rest is sperm and sperm-nourishing secretions from the seminal vesicles). The fluid secreted by the prostate also nourishes sperm and provides a medium they can move in. The muscles of the prostate and other muscles nearby contract to propel the semen down the urethra and out the penis when a man ejaculates.

At what age does the prostate start to cause problems?

Prostate problems are rare before age 55. The most common problem in older men is an enlarged prostate. This condition is usually benign and does not require treatment. In some cases, however, the enlarged organ begins to constrict the urethra, resulting in urination that is frequent, difficult to start, and slow to flow. It can also cause pain and interfere with sex. If the symptoms become severe, the usual treatment is transurethral surgery, in which the tissue pressing on the urethra is removed by means of a specially equipped cystoscope (p.127) inserted into the urethra. The procedure leaves most men sterile and a few impotent. A promising alternative involves inflating a balloon in the urethra to press aside the enlarged tissue.

Another prostate problem common in older men is cancer.

Symptoms are similar to those of an enlarged prostate; treatment is often removal of the prostate. Because the male hormone testosterone seems to play a role in causing prostate cancer, some cases are treated with estrogen therapy or by removing the testicles. Radiation therapy is used if the cancer has spread.

Doctors have traditionally relied on a rectal exam of the prostate (p.122) to screen for prostate disease. Unfortunately, by the time cancer is detected in this way, it has often spread to other parts of the body. A simple blood test that measures levels of prostate-specific antigen (PSA) is a much better screening tool. Men over 40 should undergo the rectal exam and the PSA test as part of their regular checkups. A cancer diagnosis can be confirmed with a biopsy or an ultrasound scan (pp.126–127).

What's the likely cause of painful urination in younger men?

While urination problems in older men usually result from an enlarged prostate, infection is the more likely cause in a younger man. Some sexually transmitted diseases, such as gonorrhea and chlamydial infection, can cause urination problems, usually a burning sensation when urine is passed (see *Sexually Transmitted Diseases*, p.244). Another possible cause of painful urination is prostatitis, an infection of the prostate gland that may or may not be sexually transmitted. Along with painful urination, symptoms can include pain in the lower abdomen and back, blood in the urine, and a penile discharge. A man experiencing symptoms of either prostatitis or a sexually transmitted disease should see a doctor immediately and refrain from sexual activity.

Why is one testicle usually lower than the other?

Often the left testicle is a bit heavier and larger, and hangs a little lower than the right. It's not known why, although it may be to keep the testicles from striking each other.

Sometimes a boy is born with one or both of his testicles undescended—not in their natural place in the scrotum. Although undescended testicles often drop into place on their own during infancy or early childhood, hormone therapy or surgery is necessary in some cases. If the testicles aren't in place by early childhood, they will permanently lose their ability to produce sperm. The condition may also put the individual at increased risk of testicular cancer. A boy with an undescended testicle should be seen by a doctor.

Today men are encouraged to do testicular self-exams (p.204), much as women do breast exams. Testicular cancer is the leading cause of cancer deaths in young men but is 100 percent curable if found early.

Why do so many brides develop cystitis on their honeymoon?

Cystitis is an inflammation of the urethra and bladder. The most common type, known as urinary tract infection (UTI), is usually caused by bacteria. It occurs primarily in women because their shorter urethra allows bacteria to reach the bladder more easily. A common cause of UTI is a sudden increase in sexual activity (as on a honeymoon), which increases the risk of infection. Intercourse itself may directly irritate the urethra and bladder. Also, a diaphragm that is too large may press on the bladder and urethra, and prevent the bladder from emptying completely; this allows bacteria to breed in the trapped urine.

The main symptom of UTI is a frequent, urgent need to urinate but with only a small amount of fluid passed. There is also pain and burning while urinating, pain above the pubic bone, and sometimes blood, pus, and a strong odor in the urine. Children with cystitis may run a fever with no urinary symptoms, or they may cry when urinating because of the pain.

A less common form of cystitis, called interstitial cystitis (IC), has similar symptoms, only far more severe and persistent. The condition, a chronic inflammation of the bladder, is difficult to diagnose and may require surgery. Its cause is uncertain, but it's not a bacterial infection.

What is the best way to treat cystitis? How can I keep from getting it so often?

Although some cases of UTI go away on their own, antibiotics are usually prescribed for quick relief and to rid the body of infection. Any woman with cystitis symptoms should have a urine test and possibly a urine culture so that the proper antibiotic or other medication can be prescribed. Untreated cases of cystitis may spread to the kidneys, where an infection can have serious consequences. Fever, chills, and abdominal and back pain are common signs of kidney infection.

For IC, an anti-inflamatory, muscle-relaxing, or other drug may be prescribed, not always with successful results. Although both IC and UTI require medical attention, soaking in a tub or putting a hot-water bottle on your back or lower abdomen can provide temporary relief. To

keep from aggravating the condition, avoid anything that may irritate the urinary tract, including cigarettes, coffee, alcohol, and spicy dishes as well as feminine hygiene sprays and scented douches. For UTI, drink plenty of liquids (see below).

Recurrent bouts of cystitis may be caused by repeated irritation or infection of the urethra during intercourse. If irritation is the problem, a change in your lovemaking position may help. If the problem is repeated infection, your doctor may prescribe an antibiotic, such as a sulfa drug, as a preventive measure.

FACT OR FALLACY ?

Drinking cranberry juice cures cystitis

Fallacy. This time-honored remedy—also touted as a preventive—has never been proven effective in controlled studies. The theory is that cranberry juice increases urine's acidity, which in turn discourages bacterial growth. In fact, drinking cranberry juice may be more harmful than helpful: the bacteria involved thrive in an acidic environment. The best home antidote, which seems to help clear up cystitis and to prevent new rounds of infection, is just drinking lots of nonalcoholic, caffeine-free liquids. Other preventive measures include keeping the urethral and genital area clean and urinating often, especially before and after intercourse.

What is vaginitis?

The term covers a variety of conditions, but essentially it's an inflammation of the vagina. It may be caused by an infection, an allergic reaction (to a cream, for example), a hormone deficiency, douching, a foreign body in the vagina (such as a tampon left in too long), a cut, a scrape, or irritation from intercourse without enough lubrication.

Bacterial secretions normally keep the vagina somewhat acidic; this controls the growth of yeast, fungi, and other organisms. When the acidity is disturbed, these organisms may proliferate, cause irritation and infection, and produce a discharge. A yeast infection (p. 250) is a common form of vaginitis, as is trichomoniasis (see *Sexually Transmitted Diseases*, p. 244). Many other types of vaginitis are grouped together as nonspecific vaginitis. Symptoms are a strong-smelling discharge and often back pain, cramps, swollen glands in the groin, and an urge to urinate.

Because of changing hormonal levels, pregnant and postmenopausal women are particularly susceptible to vaginitis, but any woman can develop a case. Some types are sexually transmitted; others may be picked up from a washcloth or towel. To reduce the risk of vaginitis, a woman should keep her genitals clean, using mild unscented soap and water. She should also wear clean cotton underpants (nylon retains moisture and heat, which promote bacterial growth). Keeping the intake of caffeine, alcohol, and sweets at a low level may also help to maintain the proper acidity.

Vaginitis is usually treated with antibiotic or antifungal drugs. Creams or suppositories may also be used, as the main treatment or as a supplement.

How can I avoid yeast infections?

This fungal infection, also called candidiasis, moniliasis, or thrush, produces a thick, cheeselike vaginal discharge. It may also cause discomfort during urination along with itching or burning of the vagina and external genitals, especially during arousal and intercourse. The growth of the fungus *Candida albicans* is normally controlled by bacteria in the vagina, but lowered resistance or antibiotic treatment that changes the normal bacterial balance of the vagina may encourage fungal growth. Some diseases, such as diabetes, and hormonal changes produced by pregnancy or birth control pills may have the same result. Yeast infections can appear on other moist areas of the body, such as the mouth or under the breasts. Although women make up the vast majority of cases, men may develop candidiasis on the penis; infants with diaper rash are also susceptible.

Candidiasis is best prevented by keeping the skin clean and dry, wearing cotton instead of synthetic underwear, avoiding tight clothing, maintaining overall good health, and avoiding sexual contact with an infected person. Women with repeated infections who take the pill may want to try another contraceptive. A yeast infection is usually treated with antifungal drugs or creams.

My sister got pelvic inflammatory disease after being fitted with an IUD. Are there long-term effects?

Pelvic inflammatory disease (PID) is an infection of the fallopian tubes, ovaries, uterus, or abdomen. Women who have sexual relations with a number of partners, use an intrauterine device (IUD) for birth control, have recently undergone pelvic surgery, or have had the disease before are at high risk for PID. The microorganism that causes chlamydial infections (see *Sexually Transmitted Diseases,* p. 244) is responsible for many cases of pelvic inflammatory disease. PID can also be caused by bacteria, such as the type responsible for gonorrhea. These germs reach the female organs through the vagina, as a result of sexual transmission or placement of an IUD, or through pelvic surgery.

The symptoms of pelvic inflammatory disease include severe abdominal pain, heavy and odorous vaginal discharge, abnormal vaginal bleeding, painful urination or bowel movements, fever, and nausea. A doctor makes a diagnosis by assessing a patient's history, by physical examination, and by special tests such as a culdocentesis. In this procedure, fluid taken from the area surrounding the uterus, ovaries, and fallopian tubes is analyzed. Pelvic inflammatory disease is always treated with antibiotics. If the microorganism causing the infection can be identified, which is not always the case, it's often possible to target the antibiotic more specifically at the troublesome germ.

Among the possible immediate complications of pelvic inflammatory disease are the formation of pelvic abscesses and, in rare cases, a life-threatening infection of the bloodstream. In the long run, pelvic inflammatory disease can lead to infertility, chronic abdominal pain, and scarring of the fallopian tubes. This scarring in turn can cause an ectopic, or tubal, pregnancy (p. 262), which usually requires major surgery. Having had pelvic inflammatory disease is a main risk factor for an ectopic pregnancy.

Can I still get toxic-shock syndrome from using tampons?

Toxic-shock syndrome is a potentially fatal condition caused by a bacterial toxin. It was first seen in the late 1970's; by the early 1980's hundreds of cases were being diagnosed in women using highly absorbent tampons (and in a few using a diaphragm). In the peak year of 1980, toxic-shock syndrome struck 13 of every 100,000 American women of menstrual age; out of a total of 890 cases nationwide that year, 35 women died.

Today the condition affects 1 in 100,000 women and causes few or no deaths. This dramatic improvement is due primarily to changes in the production, labeling, and use of tampons. Several highly absorbent tampons have been taken off the market. Tampons are now rated on a uniform absorbency scale (classifications such as "junior," "regular," and "super absorbent" mean the same thing on all brands). The U.S. Food and Drug Administration also requires that tampon boxes carry a warning about the risk of toxic-shock syndrome.

That risk is virtually nonexistent if you use the least-absorbent tampon for your needs and change it regularly. It's also a good idea to avoid using tampons at the beginning of your period, when 70 percent of all cases of toxic-shock syndrome occur.

The symptoms of toxic shock resemble those of the flu—high fever, aching muscles, sore throat, dizziness, vomiting, diarrhea—but they also include a sunburnlike rash and a sudden, severe drop in blood pressure. A woman who suspects she has this syndrome should seek immediate medical attention. Prompt treatment with antibiotics usually prevents serious consequences.

THE FACTS ABOUT PMS

What is it? Premenstrual syndrome, or PMS, is a collection of physical and psychological symptoms (150 have been identified) that affect a third of menstruating women 2 weeks or less before their periods. (PMS begins at or after ovulation.) For most women, PMS is simply an inconvenience, but for 5 to 10 percent it is very debilitating. Symptoms include mood swings, irritability, anxiety, fatigue, lethargy, abdominal bloating, water retention, breast swelling and tenderness, headache, back and lower abdominal pain, increased appetite, and cravings for sugary, salty, or high-carbohydrate foods. PMS is suspected when such symptoms are repeatedly associated with the menstrual cycle.

What causes it? No one really knows. Changing levels of the hormones estrogen and progesterone may play a role, but it's unclear why some women are severely affected and others aren't. Deficiencies of vitamins E and B6 and of magnesium are suspected, but

unproven, causes. Possible links between PMS and depression and PMS and thyroid disorders are being researched.

How is it treated? Treatment depends on a woman's symptoms. Relaxation techniques (pp. 206–207) can relieve tension and anxiety. Prescription diuretics sometimes prevent fluid retention. Exercise may lift spirits and reduce mild pain by stimulating the release of endorphins, the body's natural painkillers. Aspirin, ibuprofen, and prescription prostaglandin inhibitors help relieve cramps in some women. Others report benefits from taking vitamin E and avoiding caffeine, alcohol, salt, or sugar. For severe mood swings, a doctor may prescribe antidepressants or anti-anxiety drugs. Neither the hormone progesterone, which doctors often prescribe, nor vitamin B6, which many women take, has been proven effective. In a third to a half of women with PMS, the symptoms simply go away no matter what the treatment.

Why do some women have irregular periods?

There are many possible causes. Although the average woman menstruates every 28 days, a range from 22 to 35 days is considered normal. Periods may become irregular before menopause, sometimes starting in the mid-forties. A woman who loses a lot of weight or has a low body-fat percentage may have lighter or less frequent periods, or none at all (the loss of periods is called amenorrhea). Menstrual patterns can change in response to emotional stress, traveling, starting or stopping the pill, or having an IUD inserted or taken out. Medical problems, such as thyroid disorders, fibroids (p.252), or cervical cancer, can cause irregular bleeding. And, of course, a missed period may indicate pregnancy.

Women who menstruate irregularly or not at all may be at increased risk for osteoporosis, a disorder in which bones become brittle due to calcium loss (see *The Facts About Osteoporosis,* p.379). A woman who is not menstruating consistently should see her doctor and discuss the pros and cons of taking synthetic hormones to stimulate regular monthly periods.

I have a Pap test regularly. But I wonder: How accurate is it?

A Pap test, or cervical smear (p.124), is not infallible. The doctor or nurse may not collect a sample that is representative of the full cervix. Or the lab technician may misread the specimen under the microscope. In the late 1980's some labs were found to have a false negative

rate of 25 percent—that is, 1 in 4 specimens with abnormalities was judged normal. Since then the federal government has established uniform guidelines for controlling the accuracy of Pap tests, including a limit on the number of slides a technician can view during an hour and a work day. About 75 percent of all Pap tests in the United States are now done by accredited labs, facilities that are certified by private regulatory associations to meet the federal standards.

An abnormal Pap test usually does not mean that you have cancer, but the situation should be carefully monitored. Your doctor will probably order another Pap test. A second abnormal test result is usually followed by colposcopy (a detailed examination of the cervix with a vaginal endoscope, or fiberoptic tube) and, if needed, a biopsy (p.144).

GYNECOLOGICAL EXAM

A gynecological checkup is not painful, but can be an uncomfortable experience, especially for the uninitiated. If you are having this exam for the first time, let your doctor know. For the pelvic part of the exam, you lie on your back on an examination table, knees bent, with your feet in stirrups at table level. A sheet covers your legs and torso. A complete exam will overlap a regular checkup in many areas (medical history, including menstrual cycle, past pregnancies, and birth control methods used; height and weight measurements; blood tests; urinalysis; blood pressure check; stethoscope check of heart, lungs, and abdomen) but should also include:

☐ Breast examination and instructions for breast self-examination (p.203)

☐ Rectal exam

☐ Visual exam of the external genitalia, vagina, and cervix (the walls of the vagina are held apart with a device called a speculum)

☐ Manual exam of the uterus, ovaries, and fallopian tubes (the doctor, wearing a latex glove, inserts two fingers into the vagina and palpates, or presses, the lower abdomen with the other hand, feeling for signs of soreness, enlarged organs, or abnormal growths)

☐ Pap test (p.124)

☐ On a first visit, blood test for rubella (German measles) if you're of childbearing age.

How often should a woman see a doctor for a pelvic exam?

Most doctors and the American College of Obstetricians and Gynecologists recommend a yearly gynecological examination starting around the time a woman becomes sexually active, or by age 18 at the latest. More frequent exams may be necessary in order for a doctor to monitor some conditions, such as an ovarian cyst or endometriosis. Most women have their yearly pelvic exam done by their primary physician or their gynecologist. Family planning clinics also offer pelvic exams.

A friend of mine has endometriosis. How serious is this?

Endometriosis is a disorder in which the tissue lining the uterus, known as the endometrium, starts to grow in other parts of a woman's body, usually in the pelvic cavity (on the cavity wall, fallopian tubes, ovaries, vagina, intestines, bladder, or the outside of the uterus). These growths bleed each month like the uterine lining. Since the discharge has nowhere to go, it can cause inflammation and form cysts, lesions, and scar tissue. Any premenopausal woman can get endometriosis. The condition goes into abeyance during pregnancy, and the symptoms cease completely after menopause.

The symptoms of endometriosis are pelvic pain around the time of ovulation and menstruation along with painful intercourse and bowel movements. In some women, however, the condition is painless. A woman may become infertile if growths block her ovaries and tubes. Although endometriosis is sometimes detected during a regular pelvic examination, the only sure way to diagnose it is by laparoscopy—viewing the pelvic organs through an endoscope, or fiberoptic tube (p.126), put through a small incision in the abdomen.

Endometriosis is treated with drugs that suppress hormone production and allow growths to shrink. Such drugs, however, can produce unwanted side effects, including weight gain, a deepening of the voice, the growth of facial and body hair, water retention, mood swings, and irregular vaginal bleeding. New treatments based on hormones that suppress ovarian function with less serious side effects are showing promise. In some cases growths are removed surgically, with a scalpel or a laser (this procedure can be done during a laparoscopy). Surgery may bring short-term relief and improved fertility, but growths can recur.

Because pregnancy halts the disease's progress, a doctor may suggest that a woman who wants children anyway try to conceive. The benefits, however, may not outlast the pregnancy.

What are fibroids?

Fibroids are benign (noncancerous) uterine growths that occur on the inner or outer surface of the uterus or within the uterine wall. They grow either singly or in clumps and range in size from smaller than a pea to larger than a grapefruit. Any woman can get them, but they are most common in women in their thirties and forties; about 25 percent of women over 35 have them.

What causes fibroids is unknown, although some doctors think they're related to estrogen levels, since high levels of this female hormone seem to promote their growth. Fibroids tend to get bigger when a woman is pregnant and her estrogen levels are high or when she is taking high-estrogen birth control pills. The growths often shrink after a woman undergoes menopause.

Symptoms of fibroids include longer, heavier, and more painful periods; bleeding between periods; pain in the abdomen or lower back; frequent urination; and constipation. In rare cases there may be abdominal swelling or infertility. Some women have no symptoms, even with large fibroids. Symptomless fibroids may first be noticed during a routine pelvic exam. A more definitive diagnosis can be obtained with ultrasound, contrast X-rays, and endoscopic examination of the abdominal cavity or the inside of the uterus (see *Diagnostic Tests,* pp.126–127).

Will I need surgery to remove my fibroids?

A woman with few symptoms, small fibroids, or who is near menopause may not need treatment. But she should have her condition monitored with yearly pelvic exams and should see her doctor if symptoms develop. In rare cases the stem holding a fibroid to the uterus can become twisted, causing acute pain, fever, and bleeding. In less than 1 percent of cases, a fibroid can become cancerous.

There's no universally accepted medical treatment for fibroids. Hysterectomy, the removal of the uterus, was once the common treatment. But myomectomy, the surgical removal of the fibroids, is performed with increasing frequency, particularly on young women who may want to have children. A more complicated procedure than hysterectomy, myomectomy may produce scarring that can cause pain and infertility. And there's no guarantee that fibroids won't recur after the operation.

I've heard that many hysterectomies are done unnecessarily. Is this true?

Hysterectomy—the removal of the uterus and sometimes the ovaries and fallopian tubes—is one of the most frequently performed and controversial surgical procedures in the United States. Done most often to remove fibroids, it is also used to treat uterine and cervical cancer, menorrhagia (heavy menstrual bleeding), extensive and debilitating endometriosis, severe recurring infection, and prolapsed uterus. It can be performed through the abdomen or the vagina and is almost always an elective, rather than emergency, procedure.

A 25 percent jump in the number of hysterectomies in the early 1970's led many people to question whether the operation was always necessary or in the woman's best interest. Hysterectomy requires general anesthesia, a hospital stay, and several weeks' rest. Complications can include hemorrhage, infection, and urinary tract problems. A premenopausal woman becomes infertile, and if her ovaries are removed along with her uterus, she may undergo menopause, experiencing hot flashes and other menopausal symptoms. Even if a woman keeps her ovaries, she may experience some symptoms of menopause because their blood supply is often impaired.

The hysterectomy rate has fallen in recent years, but it's still a good idea to get a second opinion if your doctor proposes the operation. Except in an emergency, the decision to have this operation or not is yours to make in consultation with your doctors. It should depend on your symptoms and how much they interfere with your everyday life. When performing a hysterec-

tomy on patients over age 45, some doctors routinely—and unnecessarily—remove the ovaries as well. Find out what your doctor's policy is on this matter and make your wishes known.

What is a D and C?

The abbreviation D and C stands for dilation (or dilatation) and curettage and refers to a procedure in which the cervix is widened (dilated) with special instruments so that the lining of the uterus (endometrium) can be gently scraped clean with a device called a curette. D and C was once used as a method of abortion during the first trimester, but vacuum aspiration has replaced it for this purpose. Today, a D and C may be done to remove fetal tissue after a miscarriage or to treat heavy menstrual bleeding caused by a thickened uterine lining. The procedure is also used to diagnose other uterine disorders, such as cancer. Although often performed under general anesthesia, a D and C is a simple operation without side effects. The endometrium soon grows normally and regular menstrual periods resume.

What should a couple do to get fit before trying to conceive?

The health and habits of both parents at the time of conception and of the woman in early pregnancy may affect fetal health. Women are better able to conceive and carry to term if they are within a normal weight range, menstruate normally, and are not deficient in key vitamins or minerals. A woman on the pill who decides to conceive should switch to another form of birth control for 3 months in order to get back on self-regulated cycles. Because some commonly used

INFERTILITY: CAUSES AND TREATMENTS

The inability to conceive is a problem for as many as 1 couple in 6, and doctors can help in about half the cases. The common causes and treatments of infertility in women and in men are listed below and at right. (Infertility may also result from a combination of factors involving both partners; in some cases, the cause is never found.) Techniques used to detect the causes of infertility are described at the bottom of the chart.

WHY A WOMAN MAY BE INFERTILE

Ovarian malfunction. The ovaries fail to ovulate or to produce enough progesterone, the hormone that prepares the uterine lining for a fertilized egg. BASAL BODY TEMPERATURE CHARTING may suggest absence of ovulation or insufficient progesterone; a BLOOD TEST, an ENDOMETRIAL BIOPSY, or a URINE TEST may be used to confirm the finding. Ovulation can often be stimulated with oral or injected hormones (this treatment may result in multiple births).

Blocked fallopian tubes. An obstruction in one or both fallopian tubes prevents sperm from reaching the egg. The blockage may be a congenital defect, scar tissue from infection or surgery, or the result of endometriosis (p.252). A HYSTEROSAL-PINGOGRAM can usually detect a blockage; sometimes a LAPAROSCOPY is needed. Endometriosis can be treated with surgery or drugs. Microsurgery may correct some blockages. Otherwise, in vitro fertilization (p.257) may be recommended.

Cervical mucus problems. The cervical mucus blocks or kills sperm because it is thick and acidic, is not abundant enough, or contains antibodies to sperm. These incompatibility problems can be detected with a POSTCOITAL TEST, followed by a BLOOD TEST or, if antibodies are suspected, a SPERM ANTIBODY TEST. A couple with this problem may be advised to consider artificial insemination (p.256) or in vitro fertilization (p.257).

Uterine disorders. In a few cases, a congenital malformation or the presence of fibroids (p.252) or scar tissue may prevent implantation of a fertilized egg or cause miscarriage. The condition may be detected during a pelvic exam (p.252); a HYSTEROSALPINGOGRAM or HYSTEROSCOPY may be used to make or confirm a diagnosis. The shrinking of fibroids (p.253), removal of scar tissue with a laser, and surgical correction of certain malformations often improve fertility.

DIAGNOSTIC TESTS AND PROCEDURES

Basal body temperature (BBT) charting. A woman takes her temperature orally each morning upon waking and records it on a calendar chart. A rise in temperature in the second half of the cycle often signals the release of the hormone progesterone, which occurs after ovulation.

Blood tests. A blood sample is analyzed for signs that a woman's cervical mucus or a man's semen contains antibodies to sperm. A woman's blood may also be analyzed for the level of the hormone progesterone after ovulation and a man's, for the level of pituitary hormones, which affect sperm production.

Endometrial biopsy. A tiny piece of the uterus's lining (endometrium) is surgically removed through the cervix for

microscopic examination. This is done just before a woman's period to see if she is producing the hormone progesterone.

Hysterosalpingogram. Dye is injected through the cervix into the uterus and fallopian tubes and a contrast X-ray (p.126) is taken to reveal any malformation, fibroids, scar tissue, or other blockage.

Hysteroscopy. Under general or local anesthesia, an endo-scope (p.126) is inserted through the cervix to examine the interior of the uterus.

Laparoscopy. Under general anesthesia, an endoscope is inserted through a small incision (usually just below the navel) into the pelvic cavity to examine the ovaries and the outer surfaces of

---

substances may harm the fetus, the American College of Obstetricans and Gynecologists advises women who are trying to conceive to avoid alcohol, illicit drugs, and tobacco. A woman who uses any of these substances before she realizes she's pregnant should tell her doctor. Some doctors also recommend giving up caffeine.

Fathers who drink heavily around the time of conception may also affect the well-being of their offspring. One study reported that men who drank regu-larly (about two standard-size drinks a day) produced infants who weighed an average of 6.4 ounces less than those of fathers who drank occasionally. In another study, the offspring of male rats who derived 35 percent of their calories from alcohol (as many human alcoholics do) were less adept at running mazes than the offspring of nondrinking male rats. Moderate drinking by fathers seems to have no effect on their offspring, nor does smoking or caffeine use; the effects of illicit drug use are unknown.

Will taking extra vitamins and minerals help me conceive?

There is no evidence that taking vitamin and mineral supplements will improve either a woman's or a man's fertility. But studies indicate that supplements taken early in pregnancy (before a woman knows she's expecting) may reduce the risk of some birth defects. In one study women given folic acid were less likely to have infants with spinal-cord and brain defects. Vitamins A, C,

WHY A MAN MAY BE INFERTILE

Low sperm production. The number of sperm in semen is insufficient to insure that one will survive and fertilize an egg. Sperm count is determined by SEMEN ANALYSIS. A number of factors can reduce sperm production: use of tobacco, alcohol, and certain drugs; the presence of varicoceles (varicose veins above one or both testes); a deficiency of pituitary hormones; or an earlier infection (such as a postpubescent case of mumps that resulted in inflammation of the testicles). Avoiding tobacco, alcohol, and any drug known to interfere with a man's fertility may solve the problem for some men. If a physical examination reveals varicoceles, blocking or tying them off may help increase the production of sperm. If a BLOOD TEST reveals a low level of pituitary hormones, drugs that increase their output or replace them may spur sperm production. When a low sperm count results from an earlier infection or when the cause can't be determined, there is no treatment.

Seminal fluid problems. The volume of fluid in semen is low, making it difficult for sperm to survive in the acidic environment of the vagina. Or the fluid may fail to reliquefy, as it normally does, about a half-hour after ejaculation; this impedes the passage of sperm through the cervix. Both the volume and viscosity of seminal fluid can be checked by SEMEN ANALYSIS; if there is a problem, artificial insemination may be recommended. In some cases, a POSTCOITAL TEST reveals that the semen contains antibodies to its own sperm; a BLOOD TEST or a SPERM ANTIBODY TEST may be done to confirm the finding. The cause of this problem is unknown, and there is no treatment.

Defective sperm. Semen contains a large number of sperm that are abnormal in shape, don't move actively forward, or have some other defect that prevents them from penetrating an egg. Sperm shape and movement are checked by SEMEN ANALYSIS, and their ability to penetrate an egg by SPERM PENETRATION ASSAY. In most cases, there is no treatment.

Blocked sperm ducts. The duct system that carries sperm from a man's testes is blocked by infection (often from a sexually transmitted disease) or by scar tissue resulting from infection, injury, or surgery. Once an infection has been diagnosed, antibiotic drugs may be used to cure it if the infection is caused by bacteria or chlamydia. A blockage caused by scar tissue can be detected by an ultrasound scan (p.126) and sometimes cleared by microsurgery.

the fallopian tubes and uterus. Microsurgery for any problem found is usually performed at the same time.

Postcoital test (PCT). A sample of cervical mucus collected 2 to 12 hours after intercourse is examined microscopically to evaluate the mucus, sperm, and the interaction between them. The test is done 2 or 3 days before ovulation when the mucus should be watery, alkaline, and abundant, allowing sperm to pass through. Timing is crucial; the test may have to be repeated several times.

Semen analysis. A semen sample is examined microscopically to determine sperm count, motility (movement), and morphology (shape). Semen volume and viscosity are also assessed.

Sperm antibody test. The man's semen, the woman's cervical mucus, or either partner's blood is analyzed to determine if it contains substances that disable sperm.

Sperm penetration assay (SPA). Also known as a hamster egg penetration test. Semen is mixed with specially prepared hamster eggs to see the percentage of sperm that penetrate them. Used to see if a man's sperm has a defect that prevents it from making the changes necessary to penetrate eggs.

Urine test. Using a kit, the woman tests a sample of her urine for the presence of luteinizing hormone (LH), which stimulates the ovaries to release eggs.

D, and E may also help prevent such defects. In addition, pregnant women often need to take extra calcium and iron. It's not a good idea, however, to take supplements indiscriminately or without asking your doctor's advice first.

We've been trying to conceive for 6 months. Should we see a doctor about infertility?

Infertility is usually defined as the failure of a couple to achieve a pregnancy after a year of intercourse without using any form of contraceptive. About 90 percent of women trying to get pregnant do so within a year (80 percent for first pregnancies). Women who don't, or who twice in a row don't carry a pregnancy to full term, may be advised to seek medical help (usually with their spouses). Many couples start by visiting their primary physician, who may refer them to a gynecologist, urologist, or reproductive endocrinologist, depending on the type of suspected problem (see above).

When a couple sees a specialist, they both usually undergo a battery of tests to detect the cause of the infertility. A doctor may ask extensive questions about infections, surgery, diet, exercise, drug and alcohol use, and past infertility treatment. It's estimated that 40 to 50 percent of fertility problems involve the woman, 30 to 40 percent the man, and 10 to 15 percent either involve both partners or have an unknown cause. About half of the couples treated for infertility eventually conceive.

Is it true that drinking coffee can make a woman less fertile?

No, not according to a recent study by the Centers for Disease Control (CDC). An earlier, well-publicized government study had suggested that consuming more than a cup of regular caffeinated coffee each day reduced the fertility of some women; the chances of conceiving seemed to decline as daily caffeine consumption increased. But the much larger CDC study apparently ruled out any link between caffeine and fertility.

Researchers at the CDC analyzed the caffeine consumption of more than 2,800 pregnant women and 1,800 women who had tried unsuccessfully to conceive for a year or more. When the researchers took into consideration other factors that affect conception, such as age, smoking, and previous pregnancies, they found that delays in conceiving did not increase with caffeine intake, whether the source was coffee, tea, or cola drinks. No matter how much caffeine a woman consumed, it took her an average of 4½ months to conceive. The American College of Obstetricians and Gynecologists does not list caffeine among the substances that women should avoid when trying to conceive.

I've been told that if my husband and I relax and stop worrying about having a baby, it will be easier to conceive. Is this true?

Taking a more relaxed approach to the problem of having a baby may be good for a couple's psychological health, but it will rarely lead to conception. In 80 to 90 percent of cases, infertility has a definite physiological cause.

There is some evidence, however, that psychological stress can negatively affect the levels of hormones that make a woman fertile. Some women stop menstruating in times of stress, for example. Thus, a few infertile women who are under stress may find they are able to conceive when the source of stress is removed. Couples under stress may also have sex less often, which obviously affects their chance of achieving pregnancy.

If you are trying to conceive, it's important to share your feelings with your spouse, keep a sense of humor, and bear in mind that sex is not just for making a baby.

We can't conceive a child normally. Should we consider artificial insemination?

For couples who have tried treatment and still can't conceive by normal intercourse, artificial insemination is an option that they might want to consider and discuss with their doctor. Artificial insemination is used most often when a man has a low sperm count or a woman's cervical mucus is too acidic or produces antibodies that attack the man's sperm. Less commonly, it is used when impotence or another problem prevents intercourse or when a man might pass on a hereditary disease to his offspring. In a simple procedure—done by the woman's doctor or by a technician at a sperm bank—sperm is injected into the woman's cervix around the time when she is ovulating and most fertile. The sperm may be either her husband's (when there is a cervical-mucus incompatibility problem, for example) or, more often, a donor's. The sperm donor is usually anonymous, although some couples arrange to have sperm donated by a friend or by a relative of the husband. In cases where the husband's sperm count is marginal, his sperm may be mixed with the donor's so that there's a possibility of the husband actually being the biological father.

Most women require three to five inseminations before becoming pregnant. After five unsuccessful attempts, the success rate is very low. In more than half the states the child is the legal offspring of the husband and wife (provided the husband agreed to the procedure); the donor has no parental rights or obligations. Other states have no laws on the question, leaving all concerned in legal limbo.

Sometimes when a woman is unable to carry a child, a couple may arrange for another woman to be artificially inseminated with the husband's sperm. But using a surrogate mother is a highly controversial, emotionally risky choice; laws and court decisions governing the entire surrogate process vary widely.

How safe is it to use a sperm bank?

A sperm bank is a medical laboratory that collects and stores sperm for artificial insemination. Besides storing sperm from donors and husbands, a sperm bank can be used by a man, married or not, to store his sperm when he is about to undergo a procedure or treatment, such as vasectomy or radiation therapy, that may leave him sterile. There are about 80 sperm banks in the United States and some 30,000 artificially inseminated births a year. No federal regulations govern sperm banks, and not all states control screening. Each sperm bank sets its own guidelines. Most record a donor's family and medical history and test for sexually transmitted diseases; some do genetic screening and chromosome analysis of donors to detect hereditary disease. Donors are usually medical and dental students who are paid a small fee and allowed a limited number of donations.

When sperm is collected from donors, it is frozen for storage, then thawed just before insemination. Fresh sperm has a somewhat higher success rate than frozen sperm (60 to 70 percent for fresh versus 55 percent for frozen) and was once routinely used. However, because it's possible to transmit the viruses for AIDS and hepatitis B in semen before the donor has tested positive, the American Fertility Society now recommends that semen be frozen for 6 months and that the donor be retested and found negative before his semen is used. When the sperm is from the woman's husband, however, it is often used fresh.

When selecting donor sperm to inseminate a married woman, most sperm banks try to use sperm from a donor who matches as closely as possible the physical characteristics of her husband. Most sperm banks also follow strict procedures to keep all donors' and husbands' sperm clearly identified so that each woman receives the correct sperm.

How is a "test-tube" baby conceived? How successful is this procedure?

A so-called test-tube baby is the result of a process known as in vitro fertilization. In this procedure, an egg is taken from an ovary just before ovulation (through either the vagina or a small abdominal incision), placed in a sterile dish, and fertilized with sperm. If the egg and sperm unite and the fertilized egg starts to divide, it is inserted through the vagina into the uterus, where it's hoped the embryo will implant and grow.

In vitro (literally, "in glass") fertilization is an option for women whose fallopian tubes are blocked but whose ovaries and uterus function normally. Performed at about 200 medical centers in the United States, the procedure is costly and has a low success rate. Despite technological advances since the first test-tube baby was born in 1978, the success rate of in vitro fertilization is 25 percent at most.

An alternative procedure, GIFT (*G*amete *I*ntra*F*allopian *T*ransfer), involves placing the sperm-egg mixture in the fallopian tube for fertilization. The GIFT success rate is higher than that of in vitro fertilization.

I've miscarried once. What is my risk of having another miscarriage or a problem pregnancy?

Miscarriage, or spontaneous abortion, is the natural termination of a pregnancy before the 22nd week (in most cases, before the 12th week). As many as 1 in 6 pregnancies end in miscarriage, often without a woman realizing she is pregnant. The signs of a miscarriage are heavy bleeding and cramping that might be mistaken for a severe menstrual period. In the course of a miscarriage, the embryo or fetus is expelled along with the uterine lining. Medical attention is needed to make sure no fetal tissue is left in the body, where it can cause infection. To remove any remaining fetal tissue, the doctor may perform a D and C (p.253). Some women require a few days of bed rest after a miscarriage.

Many miscarriages result from fetal abnormalities, mainly genetic and developmental defects. Other causes include maternal infection or exposure to toxins, hormonal imbalances, fibroids, and a weak cervix. Doctors don't always know what causes a miscarriage or why certain women seem more prone to them.

The risk of miscarriage rises with age, and women who have miscarried once have a greater risk of doing so again. However, most women who miscarry eventually carry a pregnancy to full term. In most cases a woman can resume sexual relations 4 to 6 weeks after a miscarriage (when the cervix is closed), provided her doctor doesn't advise against it. A woman who has two or more miscarriages in a row should consider seeing a doctor who specializes in patients with problem pregnancies.

Sickle-cell anemia runs in my family. How can I make sure I won't have a child who inherits it?

Sickle-cell anemia is an often fatal inherited blood disease that affects primarily blacks. About 1 in 400 black infants are born with it and about 1 in 12 blacks carry the trait. If both parents have the trait, their children have a 25 percent chance of having the disease and a 50 percent chance of inheriting the trait. If one parent has the trait, a child is unlikely to be born with the disease but may carry the trait. Ask your doctor to refer you and your spouse to a genetic counselor, who can help you assess the risk to your children.

What does a genetic counselor do?

Genetic counselors are usually physicians who have a specialty in medical genetics. They work together with patients' doctors to provide information and guidance on genetic diseases, such as sickle-cell anemia and cystic fibrosis; chromosomal abnormalities, such as Down's syndrome; or birth defects, such as congenital heart disease.

Although genetic counselors rely heavily on the information that a couple supplies about relatives with genetic disorders, the rapidly developing field of genetic science can predict with increasing accuracy whether a person risks passing on a disorder to his or her children. Chromosome analysis of white blood cells can reveal defective genes or more often genetic markers (chromosomal material usually associated with a certain condition though not the cause of it). The knowledge gained from testing and counseling can help a couple make a decision about whether or not to conceive or proceed with a pregnancy. Genetic testing usually deals in possibilities rather than certainties, and education and counseling of the couple should go hand in hand with testing.

A couple should consider seeing a genetic counselor—preferably before the woman becomes pregnant—if they know or suspect that either of them has or may carry a genetic disorder or if they already have had a child born with an abnormality. Older mothers and workers with extensive exposure to radiation or chemicals may also find counseling helpful. To find a qualified counselor in your area, contact the National Society of Genetic Counselors (see Appendix), which certifies counselors, or ask your doctor for a referral.

What are the early signs of pregnancy?

Within 4 weeks after conception, a pregnant woman may notice some of the following symptoms:

STARTING A FAMILY AFTER 30

Doctors once routinely advised women to have their first child before age 30, before fertility declines and the risks of miscarriage, childbirth complications, and birth defects increase. According to a study at Mount Sinai Hospital in New York City, a woman's chance of having a cesarean rises from 22 percent in her twenties to 26 percent at 30 and to 34 percent at 35. During pregnancy, a 35-year-old has a 7 percent chance of developing diabetes and an 8 percent chance of developing high blood pressure—double the risks she had in her twenties. Her baby also has a slightly greater chance of requiring intensive care. Studies have shown that the likelihood that a child will have Down's syndrome or another genetic birth defect increases with the mother's (and possibly the father's) age.

On the positive side, the Mount Sinai study found that first babies born to mothers over 35 are at no significantly greater risk of being premature or stillborn or of having a lower Apgar score (p.265). Improved prenatal care has reduced the dangers of pregnancy-related diabetes and high blood pressure. Down's syndrome and other genetic birth defects can now be detected as early as the first trimester by chorionic villus sampling (p.261). And a recent study indicates that the incidence of many common birth defects, such as spina bifida, is not tied to maternal age.

Today, 1 in 5 first-time mothers is over 30, and her risk of having a problem pregnancy or an unhealthy baby is only slightly higher than a younger mother's. Even a woman over 40—if she's healthy and of average weight and sees her doctor regularly—can reasonably expect a normal pregnancy and a healthy baby.

☐ A missed period, or one with a shorter, less copious flow
☐ Breasts that are swollen, tender, or tingly
☐ A frequent need to urinate
☐ Fatigue
☐ Nausea, vomiting (especially in the morning)
☐ Appetite increase or decrease
☐ Constipation, heartburn
☐ Bloated sensation
☐ Abdominal cramps
☐ Mood changes

The symptoms and their degree of intensity vary from one woman to another. A woman who suspects she may be pregnant, even if she has no signs, is often advised to have a pregnancy test. Confirming a pregnancy early allows a woman to get good prenatal care in the critical early weeks of pregnancy or to terminate the pregnancy, if she so decides, during the first trimester, when the procedure is safer and simpler than it would be later on (p.245).

What's the best way to confirm a pregnancy? Are home tests as good as doctors' tests?

Most women who suspect they're pregnant have their suspicions confirmed or dismissed by means of a urine test that measures the level of the hormone human chorionic gonadotropin (HCG), which is produced by the placenta and is present only during pregnancy. A standard urine test given by doctors and clinics is accurate for most women starting about 27 days after conception, or about 2 weeks after a missed period. A newer test, known as the urine tube test, can be accurate as early as the first day after a missed period, or 2 weeks after conception.

Instead of going to a doctor or a clinic, many women prefer to use home pregnancy test kits. These over-the-counter urine test kits are basically the same as the newer tube tests given by doctors and are just as accurate when used properly. With a urine test, only about 3 to 5 percent of positive results are false positives, indicating that a woman is pregnant when she is not. But about 20 percent of all negative results are false negatives, indicating that a woman is not pregnant when she is. Reasons for the false negatives include taking a test too early in the pregnancy, using a urine sample that's contaminated or that's not from the first urination of the day, when HCG is most concentrated, and having an ectopic or other abnormal pregnancy. If a test is negative and you still suspect you're pregnant, see your doctor. He or she may suggest a blood test, which is more sensitive in detecting HCG than urine tests and can establish pregnancy within 9 to 12 days of conception. Given by doctors and clinics, blood tests are more expensive than urine tests and are generally used only when there's doubt or when a very early diagnosis of pregnancy is needed.

Starting about 6 weeks after a missed period, a doctor can detect a pregnancy by performing a pelvic exam. At this stage of a pregnancy, the uterus softens and changes size and shape, and the cervix may become bluish because of increased circulation.

FACT OR FALLACY ?

Couples are most likely to conceive in December

Fact. In our temperate climate a couple trying to have a baby has a greater chance of conceiving in December than in any other month, according to demographers. If the theory is correct, the peak month for U.S. births should be September (9 months later), and it is. There are probably many reasons for this. During the holidays couples have more time to relax and be together, for example. But temperature could also play a role. A study of men in San Antonio found their sperm counts to be significantly lower in summer than winter. The lowest U.S. birth months are April and May, 9 months after the crushing heat of July and August.

How is a baby's birth due date determined?

About 80 percent of women give birth between 38 and 42 weeks after conception; the average term for a pregnancy is 40 weeks. The due date can be calculated roughly—and only roughly—by taking the first day of the expectant mother's last normal period, adding 7 days to it, then counting back 3 months. (It's usually easier to count back than to count forward 9 months.) This method of calculation may be off for women who don't menstruate regularly or who have shorter or longer cycles. Doctors can also closely estimate the stage of pregnancy when they do a pelvic exam after the second month. An ultrasound scan of the fetus (p.261), often taken between the 16th and 18th weeks of pregnancy, allows a doctor to determine the age of the fetus even more accurately. Only 4 percent of women give birth on their predicted due date. A birth is considered premature before 37 weeks, late if the baby is born after 42 weeks.

I'm expecting my first baby. I worry all the time about what could go wrong. How can I tell what's normal and what isn't?

It's natural to worry about possible complications at this time, especially if you're a first-time mother. And if you do have some worrisome symptom, it's always better to have it assessed by your doctor than to ignore it. To lessen your anxieties, keep in touch with your doctor about physical changes and have regular medical checkups (see *Caring for Your Unborn Child,* following pages). Talk to other women who are pregnant or have recently been pregnant, and consider taking pregnancy education and childbirth preparation classes, which are offered by hospitals and clinics and through doctors.

Report symptoms that indicate possible problems to your doctor promptly. These are the main ones to watch out for:

☐ Vaginal bleeding, excessive discharge, or fluid leakage
☐ Lower abdominal cramps
☐ Excessive vomiting
☐ Burning or painful urination
☐ Fever and chills
☐ Sudden weight gain or loss
☐ Dizziness, seeing spots
☐ Little or no fetal movement (after 20 weeks)
☐ Signs of labor (p.263).

CARING FOR YOUR UNBORN CHILD

The 40 or so weeks of pregnancy are divided into three trimesters, in which the mother's body undergoes the extraordinary changes outlined below. No two women experience pregnancy in exactly the same way, and regular medical care throughout this period is critical. A doctor or a nurse-midwife can help the expectant mother anticipate and cope with her body changes, monitor fetal development with one or more of the tests described below, and discuss lifestyle issues that affect both mother and baby (facing page).

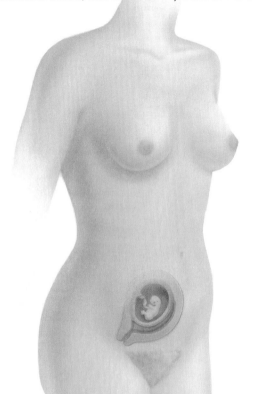

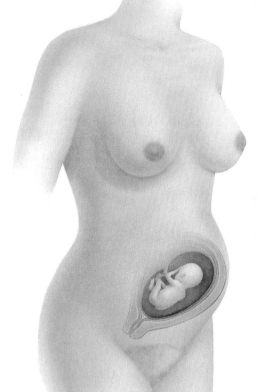

First trimester (0–14 weeks): missed periods or very short, scant bleeding . . . breast enlargement and tenderness (blue veins become visible on breasts and nipples become larger and darker) . . . nausea and vomiting, especially in the morning ("morning sickness"), heartburn, constipation . . . tiredness, lethargy, and increased sleep needs . . . frequent need to urinate . . . moderate weight gain and increase in appetite with food cravings or aversions . . . increased vaginal secretions . . . shifting moods and changes in libido . . . changes in blood pressure that may cause faintness or dizziness, especially when standing up quickly

Second trimester (15–28 weeks): swelling of the uterus . . . water retention (edema) causing ankle swelling . . . detectable movements of the fetus ("quickening") . . . breast enlargement and darkening of nipples . . . nausea and frequent urination diminish . . . return of energy . . . increased rate of weight gain . . . increased heart rate and blood volume . . . hemorrhoids . . . increased sweating and flushing . . . leg cramps, especially when sleeping or lying down, and varicose veins in the legs . . . inflammation and/or bleeding of the gums (pregnancy gingivitis, caused by changing hormone levels) . . . mood swings . . . possible backache from pressure on lower back

PRENATAL SCREENING

A woman should see her doctor as soon as she suspects she is pregnant. At the first visit, the doctor confirms the pregnancy, estimates the due date, performs a general checkup (p.122) and a pelvic examination (p.252) to detect any physical complications, and tests for blood type and Rh factor, anemia, infections, and immunity to rubella (German measles). Checkups are scheduled every month until the 28th week, every 2 weeks until the 36th week, and then weekly until delivery. Extra visits may be necessary if the mother is

over 35, has hypertension or diabetes, or if problems develop. During checkups, one or more of the following screening tests may be performed.

Alpha-fetoprotein (AFP) assay. Alpha-fetoprotein, a substance produced by the fetus, can be detected in the amniotic fluid and the mother's blood. High levels in the second trimester may indicate a brain or spinal defect, fetal death, or multiple pregnancy. An abnormal reading is followed by a second AFP, and if needed,

AMNIOCENTESIS and an ULTRASOUND SCAN. The test is recommended when there is a family history of neural defects.

Amniocentesis. Performed around the 16th week of pregnancy, this test examines fetal cells in the amniotic fluid. Amniocentesis reveals the fetus's sex; chromosomal abnormalities, such as Down's syndrome; certain metabolic disorders, such as Tay-Sachs disease; and problems in neural development, such as spina bifida. Using a local

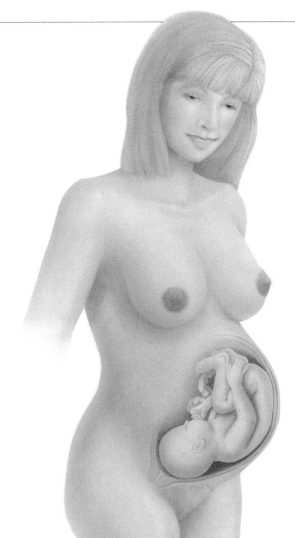

Food. For diet guidelines for pregnant women, see page 42.

Vitamin and mineral supplements. Your doctor may recommend iron, calcium, and folic acid supplements, as well as a multivitamin.

Exercise. Active women can continue to work out, but should reduce the length and intensity of sessions, minimize jarring movements, and avoid exercises done lying on the back after the fourth month. Inactive women should not start a fitness program while pregnant. For more on exercising during pregnancy, see page 105.

Weight gain. The average pregnant woman gains 24 to 30 pounds; the American College of Obstetricians and Gynecologists recommends gains of 25 to 35 pounds. Report a plateau or a sudden large increase in weight to your doctor.

🚫 **Alcohol**. Heavy drinking during pregnancy has been linked to fetal alcohol syndrome (FAS), a group of birth defects including stunted growth, physical deformity, mental retardation, heart abnormalities, and hyperactivity.

🚫 **Drugs.** Check with your doctor before taking any prescription or over-the-counter drug — even aspirin. Avoid any use of illicit drugs.

🚫 **Caffeine.** Some doctors recommend reducing or eliminating caffeine because of its effects on maternal and fetal heart rate and blood pressure.

🚫 **Smoking.** Smoking sends harmful chemicals to the fetus, limits absorption of oxygen and nutrients, and stunts growth. A smoker's baby has a higher risk of brain damage, cerebral palsy, behavioral problems, and sudden infant death syndrome (SIDS).

Third trimester (29 weeks–delivery): increase in many second-trimester symptoms . . . uterus continues to enlarge and stretch marks may appear on abdomen, breasts, thighs . . . rate of weight gain increases . . . breasts become very large and heavy and colostrum can be expressed from the nipples . . . Braxton-Hicks contractions (mild tightening of the uterus that does not signal onset of labor) . . . fatigue and shortness of breath, even with mild exertion . . . "lightening," or turning and dropping of the baby's head into the pelvis as early as the 36th week (this may relieve pressure on breathing and increase pressure on bladder) . . . indigestion, heartburn, and constipation . . . frequent urination and possible urine leakage when sneezing, coughing, or laughing . . . slight rise in body temperature (may cause flushing and sweating) . . . insomnia and increased need for rest

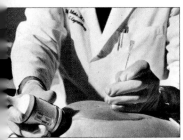

In **amniocentesis** the doctor draws 20–30 ml of amniotic fluid for analysis.

anesthetic and guided by ULTRASOUND SCAN the doctor inserts a needle through the mother's abdomen into the uterus (left) to withdraw fluid. The test increases miscarriage risk by about 0.5 percent.

Chorionic villus sampling (CVS). Performed from the 9th to the 12th week of pregnancy, this test can detect genetic disorders and the sex of the fetus earlier than AMNIOCENTESIS. A catheter inserted through the vagina into the uterus or a needle inserted through the abdomen is used to re-

move a sample of the chorionic villi (small protrusions that anchor the fetus to the placenta); results are available in a week to 10 days. CVS increases miscarriage risk by about 1 percent.

Ultrasound scan. This procedure, described on pages 126–127, may be performed after the 5th week of pregnancy to assess fetal size, position, and viability, determine due date, check the condition of the placenta, detect abnormalities, and diagnose a multiple pregnancy.

How serious is a tubal, or ectopic, pregnancy?

A tubal pregnancy, more properly called an ectopic pregnancy, results when a fertilized egg implants outside the uterus, usually in a fallopian tube. It can happen to any woman, although previous tubal surgery and pelvic infection increase the risk. The early signs of an ectopic pregnancy are similar to those of early pregnancy, notably a missed period, breast tenderness, nausea, and fatigue. An ectopic pregnancy is sometimes diagnosed at this early stage by a blood pregnancy test or an ultrasound scan. More often, the embryo begins to grow and presses on the tube, causing severe abdominal pain and sometimes bleeding. Immediate surgery is needed because a tube rupture can be fatal. In some cases the surgeon is able to remove just the embryo and save the tube, but usually the tube is removed with the embryo inside it. A woman can still conceive as long as at least one tube and ovary remain.

How far into pregnancy is it safe to have sex?

At one time obstetricians routinely advised against having intercourse during the last month of pregnancy. Although not all doctors agree, most now say that it's fine to have intercourse during the entire time the woman is pregnant as long as the pregnancy is normal with no complications. If a woman has a history of miscarriage or is having light bloody discharges or showing other signs of a possible miscarriage, her doctor may recommend abstaining from intercourse during the first few months of pregnancy. If a woman has a history of giving birth prematurely, a doctor may advise her to avoid intercourse during the last month or so. At any point a doctor may advise against sex for a few weeks if the woman develops an infection or experiences pain with intercourse.

During the last month or two, a couple may find it more comfortable to have intercourse on their sides, a position that also limits penetration and the possibility that it may trigger premature labor.

My daughter wants a midwife to deliver her baby. Is this safe?

Yes, if she is using a trained nurse-midwife and there is no sign that she might have a problem with pregnancy or labor. Like obstetricians and family practitioners, midwives care for and assist mothers and their babies during pregnancy, labor, delivery, and the period immediately afterward. When the term *midwife* is used today, it usually refers to certified nurse-midwives (C.N.M.'s)—nurses who have received postgraduate training in midwifery, obstetrics, gynecology, and newborn care. They must meet state requirements and be tested and certified by the American College of Nurse Midwives. There are about 4,000 C.N.M.'s in the United States. A few have private practices but most work for hospitals, independent birthing centers, HMO's, or public health departments. Around 80 percent of the deliveries they oversee are in hospitals, with the rest nearly always in birthing centers. Occasionally, a C.N.M. will agree to deliver a baby in the mother's home if safety standards are met.

Studies show that a woman who has a healthy pregnancy and a normal labor and delivery is as safe with a C.N.M. as with a physician. Nurse-midwives are

BIRTHING CLASSES

Education is important for expectant parents who want to be active participants in their baby's birth—a trend now encouraged by most hospitals and birthing centers. Birthing classes teach the mother how to relax and how to cope with pain during contractions. Her partner learns techniques (massage, timing contractions) designed to help her through labor. Both parents are prepared for choices they may have to face during labor (whether to have surgical instead of vaginal delivery, for example, or whether or not to use painkillers).

Your obstetrician or certified nurse-midwife can recommend a good birthing class in your area. Most are based on the works of one or more of the doctors who pioneered the field of natural childbirth:

☐ Grantly Dick-Read, a British obstetrician and author of *Childbirth Without Fear* (1943), was the first doctor to invite fathers into the delivery room. He believed that education and relaxation exercises could break the fear-tension-pain cycle that made childbirth so difficult for women.

☐ Fernand Lamaze, a French doctor influenced by the Russian behaviorist Pavlov (who conditioned dogs to salivate at the sound of a bell), developed a birthing method in the 1950's that combines education, relaxation techniques, and specific breathing exercises for women to use during the different stages of labor. Lamaze classes also teach the partner to lightly massage the mother's abdomen to relax her.

☐ Robert Bradley, an American doctor, taught fathers in the 1950's and 1960's to coach their partner during labor. His 9-month birth preparation program stresses diet, exercise, and deep breathing.

☐ Frederick Leboyer, another French physician, advocated in the 1970's that a baby be spared some of birth's trauma by keeping the delivery room quiet and dim and by immersing the newborn in a warm bath that simulates the environment of the womb.

GIVING BIRTH

As a woman's pregnancy comes to term, the first sign that labor is imminent may be what's known as the "show," a discharge of slightly bloody mucus from the vagina. (This mucus is the plug that seals the womb during pregnancy.) Another cue may be a gush—or trickle—of water ("breaking of the waters"), which indicates that the membrane holding the amniotic fluid has broken. Or uterine contractions may simply begin without warning. These early pains signal the start of the normal three-part labor process.

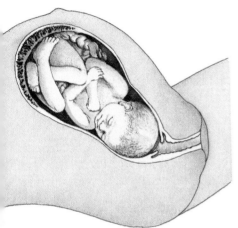

Labor follows "lightening," the baby's descent into the pelvic cavity near the birth canal. (The shift in position relieves pressure on the mother's diaphragm and allows her to breathe more easily.) The opening of the cervix, or neck of the womb, is 1.5–2 cm (0.6–0.8 in.) across.

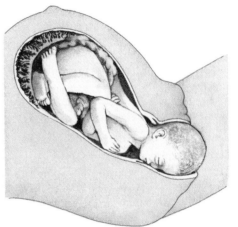

In the first stage of labor contractions stretch the cervix and dilate its opening until it is large enough for the baby to pass through—10 cm (4 in.). For first-time mothers this part of labor averages about 12 hr. Women who have had a child may dilate fully in less than 8 hr.

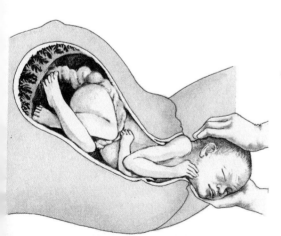

The second stage of labor, which lasts from 30 min. to 1½ hr., is marked by stronger contractions that push the baby through the birth canal. First the head, face down, passes under the pubic bone and out; then the baby turns sideways, allowing the rest of the body to slip out.

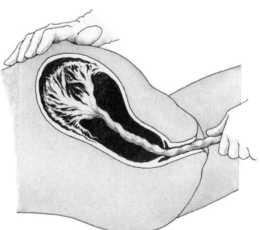

In the third stage of labor contractions expel the placenta, or afterbirth, now separated from the wall of the womb, through the birth canal. This process, which is often assisted by a doctor's gentle kneading of the mother's abdomen, takes only about 10 min.

especially effective in caring for women whose social and economic circumstances put them at high risk of bearing a child with a low birth weight; such women apparently find a midwife's care less intimidating than a doctor's and make fuller use of it. Nurse-midwives stress natural methods of childbirth and are less likely than doctors to recommend medical intervention, such as forceps delivery or cesarean section, procedures that C.N.M.'s can't perform themselves. Nurse-midwives always work in association with a physician, who can be called in if an emergency or other condition requires a doctor's attention. Besides C.N.M.'s, many uncertified (lay) midwives still serve poor rural women, although the practice is illegal in most states.

What kinds of drugs are given during labor? Do they affect the baby?

Drugs can be given to speed up or slow down labor, induce relaxation, and mask pain. When labor doesn't begin when it should or progresses too slowly, a synthetic form of the hormone that normally causes contractions may be given through an intravenous drip or by injection. Conversely, if labor starts prematurely, a doctor may try to stop it with a drug.

During labor a woman may be given any of a variety of drugs that lessen pain and anxiety and block sensation. To help her relax she may be given a tranquilizer, which has minimal effect on the baby. To relieve pain she may receive an analgesic, such as Demerol. Analgesics may make a newborn less responsive and cause respiratory problems, especially in premature infants.

The anesthetic most often used for delivery is an epidural block (see *Anesthesia*, p.145). Because the block can slow fetal heart rate, a fetal monitor is usually used when this type of anesthetic is administered. A cesarean section is usually performed with an epidural or spinal block; it can also be done under general anesthesia, but at the risk of reducing newborn responsiveness and causing respiratory problems. A local anesthetic may be injected around the vagina, with little or no risk to the baby.

Most hospitals routinely administer some drugs during labor and delivery. If you want to try to give birth without drugs or put off their use until the last stages of labor, tell your doctor during a prenatal visit. It's best for both patient and doctor to maintain a flexible attitude about pain medication. Every case is different, and no woman should ever feel guilty about needing relief for her pain.

Why are so many babies delivered by cesarean section? What are the risks?

Nearly 25 percent of American babies are delivered by cesarean section, that is, through a surgical incision in the abdomen. A cesarean is usually performed when a doctor believes the risks to the mother and baby of continued labor and vaginal delivery outweigh the risks of surgery. In some cases a cesarean can be lifesaving—for example, when the placenta detaches too soon and blood loss threatens the baby's life. Some doctors also routinely perform cesareans when there is a moderate risk of complication, as when the baby is in a breech (bottom first) position.

The rate of cesareans has increased fourfold since 1970, and there is concern that the procedure may be overused. Some hospitals have rates as low as 12 to 15 percent; others as high as 35 percent. One reason for the high rate may be doctors' fear of being sued for not having ordered the procedure if a birth has unexpected complications.

Although usually safe, a cesarean is major surgery, entailing a much higher risk than normal birth and requiring a longer hospital stay and recovery. A woman worried about having an unnecessary cesarean should discuss her concerns with her doctor and find out the doctor's rate of cesareans as well as the rate at the hospital where she'll give birth.

I've had one baby by cesarean. Must I have one for my next child?

Not necessarily. Repeat cesareans used to be standard practice because doctors feared that the old cesarean scar would rupture if the baby was delivered normally. Now, however, the American College of Obstetricians and Gynecologists advises doctors and hospitals to attempt vaginal delivery when the mother-to-be meets certain criteria. Her earlier cesarean should have been made with a horizontal incision "below the bikini line" (the type used most often today), as opposed to a higher vertical cut. She should also be carrying only one baby, who has an estimated weight of less than 14 pounds and is not in a breech position. A woman who meets these criteria—and most mothers with previous cesareans do—should try to deliver vaginally under the supervision of a doctor or midwife, who can interrupt labor if a cesarean becomes necessary. Studies show that 50 to 80 percent of such mothers are able to give birth vaginally and that the rates of maternal and infant death are lower than in repeat cesareans. The mothers also have fewer complications.

What is an episiotomy? Why is it done?

An episiotomy is a cut made in the perineum—the tissue between the vagina and anus—to ease delivery. It is usually necessary in forceps and breech deliveries and when the baby has a large head. An episiotomy is also done to speed delivery when the baby is premature or in distress. Some doctors routinely cut the perineum to keep it from tearing, which can be painful and harder to repair and slower to heal than a surgical incision. Other physicians, however, feel routine episiotomy is unnecessary. It's best to discuss this matter with your doctor during a visit before the birth.

After the delivery the episiotomy incision is usually stitched with absorbable sutures and heals without complications.

What are the risks of premature birth?

Although delivering before term presents little risk to the mother, premature birth is the major cause of health problems and death in newborns. A baby is called premature when it is born 37 weeks or less after the first day of the mother's last period. Premature babies weigh less than those carried to term and have a greater risk of jaundice, lung infection, and respiratory distress syndrome, a condition that impairs breathing. The cause of early onset of labor is not always clear, but factors that can play a role include infection, an abnormally shaped uterus, fibroids, early rupture of the amniotic sac, and a placenta that separates early or that is too low in the uterus. Stress and extreme physical exertion may play a role, but not normal exercise. Teenagers and mothers who

smoke or have high blood pressure tend to have premature babies more often than normal, as do women who are carrying twins or who have had a previous premature delivery.

If a woman starts labor early, she is carefully monitored and may be given drugs to try to stop contractions. If the contractions stop before the woman breaks water, the pregnancy can usually continue normally. But if labor is caused by a threatening condition, such as an infection, it is usually allowed to continue.

If my baby is a boy, should I have him circumcised?

Circumcision, the removal of the foreskin of the penis, is performed on some male infants for religious, cultural, or hygienic reasons. The procedure takes a few minutes in newborns and is considered safe when done by a doctor or other experienced person on a healthy infant at least 12 to 24 hours old. It is performed with a topical anesthetic, a local nerve block, or no anesthetic at all. Circumcision of an adolescent or adult—for a persistent problem with genital warts, for example—is a more complex procedure, usually requiring a general anesthetic.

For years circumcision was standard in the United States. But the number declined after many doctors and parents began to question the practice, saying it was unnecessary as long as a boy or man bathed regularly and kept the area under the foreskin clean. Recent studies, however, show that the rate of urinary tract infections among uncircumcised infants is about 10 times higher than among circumcised ones, and a urinary tract infection in a baby during the first 6 months can be serious. Studies

also suggest that uncircumcised men have a higher risk of getting a sexually transmitted disease, which in turn is linked to an increased risk of penile cancer and, in their mates, of cervical cancer.

Today circumcision is a matter of heated discussion, with strong advocates on both sides. The American Academy of Pediatrics advises parents to discuss the potential benefits and risks with their baby's future pediatrician before the baby is born and to base their decision on that discussion, taking into account religious and cultural factors. Aside from regular cleaning with soap and water, no special care is needed for a boy's penis, circumcised or not. Circumcision does not affect later sexual pleasure.

I hear new parents talking about their baby's Apgar score. What is it?

Developed by anesthesiologist Virginia Apgar, the score records an infant's condition just after birth. At 1 and 5 minutes after birth, the medical team checks the baby for five vital signs that spell out Apgar: Appearance (skin color), Pulse, Grimace (irritability reflex), Activity (muscle tone), and Respiration. Each factor is given a rating of 0, 1, or 2 points, which adds up to a total score between 0 and 10. A baby with a score below 4 is in poor condition and needs emergency care. A baby with a score between 4 and 6 is in fair condition but may require some medical attention. A score of 7 or above indicates a well baby, one the parents can touch and hold.

Some parents worry needlessly about their child's Apgar score. It is an indicator only of an infant's condition immediately after birth. It does not predict future health or intelligence.

Why do mothers feel blue after giving birth? How long does it last?

An estimated two-thirds of new mothers develop a case of the blues, usually starting 4 or 5 days after giving birth. After the drama of childbirth, many mothers feel let down, exhausted, and overwhelmed by the responsibility of baby care, especially if left alone at home with an infant. These factors together with sudden hormonal shifts may make the new mothers feel unhappy, irritable, frightened, discouraged, confused, and weepy. With the support and help of family and friends, these mild doldrums usually pass in a few days. Continuing changes in a woman's hormonal balance, however, may lead to a recurrence of symptoms during the first month or so after childbirth.

My friend became not just blue but very depressed after having her baby. Is this common?

About 10 to 15 percent of new mothers develop postpartum depression, lasting from a few weeks to a year or longer. Symptoms include constant fatigue, restlessness, insomnia, loss of appetite or binging, inability to concentrate, and loss of self-esteem, often characterized by a feeling of being unable to care for the new baby. About 1 or 2 in 1,000 women actually become psychotic (p. 175) after childbirth. They may lose their sense of reality and experience delusions, hallucinations, and rapid mood changes.

Both postpartum depression and psychosis are probably caused by underlying factors that are aggravated or brought to the surface by the birth. Depression is more likely to develop in a

FEEDING YOUR BABY: BREAST VERSUS BOTTLE

For the first 4 to 6 months of life, most babies' nutritional needs can be met with either breast milk or bottled formula. Physicians recommend breast milk because it contains the ideal balance of nutrients for a human infant plus antibodies to protect against infections, both in infancy and later; babies are also less likely to be allergic to their mothers' milk. On the other hand, formula feeding is convenient, especially for working mothers, and it allows careful regulation of the baby's nutritional intake.

About 96 percent of women can breast-feed successfully; for those who can't or prefer not to, formula provides a safe, healthy alternative. With either method, feedings should be a time of loving interaction between mother and child. Make eye contact, smile, and talk to your baby.

Breast-feeding should start right after birth so that your baby gets the nutritional and immunological benefits of colostrum, the thick, yellowish fluid that the breasts produce before milk begins to flow. Frequent nursing in the first few days encourages a consistent, plentiful supply of milk, and nursing on demand in the first few weeks maintains it. Other ways to make breast-feeding work smoothly:

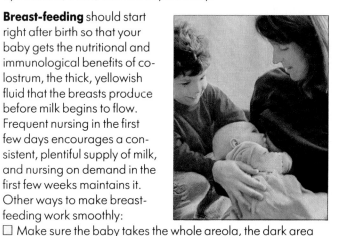

☐ Make sure the baby takes the whole areola, the dark area around the nipple. This stimulates milk flow and prevents biting of the nipple, which can cause soreness.
☐ Draw off extra milk with a breast pump to relieve engorgement (painful overfull breasts). Store breast milk in the refrigerator for bottle-feeding when you are not available. (It's a good idea to get a breast-fed baby used to a daily bottle of milk or formula.)
☐ For the nutritional needs of nursing mothers, see page 42. Check with your doctor about medications you can safely use.

Formula feeding is easy; you simply measure and mix a base with water. A few precautions ensure problem-free feedings:
☐ Make sure all equipment is scrupulously clean. Follow directions on formula cans or boxes carefully. Prepare several bottles of formula at a time, store them in a refrigerator, and then warm a bottle in a pan of hot water (not in a microwave) as needed.
☐ Don't overfeed the baby, and don't supplement formula with vitamins (it already has a good balance of vitamins and too much vitamin A or D can be toxic to an infant).
☐ Don't switch an infant to straight cow's milk before he or she is 6 months old.

woman who has a family history of mental disorder, whose relationship with her husband is strained, or who gets little or no support from family and friends. Having financial worries and being a first-time or single mother may also contribute to a new mother's depression. Postpartum depression or psychosis should be brought to the attention of a doctor as soon as possible. For more on depression and its treatment, see pages 169–174.

What's the best way to get back in shape after having a baby?

If you exercised regularly before and during pregnancy and if your doctor approves, you can plan a gradual return to your previous type and level of activity about 3 months after a normal vaginal delivery; wait 3 to 6 weeks longer after a cesarean. If you were sedentary before becoming pregnant, don't overdo it now.

Walking and swimming are considered safe postpartum exercises for most women. Because pregnancy may have weakened your back, you'll benefit from the back stretching and strengthening exercises described on pages 218–219. There are also low-impact aerobics routines designed for new mothers; you can practice them at home with a videotape or by enrolling in an exercise class (p.77).

At first, all new mothers should avoid jarring exercises such as jogging and high-impact aerobics; such activities can damage joints softened for childbirth and cause pain if there are incisions or tears around the vagina. Whatever exercise you decide to take up, be sure to consult your doctor before you start.

Don't try to cut calories in the postpartum period. If you eat sensibly the extra weight (20–30 pounds) that you gained during pregnancy will usually come off by itself within 2 months without dieting. It's important for new mothers, particularly if they are breast-feeding, to keep up their caloric intake and energy levels during the baby's first months.

Since giving birth, I've been bombarded with child-care advice. Whom should I listen to, and how do I get over feeling incompetent?

It's not uncommon for first-time parents to be overwhelmed by conflicting advice from family, friends, doctors, and books. Feeling unprepared for parenthood, many new mothers and fathers become dependent on "old hands" or books and magazines for expertise. But much so-called baby and child-care wisdom is just folklore, fad, hearsay, or complete myth. The best advice is to experiment judiciously and use common sense in evaluating advice from family, friends, and books. Every baby is unique, and getting to know yours is a process that takes time. Concentrate on finding out what works best for you and your baby.

Good parenting isn't as instinctive as many would like to believe. Getting a baby to feed comfortably at the breast, for example, often takes a lot of frustrating trial and error for both mother and baby. Skills such as changing a diaper and bringing up a burp must be learned. Ask questions of people you trust— your pediatrician, your parents, or other parents—and consult a child-care book that seems reasonable to you. All parents make mistakes at first, but you'll gain confidence with experience. And you will come to see that there are many "right" ways to take care of a baby.

When is it all right to start having sex again after having a baby?

The standard advice used to be to refrain from intercourse for 6 weeks after delivery, in order to give vaginal muscles, cuts, and tears time to heal and to reduce the risk of infection. Many doctors now tell parents to resume sex whenever they feel physically and emotionally ready, which for some couples is as early as 4 weeks after childbirth.

Some women, however, may feel soreness and discomfort for much longer than that (in one study 40 percent of women said intercourse was sometimes painful a year after delivery). The area around an episiotomy is particularly sensitive.

Hormonal changes triggered by childbirth and lasting about 6 weeks sometimes cause vaginal dryness and vaginitis (p.249)— conditions that can make intercourse uncomfortable for a woman. The same hormonal changes may also lower libido. It's not surprising that studies by the renowned sex researchers Masters and Johnson found that about half of new mothers had little or no interest in sex 3 months after giving birth.

A husband's sexual feelings also may change when he first perceives his wife as a mother as well as a sex partner. Some couples with newborns are simply too tired, busy, and distracted for frequent, passionate lovemaking. All these reactions to parenthood don't mean the end of sex. Having a child often strengthens a couple's bond, and some new parents report feeling more playful and intimate than before. Experiencing new emotions is normal for new parents, so it's important for both to communicate their needs and desires to each other.

CARING FOR A HANDICAPPED INFANT

When parents first learn that their baby has been born with a defect, they typically experience a mix of contradictory feelings—love and protectiveness (we will go to any length to make our child right), anger (how could this happen to us?), guilt (what did we do wrong?), and fear (will the baby live?). After months of happy expectation, learning to accept an infant with serious problems is not easy. Here are some guidelines for smoothing the process.

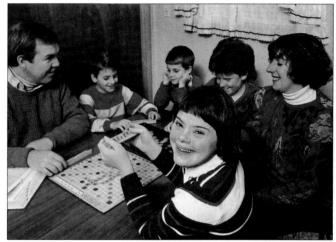

☐ Talk out your feelings about your handicapped child with each other and with a counselor or therapist.

☐ Accept your child and be honest with friends about the problems. When family and friends see how you love the baby (and you will), they too will be able to accept him.

☐ Join a parents' group; you'll find support as well as information about services and treatment programs that may benefit your child. The March of Dimes Birth Defects Foundation, among others, sponsors such groups in many areas (see Appendix).

☐ Encourage your youngster in training and therapy pro-grams, even if they are difficult or painful for the child.

☐ If you have other children, don't expect too much from them just because they aren't handicapped. Be sensitive to *their* needs; they may feel guilty about being normal or resent the attention given to the handicapped sibling.

However overwhelmed and isolated they may feel at first, the new parents of a baby with a birth defect should never feel that they are alone. One out of every 14 babies born in the United States—some 250,000 infants a year—has a birth defect. Fortunately, the prospects for many of these infants and their parents have improved considerably in recent years.

The medical outlook. Advances in neonatal care enable many endangered babies not only to survive but to develop normally. Surgeons can now correct some structural defects that were once untreatable. High-tech artificial limbs give mobility and dexterity to children without arms or legs. Special diets can correct chemical imbalances like PKU (phenylketonuria), an inherited enzyme disorder that can cause severe retardation. Early medical intervention and therapy make it possible for many more youngsters than ever before to overcome handicaps and live full lives. And research into the causes and prevention of birth defects continues, offering hope for the future.

The social outlook. Public sympathy for the problems of the handicapped has grown in recent decades. By federal law, U.S. public schools must provide education that meets the needs of *all* children. "Mainstreaming" of handicapped children in many public school systems has made it easier for normal children to accept and interact with their handicapped peers. Cities are beginning to comply with federal laws requiring access by the handicapped to transportation, walkways, and all public and many private buildings. The group home movement offers the possibility of supervised residential living for many handicapped youngsters when they become adults.

Has the cause of sudden infant death syndrome (SIDS) been found?

SIDS (also known as crib death) is the unexpected death of an apparently healthy baby, usually during sleep. It is the major killer of infants between ages 2 weeks and a year, and its causes are still not known. Abnormal breathing and heart rate are thought to play a role in most SIDS cases. Sudden major respiratory infections and congenital metabolic problems are among the possible causes that are now being investigated.

Risk factors associated with SIDS include prematurity, low birth weight, cold weather, low socioeconomic status, death of a sibling from SIDS, and a mother who is young or anemic or who smokes or uses drugs. Babies who have suffered apnea (interrupted breathing) once and been resuscitated are also at high risk for SIDS.

Prevention so far rests in good prenatal and postnatal care, avoidance of smoking and drug-taking during pregnancy and breast-feeding, and careful monitoring of the baby during and after any illness. For children who've had an episode of apnea or have heart-lung problems, doctors may recommend a home alarm system that sounds when a baby stops breathing. Many hospitals have medical teams that train parents to use the alarm and that will respond to an emergency call. The alarm, however, is a mixed blessing: it may allay anxiety, but it doesn't seem to lower the risk of death, and false alarms occur frequently.

The family response to an infant's sudden death is usually intense grief; parents often feel guilty while siblings, fearing they will die the same way, may have nightmares or go through periods of bed-wetting. Counseling by a family physician, pediatrician, social worker, family therapist, or clergy member may help deal with the misplaced blame and loss of confidence many parents and siblings experience. Joining a support group of other families who have had babies with SIDS may also help.

When do babies finally start sleeping through the night?

Every child is different. Most infants sleep through the night by 3 months, but some may waken (for a feeding or just to cry and fuss) for a year or longer. Following are a few things parents can do to help establish all-night sleep habits:

□ Never wake a sleeping baby. Infants set their own sleep-wake schedules; interfering tends to make the pattern erratic. If a baby wakes up for a feeding every 2 to 4 hours, parents may be tempted to rouse the child to suit their own needs, but this is not a good idea. Waking an infant interrupts—and prolongs—a natural progression toward sleeping through the night.

□ Put a baby to bed full and dry. Make sure the infant gets enough milk at the late-evening feeding and has a dry diaper.

□ Make nighttime feedings low key. Keep lights dim and nurse without a lot of cooing, talking, and eye contact. Change the baby's diaper if necessary.

□ Provide daytime stimulation. In contrast to night feedings, make nursing during the day an opportunity for interaction—eye contact, talking, singing, cooing, and as the baby grows, movement and play.

□ Soothe, but don't pamper, a fussy baby. A baby who awakens not to feed but to cry and fuss may just need a minute of comforting. In many cases a baby will stop crying after a few minutes; if not, look for signs of sickness or discomfort. Rub the baby's back, and make sure the baby is covered, doesn't feel feverish, and is lying comfortably. Try to avoid picking the infant up.

□ When the baby is between 9 and 12 months, try breaking the night feeding habit by letting the baby cry until he exhausts himself (the crying usually lasts only 10 to 20 minutes). Some babies will sleep through the next night, but others may wake up crying 2 or 3 nights more.

What are the signs of teething, and how do I make my baby more comfortable?

The period when the first set of teeth erupts (usually at 6 to 8 months of age) is a painful time for many babies. A teething child may fuss, cry, cling, pull at an ear, rub a cheek, have trouble sleeping, or experience a combination of such symptoms. Most teething infants drool and chew on anything they can get their hands on for months before the first teeth actually emerge. Signs that a tooth is about to come in—red, swollen gums or a hard lump or ridge felt under the gum—vary widely among babies; in some infants teeth simply appear with no fuss or warning.

For relief you can give a baby something firm to bite, such as a plastic or rubber teething ring. (Biting on a hard surface creates a counterpressure on the gum, which temporarily stops the pain.) Teething rings that you keep in the refrigerator add the numbing effect of cold. Cold food (a small frozen bagel, for example) can also be soothing, but should be given only to a baby who is sitting up (to prevent choking). A doctor may suggest a

WHY A BABY CRIES

Babies sometimes cry for no obvious reason, but often it is because they are hungry, lonely, uncomfortable, or in pain. Although the crying usually stops when you correct the problem, figuring out what that is takes time and patience. (Often the only way to find the cause of a crying jag is to discover what stops it.) Remember, too, that a jumpy or overtired parent can further aggravate a crying baby.

Cause	How you can tell	Remedy
Habit	Routine nighttime crying that stops when you enter room.	Wait before going in; baby may fall asleep. Hold baby for a few minutes; sing a lullaby. You can take baby to bed with you, but this may start a difficult-to-break habit.
Hunger	Long time since feeding, or small last feeding. Rhythmic brief cries that intensify.	Offer food or increase regular amount.
Discomfort	Diaper rash, eczema, wet or soiled diaper, cold fingers and toes.	Treat condition or remove source of discomfort. Cover baby.
Colic	Restless; draws up legs. Severe crying spells that do not respond to comforting. May pass gas. Occurs when baby is between ages 2 weeks and 3 months.	Cuddle, carry, or rock baby. Put baby on his abdomen on your lap, over your arm, or on a warm hot-water bottle. With bottle-fed baby, make sure nipple hole is not too small.
Loneliness or boredom	Cries when alone; stops when you talk to him or pick him up.	Carry or keep baby with you. Talk to him for a while or offer him a toy. Prop him up so that he can see you and other family members.
Tiredness	A distinctive moaning cry. Irritable. Red or swollen eyelids. Has missed a nap.	Try to calm baby and get him to go to sleep.
Thirst	Overheated, flushed, or sweating. Hot room or weather.	Give baby a bottle of water. Don't let baby get overheated.
Teething	Fretful. Has trouble sleeping. Increased crying and salivating. Begins about age 6 months.	Give baby something to chew (p.269).
Urinating	A sudden shriek.	Change diaper.
Illness	Poor appetite. Fever. Signs of a cold. Diarrhea. Baby pulls at ear; vomits. Pain is suggested if crying is severe, won't stop when you pick baby up, or is accompanied by pale skin or drawing up of legs.	To determine the best course of action, see *Identifying Childhood Illnesses*, pp.274–275.

mild analgesic such as acetaminophen or a pain-relieving cream or gel to rub on the gums.

As difficult as teething can be, don't assume that it is behind all of a baby's unusual symptoms. If your child runs a high fever, suffers a prolonged loss of appetite, or has diarrhea for more than 24 hours, check with your doctor.

What are the effects on a child of care by someone other than parents?

This is an increasingly important question: 65 percent of mothers with children under age 18 in the United States work outside the home and most depend on

some form of child care. (And 70 percent of single parents work.) A number of studies have shown that toddlers cared for outside the home in well-managed day-care programs are more independent, better able to make friends, and possibly more intellectually competent than other children. When they enter school, they are better adjusted, more persistent in their work, and more likely to be leaders. While they may form attachments to outside care givers, they seem to maintain strong bonds with their parents.

Clearly, young children can thrive in good child-care programs. The research on infants (under a year old) is more controversial, however. The studies suggest that babies who receive more than 20 hours a week of nonmaternal care suffer emotionally as a result and display behavioral problems later. Mothers may be wise to work part-time for the baby's first year if it's financially possible to do so.

At what age should a child be toilet trained? What's a good strategy?

There is no set age. The most important rule is not to rush the child (many perfectly normal youngsters are not ready for toilet training until age 3). Children under a year have no bladder or bowel control. Between 18 and 24 months of age, a child usually starts showing signs that he may be ready for training: he can follow simple verbal instructions, can handle the basics of dressing and undressing himself, remains dry and unsoiled for at least 2 hours at a time during the day, and signals through expression, posture, or words that he's about to urinate or defecate.

Because using a toilet involves many skills, concepts, and emotions, it helps to break the process down into steps. Start by placing the fully clothed child on a potty chair or seat and explaining its purpose. Parents and older siblings can tell a child when they are "going potty" and have the child watch (the idea that this is usually done in private can be instilled later). Also watch for

FINDING GOOD CHILD CARE

For parents of infants, toddlers, and preschool children, finding affordable, high-quality child care is a challenge. Child-care facilities are not regulated by federal law, and state guidelines vary. Check with family and friends, your physician, your church or synagogue, and the local elementary school for possibilities. Give yourselves several months to find the right arrangement. And before committing to one, make sure that you and the care givers are in general agreement on basic values and such particulars as feeding, hygiene, discipline, and activities. Start any arrangement with a trial period.

There are three basic child-care options available to you: care in your home, care in another person's home, or group care in a center. Each has its advantages and disadvantages.

☐ In-home care can offer the consistency that's important for infants and very young children. In his home environment, your baby can enjoy the complete attention of the care giver, with whom a close relationship often develops. However, in-home care can be costly. And changing an in-home care giver, for whatever reason, will be difficult for the child to accept.

☐ Care in another person's home (often called family day care) is usually less expensive than in-home care but subjects your child to another family's standards. In some states such care givers are licensed; ask to see the license. Check references and ask questions. Make sure that the care giver doesn't take in too many children (more than 6 preschool children, fewer toddlers); that your standards for activities and discipline are close; and that conditions in the house are safe and sanitary. Visit often before making a commitment. The care giver should be loving, warm, and patient; the atmosphere relaxed; and the other children cheerful and busy.

☐ Group care in a center offers the stimulation of other children, games, and play facilities in an organized program for toddlers and preschoolers (many do not accept infants). Features to look for in a child-care center include a state license (for health and safety standards), a low ratio of children to staff, a head teacher with a degree in early childhood education, a loving atmosphere, and some form of parental involvement in the institution (a parent's seat on the board, for example, or evening parenting classes).

After finding a good child-care arrangement, remember that you'll also need a backup sitter for occasions when your child (or in-home care giver) is sick or when other contingencies arise.

As tough as it may be for parents to turn their children over to someone else for daily care, the parents' attitude has a lot to do with how well the arrangement works. If you approach sharing child care with outsiders positively, your child is likely to react positively as well. Let your child know that while parenthood is important to you, other things, such as holding a job, are too.

signs that a child is urinating or defecating (a grunt or a distracted look, for example), and remark on what is happening.

The next step is to encourage the child to tell someone when he has to use the toilet. Many children first speak up after the fact; this is progress and should be praised, while you also gently remind the child to give notice sooner next time. It often helps to sit the child on the potty for a few minutes at a regular time each day (don't leave him unattended); a child who protests may not be ready. Never scold a child who asks to use the toilet and then doesn't go, or who goes immediately after being taken off; this is common.

Children can be taught proper hygiene—wiping, flushing, washing hands—at the same time. While you want children to regard urine and feces as normal and natural, you also want them to know that such wastes are not to be played with.

With some toilet-training success, a child can start wearing training pants instead of diapers, although there will still be accidents. Most children learn bowel control before bladder control; it may take a year or more for a child to stay dry at night. If daytime soiling or wetting persists after age 5, discuss the matter with the child's doctor.

My son wets the bed. How can I help him stop?

Bed-wetting (enuresis) is common in children, seemingly more so in boys and in children whose parents also wet the bed as youngsters. Nearly 20 percent of 5-year-olds and more than 10 percent of 6-year-olds have wet nights occasionally. Almost all children outgrow the problem by adolescence. Six-year-olds who wet the bed may just have a

slower-than-average rate of development, possibly caused by a deep sleep pattern, small bladder capacity, or combination of the two. If wetting continues much longer, tell the child's doctor, who will either make an appointment or refer you to a urologist. It may be that your child isn't producing enough of the hormone that regulates urine production. If that's the case, the doctor may prescribe a synthetic form of the hormone, desmopressin acetate.

Psychological factors should also be considered, especially if a previously dry child suddenly starts wetting. Bed-wetting can be an expression of anger, confusion, anxiety, hostility, or a cry for attention; when the underlying issues are addressed, the problem often clears up. The sudden onset of bed-wetting could also indicate an allergy, a bladder infection, or even sexual abuse.

Many children, however, wet the bed for no apparent reason. Parents should treat these episodes matter-of-factly, realizing that the child probably feels worse than (and wants the problem to go away as much as) they do; after all, bed-wetting may keep the child from spending the night with friends, going to camp and otherwise feeling grown up. Restricting evening fluid intake and having the child make a late-night trip to the bathroom may help. Humiliating him or making him clean up the mess does more harm than good.

Tonsillitis keeps my daughter out of nursery school a lot. Should her tonsils be removed?

Tonsillectomy—surgical removal of the tonsils—used to be recommended routinely as the cure for childhood tonsillitis (tonsil infections). Now the procedure is performed only as a last resort.

Tonsils consist of infection-fighting lymph nodes. Along with the adenoids above them, tonsils normally protect young children from respiratory tract and lung infections. (Tonsils reach their maximum size at about age 7, and then begin to shrink.) This function makes doctors reluctant to remove even infected tonsils unless tonsillitis attacks are frequent and quite severe or an abscess develops.

Tonsillectomy is a relatively simple operation, usually performed under general anesthesia in a hospital, where any complications can be treated more easily (complications are rare but can be serious). After the surgery the child rests, avoids food any more solid than ice cream for a few days, and is given analgesics (such as acetaminophen) as needed for pain relief.

Adenoids are often removed at the same time as the tonsils. In most youngsters adenoids begin to shrink at about age 5 and disappear by puberty. In some cases, however, they enlarge and obstruct the flow of secretions from the nose and middle ear, causing recurring respiratory and ear infections and even deafness.

Can kids be protected from head lice?

Yes; good grooming and avoiding contact with lice-infested children is the best prevention. The head louse (*Pediculus humanus capitis*) is a flat wingless insect about ⅛-inch wide that lives by sucking blood from scalps. The resulting itchy red spots can become inflamed and infected. Although children are most at risk, anyone can become infested by coming into contact with the insects themselves or with the small pale eggs (nits) that the females lay in the hair close to the scalp.

Lice are easily treated with over-the-counter lotions or shampoos containing nontoxic pyrethrins or piperonyl butoxide. Running a fine-tooth comb through the hair removes dead lice and nits. To keep an infestation from recurring, wash combs and brushes in very hot water or soak them in rubbing alcohol for 5 to 10 minutes to kill live eggs. Wash clothing and linen in hot soapy water and dry in the dryer for at least 20 minutes. Clothes that are dry-cleaned should be kept sealed in plastic for 2 weeks to ensure that the nits are dead. Upholstery, carpets, curtains, mattresses, and plush toys should be vacuumed thoroughly and the vacuum bag thrown away immediately. You may also need to wash and vacuum your car's interior.

What is scoliosis and how is it treated?

Scoliosis is an S-shaped curvature of the spine that affects about 2 to 3 percent of children, boys and girls equally. It usually begins in childhood and becomes more pronounced during adolescent growth. In its early stages, scoliosis causes no pain and may be barely noticeable. Left untreated, an advanced case may result in deformity, back pain, disc deterioration, and breathing difficulties in adulthood.

Scoliosis is often diagnosed during a routine checkup or school screening (usually done in the fifth, sixth, or seventh grade). Parents should be alert to such signs as ill-fitting clothes, uneven hemlines or trouser legs, one hip or shoulder (usually the right) higher than the other, a shoulder blade that sticks out, or one arm that hangs further down or out from the body. If you suspect your child might have scoliosis, see a doctor.

FACT OR FALLACY ?

An only child inevitably grows up selfish, dependent, and maladjusted

Fallacy. This stereotype wasn't borne out by child development experts who reviewed 141 studies comparing only children and children who have siblings. The researchers found no significant differences between the two groups in maturity, self-control, flexibility, generosity, leadership, and happiness. Only children, however, did rate higher in self-esteem and motivation to achieve. Credit for these qualities goes to parents who give their only child lots of encouragement and attention. A later study suggests that first-born children and both children from two-child families reap the same benefits—good news for youngsters in today's smaller families.

To correct a slight curve in the spine, the doctor may prescribe a regimen of exercises to strengthen the abdominal muscles. In such cases, a child's progress is monitored by frequent examinations and X-rays. More severe cases may require wearing a brace 24 hours a day (except when bathing or exercising) to keep the curve from worsening during adolescent growth. In rare cases, a child must wear a body cast for 3 to 6 months or be placed in traction for 7 to 10 days before undergoing spinal-fusion surgery.

My child is always in motion—being around him for 5 minutes exhausts me. Could he be hyperactive?

It's possible; the best way to find out is to make an appointment with the child's doctor. Sometimes normal children who are merely overactive or just more energetic than an adult feels up to coping with are misclassified as hyperactive by parents and other observers. True hyperactivity, which is medically known as attention deficit hyperactivity disorder (ADHD), is characterized by frequent bouts of excessive, inappropriate activity that cannot easily be calmed. In addition to having a short attention span (or attention deficit), children with ADHD tend to be restless and impulsive. They may throw tantrums and be emotionally unstable, disruptive, and difficult to discipline. Their memory and muscle coordination may be poor.

Hyperactivity is a complex condition with a number of possible causes, including brain and central nervous system problems due to birth trauma, food allergies, vitamin deficiencies, lead poisoning, or exposure to radiation. Symptoms usually appear by age 5, although ADHD may go undiagnosed until the child starts having difficulties at school, usually in the form of both poor grades and discipline problems. Some children outgrow the disorder, but many continue to exhibit symptoms through adolescence into early adulthood.

The treatment for ADHD usually involves a combination of behavior-modification therapy, which helps a child learn how to concentrate and act less impulsively, and drug therapy. The drugs used are central nervous system stimulants, which para-

Continued on page 276

IDENTIFYING CHILDHOOD ILLNESSES

If you can answer yes to any of the five questions in this box, CALL DOCTOR IMMEDIATELY. If you can answer no to all of them, pick the most appropriate of the major symptom charts on these pages, then read down the list of questions on the left side of the chart until you find the set of symptoms that most closely resembles those of your child. You'll find possible causes and treatments in the corresponding box on the right. If you don't find a satisfactory answer, call your doctor.

Is child not fully conscious or unnaturally drowsy?

Has child's color become very pale and stayed that way?

Is there blueness around child's face or lips?

Does child have serious difficulty in breathing?

Is there a rash that looks like bleeding under the skin and that does not turn pale when you press firmly?

RUNNY NOSE AND FEVER

If a fever is over 105° F rectally, accompanied by signs of heatstroke or other serious illness, or occurs in a child under 2 months old, CALL DOCTOR IMMEDIATELY. Call a doctor as soon as practical for a fever over 102° F, a low-grade fever lasting more than 3 days, or if child is 2 to 6 months old. When treating a fever, give the child acetaminophen and cool liquids, such as diluted fruit juice.

Any of these symptoms: not fully alert, stiff neck, extremely pale, a rash that looks like bleeding under the skin and does not go pale when you press firmly?	Possible major illness (septicemia, meningitis). CALL DOCTOR IMMEDIATELY.
Rash of flat, irregularly shaped pink spots, merging together? Eyes sore? Cough?	Possibly measles. Treat fever. Consult doctor.
Rash of tiny pink spots on face, trunk, and limbs? Enlarged lymph nodes behind ears? Not very ill?	Possibly rubella (German measles). Treat fever. Consult doctor. Keep child away from pregnant women.
Rash of blisters in clusters?	Possibly chicken pox. Treat fever; use calamine lotion on skin. Consult doctor.
Any swelling under the jaw?	Possibly mumps. Treat fever. Consult doctor.
Aching limbs? Headache? No rash?	Possibly flu. Treat fever. Consult doctor.
Any ear pain?	Possibly ear infection. Treat fever. Consult doctor.
Sore throat? Tonsils very red with tiny yellow-white patches?	Possibly tonsillitis. Treat fever. Consult doctor.
Sore throat? Sneezing? Nasal congestion?	Possibly common cold. Treat fever.

RASH FOR MORE THAN A WEEK

Rash in diaper area of a child in diapers?	Probably diaper rash. Apply water-repellant cream. Change diapers often or leave off. Don't use plastic pants.
Rash in or around mouth of child who is out of diapers? (Or diaper-area rash won't go away despite treatment?)	Possibly thrush. Make appointment with doctor.
Rash located mostly around mouth and chin, behind ears, or on elbows, backs of knees, or neck? Itchy, dry, and scaly? Or oozing pimples?	Possibly eczema. Make appointment with doctor.
Itchy blisters with yellow, crusty scabs?	Possibly impetigo. Make appointment with doctor for same or next day. Use separate washcloth and towel for child.
Very itchy raised red lines between fingers, in elbow or knee creases, on arms, legs, or trunk, but not on head?	Possibly scabies. Make appointment with doctor.

ABDOMINAL PAIN AND/OR DIARRHEA

Any of these symptoms: listlessness, sunken eyes, dry mouth, infrequent urination, dark urine, not fully alert?	Possible major illness (meningitis, gastroenteritis with dehydration). CALL DOCTOR IMMEDIATELY.
Pain persists or becomes worse? Possibly a fever?	Possibly appendicitis. CALL DOCTOR IMMEDIATELY.
Sore throat, aching muscles, or headache? Fever?	Possibly flu. Treat fever. Consult doctor.
Appetite loss, nausea, vomiting, or cramps?	Possibly gastroenteritis. Give fluids, but not milk. CALL DOCTOR IMMEDIATELY if condition persists or worsens.
Severe crying? Passes gas? Age under 3 months?	Possibly colic. Treat as described on p.270. Consult doctor.
Similar pain occurred three or more times in last year?	Recurrent abdominal pain. May be stress-related. Make appointment with doctor.

ABNORMAL BREATHING

Very rapid breathing with high temperature or chest pain?	Possibly pneumonia. CALL DOCTOR IMMEDIATELY.
Severe paroxysms of coughing, which may cause vomiting or going blue in the face?	Possibly whooping cough. CALL DOCTOR IMMEDIATELY.
Difficulty breathing and swallowing? Wheezing? Muffled voice? Possibly drooling? Turning blue?	Possibly epiglottitis (an infection of flap protecting larynx). CALL DOCTOR IMMEDIATELY.
Hoarseness? Noisy breathing or wheezing with ringing or barking cough? Does not act very sick?	Possibly croup. Keep child in a steam-filled room. Call doctor if steam brings no relief.
Noisy, musical-sounding breathing that is rapid or accompanied by cough? Has child had this before?	Possibly asthma. Use child's regular asthma medicine. CALL DOCTOR IMMEDIATELY unless the wheezing is very mild.
Noisy breathing with no other symptoms?	Possibly bronchitis or asthma. Consult doctor, or CALL IMMEDIATELY if symptoms are severe or if child is less than 2 years old.

JERKY MOVEMENT OF LIMBS

If convulsions last longer than 5 min. or if convulsions recur, CALL DOCTOR IMMEDIATELY. During a seizure, do not restrain the child or put anything in the mouth. Afterward, put the child in the recovery position (p.425), that is, on his or her stomach with the head to the side.

Unconscious or not fully alert afterward? No fever?	Possibly epileptic seizure. CALL DOCTOR IMMEDIATELY. If child has history of epilepsy, follow doctor's earlier advice.
Not fully alert? Fever, possibly headache?	Possible major illness (meningitis or encephalitis). CALL DOCTOR IMMEDIATELY.
Fever? Possibly briefly unconscious?	Possibly febrile convulsion related to infectious disease. Sponge body with lukewarm water; give acetaminophen. If first attack, CALL DOCTOR IMMEDIATELY. If child has a history of febrile convulsions, follow doctor's earlier advice.
Abdominal pain, diarrhea, or vomiting?	Possibly gastroenteritis. Give fluids, but not milk. If there is listlessness, sunken eyes, or very dry mouth, or if condition persists or worsens, CALL DOCTOR IMMEDIATELY.
Severe crying? Passes gas? Age under 3 months?	Possibly colic. Treat as described on p.270. Consult doctor.
Just one brief convulsive bout?	Call doctor and make appointment.

doxically have a calming effect on hyperactive children. Although the drugs do have side effects, such as wakefulness at night and loss of appetite, these effects are reversible and rarely serious.

Also important in the treatment of hyperactivity are proper classroom placement and remedial instruction to help the child cope with his learning difficulties, as well as some kind of physical education or sports program to help him develop poise and coordination. Children with ADHD do best in a stable, structured home environment. Although parents should discipline unruly behavior by a child, they should avoid resorting to physical or verbal abuse no matter how exasperating the child becomes.

We are about to have a second child. How can we prepare our daughter for the new baby?

To minimize feelings of shock, confusion, and abandonment, it's important to prepare young children in advance for the arrival of a sibling (perhaps when the signs of your pregnancy first become visible). Talk about the role of an older sister or brother and, depending on her age and temperament, let your youngster help you get ready for the baby. Some children like having their own baby doll to take care of before the birth. (It will help you talk about the new baby, too.)

Also avoid making any major changes in your child's life in the weeks just before or just after the new baby's birth. Don't start toilet training her, for example, or move her from a crib to a bed just when you expect the new baby. Her world will become topsy-turvy enough with a new sibling diverting your attention. If you plan to have your daughter stay with a relative or friend

while you are in the hospital giving birth, it may help to have a dry run a few weeks before the event, so that she won't associate the new baby with fear and separation from her parents.

Once the new baby is born, concentrate on reassuring your daughter that both her parents love her as much as ever:
☐ Talk to her by phone soon after the birth, and allow her to see you and her new sibling as soon as possible.
☐ Give her frequent hugs, smiles, and other physical signs of affection.
☐ Involve her in (or allow her to watch) diapering, nursing, and bathing the baby.
☐ Encourage family and friends to pay attention to all the children, not just the new baby, and to congratulate the big sister on her new status.
☐ Remember that the older child needs tolerance and understanding as she comes to terms with a big change in her life. You may notice regression in toilet training, for example, or babyish behavior in other areas for a while. If you are supportive, this phase will probably pass quickly.

How can I talk to my children about sexual abuse without really frightening them?

Talking about sexual abuse should be part of your children's general sex education. Including this difficult issue in an overall discussion of healthy sexuality helps make the topic less scary.

Children under 3 can be taught the names of body parts, including the genitals. Between ages 3 and 5, a child can be told that the genitals are private and shouldn't be touched by another person. State this in a calm, nonthreatening way, and remind the child of it every so often.

Children ages 5 to 8 should be taught safety rules for outside the home (don't talk to, accept presents from, or get in a car with a stranger). They should also learn the differences between a "good touch" and a "bad touch." Encourage your children to talk to you about experiences they find bewildering or frightening.

You can have more specific discussions about what constitutes sexual abuse with children in their preteen years. Teenagers should be also be warned about date rape (p. 243), sexually transmitted diseases (p. 244), and unplanned pregnancy.

The main message to get across to children of all ages is that they can and should say "no" to any threatening sexual conduct. They should tell an adult (a parent or a teacher, for example) about any inappropriate touching, talk, or other activity with an adult or an older child—no matter who it is—and about abuse of another child.

Maintaining open communication with children in all areas of their lives makes it easier to discuss sexual abuse, too, and encourages children to talk about their fears and concerns. It's also important to give youngsters plenty of individual attention and to get to know the adults and older children with whom your child spends time.

Many schools have abuse education and prevention programs. Find out about your school's plans so that you can coordinate discussions at home with them.

What are signs that a child has been abused sexually? What should I do if I suspect it?

Sexual abuse of a child encompasses more than sexual contact. Any sex-related act between a child and an adult or an older

WHEN CHILDREN ASK ABOUT SEX

Sex education is more than a talk about "the facts of life." A child needs to learn gradually about the sexes' physical differences, privacy, reproduction and birth, puberty changes, masturbation, contraception, and sexually transmitted diseases. Here are some guidelines for handling the subject.

 Review the facts. Read sex education books for children and for parents to find an approach that you like. Keep informed as your children grow older to correct misinformation from peers.

Get comfortable talking about sex. Rehearse with your spouse or attend a workshop (see Appendix). If you still feel ill at ease, tell your child that you feel awkward but that you think discussing sex is important.

 Find out what a child is really asking. At age 2 or 3, a toddler may want to know what the genitals are, why girls and boys are different, and where babies come from. But find out what a child really wants to know first. When your 2-year-old asks, "Where did I come from?" she may want to know if she was born in a hospital or in another city. Ask, "Where do *you* think you came from?" to discover what's on her mind. If she is asking where babies come from, you can explain or correct a misconception ("Joey said I came out of your belly button").

Coordinate your efforts with those at school. Plan discussions at home to follow up on sex education programs at school.

 Keep it simple and honest. Give clear, straightforward answers with accurate names (penis, vagina). Relax and use a conversational tone. Remember toddlers are literal; told that babies grow "in Mommy's tummy," a child may think babies have something to do with food and eating. Instead, try, "Babies grow in a special place in Mommy's body." Don't overexplain. A sentence or two may satisfy a preschooler.

Take the initiative. Raise issues yourself: "Do you know why Mrs. Jones' stomach is so big? She's going to have a baby." Children often get wrong or incomplete ideas from friends. Check occasionally to see if your child has a clear grasp of basic facts. At puberty, for example, clarify what a child knows about sexually transmitted diseases (p.244).

Make sex education a joint responsibility. Both parents should be involved and impart the same clear, consistent expressions of their values. If Dad answers boys' questions and Mom girls', children may assume that one sex's interests don't concern the other.

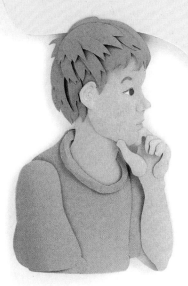

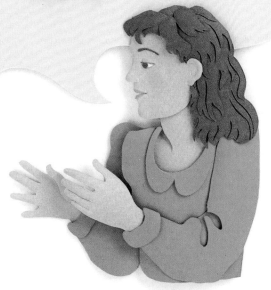

child is considered abusive. Displaying the genitals to a youngster, showing a child a sexually explicit picture, and photographing a child for pornographic purposes are all forms of abuse. It's estimated that 1 in 4 girls and 1 in 7 boys in the United States are sexually abused at some point in their childhood or adolescence. And most cases involve someone the child knows, often a relative or friend of the family.

Because many abusers tell children not to reveal their "secret," the signs of child sexual abuse may be subtle. These include fear of a certain place or person, fear of a physical examination, disturbed-looking drawings, acute awareness of the genitals or of sexual words and acts, overreaction to questions about touching by another person, nightmares, and sudden changes in mood, behavior, or school performance. Physical signs include sexually transmitted diseases and changes in the genital or anal area. Children who try to talk about abuse may reveal only vague, sketchy details. Some tell a friend or a sibling, who may tell an adult.

Teachers, school officials, doctors, nurses, social workers, counselors, clergy, and police officers are all required by law to report cases of known or suspected child sexual abuse. If you know of a case of abuse or strongly suspect that abuse is happening, it's a good idea to tell someone in one of these fields. Cases are checked by the police or a social service agency; their action is geared primarily toward protecting the child and preventing further abuse.

If your suspicions are less strong, or you have few details, you may want to talk with the child first. Be calm and make it clear that the abuse isn't the child's fault and that he or she

won't be harmed by telling. Take what the child says seriously and contact a professional as soon as possible. In the meantime keep the youngster safe. Sexually abused children who are ignored or doubted may remain victims for years. If the child isn't yours, tell his or her parents or caretaker if this won't put the child in danger. Otherwise, notify your city or state social service agency; its child protection service can do a proper evaluation.

My mother just died. Should we take our 4-year-old daughter to the funeral?

Children vary in their ability to fathom death, depending largely on how old they are. They comprehend it on some level by age 3, and by 6 or 7, they will feel some loss briefly if a close relative or friend dies. But most children don't develop a real understanding of death until around 9. Before that, they usually don't fully grasp that death is irreversible and often confuse it with a long absence. They may understand it better if they have experienced the death of a pet.

Experts disagree on the age at which it's appropriate for children to attend a funeral, although there are some who advise against it for children under 6 or 7. It's important to maintain your daughter's routine as much as possible and not to force her to mourn or go to the service if she doesn't want to. If your daughter wants to talk about her grandmother or about death itself, make time to discuss the subject with her. Young children are probably better off without long, complicated explanations of death. A clear, matter-of-fact discussion is usually best. Don't lie to your daughter ("Grandma's gone on a trip") or discourage

her from asking questions. Be open about your grief so that your child sees it as a natural reaction to death.

My husband says it's OK to let the kids have an occasional sip of beer or wine. Is this healthy?

Alcohol consumption is illegal in all states for anyone under age 21 and contrary to the beliefs of many religious groups. But it's not uncommon for parents who do drink to allow children to sample alcohol (watered wine, for example) at family celebrations and occasional meals. There's some evidence that children introduced to alcohol in a responsible family setting have fewer problems with it throughout life than children who first drink on the sly with their friends. Keep in mind that alcohol's effects depend on the size of a person, so any amount consumed by a child will have a greater impact than in an adult.

More important, parents who drink can encourage responsible drinking by setting a good example: drinking in moderation and never when driving or operating machinery, not treating alcohol as a way to deal with problems, and not seeing drunkenness as entertaining or funny. Show children from an early age that celebrations and happy times, while they may include alcohol, don't depend on it. Explain the effects of excessive drinking (p. 163), including problems associated with alcoholism. Children who have family members with a history of alcohol abuse are more at risk than others of becoming alcoholics, and they should learn about the possibility of addiction. When children reach their teen years, it's unrealistic to expect that they won't be tempted to experiment with alcohol. Those with good role models and education may have a better chance of dealing effectively with situations involving alcohol.

My children fight and argue constantly. What can I do?

Fighting with siblings is a way of learning how to assert oneself and work out differences. If the children are the same sex and about the same age, the fighting is likely to be even more intense, as children try to distinguish themselves from each other.

While such competition is normal, parents should watch for signs of extreme aggression, such as unprovoked attacks or excessive verbal abuse, that may be symptoms of a serious emotional problem. As a general rule, it's best to intervene as little as possible in sibling disputes in order to avoid taking sides (or at least seeming to). Let your children settle their own differences. If you do intervene, encourage children to work out a compromise (sharing, for example, or taking turns) rather than dictating a solution. Try not to assign blame unless one child

is flagrantly at fault (which is seldom the case, despite claims that "*She* started it!"). Often simply threatening to separate bickering children will encourage a resolution. Notice how you and your spouse argue; children learn by example. Also, an increase in tensions between parents may spur an increase in the amount of fighting between children.

Should I push my child to make friends?

Making friends is an important part of a child's social development, but there is rarely a need

GENDER DIFFERENCES: INBORN OR LEARNED?

For all the hundreds of studies that have examined this question, the answer remains elusive. Beyond the obvious physical differences between the sexes, most aspects of what we deem male and female traits seem to be determined by environment— signals picked up from parents, from other male and female role models in a child's life, from friends and siblings, and from books, movies, television, and other media.

Or are they? Newborn boys and girls have similar activity levels; between ages 1 and 2, both sexes are equally likely to fuss in the bathtub, explore strange rooms, and fidget while being dressed. At age 3, however, a few studies show boys beginning to be more active than girls. This could imply either that parents encourage boys to move around more than girls or that an inborn tendency begins to manifest itself at this stage.

Similarly, some studies find that before age 2 both sexes are equally aggressive, but that between ages 2 and 3 boys begin to show more aggression. This suggests to some researchers that aggressive behavior may be subtly encouraged in boys and discouraged in girls. Without realizing it, parents may be giving different messages to each. A boy, for example, may be admonished for hitting a girl, but chided less harshly for striking

another boy. His sister may be equally rebuked for striking anyone, girl or boy. Other researchers, however, maintain that such tendencies result from subtle differences in the physiology of the brains of males and females.

The nature-nurture debate also continues in the area of male and female aptitudes. Psychologists and educators have long believed (and test scores back them up) that girls are naturally better at verbal skills (reading and writing) while boys are superior in mathematical and spatial-visual abilities. These verbal and mathematical differences become especially noticeable during adolescence. Nature-supporters say they result from the increased production of sex hormones at that age; nurture-supporters again point to differences in upbringing.

Whatever explains the distinctions between male and female aptitudes in general, statistical differences between groups of people cannot predict any individual's capabilities. Just as there are many women who are taller than most men—even though men in general are taller than women—there are many women who excel at math and many men who possess superior verbal skills. Parents should never discourage any child— boy or girl—from following an interest or a profession just because of his or her sex.

to push children to do it. Most toddlers play by themselves, although they may spend hours in the company of other children. Play becomes interactive at about age 3. In their preschool and early school years, children are generally attracted to children with a similar style of play. Quiet children, for example, prefer other quiet children, and active youngsters tend to team up with more active playmates. By age 10, shared interests become more important. Teenagers seek out friends who can help them to solve problems and make sense of the world. In general, boys have more friends than girls, but girls' friendships tend to be more intimate, placing greater emphasis on shared secrets and one "best" friend.

Parents can encourage their children to make friends by exposing them to other children from an early age, asking questions about their friends, and listening to them talk about their friends. A child who's slow to make friends or prefers playing alone shouldn't be pushed, as long as he or she seems otherwise happy and doesn't fight or bully other children. A solitary child who seems unhappy may be under stress, may have been rejected by others at school, or could have an emotional disorder. If you suspect a problem, talk it over with your child and consider seeking therapy. Like many adults, however, some kids simply prefer their own company, and in general this is no cause for worry.

Many children have an imaginary friend whom they talk to, play with, blame for misbehavior, and ask parents to set a place for at the table. This is normal; parents should play along without overdoing it, since the child usually knows, as a practical fact, that the friend isn't real.

Does seeing violence on TV inspire violent behavior in children?

It may. Studies show that children exposed to violence on TV may become more hostile and impatient. They're also prone to be more aggressive, tense, and irritable and are less likely to obey rules. Unfortunately, American children are exposed to a lot of violence. They watch an average of 3 to 5 hours of television a day and view an estimated 12,000 violent acts a year.

Although sexually explicit material can be blocked out on most cable systems, it's hard for parents to keep their children from watching violent shows on regular broadcast television. The American Academy of Pediatrics recommends that children watch TV no more than 2 hours a day. Parents should find out what their children are watching and ban shows and movies they find inappropriate. It's also important to provide alternative activities, such as reading and games, that encourage children to use their minds and imagination instead of passively staring at the television screen.

My son often doesn't go to sleep until 10 or 11 o'clock at night. Is this bad for his health?

Like adults, children vary in their sleep needs. A child who is alert and happy during the day and doesn't seem to get sick more often than normal is probably getting enough sleep. Many children today stay up later than their parents did, possibly because parents work longer hours and otherwise wouldn't get to see much of them.

Child-study experts suggest that parents establish and enforce bedtime rules and proce-

dures. Bedtime rituals such as brushing teeth, reading stories, having a drink of water, and saying prayers help children feel secure, but parents shouldn't give in to tactics that postpone bedtime too long. For an overtired child who has trouble going to sleep, try having a quiet time before bedtime. A scared child should be reassured but not pampered; leaving a lamp or a night light on may help, but sleeping with parents is usually not a good idea. Children tend to sleep better if they get a reasonable amount of physical activity during the day, so a parent should encourage active daytime play.

How should I prepare my daughter for her first period?

Girls in the United States start menstruating between ages 12 and 13. Some girls start at 9 or younger, so you shouldn't wait too long to discuss the subject with your daughter. The health curriculum of many schools includes classes for girls on menstruation; you may want to find out if and when your daughter's school plans to do this so that you can have your talk with her around the same time. This is also a good opportunity to discuss other changes associated with puberty—the appearance of pubic and underarm hair, the development of breasts, a growth spurt—which actually precede most girls' first period.

At this preliminary stage it's enough to tell a girl that special pads and tampons handle the flow; she can be instructed in their specific use when her first period begins.

Try to communicate to your daughter that menstruation is a natural part of the maturing process, not something painful or dangerous. Help her to understand that menstruation is a sign of a reproductive capability that entails responsibility. Before she becomes sexually active, she should understand that as a menstruating woman she is physically capable of becoming pregnant.

A girl's mother is usually the best person to tell her about menstruation; friends and siblings don't always have all the facts. When the mother is absent or can't do the job, another woman close to the girl should be asked to step in.

When should a girl go to a doctor for her first gynecological exam?

The American College of Obstetricians and Gynecologists suggests that a girl see a gynecologist at age 18 or at the onset of sexual activity, whichever comes first. It's not necessary to have a gynecological exam at the first menstrual period; most menstruation problems can be handled by a family doctor or pediatrician. Irregular periods and mild cramping, which are common in girls, rarely require medical attention. Severe cramping, however, may indicate some kind of problem and should prompt a visit to a gynecologist.

Telling a girl what to expect at her first exam (p. 252) will help allay anxiety and prepare her for the intimate nature of the procedures. She should understand why a pelvic exam and tests such as the Pap smear are done. She should know that some procedures may be uncomfortable but won't hurt. And she should be encouraged to ask the doctor any questions she may have about sexuality or reproduction.

Whether anyone accompanies a girl to the exam should be up to her. A girl who is nervous may appreciate the presence of her mother, older sister, or a friend.

(Having a relative or friend present should be cleared with the doctor beforehand.) Other girls see the first exam as a private matter and a step toward independence, and prefer to go alone. In either case, the girl should know that her records and any exchange between her and the doctor are confidential.

When do boys enter puberty? What are the physical signs?

Male puberty is a series of gradual changes that take place over several years, usually between ages 10 and 18. The first sign of puberty is usually growth of the testes and scrotum; then a year later the penis starts growing at a faster rate and reaches adult size by age 16. Pubic hair usually appears during the same period. Most boys will have their first ejaculation in their early teens, often as a nocturnal emission ("wet dream"). Other changes include the growth of underarm, facial, and chest hair, a deepening of the voice, and a sharp increase in height, weight, and muscle mass. Like girls, boys should learn about the changes before or as they start to experience them. It's important to stress that the timing and rate of changes vary widely, and to reassure a boy that he is normal even though he may be ahead of or behind his peers.

My daughter, who's 15, is going steady and I'm worried she might have sex. How can I convey my feelings to her?

Many parents have religious and moral objections to sex before marriage. But even if you don't, it's natural for a parent to want a child—girl or boy—to delay sexual activity until she or he is

emotionally mature enough to handle the consequences. Your child may already be well aware of your feelings from just having been around you all her life. But it's still a good idea to have an honest one-on-one talk with her about the subject now that she's dating seriously. Make it clear to your daughter that it is OK to postpone sex even if "everyone is doing it" and even if she feels pressure from her boyfriend or peers. Explain that there are emotional risks in becoming sexually intimate with someone before she is old enough to handle the potential problems of a close relationship. Of course, the risks of becoming pregnant or of contracting a sexually transmitted disease (p. 244) should also be discussed.

On the other hand, parents should be aware that they can't hold back a teenager's emerging sexuality. It is natural for teenagers to be curious about sex and the changes in their bodies. Even if they do avoid full intercourse, dating couples are likely to become involved in some types of sexual experimentation. Parents should make sure their teenage children have access to reliable information about birth control and disease prevention. The source of this information can be a doctor, the child's school, organizations such as Planned Parenthood (see Appendix), or the parents themselves.

My teenage son has told me he's gay. How should I counsel him?

The first thought of many parents in this situation is: Why? Years of research have not found a cause or set of causes for homosexuality (the word comes from the Greek *homo*, meaning same, and is defined as sexual attraction to and activity between persons of the same sex). Psychological, biological, and cultural factors probably all play roles. Homosexuality has not been linked to any psychological problems or abnormalities—in other words, your son isn't crazy. There's also no reason to blame yourself and how you raised your child; few psychologists today believe that upbringing is the main determinant of sexual orientation.

What you say to your son depends on your own feelings about the issue, but it's a rare parent who has no trouble accepting a child's homosexuality. Most major religions officially consider homosexuality a sin, although many individual members of the clergy disagree. It was only in 1974 that the American Psychiatric Association reclassified homosexuality from a mental illness to "an alternate choice of sexual experience." Society's general attitude toward it ranges from outright condemnation to an uneasy tolerance at best. Even though homosexuality is more accepted today than it once was, it's not easy for many gay people to be open about their sexual orientation, and it was probably very difficult for your son to tell you that he is gay.

Even if your son's announcement is painful to you, it's important for you to be as supportive as possible. Try to help him find counseling if he needs it. Adolescence is a time of great confusion about many things, and your son may be signaling sexual confusion rather than a firm commitment to a homosexual lifestyle. A skilled therapist can help him sort through and resolve these issues. Assuming your son is gay, remind him (and yourself) that he isn't alone—estimates suggest that 5 to 10 percent of men and 3 to 5 percent of women are primarily or exclusively homosexual—and that most gay people lead ordinary, stable lives, frequently in committed relationships. Of course, make sure that your child is thoroughly aware of the perils of AIDS and how to avoid it (pp. 242–243).

How can parents help children handle the stress of divorce?

More than a million children are affected by divorce each year in the United States, and no matter how the breakup is handled, the impact on their lives is enormous. Researchers say that the short-term effects can range from bed-wetting and aggressive behavior to poor schoolwork. The long-term effects may include depression and underachievement. Years and even decades later children may still be coping with the emotional aftermath of their parents' divorce. But the evidence also suggests that living in a conflict-filled household can be more damaging for a child than witnessing a divorce. And the effects of a divorce aren't all negative. According to one study, children of divorced parents were more determined than others to establish a committed relationship and to avoid divorce.

Although most children sense when a marriage is unhappy, the decision to divorce should be communicated clearly and directly. Children who are lied to (told that one parent is going away for a while, for example) will usually figure things out and lose trust in what you tell them. Make it clear that the divorce isn't the child's fault; this is important with young children who may be testing parents with declarations like "I hate you! Go away!" and then see the divorce as a fulfillment of that wish.

Keep children's routines as stable as you can. Try to make arrangements that don't require them to move or spend too much time with grandparents, other relatives, or sitters. Also don't overlook older children's needs. The disappearance of a stable family structure can be very hard on teenagers, more so, according to some studies, than on their younger siblings. Overloading your teenage children with new responsibilities or making unrealistic emotional demands on them in the wake of a divorce only adds to their stress.

Make sure that both you and your former spouse have regular contact with all your children. Both of you should attend important events, such as school plays, concerts, and graduations, sitting together if possible. Studies show that the single most important indicator that a child will handle a divorce successfully is a good relationship with both parents. Don't encourage children to take sides or to act as go-betweens. Pumping a child for information about your former mate can lead to sullen, withdrawn behavior. Some anger toward your ex-spouse is natural, but it should not be acted out in front of your children.

Do children in single-parent households face special problems?

They probably do, but the research on the subject doesn't provide a clear answer. According to the Census Bureau, there are nearly 10 million one-parent households in the United States and 1 out of 4 children under age 18 lives in one. However, since a majority of these children are in one-parent homes as a result of divorce or separation, it's difficult to tell whether any out-of-the-ordinary problems they may have are caused by the emotional turmoil and dislocation of divorce, by the strains of living without

STEPPARENTING

Although 7 million American children under age 18 live in households where one or both parents were married before, the dynamics of stepfamilies didn't receive serious research attention until the 1970's. What has been found is not surprising: a stepfamily (also called a remarried or blended family) presents tough challenges for both the natural parent and the stepparent (some 60 percent of second marriages with children involved fail). Important lessons can be learned from stepfamilies that have succeeded.

Be a couple first. The natural parent and stepparent sometimes concentrate so hard on forging new parent-child ties that they ignore their own bond. This weakens the structure of the whole family. If your marriage is solid, in time the other stepfamily relationships will fall into place.

Make a fresh start. Settle the new family into a new home if you possibly can. It eliminates the perception that one family has invaded the other's territory and puts everyone on an equal footing. If you must stay in one parent's residence, renovate and redecorate to give everyone the sense of a new beginning.

Keep expectations reasonable. It's natural for adults who have suffered through a divorce or the death of a spouse to want to create a perfect new family as quickly as possible. But children will have mixed feelings at best about accepting another parent. They will find sharing parental affection with new siblings very difficult. Jealousy, fear, anger, and resentment are much more likely than a "Brady Bunch" scenario.

Accept the limits of stepparenting. Stepparents and stepchildren may over time form satisfying attachments. But a child's natural parent (even a negligent one) will almost always come first. In most states, unless you adopt your stepchildren (with the natural parent's consent), you have no legal rights (you can't even authorize emergency medical treatment).

Be patient. Psychologists suggest that a realistic timetable for a stepfamily to coalesce is at least 4 years—even with all the advantages of open communication, family counseling, and the help of a support group such as the Stepfamily Association of America (see Appendix).

Less is better. This adage applies to discipline and forced "togetherness," especially in the early stages. Parents and stepparents should agree on and set rules, but psychologists suggest that in the beginning each birth parent do the enforcing with his or her own children. Later both parents can slowly move toward sharing authority. Adolescents and teenagers who are moving to become more independent may resist having to focus on the new family. Their feelings should be respected.

the daily presence of a father or a mother, or by some combination of the two conditions.

There is no question that raising children alone is stressful to the parent, who in addition to managing the household and in many cases holding down a full-time job, has to provide discipline and emotional support for the children, serve as both mother and father when the situation calls for it, and somehow try to squeeze in a personal life as well. Even if the absent parent helps support the family financially, a lack of money is often a strain on single-parent homes. About 85 percent of them are headed by the mother, and households headed by females generally have lower incomes than others.

Whether and how the single parent's stress affects the children depends a great deal on the personalities involved. But even if a one-parent home functions smoothly and with a minimum of stress, the absence of one parent may cause the children to feel emotionally deprived; this is especially true of boys who lack a proper male role model.

In general, however, research suggests that children will thrive despite the absence of a parent as long as they are raised in a warm, loving environment. Indeed, a child is nearly always better off in a single-parent home than in a conventional situation in which one parent is abusive or misuses drugs or alcohol.

How can a busy family like ours make the most of the time that we spend together?

With more and more two-career couples, electronic diversions, and hectic schedules for parents and children, a family today can easily fall into a pattern of coexisting without meaningful interaction. Experts agree that the loss can have negative effects on individual development, leading to feelings of isolation, loneliness, and alienation in adults and children alike. Family time, they say, is not a luxury, it's a necessity. Here are some tips for making the most of the time you spend together:

☐ Go for quantity and quality. Both the amount of time families spend together and how they spend it count. Parents should set aside a time to give their children undivided attention every day, perhaps after school, at dinner, or right before bed. (A couple should also reserve time for each other.) Celebrating holidays and birthdays together and taking recreation as a family—whether it's going to a zoo, museum, or baseball game—are other ways that a family can make the most of their time together. On the other hand, many feelings are shared and lessons are learned when parents and children are simply together—doing chores, getting ready for school and work, and doing other everyday activities at home.

☐ Be realistic. Accept that working full-time may sometimes mean missing certain special moments in your children's lives and that not every meaningful family moment has to involve the whole family. By all means set goals for family togetherness, but don't expect to meet them all.

☐ Focus on the moment. Concentrate on what's going on when you're with family members. Leave work concerns at work. When you ask your child a question, listen to the answer. A child can tell whether you are really paying attention or not.

☐ Get everyone's input. Not every family activity will delight all its members, but ignoring the wishes of some virtually ensures that they'll resist joining in.

☐ Put the children to work. Start delegating early—and don't worry if the results don't meet your normal standards. An imperfectly folded pile of laundry still gives a child a sense of accomplishment—and lets you visit while you do the ironing. Even toddlers can help with simple meal preparation, yardwork, shopping, and cleaning jobs.

☐ Make meals a priority. Families who eat their main meal together find it is possible to juggle work, school, lessons, play, and other commitments around this binding experience. Meals offer a chance to share the day's events and impressions, voice opinions, coordinate schedules, and circumvent brewing crises.

☐ Respect privacy and individual needs. Teenagers have more outside commitments than younger children and may resist spending excessive amounts of time with the family. Know when to stop pushing.

☐ Protect your family time. Let friends and co-workers know that your family is a priority. Set guidelines for when you can and can't work late, and avoid working on the weekends.

Is family still as important to most people as it once was?

In surveys asking people to name what they consider the most important things in life, family typically rates ahead of money, sex, fame, power, career success, friends, and a clean environment. In one Harris poll, happy family life was considered essential or very important by 97 percent of the people who responded.

The family is vital for many reasons. Chief among them is meeting the needs of children, who are born helpless and dependent on parents. In most societies the family is the basic economic unit, usually providing for those too young, old, sick, or otherwise unable to support themselves. The family also offers a place for children to develop emotionally; ideally they are able to test their growing sense of self without fear of disgrace or rejection, while at the same time learning the limits of acceptable conduct. Parents pass on to children their values, opinions, and modes of behavior. For many people the family is a lifelong haven and refuge, a place to return to when the outside world becomes hard and cold.

Definitions of family change, depending on society's norms. While the basic unit in America today is still the nuclear family of a father, a mother, and their children, families may be headed by a single parent or they may contain step- or adopted children, aging relatives, or nonrelatives. A married couple without children is still a family and so is an "empty nest" couple whose grown children have left home. A mutually committed unmarried couple or even friends living communally may call themselves a family. Indeed, the family unit we imagine most often—a married couple with growing children—now makes up only about one-quarter of U.S. households. The main criterion for family seems to be members who are committed to one another in a supportive and loving relationship.

The family has survived historical upheavals and challenges to its crucial place in the fabric of society. As much as we all find our particular families at times hard to deal with, the institution is probably here to stay.

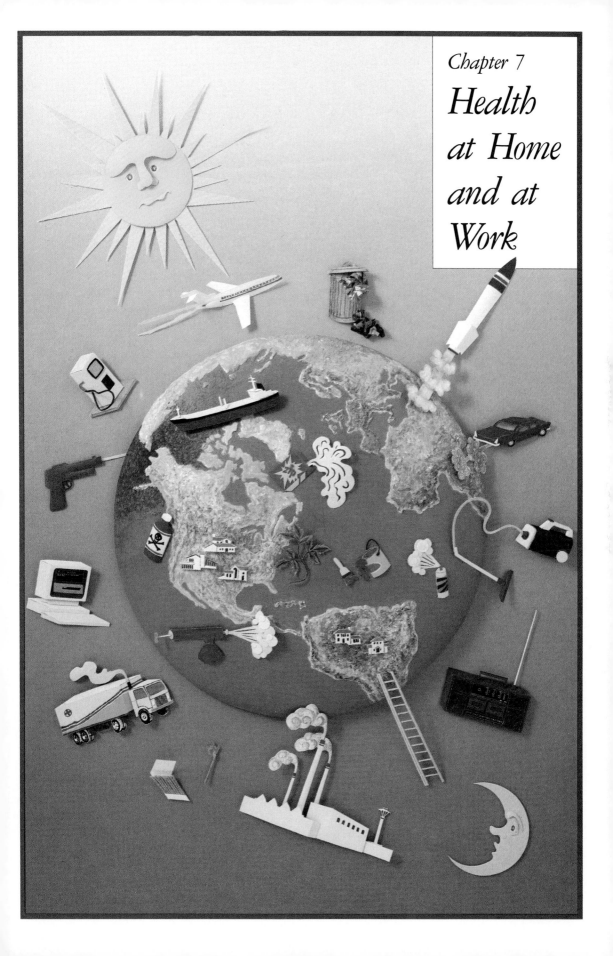

Chapter 7

Health at Home and at Work

Poisoned Walls

The pride of Frank and Sally F.'s lives was their two-year-old daughter, Kate, and the work they were putting into the renovation of their century-old house. About a year after starting the job, Frank read an article about the dangers of lead poisoning in children when paint is stripped in old houses. Except for a slight appetite loss, Kate showed none of the symptoms of lead poisoning mentioned in the article, but even so, Frank and Sally were alarmed. At their insistence, Kate's pediatrician tested her blood for lead content. The results were an astounding 70 micrograms of lead per deciliter of blood (the average is 5 to 10 micrograms).

How could this be? Kate had never eaten paint chips. Frank and Sally had been careful about sealing off rooms and disposing of debris. But despite their efforts, they couldn't shield Kate from the minute lead particles that had permeated her environment. After months of intensive chelation therapy to cleanse her blood, Kate's lead level dropped to about 25 micrograms. Not only is this still high, but lead remains trapped in her bones and may continue leaching into her system for the rest of her life.

As for the house, after hiring professionals to remove the lead paint, Frank and Sally put it up for sale, knowing at least that it would never harm another child as it had their own daughter.

A Lucky Hunch

Marion P., 72, was an active woman and avid gardener who loved the outdoors. But over the course of several months her daughter, Wendy, noticed that Marion was slowing down. Even worse, she seemed confused and less mentally sharp. Marion herself realized that something was wrong, but wrote it off to old age. Wendy wasn't so sure. While pondering the many possible reasons for her mother's decline, Wendy hit upon the idea of Lyme disease. After all, the ticks that spread the infection were common in the area, and Marion was often outdoors.

At her daughter's urging, Marion had her blood tested. Not only did she have Lyme disease, but her symptoms suggested an advanced case. A spinal tap performed at a Lyme disease clinic showed that the infection had affected Marion's central nervous system. Relieved to know that she wasn't growing senile, Marion was treated for two weeks with daily intravenous doses of a powerful antibiotic. Within six months she was herself again, tending to her garden. Only now, Marion makes sure to cover her arms, legs, and feet outdoors and to check for ticks before going back into the house.

Allergic to Work

For Jessica M., being at work often meant teary eyes, a runny nose, a sore throat, headache, and fatigue. Some of her colleagues at the small publishing firm complained of similar problems. Yet all of them swore that when they were away from the office for a few days, the symptoms disappeared. Reacting to a rise in absenteeism and a drop in productivity, management called in the National Institute for Occupational Safety and Health (NIOSH) to check out the building.

NIOSH inspectors evaluated the ventilation system and tested the air with an organic vapor sniffer. Near the copy machine, the sniffer's needle jumped, indicating a vapor buildup. The inspectors took samples of the air and of the copier's toner fluid for analysis at a NIOSH lab.

The culprit was the copier, which used too much toner and created too much vapor. Poor ventilation allowed the vapor to build up and spread through the building. Once these problems were fixed, the allergies disappeared.

Controlling Environmental Risk

The words *environment* and *pollution* conjure up images of oil spills, dwindling rain forests, and nuclear disasters. Unfortunately, the price we pay for technological progress is a world that's perceived to be fraught with environmental danger. Whether it actually is or not, however, is a matter of continuing debate. This chapter has been designed to help you assess the risks of modern life and take steps to reduce them. As a first step, pick the phrase or phrases that most accurately complete the environmental-health statements below.

1 The most common environmental cause of cancer death is _____ .

A. asbestos
B. tobacco
C. pesticides in water and on food

2 Ozone is _____ .

A. a form of oxygen
B. a component of smog
C. an atmospheric gas that protects the earth from harmful solar rays
D. an ingredient in spray propellants

3 The _____ gas sometimes emitted by new carpeting and furniture can cause headache, dizziness, eye irritation, and other symptoms.

A. radon
B. carbon monoxide
C. nitrogen dioxide
D. formaldehyde

4 If you find intact asbestos insulation in your home, it is best to _____ .

A. remove it yourself right away
B. hire a contractor to remove it
C. leave it in place

5 The usual treatment for a radon problem is _____ .

A. sealing radon entry points
B. installing a proper ventilation system
C. there is no way to rid a home of radon

6 The first sign that continual exposure to loud noises is affecting hearing usually is _____ .

A. a constant ringing in the ears
B. difficulty understanding speech
C. music sounding off-key

7 According to some studies, radiation from electric blankets may increase cancer risk among _____ .

A. the elderly
B. people with chronic illnesses
C. children whose mothers used electric blankets during pregnancy

8 To put out an oil fire, use a _____ fire extinguisher.

A. Class A
B. Class B
C. Class C
D. Class ABC

9 Your best protection in an auto accident is _____ .

A. an air bag
B. a buckled seat belt
C. an air bag and a buckled lap/shoulder belt

Answers
For more information on any of the quiz topics turn to the pages listed next to the answers.

1. B, p.288	4. C, p.294	7. C, p.303
2. A,B,C, p.293	5. A,B, p.296	8. B,D, p.310
3. D, p.293	6. B, p.299	9. C, p.317

It seems that almost every day I read another story about pollution. Are the air, water, and land really as contaminated as the media say they are?

The media have done a valuable service by bringing environmental issues to the attention of the American people. During the 1970's informed citizens demanded environmental reforms of Congress, and the result was landmark legislation—the Clean Air and Clean Water acts, which placed severe restrictions on the amount and kinds of wastes that industry could release into the air or water.

A great deal of progress has been made since then. By 1990 lead levels in urban air were down 87 percent from 1977. More than 127 million people (compared with 85 million in 1972) are now served by adequate sewage-treatment programs. And since bans against certain pesticides, including DDT, were enacted in the early 1970's, once-endangered species like the bald eagle have made a comeback.

The cleanup is far from over, however, and the media continue to focus attention on environmental hazards. Pictures of sewage washing up on beaches or of overflowing landfills, for example, underline the need for better solid waste disposal.

Of course, news reports tend to focus on the worst-case scenarios—Love Canal, Chernobyl, oil spills polluting the Alaska and Texas coastlines. Because media coverage is dramatic and compelling—particularly when an environmental catastrophe is shown on TV—the chance of a similar event occurring closer to home may seem greater than is statistically the case. An analogy can be made to flying and

driving. Graphic media coverage of airline disasters causes some people to feel that flying in an airplane is more dangerous than driving in an automobile, whereas the reverse is true. Similarly, not all beaches have been contaminated with medical wastes, but after intensive media concentration on the problem, many people may think that every beach is in trouble.

Does that mean you should ignore or discount what you read in newspapers or see on TV? Not at all. The prudent course is to use the information as a starting point; then ask questions of your local officials to determine whether there is a problem in your community.

There have been many warnings about carcinogens in our environment. How much of a threat to the average person are these substances?

The most common environmental cause of cancer deaths is also the most preventable—the use of tobacco. The toxic materials that people tend to worry about—pesticides, benzene, or asbestos—are responsible for only about 6 percent of cancer deaths. And the risk is greatest for people whose work exposes them directly to these industrial carcinogens. For example, a farm worker who frequently handles pesticides has a far greater cancer risk than the person who eats fresh fruit and vegetables that may contain some pesticide residues, assuming that all other factors, such as tobacco use and diet, are equal.

It's worth remembering that exposure to a carcinogen does not necessarily mean you'll develop cancer. Many factors—including genes, gender, diet, al-

cohol and tobacco use, viruses, sexual and reproductive history, as well as environmental pollutants—help determine susceptibility to cancer (see *Common Cancers: Assessing Your Risk,* p. 204). And while there's little you can do about genes and gender, many of the other factors are subject to your control.

How safe is our water supply? How can I tell what's in my tap water?

Most public water systems in the United States are regulated by the U.S. Environmental Protection Agency (EPA) under the Safe Drinking Water Act and are relatively safe. Thanks to chlorination and government regulation, the waterborne plagues of the past—such mass killers as cholera, typhoid, and dysentery—have been eliminated. However, perils of a different nature still lurk in the national water supply. The following are among the most serious:

☐ Lead enters tap water from corroded lead pipes and solder; the alloys in many faucets also leach lead into the water flowing through them. Whether drunk, eaten, or inhaled, lead can cause major health problems, especially in the young (p. 298).

☐ Radionuclides are radioactive atoms that emit cancer-causing radiation as they decay. Naturally occurring deposits of different radionuclides pose a threat to underground water sources in different parts of the country, with radium most often a problem in the Midwest and Appalachian regions, uranium in the Rockies, and radon gas in the Northeast (see *The Facts About Radon,* p. 296).

☐ Disease-causing bacteria and viruses are still transmitted by tap water, despite preventive measures such as chlorination.

CREATING A HEALTHIER PLANET

As disheartening as the world's pollution problems appear to be, many Americans, working individually and in groups, have decided to "do something about it." Their stories prove that people *can* make a difference in the fight to clean up our soil, water, and air.

A student revolt. In 1986, sixth-grade students at the Jackson Elementary School in Salt Lake City discovered that an abandoned lot three blocks from their school was a toxic waste site. With the help of their teacher, they wrote the Utah Department of Health to ask when the lot would be cleaned up. Informed that it wasn't slated for cleanup, the students sprang into action. A telephone and letter-writing campaign aimed at the mayor, the state health department, the Environmental Protection Agency, and the company whose barrels littered the site got results: the barrels of toxic chemicals were removed from the lot.

But the battle still wasn't over; the state now claimed it had no money to restore the contaminated land. Undaunted, the children appealed to corporations for money—only to discover that the state couldn't accept private funds for this purpose. The students drafted their own bill to get around that snag and lobbied the state legislature for its passage. The measure sailed through both houses. Thanks to the persistence of sixth-graders, a once toxic site is no longer a threat to an entire community.

Wetlands waste treatment. Worried about the high costs of buying into a new regional sewage treatment plant, the town of Arcata in northern California built itself a natural waste-processing system for less money. The payoff was more than cheap clean water; the town also gained a scenic 154-acre wetlands park that attracts some 200 species of birds.

Dug out of abandoned waterfront land where the town dump had once stood, the man-made wetlands use the ecology of marshes to purify sewage, which in turn helps nourish the plant and animal life of the marsh park. First, solid sludge is separated out of the sewage in a holding tank (plans call for the sludge to be used as compost). The remaining waste water flows through two oxidation ponds and then is treated with chlorine (to kill germs) before it enters the microbe-rich wetland marshes. By the time it empties into Humboldt Bay, Arcata's sewage has been transformed into clean water.

Tree power. Trees—if there are enough of them—can fight pollution: directly by using up carbon dioxide and creating oxygen, and indirectly by protecting buildings from heat and cold and cutting down on fuel use. The need for trees is most acute in smog-smothered cities like Los Angeles. Andy Lipkis, founder of the nonprofit corporation Tree-People, has overseen the planting of more than 2 million trees in his home town of Los Angeles and more than 200 million around the world. On his agenda for the 1990's is planting several million more trees in Los Angeles and educating schoolchildren to become caring stewards of their city's trees.

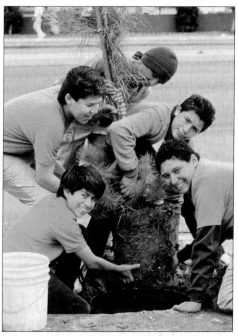

A new breed of Johnny Appleseed is emerging in America. In Los Angeles, environmentally conscious youngsters plant another tree for their city.

☐ Ironically, the chlorination process used to clean up the water supply creates organic chemical by-products that are potentially cancer-causing.

To determine the quality of your tap water, begin by making inquiries at your local water department. Suppliers of drinking water are required to make periodic tests to ensure that the legal limits set by the EPA for drinking water contaminants are being met, and you have a legal right to those test results.

However, not all suppliers perform these tests, and your water could be tainted by a substance that the EPA doesn't regulate or by a problem in your home plumbing. If you have doubts about the safety of your drinking water, consider sending a sample of it to a water-testing laboratory. For a fee that is usually under $100, the lab should provide you with a special mailing container and send you an analysis of the water, along with suggestions for improving it, if necessary. To find a water-testing lab in your area, check with your local or state health, water, or environmental resources department.

Which is safer, surface water or water from underground sources?

As long as it's adequately monitored and treated, water can be safe to drink whether it comes from surface sources, such as lakes and rivers, or from underground wells, springs, and aquifers (huge reservoirs made of porous layers of sand, gravel, and rock). Conversely, water from both types of sources is subject to contamination.

Federal regulations have set strict limits on what industry can discharge into surface waterways. And even though a manufacturer sometimes wantonly or

CLEANING UP YOUR DRINKING WATER

There are many water treatment devices on the market—ranging from useless to very effective. No system removes all the possible contaminants that water might contain. Have your water tested (see left) and know which pollutants you want to remove before buying a water purifier. Also, before deciding on a particular model, read the manufacturer's instructions and claims carefully. Avoid devices that promise to remove 100 percent of anything. And bear in mind that if you don't properly install and scrupulously maintain a purifier, you risk contaminating your water with trapped bacteria.

Water-softening units remove calcium, magnesium, and other minerals that make water hard and leave deposits inside water heaters and pipes as well as on bathtubs and clothes. As water comes into contact with sodium pellets in the unit, a chemical exchange occurs, and sodium is substituted for the calcium and magnesium in the water. (For people on sodium-restricted diets, there are units that use potassium pellets.) Claims that water softeners remove other toxic metals may be exaggerated. The units' main purpose is to make the water softer, not safer.

Activated carbon filters are the most popular, least expensive water purifiers. They absorb certain organic chemicals that give water unpleasant tastes and odors, but don't remove bacteria or most inorganic chemicals, such as salts or metals (some specially prepared models do remove lead). Unless carbon filters are maintained and replaced regularly, they can harbor bacteria. The filters come in three forms: whole-house models that are installed in the basement or outside the house, under-the-sink filters, and, least effective of all, faucet-attached devices.

Reverse osmosis (RO) units have a pre-filter, which removes rust, silt, and sediment. The filtered water is then forced under pressure through a semipermeable membrane, which blocks most inorganic chemicals (including iron, lead, salts, asbestos, and nitrates). A carbon filter gives the water a final cleansing. RO units waste water and are not recommended for areas with low water pressure or where water has a high bacteria count. Filters and membranes must be replaced often.

Distillation units remove impurities by vaporizing and then condensing water; the process kills most bacteria and viruses and leaves behind (in the boiling chamber) anything that won't boil or evaporate, including sediments, minerals, and metals. A carbon filter helps remove any lingering organic chemicals. Distillers do not remove all chemical pollutants, nor do they always kill all bacteria. (Because bacteria can proliferate in distilled water, it should be kept in a refrigerator for no more than a week.) Most units must be filled manually and use a lot of electricity. The boiling chamber must be cleaned often to avoid corrosion.

accidentally discharges illegal wastes into a body of water, such cases are easier to detect and correct than instances of groundwater pollution.

Water from underground sources—used by about half of the U.S. population—can be contaminated by chemicals leaking from hazardous waste sites or from corroding underground storage tanks. Agricultural pesticides and fertilizers are a threat to public and private wells in many parts of the country, especially the Midwest.

When such tainting occurs underground, however, it may take a long time for people to realize that the water is polluted and even longer to identify the chemicals and the source. Also, 46 million Americans get their water from private wells outside the EPA's jurisdiction, and unless a well owner is diligent and tests the water often, contamination may not be detected immediately.

Can fluoridated water be harmful?

The debate over fluoride has been raging ever since state and local governments began to fluoridate public water sources in 1945. Fluoride is added to water supplies and dental products because it hardens tooth enamel, making it more resistant to cavities. Research has shown that 40 to 60 percent of the reduction in tooth decay in children since 1945 is directly linked to fluoridated water.

While 9 million Americans drink from water supplies containing natural fluoride, 121 million drink artificially fluoridated water. Forty-two of the 50 largest cities in the United States fluoridate their water; two that do not are Los Angeles and San Diego.

Early opponents of fluoridation labeled the practice "forced medication" or worse. In 1990 the controversy flared up again when the National Toxicology Program (NTP) released a study which found that rats given fluoridated water developed osteosarcoma, a rare form of bone cancer.

Advocates of fluoridation point out that a person would have to drink between 360 and 700 glasses of fluoridated water per day to ingest amounts of fluoride equivalent to those given the rats in the NTP study, and that in more than 45 years scientists have failed to find a definitive link between fluoridated water and bone cancer in people. Although ingesting too much fluoride may cause fluorosis, or tooth staining, there is still no solid evidence that fluoridation at the limits set by the Environmental Protection Agency is harmful. (For more on fluoridation, see p.36.)

What other steps can I take to clean up my water supply?

Lead that leaches into drinking water from lead pipes or solder is a serious health hazard, especially in large cities. Because hot water absorbs lead and other metals more readily than cold, use only water from the cold-water tap for drinking purposes. Water that sits undisturbed in pipes overnight tends to accumulate lead. Each morning before you drink any water from the tap, flush out the system by letting the cold water run full force for a few minutes or until it is as cold as it gets. Save the runoff water for household cleaning. During the day, just let the cold water run briefly before you use it, to be on the safe side.

Either at home or when you're traveling, if you must drink water that is cloudy or that comes from a suspect source, make sure it has been boiled for at least 20 minutes or sterilized with chlorine or iodine purifying tablets. Let sterilized water stand for about half an hour after treatment before drinking it.

Farms and factories are not the only sources of water-polluting waste. If poured down drains or dumped on the ground, many common household products pose a threat to underground water supplies. Take leftover oil-based paints, paint removers and thinners, and chemical cleaning agents and lawn products to a waste collection center. Have a local service station dispose of waste oil and other automotive fluids. Take auto batteries to a battery dealer for recycling.

On a community level, check to make sure that your local government regularly tests drinking water supplies as required by the U.S. Environmental Protection Agency. If you find that your local government is not testing the water supply adequately or is lax about enforcing standards, contact the regional office of the EPA or join a local action group such as the Clean Water Action Project (see Appendix). Do not assume that you as an individual cannot effect change; there have been many cases in which grass-roots campaigns have prompted local, state, and even federal action to clean up water supplies.

Are bottled waters any purer than tap water?

Some bottled waters may not even be as clean as your tap water, and they are certainly more expensive. In 1990 a prestigious European brand was pulled off supermarket shelves when traces of benzene were found to have been introduced during bottling. Other bottled waters have been found to be tainted with bacteria, as well as with such chemicals as arsenic, toluene, and trichloroethane.

Before you decide to switch to a bottled water, make sure you know what you're buying. *Seltzer* is simply tap water that has been injected with carbon dioxide. *Club soda* is also carbonated tap water, with sodium and other minerals added. *Mineral water* is any water that contains minerals; it usually has a higher mineral content than ordinary tap water. *Sparkling water* is any carbonated water (some are naturally carbonated, others are injected with carbon dioxide). *Spring water* must reach the earth's surface naturally from a spring, but this by itself is no guarantee of purity.

Read bottle labels or contact the manufacturer to find out where a water comes from, how it's processed, and what's in it; ask the manufacturer to send you recent test results. The International Bottled Water Association (see Appendix) can also tell you whether a particular brand meets their standards.

Pay special attention to a water's sodium content; it's high in many brands. Try to buy water in glass rather than plastic bottles; the latter can leach undesirable chemicals into the water.

How do I know if our local beach is safe for swimming?

Call your city or county health department, which should conduct a water-sampling program throughout the swimming season and issue periodic lists of areas that are considered unsafe. Avoid beaches that have been tainted with sewage or medical waste until the health department has declared them safe.

Heavy rainfall may cause significant amounts of untreated sewage to be discharged into certain rivers and coastal waters. Refrain from swimming in areas known to be affected in this way for at least 2 days following heavy rains.

Is the air outdoors generally safe to breathe?

It depends on where you live and on pollution levels and weather conditions on any given day. The air over large, industrialized urban centers is often tainted by vast quantities of toxic gases and particulates (minute particles of liquid or solid matter), most of which are by-products of the burning of fossil fuels. State and local governments, under U.S. Environmental Protection Agency guidelines, monitor the air in all major metropolitan areas for six principal pollutants: ozone, particulate matter, carbon monoxide, nitrogen dioxide, lead, and sulfur dioxide; on the basis of these readings the air is graded acceptable, unhealthy, unacceptable, or hazardous.

Although winds scatter pollutants, and rain and snow wash them out of the air, weather conditions sometimes conspire to create air pollution emergencies. In a phenomenon known as thermal inversion, a layer of warm air covers a layer of cold air, preventing pollutants near the ground from rising and scattering. Thermal inversions over New York City resulted in the deaths of hundreds of people from respiratory diseases in 1953 and again in 1963. It is estimated that air pollution today costs the United States some $40 billion a year, or about $160 per person, in premature loss of life, reduced productivity, and increased health care costs.

Most vulnerable to the effects of air pollution are children, the elderly, smokers, and those suf-

FACT OR FALLACY ?

Biodegradable packaging benefits our environment

Fallacy. "Biodegradable" plastic is bad news on every count. It never really breaks down (microorganisms eat only the cornstarch and sugar added to it). And in landfills, where waste plastic usually ends up, it may leach lead and other toxic metals into groundwater. Paper isn't a very good alternative: its manufacture creates as much air and water pollution as that of plastic. In airless landfills, paper doesn't degrade very quickly either. The real problem with all packaging is simply the enormous quantity that is made and discarded after a single use. Paper products have the advantage here: they can be recycled more effectively than plastics can. How can you help? Choose only recyclable packaging. Reuse whatever plastic or paper you already have. Bring a tote bag when you shop to carry purchases home.

fering from respiratory and heart diseases. But when air quality is designated unacceptable, even the young and healthy can experience such symptoms as dizziness, headaches, eye irritation, coughing, sneezing, shortness of breath, and nausea. When air pollution levels rise, avoid strenuous work or exercise outdoors. If you are in one of the risk groups mentioned above, stay indoors.

What is ozone and how does it affect us?

Ozone is a form of oxygen whose molecules contain three oxygen atoms rather than the two that make up ordinary oxygen molecules. Constantly replenished through natural processes, ozone circles the earth in a protective layer that blocks out the sun's harmful ultraviolet rays. Without the ozone layer, there would be more cases of skin cancer, and the earth's land and oceans would be hotter.

Unfortunately, man-made industrial chemicals—primarily chlorofluorocarbons, methyl chloroform, and carbon tetrachloride—are now depleting the atmosphere of ozone faster than it is being replaced. In 1984 scientists discovered a "hole" in the ozone layer over the Antarctic, which by 1987 had grown to an area as large as the United States. In the temperate zone of the northern hemisphere, ozone is being lost more than twice as fast as scientists had expected.

Although some steps have been taken to phase out production of chlorofluorocarbons, critics contend that the remedial actions are not aggressive enough to deal with what may be an environmental crisis.

Paradoxically, ozone is a danger to humans at ground level, where it is produced commercially for bleaching, deodorization, and disinfecting and as a by-product of the interaction between automobile exhaust fumes and sunlight. A major component of smog, ozone can weaken the body's immune system and attack lung tissue. Air containing 0.14 parts per million is harmful to people who are active outdoors most of the day, such as children or construction workers, and to people who exercise during hours of peak pollution, such as joggers.

My home is well insulated. Now I'm told that a tightly sealed building may be a health hazard. What are the risks?

The good news is that by tightly insulating your home you have reduced your energy costs. The bad news is that by reducing the ventilation you risk breathing higher concentrations of various air pollutants. These include:
□ Cigarette smoke, which may account for some 400,000 deaths a year—including 50,000 deaths linked to the inhalation of secondhand smoke.
□ Radon, a colorless, odorless natural gas that seeps from the earth into buildings in some areas in the United States. According to the National Academy of Sciences, the risk of developing lung cancer is at least 10 times greater for smokers who are also exposed to high concentrations of radon.
□ Asbestos, a fibrous mineral that was often used as insulation around hot-water pipes and furnaces as well as in floor tiles, ceiling panels, siding, shingles, sound barriers, and fireproofing materials. If the tiny asbestos fibers are ingested or inhaled, they may lodge in body tissue and cause cancer.
□ Lead, a major polluter of water that can also cause health problems when inhaled as dust or fumes. Lead affects the nervous system, kidneys, and blood cell production, and can cause hypertension, fatigue, loss of appetite, and impaired mental capacity in adults. It is especially dangerous to fetuses and children.
□ Formaldehyde, which is used in more than 3,000 products, including cosmetics and toothpaste, and is a main component of the adhesive used to bond the particleboard and plywood so of-

ten found in paneling, floors, and kitchen countertops and cabinets. When these adhesives break down, they emit formaldehyde gas, which can impede breathing, irritate the eyes and skin, and induce nosebleeds, headaches, fatigue, and nausea. (It takes about 8 years for the formaldehyde gas in pressed-wood products to dissipate, so the problem is most acute in newer homes.)
□ Carbon monoxide, an element in cigarette smoke that may also be emitted by fireplaces, kerosene space heaters, furnaces, and gas stoves that are not in top working condition. This odorless, colorless gas can cause nausea, severe headaches, dizziness, or confusion, and may be fatal in high concentrations.
□ Nitrogen dioxide, a severe lung irritant produced by the same sources as carbon monoxide.

How can I tell if my home is sealed too tightly?

You may have an indoor pollution problem if you or members of your family are experiencing otherwise unexplainable headaches, dizziness, fatigue, or irritation of the eyes, nose, and throat—especially if the symptoms subside when you are away from home for a time and recur when you return.

If your health problems developed shortly after you redecorated your house or moved into a new one, the cause may be formaldehyde and other gases emitted by carpeting or new furnishings. The effects of these pollutants are most acute during the coldest and warmest seasons of the year, when windows are often kept closed.

It may sound simplistic, but the best way to reduce indoor air pollution is to maintain good ventilation in the house by keeping some windows partly open or using an exhaust fan to draw in outside air. Even in winter, cracking open a window won't add too much to your electricity bills and may help cut down the amount of pollutants you inhale.

If possible, schedule extensive painting or cleaning in the spring and fall, when doors and windows can be left open. Pick these times, too, for moving in new furniture or carpeting.

For more on cleaning the air inside your home, see page 297.

The insulation on the hot-water pipes in my basement contains asbestos. Should I have it removed?

Not necessarily. Asbestos usually isn't a hazard unless it's broken up, in which case it can release inhalable microscopic fibers. Have asbestos removed only when it is damaged or crumbling, or if it will be disturbed during remodeling or demolition. If it is undamaged, leave it in place. If you are not sure whether a product in your home contains asbestos, ask the manufacturer or hire an experienced asbestos consultant to do a survey of your home. Do not attempt to remove asbestos yourself.

What's the best way to remove asbestos?

Hire a contractor who has had special training in this area. Since 1985 the U.S. Environmental Protection Agency has funded training centers around the country, which have turned out more than 10,000 specialists in asbestos control. Ask to see the contractor's certificate verifying training, and ask for references from previous clients. Make sure the asbestos contractor you hire

---

FACT OR FALLACY?

Sidestream smoke from low-tar cigarettes is safer than smoke from regular cigarettes

Fallacy. A study by the U.S. Department of Agriculture has found that the smoke from low-tar cigarettes may actually be *more* harmful. Tests performed by the USDA's Tobacco Quality and Safety Research Lab in Athens, Georgia, found that while low-tar smoke was less harmful to smokers, the effects were reversed for people inhaling sidestream smoke (the smoke that gets into the air as cigarettes burn between puffs). The reason may be that low-tar cigarettes release more toxic fumes through the burning end than through the filter end.

---

takes the following precautions:
☐ Closes the heating and air-conditioning system before any work begins.
☐ Seals off the work site from the rest of the house and clearly marks the site as a danger area.
☐ Provides workers with protective clothing, including respirators, gloves, and hats, and disposes of them after use.
☐ Wets down all asbestos-containing material with a hand sprayer before cleaning up, to keep fibers from becoming airborne.
☐ Drills or cuts asbestos-containing material in a special containment room. The material should be wet down before it is drilled or cut.
☐ Removes materials in com-

---

plete pieces whenever possible; if large pieces are broken up for easy removal, they are more apt to release asbestos into the air.
☐ Supplies thick, leakproof plastic bags to contain debris and any materials that are removed. The bags should be sealed, labeled, and taken to an approved landfill.
☐ Thoroughly cleans the work area with wet rags, mops, or sponges when the job is completed; cleaning materials should be removed in sealed plastic bags.
Caution. Never sweep or dust materials or debris that might contain asbestos. Don't try to vacuum them. Asbestos fibers are so tiny that they are not captured in a vacuum cleaner, but pass through the filter and return to the air.

My husband smokes. How harmful is his habit for the rest of the family?

Very harmful. According to the Environmental Protection Agency, "passive smoking"—inhaling smoke from other people's cigarettes—may cause more than 3,800 lung cancer deaths annually and has been linked to an increased risk of heart disease. Children of smokers have respiratory and middle ear infections, bronchitis, and pneumonia more often than other children and miss more school days because of illness. Passive smoking may be even more dangerous to babies, because their immune systems are still immature.

So serious are the risks of passive smoking that the EPA has proposed declaring secondhand tobacco smoke a Class A human carcinogen, on a par with nine other pollutants such as asbestos and radon. Another federal agency, the Occupational Safety and Health Administration (OSHA), is considering labeling passive smoke a work hazard. OSHA's recommendations are likely to influence the workplace smoking policies of state and local governments as well as private employers.

I have a gas stove, and the kitchen isn't well ventilated. Are there any precautions I should take?

Smoke and fumes from combustion devices, including gas stoves and ovens, contain carbon monoxide and nitrogen dioxide, both common pollutants of indoor air (p.293). To minimize the problem, make sure that your stove is operating efficiently (burner flames should be blue; if they are yellow, too high, or noisy, have your utility company inspect the stove). Make sure, too, that the range hood is vented to the outdoors. Keep some air circulating in the kitchen by opening a window or using a window fan. Never use a kitchen stove or oven to heat a room.

Inhaling gas from a gas stove won't kill you, but it can make you sick, and if the gas builds up in an enclosed space, the result can be a deadly explosion or fire. Before buying a gas stove, make sure that it bears the seal of the American Gas Association. Have all gas appliances—stoves, water heaters, and dryers—installed by a professional plumber or appliance repair person. If you are moving into a house with used gas appliances, have the local utility check them for safety. The inspector can also show you where the gas cutoff valves are (they're usually under the burner top in gas stoves or under the broiler in ovens).

Gas appliances that are ignited by pilot lights (some stoves have an electric spark ignition instead) are usually equipped with automatic shutoff valves that stop the flow of gas when the pilot light goes out. If you smell a faint gas odor in the kitchen, check for a blown-out pilot light or burner flame on the stove or in the oven. Turn off the burner and air out the room (natural gas is lighter than air, so opening an upper window works best). When the smell has abated, you can safely relight the pilot lights.

A heavy gas odor is a serious danger signal. Immediately turn off burners, put out any flames in the house (candles on the dinner table, for example, or a cigarette), open windows and doors in the kitchen, and get everyone out of the house. If you can easily reach the gas cutoff valve in the stove, turn it off. Otherwise turn off the main gas supply at the meter. Don't touch a light switch, lamp, telephone, or anything else that could create a spark. Telephone the gas company from a neighbor's house and don't return home until the gas company gives you an all clear.

If you use bottled propane (liquefied petroleum gas) to fuel your stove, the same safety rules apply. Call your supplier or fire department for help if you smell a heavy odor of gas. When ventilating a room, however, bear in mind that propane is heavier than air and sinks to the floor.

Do wood-burning stoves pollute the air?

Old models do. Concern about this problem in the 1970's led to community, then state, and now national standards for smoke emissions from wood stoves. New stove designs introduced in the 1980's not only met the strict emissions standards set by Colorado and Oregon, but also burned fuel more efficiently, making them cheaper and safer to use (clean burning also mini-

mizes creosote buildup in the chimney, a major fire hazard with old stoves).

Since 1990 all wood-burning stoves sold in the United States have had to meet Environmental Protection Agency standards. Some approved stoves have an insulated secondary combustion chamber in which the unburned waste gases that make up smoke are ignited and burned off at temperatures above 1,000°F. A second type of clean-burning stove relies on a catalytic combustor, a device that facilitates the burning of waste gases at a lower temperature than is normally required for such combustion (500°F rather than 1,200°F). Some highly efficient stoves combine a secondary combustion chamber and a catalytic combustor.

Another EPA-approved option is a stove specially designed to burn wood pellets, a processed wood product whose low moisture content makes for a very clean-burning fuel. Some approved stoves are simply more efficient versions of the old airtight stoves, designed with smaller, better-insulated fireboxes.

If you have a wood-burning stove that predates the new standards, you may be able to add a catalytic combustor to its stovepipe, but retrofitting doesn't always work well and may not even be cost-effective. You can usually save enough in fuel and chimney-cleaning costs with an EPA-approved stove to recoup its price in 2 or 3 years.

A related source of pollution is the traditional wood-burning fireplace. Some communities already limit fireplace use. Others require that new fireplaces be equipped with glass doors and an outside air source. A fireplace insert, a stovelike device that fits into an existing masonry fireplace and is vented through

THE FACTS ABOUT RADON

What is it? Radon is a colorless, odorless natural gas formed by the breakdown of uranium in the earth. Found in varying concentrations all over the world, radon is dangerous to human beings only when it seeps out of the ground and becomes trapped in an enclosed space, such as a tightly sealed house.

Why is radon dangerous? Radon gas quickly breaks down into radioactive by-products, which if inhaled can lodge in the lungs and cause serious damage. The Environmental Protection Agency has estimated that as many as 16,000 lung cancer deaths each year (about 11 percent of the total) may be attributable to radon exposure in homes and in mines.

Whose homes are most at risk? Tightly sealed homes built in areas with rich uranium deposits are likely candidates (see map). The gas can enter a house through many pathways—dirt floors, cracked walls, joints, drains, and sumps. Every building has low-pressure areas that can draw radon indoors. Seepage is usually worse in winter (furnace-heated air rises, leaving a slight vacuum near the floor, which helps draw in radon).

Measuring radon. Two types of radon detectors are sold at hardware stores— the charcoal canister and the alpha track. Either is placed in a room for a specified time (3 to 7 days for the charcoal canister, 2 to 4 weeks for the alpha track detector) and is then sent to the manufacturer or a laboratory for analysis. A detector and the analysis generally cost less than $50. (Some state and local governments in high-radon areas provide detectors free to homeowners.)

Especially if you live in a high-radon area, have your home tested twice a year. Test heavily used areas of your house as well as the basement, if you have one. Close windows and doors in the rooms being tested for 12 hours prior to the test, and keep them closed during the test. Results are reported in either *working levels* (WL) or *picocuries per liter* (pCi/l). If the reading exceeds 0.02 WL or 4 pCi/l, your home has too much radon.

Radon remedies. If your home's radon levels are high, bring in an experienced contractor to assess the situation and recommend solutions. Ask the nearest EPA office or your state radiation agency for names of firms that have participated in the EPA's Radon Proficiency Program. (Fraud abounds in this field.) Sealing radon entry points and proper ventilation are the usual solutions to a radon problem. But since every house is different, it's best to have a professional devise a system tailored to your home. In the meantime, don't smoke or allow smoking in your house (smoking makes radon deadlier).

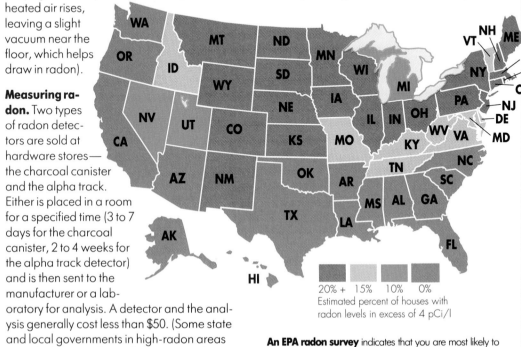

20% + 15% 10% 0%
Estimated percent of houses with
radon levels in excess of 4 pCi/l

An EPA radon survey indicates that you are most likely to have a radon problem if you live in the Northeast or Midwest.

the chimney, can reduce the pollution emitted by a fireplace while enhancing its efficiency.

I'm buying a room heater. What safety and pollution factors should I keep in mind?

You must take certain safety precautions with any room or space heater: Do not place it where it can be knocked over; keep it away from curtains, upholstery, papers, and other combustible materials (never use the heater to dry clothing); and do not leave small children alone in a room with a heater.

Space heaters are fueled by gas, kerosene, or electricity. To be safe, gas and kerosene heaters must be installed with outside vents to draw in fresh air for combustion and to exhaust wastes. Unvented gas and kerosene heaters are dangerous and have been banned in certain parts of the country; they can use up a room's supply of oxygen without warning, leaving occupants breathing a lethal dose of carbon monoxide. Although vented gas and kerosene heaters are more expensive to buy and to install than electric heaters, both are cheaper to run.

Clean and convenient, electric heaters come in two basic types: convection and radiant heaters. Convection heaters warm a whole room; radiant heaters spot-heat, warming you or a piece of furniture, not the air.

How effective an air cleaner is an air conditioner?

Air conditioning—whether it is a centralized system or a window unit—can improve the air quality in your home in two ways: it reduces humidity, cutting down on the growth of molds and fungi, and it filters pollen and spores from outside air before they are drawn in. However, you must keep the system scrubbed and vacuumed to prevent it from becoming a breeding ground for microorganisms. A central system and its ducts should be professionally cleaned every year. If you have a window unit, remove the front panel every month or so during the warm season and wash the metal coils in tepid water and borax. Remove the filter and wash it in a basin of detergent and water. Vacuum all accessible surfaces.

What steps can I take to clean up the air in my home?

The old-fashioned way is still the best: open windows at opposite ends of the house for natural cross ventilation. Use exhaust fans to vent kitchen and bathroom fumes and condensation. Airing out is particularly important in a weathertight house. Before fuel-conscious Americans began insulating and sealing their homes, the air in an average house would be exchanged for outdoor air every hour. Now, it may take 4 to 10 hours.

If there is a smoker in the house or if you question the quality of the outdoor air in your area, consider using an air purifier. It won't remove dangerous gases or odors or dust and other particles that have settled on room surfaces, but it can dilute heavy concentrations of irritating smoke and remove dust and pollen suspended in the air. There are four basic types of air cleaner:
☐ In straight filter models, a fan draws air through densely packed fibers, which trap particulate matter in the air. The best types use high-efficiency particulate-arresting (HEPA) filters. Filters must be replaced periodically.

☐ Electrostatic precipitators charge the air and its particles as they are drawn in by a fan. A polarized plate attracts and holds the charged particles, much as a magnet attracts metal filings. The plate must be removed and washed (in a dishwasher or bathtub) once a month. A whole-house unit can be installed in a forced-air heating and cooling system (prolonging its life), or you can plug in a room model.
☐ "Electret" filter units draw air through an electrically charged polyester mesh filter that traps the particles. Found most often in tabletop units designed for small spaces, electret filters must be replaced periodically.
☐ Ionizers charge the surrounding air with high voltage. The charged air molecules then attract airborne particles, which, in better models, are drawn by a fan through a replaceable filter (without the filter and fan, particles will stick to the wall nearest to the ionizer).

The National Air and Space Administration has done interesting research on the value of houseplants as pollution fighters in closed quarters. Spider plants, English ivy, ficus, and potted mums, for example, have been found to absorb three volatile organic chemicals: benzene, trichloroethylene (TCE), and formaldehyde. Homeowners who enjoy raising houseplants can take pleasure in their hobby's contribution to a healthy indoor environment. However, the number of plants needed to purify a room would daunt anyone without a green thumb.

What can I do to reduce pollution from my car?

Air pollution from automobiles is caused chiefly by gasoline exhaust fumes. The most important thing you can do is to burn less fuel. (Of course, this will save you money too.)

☐ Make fuel efficiency your number-one priority when you shop for a new car.

☐ Buy unleaded gasoline or one of the new gasolines, formulated for older cars and trucks, that have a reduced lead content.

☐ Use public transportation or a carpool whenever you can. For short trips, walk or ride a bicycle. Your car emits more toxic fumes and burns more than twice as much gasoline during the first few minutes of starting up than during normal operation.

☐ Take your automobile in for regular tune-ups and schedule periodic checks for your emissions system too.

☐ Replace your air filter at 15,000-mile intervals or sooner.

☐ Use radial tires, which if kept properly inflated can improve fuel economy by as much as 1 mile per gallon. Any type of tire that doesn't have enough air will drag, which can increase fuel consumption by up to 6 percent.

☐ Drive at a steady, moderate speed, avoiding sudden starts and stops. A car burns less gasoline at 55 mph than at 65 mph.

☐ If your car must be in idle for more than a minute, you'll conserve fuel by shutting off the engine. For less than 60 seconds, leave the engine running.

How serious a threat to young children is lead poisoning?

It is one of the most pervasive environmental threats to children's health today. Although federal regulations have cut overall lead pollution from automobiles, smelters, and factories by more than 90 percent since 1978, the lead that has already been released into the environment still contaminates our air, water, and soil. In addition,

FACT OR FALLACY?

Lead crystal containers pose a health risk

Fact. Lead crystal goblets and decanters, treasured for their sparkle, have recently been found to leach lead into the liquids they contain. Drinking wine from a crystal goblet now and then won't hurt you, although daily use is not recommended. But wines and liquors stored in lead crystal decanters acquire toxic levels of lead within 3 or 4 months; even a week or two may be too long, according to the Food and Drug Administration.

Amalgam tooth fillings cause mercury poisoning

Fallacy. News reports in 1990 raised doubts about the safety of the inexpensive silver-colored amalgam fillings dentists have used for over 150 years. The stories also suggested that taking out the fillings would relieve symptoms of diseases ranging from arthritis to multiple sclerosis. The American Dental Association disputes these claims, pointing out that no scientifically reliable study has found the mercury in amalgam to cause adverse health effects in the general population. Removing an old filling, the ADA adds, can jeopardize the soundness of a tooth, creating more problems for the patient.

the interior surfaces of about 57 million U.S. households are covered with lead-based paint, manufactured before the lead content in residential paint was controlled by law in the 1970's. Lead-based paint is still available to industry and the military, and sometimes winds up in private homes today.

Even moderately high levels of lead in a child's system may be enough to cause neurological damage that persists into and beyond adolescence. In a study conducted by researchers at the University of Pittsburgh between 1975 and 1978, a group of 270 first- and second-graders from a sampling of 2,335 children were identified as having elevated lead levels in their bodies. Of this group, 132 were retested in 1988, and although their blood lead levels were normal, the teenagers had lower grades, lower scores in reading and vocabulary tests, and poorer hand-eye coordination than other students in their age group.

How can I keep my child from ingesting lead?

Familiarize yourself with the common sources of lead exposure and try to eliminate them. A child can ingest lead by drinking water with a high lead content, by playing in soil containing lead dust, by eating food packed in lead-soldered cans, by eating lead-based paint chips, or by inhaling lead dust and fumes indoors. Make sure that your drinking water does not contain unhealthy levels of lead (p. 288). Since young children will put almost anything in their mouths, take care that they don't eat soil. A can with spots of solder visible on the seam is probably lead-soldered. Avoid such cans, or if you do buy them, don't leave leftover food in them.

The principal source of lead poisoning in children continues to be lead-based paint (the biggest problem comes from inhaling paint dust, rather than from eating paint chips). Your local health department or housing authority can give you the names of companies that will test your paint for lead content.

If there is suspect paint on your walls, cover it over with wallpaper or new paint; scraping or sanding the old paint off will simply put more lead dust into the air. Frequently washing walls, floors, and woodwork minimizes the risk of exposure to dust. Also check to see that your children's school and any homes they visit often (those of relatives, friends, babysitters) do not contain old, flaking paint.

If your children seem chronically fatigued or if they often have abdominal pains you can't account for, tell your pediatrician that you are concerned about their blood levels of lead. In its early stages, lead poisoning is treatable and can be reversed.

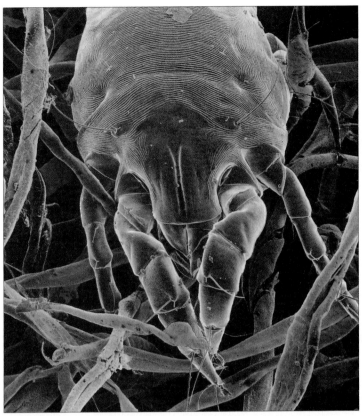

As tiny as grains of sand, dust mites by the millions lurk in bedding and carpets.

What is dust made of? Can dust be bad for your health?

Dust consists of tiny particles of solid matter, including specks of minerals picked up by the wind, mold and bacterial spores, pollen, and, in vast quantities, the fecal pellets of house dust mites, microscopic creatures that thrive in carpets and bedding by feeding on sloughed-off human skin cells.

Dust can serve as a carrier for infectious diseases and is a major trigger of allergic reactions. It may also contain toxic substances, such as insecticide residues, lead, and asbestos fibers, which can cause serious health problems if they are inhaled in sufficient quantities.

To minimize dust, vacuum your house often. However, since vacuuming stirs dust and other allergens into the air, have someone else do the job if you are allergic and stay out of recently vacuumed rooms for at least an hour, until the dust settles. If this is not practical, wear a disposable dust mask while vacuuming. Bear in mind that most dust particles are too large to remain airborne for long, and consequently are seldom affected by air purifiers (p. 297).

To reduce the dust mite population in your home, wash blankets and bed linens often in hot water. If you are allergic to dust mites and their droppings, you can buy miteproof pillowcases and mattress covers at surgical supply stores; vinyl coverings are available at some department stores.

I live in a noisy urban neighborhood, plagued by loud radios and blaring horns. Can this hurt my hearing?

It certainly can. A single very loud noise or, more commonly, continual exposure to noise above 90 decibels (see *Living in a Noisy World*, p. 300) can damage delicate cells in the inner ear known as hair cells and lead to loss of hearing.

High-frequency hearing, which detects the consonant sounds in words, is the first to suffer. That is why a person who is experiencing hearing loss can hear voices but has trouble understanding what is being said.

About 60 million people are exposed to more noise from city traffic than the EPA considers safe. In addition to causing hear-

LIVING IN A NOISY WORLD

Taking steps to turn your home into a peaceful haven will not only protect the hearing of all family members but will reduce stress levels too. Listed below at left are common sources of noise and their average decibel ratings. At right are tips for keeping things quiet in and around the house.

HOW LOUD IS LOUD?

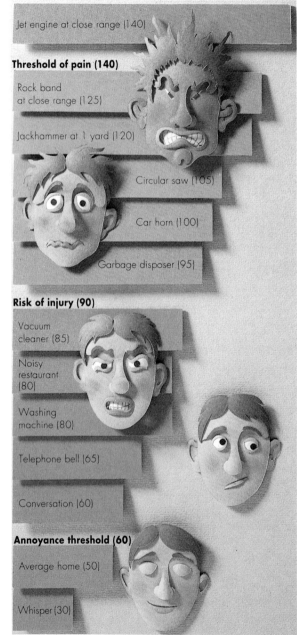

Jet engine at close range (140)

Threshold of pain (140)

Rock band
at close range (125)

Jackhammer at 1 yard (120)

Circular saw (105)

Car horn (100)

Garbage disposer (95)

Risk of injury (90)

Vacuum
cleaner (85)

Noisy
restaurant
(80)

Washing
machine (80)

Telephone bell (65)

Conversation (60)

Annoyance threshold (60)

Average home (50)

Whisper (30)

The relative loudness of sounds is measured in decibels. Continual exposure to sounds above 90 decibels can damage hearing.

Dampening indoor noise

☐ Start by selecting quiet household appliances. Before you buy any equipment, listen to various models to determine which emits the least noise.

☐ If you already have a noisy appliance, balance rotating parts and lubricate moving ones. Cover vibrating surfaces, such as the sides of a dishwasher or laundry machine, with large self-adhesive foam pads. Set a noisy furnace on resilient rubber or cork pads.

☐ Heavy lined draperies, thick padded carpeting, and upholstered furniture will soak up indoor noise. Soft, porous materials such as wool and felt are especially effective noise mufflers.

☐ You can muffle sound on indoor walls with a covering of plaster, wallboard, or cork-covered tile. Although they take up floor space, bookshelves help too.

Blocking outdoor noise

☐ Help mute incoming sounds by insulating exterior walls and under the roof.

☐ Use weatherstripping or putty to seal any cracks or holes that admit sound. Caulk around windows, doors, and electrical oulets on outside walls.

☐ Room air conditioners should be surrounded by gaskets, available at hardware stores and home centers, so that their vibration will not travel through the walls.

☐ Double-paned windows, designed to insulate, also reduce sound significantly. Or install interior storm windows.

☐ Entrance doors should fit snugly when they are closed. Avoid hollow-core doors, which admit up to four times as much noise as solid ones. Use solid doors inside, too, for especially noisy rooms, such as a workshop or laundry.

ing loss, noise is physically and psychologically stressful. It can disrupt sleep and make you tired and tense. It can also have a negative impact on children's learning skills.

We are expecting our first child in 6 months. Can noise pollution harm unborn children?

It may. The National Research Council has investigated reports of a higher rate of birth defects and low birth weight in babies born to women living near large airports. Although the evidence was not strong enough to establish a direct cause-and-effect relationship between fetal damage and noise, the council did recommend that pregnant women avoid long exposure to very loud sounds.

What is radiation and how dangerous is it?

Radiation is energy that travels through space or matter in the form of electromagnetic waves or high-energy particles. There is no way to escape radiation; whether natural (from the sun, other objects in space, or rocks and minerals in the earth) or man-made (microwaves and radio waves, for example), radiation is literally everywhere.

Radiation can be divided into two basic categories. *Ionizing radiation* is powerful enough to knock one or more electrons out of an atom, converting the atom into a charged particle called an ion. X-rays, gamma rays, and nuclear radiation are forms of ionizing radiation. Less powerful *nonionizing radiation* (ultraviolet light, microwaves, and radio waves, for example) leaves atoms intact but increases the rate at which molecules vibrate, thereby generating heat.

From a health point of view, radiation is a two-edged sword. We rely on light and heat from the sun for our very survival, yet overexposure to the sun's ultraviolet light is the leading cause of skin cancer. X-rays and other forms of ionizing radiation are extremely beneficial when they are used in controlled doses for diagnostic tests (pp. 126–127) or for therapeutic purposes (to destroy malignant tumors, for example). But in high doses, this type of radiation can kill quickly or seriously damage body tissues and cells, especially reproductive cells.

Although accidents at Three Mile Island and Chernobyl have focused public concern on the dangers of ionizing radiation, increasing attention is being paid to the potential hazards of a much more pervasive form of radiation. Microwaves are nonionizing radio waves with very short wavelengths. They are emitted by radar installations, TV transmitters, CB radios, satellites, telephone relay systems, and of course, microwave ovens. Direct exposure to intense microwave radiation can burn human body tissue just as readily as it can cook a steak. But although the evidence is still being gathered and debated, prolonged exposure to low levels of microwaves, such as those emitted by radar and telecommunications installations, has been linked to an increased risk of cancer and sterility.

I bought a microwave oven recently. What precautions should I take in using it, if any?

The U.S. Food and Drug Administration has set radiation leakage standards for microwave ovens manufactured after October 6, 1971. But if an oven's door interlock system, which cuts off microwave production when the door is open, isn't working properly, the unit can leak radiation. When you buy a microwave oven, make sure it hasn't been damaged in shipping, place it in a low-traffic area of the kitchen, and follow the manufacturer's directions carefully. Check the unit periodically to see that door hinges and latches are working properly. If you suspect a problem, have the oven tested for leakage by a qualified dealer, service center, or government testing service (or buy a microwave leakage tester at a hardware or electronics store).

Don't turn on the microwave before the food has been placed inside. During operation, do not tamper with the interlock system or try to pry open the door. (If your oven was made before 1971 and doesn't have this system, take care not to operate it with the door open and stay at least 2 feet away when it's on.)

Clean the door seal regularly with mild soap and water so that the door remains absolutely flush with the oven; also use a mild soap solution—not abrasives—to clean the interior.

Aside from leakage hazards, there are other safety considerations to keep in mind. Sugar heats rapidly in a microwave and sometimes burns. (Dishes containing metal also flash and spark in a microwave and should never be used for this purpose.) If a fire does start in your oven, don't try to put it out yourself. Leave the door closed, unplug the unit, and wait for the fire to go out before you open the door again.

It's also easy to be burned by steam that escapes as you remove plastic wrap from a microwavable container. For this reason, and because some scientists now claim that small quantities of the carcinogens benzene, toluene, and PVC may leach from "microwave safe" plastic wraps and cookware, it's prudent to use glass containers for microwave cooking. Remove any dish, even a glass one, with pot holders. Although the microwave oven doesn't heat the dish, the cooked food it contains may make it too hot to handle.

Food tends to cook unevenly in a microwave oven. While one section may turn out just right, another may be under-cooked, creating the risk of food poisoning. To ensure that microwaved food cooks thor-oughly, let it stand after cooking for the time specified in the cooking directions.

Children enjoy using micro-wave ovens, and many microwa-vable food products are being marketed for young consumers. Yet children are particularly vul-nerable to hazards created by mi-crowaves. Watching foods cook through the glass door, for ex-ample, may damage a child's eyes if radiation is leaking through the door seal. Some chil-dren have been injured by the jelly-doughnut effect—while the doughnut may be lukewarm out-side, the jelly inside may be hot enough to burn the mouth and throat. To be on the safe side, don't allow children under 7 to operate the oven, and make sure that older children know and observe all the safety rules listed above. Teach them that a micro-wave oven is not a toy but a serious adult appliance.

I've heard that radiation from home appliances can be a health hazard. Is this true?

It may be. There is concern about the electromagnetic fields generated by electricity (see *Electromagnetic Pollution,* right). How such fields affect body tis-sues is not fully understood, but

ELECTROMAGNETIC POLLUTION

We take electricity for granted in our lives. But there is growing evidence that exposure to "electric smog" could also be making us sick. When an electric current passes through wires, it affects electrons in the air around the wire, creating what is known as an electromagnetic field. The fields surrounding electrical appli-ances, electrical substations and transformers, and high-volt-age power lines are called ELF fields because their currents oscillate at extremely low frequencies (about 60 hertz).

Initial U.S. and European studies suggested that people ex-posed to ELF fields for a prolonged period had slower reaction times and motor responses, disturbed circadian rhythms, a weakening of the immune system's ability to ward off disease, and in men, lower fertility. But the early research was consid-ered inconclusive because of flaws in the way it was carried out. Then in 1987 a 5-year study by the New York Power Line Research Project found that homes near power distribution lines suffered an incidence of childhood cancer from 1.4 to 2 times that in homes farther away. In 1990 the Environmental Protec-tion Agency concluded that there is a "possible but not proven" correlation between electromagnetic fields and cancer.

Levels of electromagnetic radiation are measured in milli-gauss (0.3 milligauss is thought to be harmless; more than 3 milligauss may not be). Some utility companies will make free surveys in homes and schools, and commercial testing firms offer inspections for a fee. Magnetic-field meters can also be bought or rented. While research and debate continue, some scientists recommend "prudent avoidance" of ELF fields, which drop swiftly within a few feet or yards of the source. It may be wise to keep your children from playing directly under electrical transformers and power lines outdoors; and don't place their beds near the point where electricity enters your house.

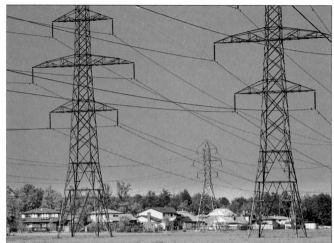

Concern about the potential hazards of electromagnetic fields has led some states to limit magnetic-field strength around transmission lines.

a growing number of studies are showing a correlation between exposure to electromagnetic fields— whether from high-power lines or from household appliances—and increased cancer risk.

The amount of exposure people get from most small appliances (toasters or hair dryers, for example) is thought to be limited, because an appliance's electromagnetic field usually drops sharply within a few inches of the motor, and the time a person remains in its sphere is brief.

However, when exposure to electromagnetic fields lasts longer, as is the case with electric blankets and water-bed heaters, the danger may be greater. Some studies have detected an increased risk of birth defects and cancer among children of women who used electric blankets during their pregnancy.

While the health effects of electromagnetic fields are being investigated and debated, you can limit your direct exposure at home by taking these steps:

☐ If you have an electric blanket or an electric mattress pad, use it to preheat the bed and then unplug it before you retire. This precaution seems especially advisable for pregnant women.

☐ Don't use an electrically heated water bed.

☐ Keep electric clocks at least a yard away from your bed.

☐ If you use a video display terminal, sit at least 24 inches away from it (p.321).

What common household products should be handled with care?

Home Sweet Home is not always Home Safe Home. Many of the everyday products we use to do the laundry and clean the house can be dangerous both to the environment and to health.

☐ Laundry detergents are usually nonbiodegradable and may contain ammonia (a powerful toxin and lung irritant), phenol (which can cause liver, kidney, and neurological damage), and other noxious chemicals.

☐ Fabric softeners contain substances that can irritate the skin and cause allergic reactions in some people.

☐ Spray starch may contain phenol, formaldehyde (p.293), and other toxic chemicals.

☐ Disinfectants contain a number of very toxic ingredients, including ammonia, phenol, and cresol (a compound with health hazards similar to those of phenol).

☐ Dishwashing liquids contain nonbiodegradable detergents and potentially harmful dyes and fragrances. They are a major cause of poisoning in children.

☐ Drain, toilet bowl, and oven cleaners may contain lye and/or hydrochloric acid. Both are powerful toxins that can burn the skin, burn internal organs if swallowed, or cause blindness if the product should come into contact with the eyes.

☐ Glass cleaners and metal polishes contain ammonia and other toxic substances.

☐ Floor and furniture polishes may contain phenol as well as volatile toxic solvents that can linger in the air for days.

☐ Paint, paint thinners, and varnishes contain hundreds of toxins and carcinogens. Toxic vapors from varnishes can linger in the air for months.

☐ Pesticides are poisons that should be avoided whenever possible (p.315), or at least not used where food is prepared.

☐ Aerosol sprays have been reformulated to avoid damaging the earth's ozone layer (p.293). Unfortunately, the new propellants (propane, nitrous oxide, and worst of all, methylene chloride) are highly flammable, probably carcinogenic, and harmful to the nervous system. Potentially toxic if inhaled, aerosol sprays can burn the eyes if sprayed in the wrong direction.

Is there any way to reduce the danger of toxic household products?

The best way is to avoid them altogether by using nontoxic alternative cleaning products (see *A Green Shopping Guide*, p.304). If you do use commercial cleaners, handle and store them with care. Become familiar with their contents, and be sure you know exactly how to use each product. Reread directions and warning labels from time to time, even if you think you know what they say. When buying spray products, look for pump dispensers; avoid aerosol cans.

When using a caustic agent, such as an oven cleaner, wear rubber gloves, long-sleeved clothing, and safety goggles. If you are working with paints or other substances that give off toxic fumes, make sure that your work area is well ventilated.

Caution. Never mix ammonia and bleach or products containing them. The combination creates toxic chloramine gas. Also highly dangerous is the combination of bleach and the acid in toilet bowl cleaners; the result of this mix is deadly chlorine gas.

Although household chemicals can harm anyone, children are most at risk. A child may be drawn to a toxic product because of its attractive packaging and touch or ingest it before you can intervene. If you have a child in the house, keep household cleaning items under lock and key. And when you use such products, never allow yourself to be distracted and leave a child unattended near them, not even for a few minutes.

A GREEN SHOPPING GUIDE

To keep your home healthy and safe, limit the toxic materials you bring into it. Think twice about the everyday products you buy at the grocery. Some items that you take for granted (chlorine bleach or disinfectants with phenol, for example) give off potentially cancer-causing fumes; others pose a threat to your immediate environment (solvents and nonbiodegradable detergents flushed down your drain can harm local water supplies). Listed below are non- or less-toxic alternatives to common household products.

Household cleaners. An effective nontoxic cleaning kit will include baking soda, salt, distilled white vinegar, and lemon juice. Dilute ½ cup white vinegar with 2 cups water to clean spots (even animal urine) out of the carpet. Pour table salt on red wine to soak it up. Lemon juice will remove rust spots and added to water will cut grease on counters and cabinets. Instead of a caustic drain cleaner, use a mixture of ¼ cup baking soda with ½ cup vinegar. Pour the solution down the drain, and stopper it tightly for 2 or 3 minutes. Then flush with hot water.

Personal hygiene products. Use shaving soap and a brush instead of commercial shaving creams. The latter often contain ammonia and ethanol, and while the spray cans that many shaving creams come in no longer use ozone-destroying chlorofluorocarbons, they now emit hydrocarbons, which pollute the air and create smog. For an effective homemade deodorant, combine equal parts of baking soda and cornstarch. And substitute cornstarch for talcum powder, which may be harmful if inhaled.

Laundry products. Use a soap powder or a phosphate-free liquid detergent to wash clothes. The phosphates in many powdered detergents pollute and clog waterways. If you like to add fabric softener to your wash, try using a cup of vinegar in the final rinse. (Natural fibers generally don't need a softener.) Instead of buying an aerosol spray starch, make your own natural spray by adding 2 tablespoons of cornstarch to a pint of water in a reusable spray bottle.

Air fresheners. Commercial air fresheners keep you from detecting offensive odors by coating your nasal passages, not by dispersing the smell. Your house will be fresher if you stick to natural remedies. Keep bathrooms and kitchens spotlessly clean. To freshen the air, leave small bowls of vinegar or baking soda on a counter in the kitchen or bathroom, or simmer some cloves, a piece of cinnamon stick, and the peel of a lemon, orange, or apple in water to create a natural fragrance.

Pest control products for pets. Commercial flea and tick sprays, dips, and powders are dangerous pesticides, which your cat or dog may ingest while grooming itself (and which children may pick up by petting the animal). Use flea and tick collars instead, or try stuffing a pillow with cedar chips to make a flea-repellent pet bed. The best defenses against pests, however, are good nutrition and hygiene. Wash your pet with soap, and check daily for fleas and ticks with a fine-tooth comb.

Are cockroaches a health hazard? What's the best way to get rid of them?

A cockroach may have spent time in a sewer or other unsanitary locale before arriving in your kitchen. It may carry salmonella (p.50) and other disease-causing microbes, and pass them on to you via the cooking utensils or food it touches. Roaches molt often while they grow, and the skin particles become airborne; an estimated 10 to 15 million Americans experience runny noses, skin irritation, and asthmatic symptoms or attacks when cockroaches are near.

The way to discourage roaches is to deprive them of their dwelling places, food, and water. Fill in the crevices where they hide with caulk; don't forget openings around incoming pipes and electrical outlets. Keep all food in closed containers or the refrigerator; don't leave uneaten pet food out either. Eliminate clutter and any source of moisture: wring out wet mops and sponges. Since roaches like stagnant air, good ventilation may encourage them to move on.

The new roach killers and

traps on the market, which contain amidinohydrazones, are very effective, and roaches have not developed an immunity to them. For an inexpensive and less toxic alternative, try sprinkling 99 percent boric acid dust in a thin layer wherever roaches have been seen. The insects ingest the dust when they groom themselves and die within a few days. Don't use boric acid, however, if you have young children who might put it in their mouths; it will make them ill.

How can I keep other household pests under control?

☐ To keep clothing moth free, be sure it is clean before storing it in airtight boxes or bags. Add cedar chips or dried lavender—they repel moths and leave clothes smelling fresh.

☐ Want to ward off ants? Try putting coffee grounds around doors and windows. Peppermint plants or crushed mint placed near entryways also will work.

☐ Proper sanitation is the key to fly control. Keep all your garbage cans clean and tightly shut. A garbage can should have a lid with a fastener to keep dogs or raccoons from opening it, and there should be no holes on the bottom or sides of the can. Tie garbage bags securely.

Don't let organic wastes accumulate in your kitchen. Check your fruit bowls often and throw out any pieces that are beginning to soften. Dispose of uneaten pet food promptly.

Use a scooper or plastic bag to remove and dispose of pet feces, which can serve as a breeding site for flies.

Placing pots of sweet basil outdoors or in window boxes or hanging bunches of dried tansy outdoors may keep flies from coming into your home.

☐ To keep mosquitoes away, screen all doors and windows, and use a yellow bug light outside entrances. (Electronic zappers kill beneficial insects, but are not very effective against mosquitoes.) Since mosquito larvae hatch in standing water, use an old broom or mop to disperse puddles that collect around your house after a rain. Try planting garlic or marigolds around your house; mosquitoes seem to find these plants repellent.

There are a number of insect repellents on the market that will discourage flies and mosquitoes. Spray them on your clothes and around doors and windows. If you prefer a noncommercial repellent, try rubbing a bit of vinegar on your exposed skin. To avoid attracting the attention of insects, don't wear perfumes or perfumed products.

Should homeowners worry about seeing an occasional mouse?

Mice do carry diseases, but the compounds made to kill them are far more dangerous. They include some of the deadliest pesticides made today and often contain such fast-acting poisons as arsenic, strychnine, or phosphorus.

As with roaches (see facing page), cleanliness and proper food storage are essential to keeping mice out of your house. Make sure, too, that all mouse holes are plugged with steel wool, plaster, or sheet metal.

Although a cat can help reduce your mouse population, the best way to get rid of rodents is still a snap-back mousetrap baited with peanut butter. Place the traps with the trigger end touching the baseboards along which mice tend to travel. Change the traps' location and the bait frequently so that mice don't learn to avoid them. Glue traps

are very effective and don't require bait, but they strike many people as inhumane. Nonlethal traps are humane and safe around children and pets, but leave you with the problem of disposing of live vermin (preferably in the wild, far from housing).

We are moving into a new house. What health factors should I keep in mind before I buy furnishings?

Furniture that is made of pressed-wood products or covered with synthetic fabrics may contribute to indoor air pollution by giving off formaldehyde fumes. Mobile homes are most affected by this because they make greater use of synthetics within a smaller area. In the event of a fire, smoke from synthetic fabrics and stuffing may emit lethal gases, such as carbon monoxide.

For your new home, use as much wood furniture (not wood veneer or particleboard) as is practical. Another nonpolluting material is metal, favored by people who like a modern look as well as durability in their furnishings. Of course, both wood and metal are also excellent shelving materials. Don't hesitate to buy used furniture if you see something that appeals to you; older furniture is generally made with fewer synthetics, and any that were used are apt to have emitted their undesirable fumes.

Most no-iron bed linens and permanent-press clothes have been treated with formaldehyde finishes. As long as you don't mind ironing them, unfinished natural fabrics are preferable. (Certain fabrics, such as wool or cotton flannel, tend to resist wrinkling naturally, without the use of a no-iron finish.) If the convenience of no-iron fabrics is important to you, at least put the

Continued on page 308

The serious health consequences of many common environmental problems should make you think twice about where you choose to live. If you have any concerns about the safety of a house, have the water supply tested (pp.288,290) and contact the local health department or environmental agency about the area's air quality (p.292) and the lead content of its soil (p.298). You cannot control all the potential hazards that a house is subject to, but you can oppose policies and practices that create pollution and support efforts to improve your local environment (see *Creating a Healthier Planet*, p.289).

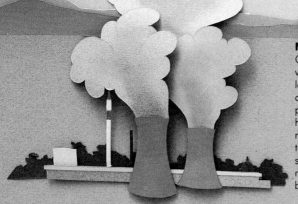

Near a nuclear power plant. Check radiation levels of the local water supply and air (even low levels can cause cancer). The risk of radiation exposure from the plant's operation is not statistically high, but how the plant handles its nuclear wastes, which can contaminate nearby air and water supplies, should concern you. A major nuclear accident is unlikely, but the effects could be lethal.

Near a medical facility. Have the water tested and find out if local beaches are safe for recreation (p.292). In recent years millions of pounds of infectious hospital wastes — which include body fluids from hepatitis, cancer, and AIDS patients, as well as used needles, linens, and bandages — have found their way illegally into city sewer systems and into the ocean. Medical radioactive wastes are less toxic and break down faster than radioactive industrial wastes.

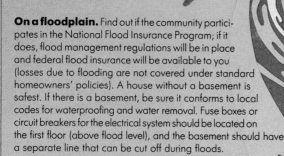

On a floodplain. Find out if the community participates in the National Flood Insurance Program; if it does, flood management regulations will be in place and federal flood insurance will be available to you (losses due to flooding are not covered under standard homeowners' policies). A house without a basement is safest. If there is a basement, be sure it conforms to local codes for waterproofing and water removal. Fuse boxes or circuit breakers for the electrical system should be located on the first floor (above flood level), and the basement should have a separate line that can be cut off during floods.

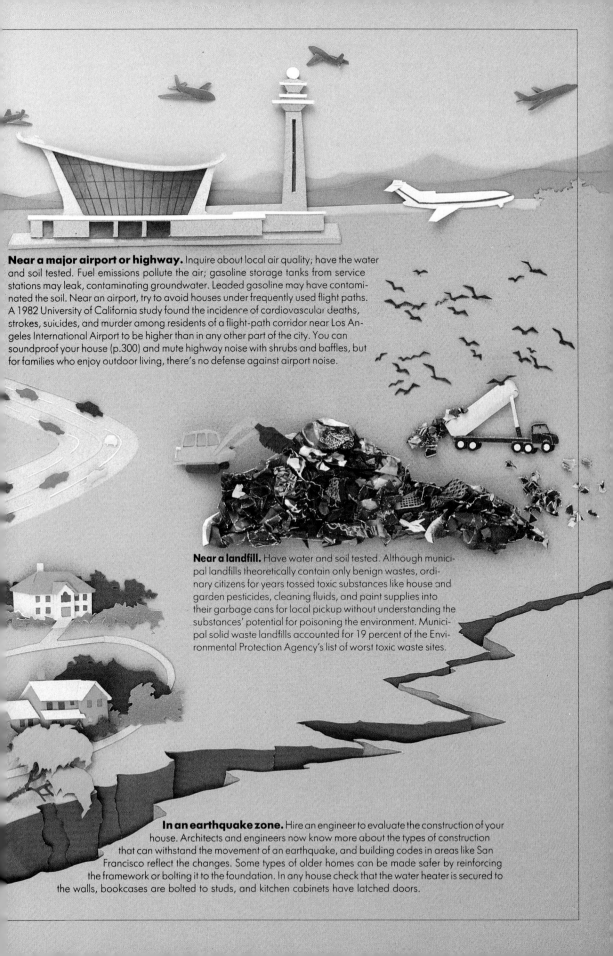

Near a major airport or highway. Inquire about local air quality; have the water and soil tested. Fuel emissions pollute the air; gasoline storage tanks from service stations may leak, contaminating groundwater. Leaded gasoline may have contaminated the soil. Near an airport, try to avoid houses under frequently used flight paths. A 1982 University of California study found the incidence of cardiovascular deaths, strokes, suicides, and murder among residents of a flight-path corridor near Los Angeles International Airport to be higher than in any other part of the city. You can soundproof your house (p.300) and mute highway noise with shrubs and baffles, but for families who enjoy outdoor living, there's no defense against airport noise.

Near a landfill. Have water and soil tested. Although municipal landfills theoretically contain only benign wastes, ordinary citizens for years tossed toxic substances like house and garden pesticides, cleaning fluids, and paint supplies into their garbage cans for local pickup without understanding the substances' potential for poisoning the environment. Municipal solid waste landfills accounted for 19 percent of the Environmental Protection Agency's list of worst toxic waste sites.

In an earthquake zone. Hire an engineer to evaluate the construction of your house. Architects and engineers now know more about the types of construction that can withstand the movement of an earthquake, and building codes in areas like San Francisco reflect the changes. Some types of older homes can be made safer by reinforcing the framework or bolting it to the foundation. In any house check that the water heater is secured to the walls, bookcases are bolted to studs, and kitchen cabinets have latched doors.

garment or sheet through a laundering or two before you use it.

Most new carpeting, especially new padding, has been treated with acrylic finishes that can produce eye and throat irritation and nausea in some people. Your dealer may be willing to air out the carpet before it is delivered. In any case, see that there is adequate ventilation when new carpeting is being installed. Then leave the windows open and shut the room for 48 hours after the rugs are down.

I've heard that a lot of home accidents happen in the bathroom. How can I prevent them?

Thousands of injuries and drownings occur in U.S. bathrooms every year; most could have been avoided with some simple safety measures.

Use a mat with suction pads or paste down decals to provide nonslip flooring for a shower or tub. Install a grab bar on the side of the tub or on a wall where needed (anchor wall-mounted bars into studs). Mop up puddles right away, and be sure that rugs have nonskid backings.

Keep breakable items out of the bathroom. Drinking glasses should be shatterproof. Shower doors should be of heavy-duty plastic or safety glass.

Make sure that the bathroom has adequate lighting, including a night light. To avoid shock, never touch electrical appliances while your hands are wet or you're standing on a wet floor. Put personal care appliances, such as hair dryers and shavers, where they cannot fall into the tub, shower, or toilet. Unplug all electrical appliances not in use. Ground fault circuit interrupters (p.309) are required on all bathroom, garage, and outdoor electrical outlets; they are also

recommended for kitchens, laundries, workshops, and wherever water and current come together.

To prevent accidental scalding to a child or yourself, run cold bath water first, then add hot; or test the temperature of the running water with the inside of your wrist. Never leave a young child unattended in a bathroom even momentarily. A child can accidentally fall into a tub or toilet and drown in a few inches of water. If you must leave the room when bathing your child, wrap him in a towel and bring him with you.

My neighbor recently took a nasty spill from a ladder. How can such accidents be avoided?

First, don't settle for anything less than the best ladder you can buy—your life may depend on it.

FACT OR FALLACY ?

Fire is the most common cause of accidental death in the home

Fallacy. According to the National Safety Council, falls—from stairs, ladders, and roofs as well as on the floor, ground, or sidewalk around the house—are by far the leading cause of home accidental deaths. In 1989, poisoning came in second, followed by fire, choking, suffocation, gun accidents, and drowning. People over 75 are most at risk of suffering a fatal fall. For more on ladder and stair safety, see above and page 310. For ways to prevent other falls in the home, see page 403.

Look for a sturdy model; if you want a wooden ladder, choose unpainted wood so that you can easily detect developing cracks or weak spots. Check that the rungs are solid and have nonslip treads. Always keep your ladder in good repair.

Whenever you set up a ladder, check that there is no electrical wiring nearby. A metal ladder is an obvious conductor of electricity, but even a wooden one can give you a shock if it's wet and cause you to fall.

When you climb up or down, always face the ladder and hold on to it with both hands.

Don't climb a ladder while carrying a heavy load in one hand. Tie the load to a rope and pull it up when you are in position. While working, keep your body within the span of the side rails; rather than leaning sideways to reach the work, climb down and move the ladder closer.

Never stand on the last rung or top platform of a ladder. If you can, have another person hold onto the base of the ladder while you're using it. If you're going to work near a door, make sure the door is locked.

Outdooor ladders are taller and therefore more dangerous than indoor models. Check that the bottom of the ladder is far enough away from the house to provide you with solid support. A rule of thumb: the ladder base should be 1 foot away from the house for each 4 feet of height that you climb.

Don't rest the top of the ladder against a surface that might crumble or wobble; roof gutters, for example, are quite fragile. For extra security, drive two stakes into the ground on either side of the ladder and tie the foot of the ladder to the stakes. If the ladder is near an open window, you may also be able to lash it to a piece of heavy furniture.

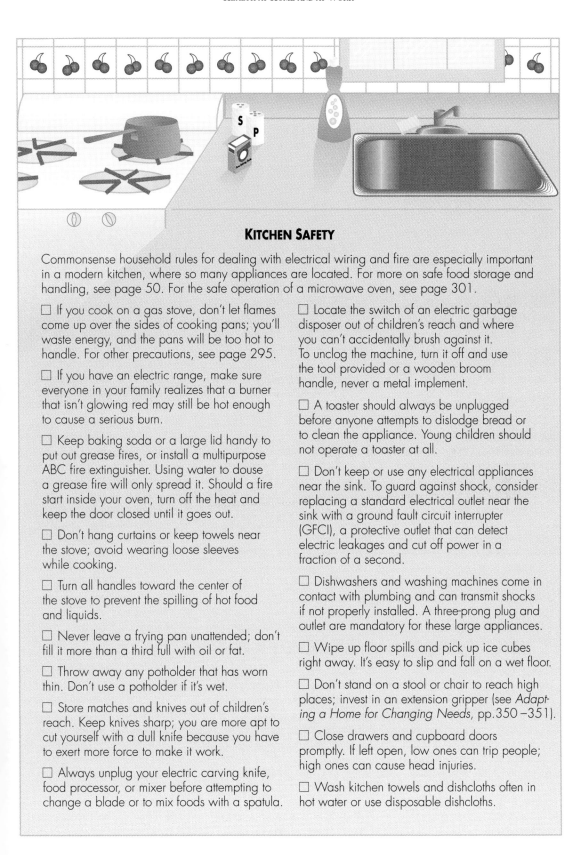

KITCHEN SAFETY

Commonsense household rules for dealing with electrical wiring and fire are especially important in a modern kitchen, where so many appliances are located. For more on safe food storage and handling, see page 50. For the safe operation of a microwave oven, see page 301.

☐ If you cook on a gas stove, don't let flames come up over the sides of cooking pans; you'll waste energy, and the pans will be too hot to handle. For other precautions, see page 295.

☐ If you have an electric range, make sure everyone in your family realizes that a burner that isn't glowing red may still be hot enough to cause a serious burn.

☐ Keep baking soda or a large lid handy to put out grease fires, or install a multipurpose ABC fire extinguisher. Using water to douse a grease fire will only spread it. Should a fire start inside your oven, turn off the heat and keep the door closed until it goes out.

☐ Don't hang curtains or keep towels near the stove; avoid wearing loose sleeves while cooking.

☐ Turn all handles toward the center of the stove to prevent the spilling of hot food and liquids.

☐ Never leave a frying pan unattended; don't fill it more than a third full with oil or fat.

☐ Throw away any potholder that has worn thin. Don't use a potholder if it's wet.

☐ Store matches and knives out of children's reach. Keep knives sharp; you are more apt to cut yourself with a dull knife because you have to exert more force to make it work.

☐ Always unplug your electric carving knife, food processor, or mixer before attempting to change a blade or to mix foods with a spatula.

☐ Locate the switch of an electric garbage disposer out of children's reach and where you can't accidentally brush against it. To unclog the machine, turn it off and use the tool provided or a wooden broom handle, never a metal implement.

☐ A toaster should always be unplugged before anyone attempts to dislodge bread or to clean the appliance. Young children should not operate a toaster at all.

☐ Don't keep or use any electrical appliances near the sink. To guard against shock, consider replacing a standard electrical outlet near the sink with a ground fault circuit interrupter (GFCI), a protective outlet that can detect electric leakages and cut off power in a fraction of a second.

☐ Dishwashers and washing machines come in contact with plumbing and can transmit shocks if not properly installed. A three-prong plug and outlet are mandatory for these large appliances.

☐ Wipe up floor spills and pick up ice cubes right away. It's easy to slip and fall on a wet floor.

☐ Don't stand on a stool or chair to reach high places; invest in an extension gripper (see *Adapting a Home for Changing Needs*, pp.350–351).

☐ Close drawers and cupboard doors promptly. If left open, low ones can trip people; high ones can cause head injuries.

☐ Wash kitchen towels and dishcloths often in hot water or use disposable dishcloths.

I'd like to be sure the stairs in my home are safe. What precautions should I take?

Stairs are the site of about 35,000 serious accidents every year. Taking the following precautions will help you and your family avoid mishaps.

☐ See that your stairways—whether to the second floor or to a basement—are brightly but not glaringly lit and that the lights can be controlled from both the top and bottom of the stairs.

☐ Make it a family rule never to leave toys, clothing, or any other item on the stairs, where someone could stumble over them.

☐ Check that all stair surfaces are nonskid. If you install carpeting, be sure that it is fastened firmly in place.

☐ Stick a strip of tape in a contrasting color along the edges of the top and bottom steps. (It's easy to fall by mistaking the next to the last step for the last one.)

☐ Imagine someone falling down your staircase; then remove anything near the bottom that might compound an injury. This includes glass doors as well as furniture that has sharp corners or tips over easily.

☐ Remember to wear safe footwear indoors. Worn slippers and socks or high-heeled shoes can lead to spills.

☐ If you must carry heavy packages on stairways, be especially careful of your balance, and don't allow a very large package to obscure your vision. Rather than carrying everything at once, make two trips.

☐ If you have young children, install and use safety gates at the top and bottom of the stairs to prevent toddlers from climbing stairs without supervision or falling down the staircase.

☐ Teach toddlers to climb downstairs backward, on all fours.

☐ Check that the rungs on handrails are not spaced so that a child's head might become wedged between them. Similarly, the gaps between open-riser stairs can be made safe by fitting boards across them until your children are older.

☐ Install solid handrails, on both sides if possible. (This is particularly important outdoors, where stairs are often made of concrete or other extra-hard material.)

☐ During the winter, put plenty of sand or rock salt on icy outdoor steps to ensure better footing.

What should I do to protect my family from a fire?

First, inspect your house for fire hazards. Your local fire department may be willing to help you with the inspection. Correct dangerous conditions and set up an annual maintenance and repair schedule for your heating system, gas and electrical appliances, fireplace, and chimneys.

Here are points to keep in mind as you do your audit.

☐ Matches and lighters should be kept out of children's reach.

☐ If you smoke, don't smoke in bed. Elsewhere in the house, use deep, heavy ashtrays.

☐ Store flammable substances (gas, kerosene, paint solvents) out of children's reach and away from heat-producing appliances in approved fireproof containers (be sure they are properly labeled). A separate tool shed is a good place to store flammable material; another option is a high shelf against the outside wall of the garage.

☐ Replace frayed electrical cords as you find them and never run cords or wires under rugs.

☐ Use the fire screen whenever you have a flame going in the fireplace; close the glass doors when you go to bed.

☐ Keep combustible materials (rugs, furniture, pillows, curtains, books, magazines) at least 3 feet away from fireplaces and space heaters.

☐ Never leave a portable heater running in an unoccupied room.

☐ Don't overload electrical circuits (see facing page) and don't use 100-watt bulbs in lamps designed for 60 watts or less.

☐ Follow fire safety rules in the kitchen (p.309).

Take these steps to protect your home and prepare your family to survive a fire:

☐ Install smoke detectors on each level of your house, outside sleeping areas, and at the heads of stairs leading to living areas. Test the equipment at least once a month; clean it and replace batteries at least once a year.

☐ Equip potential fire areas with an appropriate fire extinguisher: Class A extinguishers for paper, wood, cloth, or trash fires (keep one by the living room fireplace); Class B for oil or flammable liquids fires (keep one in the garage); Class C for electrical fires. An ABC extinguisher is a good general-purpose choice. Buy an extinguisher with a UL (Underwriters Laboratory) or FM (Factory Mutual) seal. Follow the manufacturer's directions for installation, testing, and maintenance.

☐ Work out an emergency escape plan. Find the most direct escape route from each bedroom. Also map out alternative routes in case fire blocks the primary one.

☐ Equip each upstairs bedroom with a chain or rope ladder and make it a family project to learn to climb down the ladders (they are tricky).

☐ Designate a spot where everyone will gather after leaving the house.

☐ Teach family members how to feel a door before opening it (if it is hot, they should take the alternate route out). Make sure everyone is aware of the danger of fumes generated during a fire (carbon monoxide, for example, is lethal). In a smoky fire, exposure can be minimized if you stay close to the floor and crawl to exits.

☐ Rehearse the escape plan from time to time with family fire drills.

☐ Post the fire emergency number near the telephone and find out the location of the nearest fire alarm box.

We have bought several labor-saving appliances over the years. How can we be sure that our household wiring is still adequate?

The best way is to hire a licensed electrician to check. And plan to repeat the inspection every 5 years. Too much of a house's wiring is hidden for you to attempt the job yourself.

However, there are safety precautions you can and should take yourself. The hazards of electricity for the homeowner are primarily fire and shock.

To avoid fire:

☐ Don't overload circuits. Signs that you are plugging too many lamps and appliances into a circuit are circuit breakers or fuses that trip or blow often, lights that flicker, and a TV image that shrinks when an appliance is turned on.

☐ Don't replace a fuse or reset a circuit breaker until you have taken care of the electrical problem (the purpose of fuses and circuit breakers is to cut off power *before* an overload or a short in the wiring causes a fire). If you think a circuit is overloaded, unplug appliances from it. If that doesn't solve the problem, call an electrician.

IF A FIRE BREAKS OUT

Ring an alarm. You want to make sure all the occupants of the house have heard the warning and understand that they must get up and out of the house because of a fire.

Get everyone out. Use the emergency evacuation plan (see facing page) that you and your family have worked out.

Don't delay to gather up personal belongings; things can be replaced, but people can't.

Get down on the floor and crawl to minimize your exposure to possibly dangerous gases. Fumes generated during a fire, including carbon monoxide, are killers. Stay low, but get out as fast as you can.

If your clothes catch fire, stop immediately and lie down. Put your hands over your face and roll slowly to smother the flames (running feeds the flames with oxygen).

Meet at your designated gathering site and count heads. If someone is missing, keep calling and encouraging that person to come out; don't, under any circumstances, go back into a blazing house. (Let the firefighters do the rescuing.)

Call the fire department from a fire alarm box or from a neighbor's telephone.

If the fire is localized and you think you can bring it under control by yourself, evacuate the house first and then use the proper fire extinguisher for the type of fire (see facing page). If the fire doesn't go out immediately, get out of the house.

If you extinguish a small fire, check that no upholstery is still smoldering. If you have doubts, call the fire department.

☐ Always replace a blown fuse with one of the same amperage (using a higher amperage fuse can cause overheating and fire).

☐ Check the condition of all your visible household wiring, including the cords on appliances and lamps. Have any wires that look worn replaced. To avoid damaging a cord, always pull on the plug, not on the cord, when unplugging a lamp or appliance.

☐ Use extension cords of the same gauge as the cord on the appliance and use them only on a temporary basis. Never run a cord under a rug or through a traffic pattern.

To avoid electrical shocks:

☐ Before doing electrical work, turn off power to the circuit you're working on by tripping the circuit breaker or removing the fuse that controls the circuit.

☐ Always unplug a lamp or appliance before working on it. A television set, even if unplugged, can give a shock; take it to a service repair person.

☐ Never stand on a wet or damp floor when changing a fuse, using an appliance, or doing any sort of electrical work. Cover a damp floor with rubber mats or stand on a dry board.

☐ Don't touch plumbing pipes,

plumbing fixtures, or gas pipes when working with electricity.
☐ Never immerse any part of an electrical appliance in water unless the manufacturer says it's all right to do so.
☐ Install safety covers in unused electrical outlets to keep children from poking into them. Don't poke inside an appliance yourself with anything made of metal.
☐ Outside, never use an aluminum or a wet wooden ladder near overhead wires.

I enjoy hunting and keep several guns in my home. What is the safest way to store and handle them?

You are right to be concerned about safety, since 200 children die each year while playing with guns. Store your firearms unloaded in locked cabinets. Keep your ammunition in a locked drawer at a separate location, away from heat or electrical sources. Keep keys to storage areas where children can't get at them.

Never accept anyone's assurance that a gun isn't loaded; open the action and check for yourself that the firing chamber is empty. Always point the muzzle in a safe direction; never aim a gun (even an unloaded one) at anything you don't intend to shoot. Don't engage in or tolerate horseplay with guns. Children should be forbidden to touch firearms at all.

We are adopting a 2-year-old girl. How can we make sure our home is safe for a young child?

More American children die from preventable injuries each year than from all childhood diseases combined. Making your house physically safer for a toddler is

important (and will make parenting easier), but there is no substitute for continuous adult supervision of young children.

Begin by getting down on the floor to see the world as your child will. Note dangerous temptations on low shelves or tables (breakable figurines in the living room, poisonous cleaning supplies in the cabinet under the kitchen sink). Every house is different, but making any space safe for youngsters is a matter of looking at it with fresh, child-aware eyes and using common sense; the following list can get you started:
☐ Place electrical appliances (fans, heaters, TV sets) out of the reach of children's fingers.
☐ Dangerous items like pins, needles, matches, lighters, scissors, knives, medications, and poisonous substances should be locked up.
☐ Put collections of coins, buttons, or other small items that children could choke on out of sight. Children will put anything in their mouths.
☐ Take up slippery throw rugs.
☐ Keep drapery or venetian blind cords tied up. Children can choke by wrapping a cord around their necks.
☐ Put safety plugs in open electrical outlets and remove extension cords that run along the floor.
☐ Remove furniture that tips easily; toddlers like to climb on everything. Put bumpers on sharp table corners.
☐ Limit access to aquariums or other large containers of water. Children can drown in even a pail of water.
☐ Sash windows are safe if you open them from the top only; put safety guards on other windows.
☐ Keep plastic bags for trash or from the dry cleaners away from children (a child who puts his head in one can suffocate).

☐ If your house is old, have any flaking paint tested for lead content (p. 298).
☐ Buy medicines in childproof bottles, and never tell children that medicine is candy.
☐ Install sturdy gates across stairways.
☐ Use a fire screen in front of the fireplace and, if you have a wood or coal stove, put a child guard around it.
☐ Keep poisonous plants out of a child's reach (see *Houseplants: Hazardous to Your Health?*, facing page).
☐ For kitchen and bathroom safety tips pertaining to children, see pages 308 and 309.

What potential hazards should I be aware of when I buy toys for my children?

Every year some 166,000 children are treated in hospital emergency rooms for toy-related accidents. To reduce your children's risk of injury, select playthings that are appropriate for their age group. Avoid toys with sharp edges. Play with a child and a new toy for the first half hour to detect any problems.

Toys for infants and toddlers should, most importantly, not have any small pieces that can be swallowed and choked on (button eyes on stuffed animals, bells, snap-together beads). Also avoid tippable hobby horses and hinged toy boxes that can snap shut on fingers. For preschoolers, buy well-balanced, sturdy wagons and scooters. Look for nonflammable dress-ups and doll's clothes, and check for pins (which you should remove). Check labels on art materials to be sure they are nontoxic. Preschool children need supervision to play with electrical toys or toys that shoot projectiles.

As children reach school age,

invest in high-quality equipment. Buy a good bike and a real safety helmet, for example, not a toy football helmet. Buy skates and skis that fit the child properly and supervise their use.

Always read the instructions that come with a toy, and teach your child to use it safely. If your child refuses, take the toy away. A temporarily unhappy child is better than an injured one.

Is there any harm in having pets around very young children?

America's love affair with pets is not without its problems. Dogs bite 500,000 people every year, and household pets can cause allergic reactions and sometimes transmit disease.

Because dogs may become jealous of infants and attack them, it may be prudent to postpone buying a dog if you have a child under 3. If you already own a dog (particularly a large one), never leave it alone with a baby.

Young children may unknowingly provoke a dog or cat by pulling its tail or ears, suddenly awakening it, or interfering with the animal while it is eating. Teach children to treat all animals gently. Tell them to back away if a dog growls or snarls, and to avoid strange dogs or cats altogether.

How do children catch diseases from animals? How can I best protect my children?

Some children are allergic to animal dander or to feathers. If your child is constantly wheezing or sneezing when near a pet, removing the animal from your home may be the only solution.

Children don't often catch diseases from animals, and when they do it's usually through con-

HOUSEPLANTS: HAZARDOUS TO YOUR HEALTH?

The greenery around your house—both indoors and out— may be more dangerous than decorative. Many popular garden and house plants are poisonous to humans and pets. Children, who are prone to putting just about anything in their mouths, are particularly vulnerable. Keep toxic houseplants out of their reach. Teach your child not to touch plants (many cause rashes) or to eat berries, flowers, bulbs, or leaves without checking with you. If a child does eat a part of a toxic plant, call your local poison control center.

Poisonous plants (should not be eaten): anthuriums ... azaleas ... Boston ivy, boxwood ... calla lilies ... chrysanthemums ... crocuses...dieffenbachias ... hemlocks ... hydrangeas ... lilies-of-the-valley ...mistletoe ...morning glories ... oleanders ... philodendrons ... pothos ... privet berries ... rhododendrons ... shamrocks ... spathiphyllums ... yews.

Irritant plants (may cause a rash in some people): amaryllises ... butter cups ... carnations ... cyclamens ... daffodils ... daisies ... ficus benjaminas... geraniums ... holly berries ... hyacinths ... irises ... poinsettias ... pyracantha berries ... tulip bulbs.

Safe plants (a partial listing of plants that won't do harm if touched or ingested): African violets ... asparagus ferns ... baby's breath ... Boston ferns ... California poppies ... camellias ... coleus ... dahlias ... Easter lilies ... forget-me-nots ... fuchsias ... gardenias ... gloxinias ... grape ivy ... hibiscus ... impatiens ... jade plants... maidenhair ferns ... marigolds ... orchids ... peonies ... petunias ... roses ... rubber plants ... scheffleras ... snapdragons ... spider plants ... wandering Jews ... zinnias. (Some mainly decorative plants, such as nasturtiums, pansies, and violets, are also edible.)

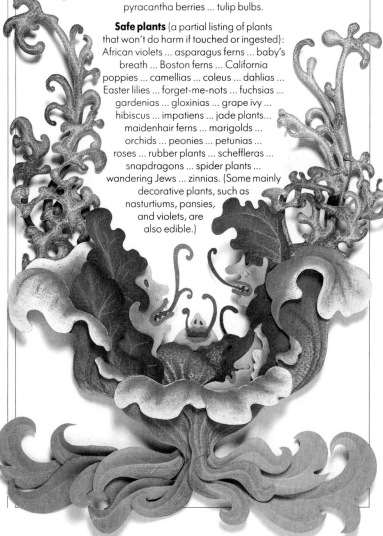

THE FACTS ABOUT LYME DISEASE

What is it? Lyme disease (named for the Connecticut town where the first cases were discovered) is a bacterial infection transmitted primarily by the bite of the deer tick. Early symptoms include a characteristic skin rash and in some cases, headaches, muscle aches, fatigue, and fever. Occasionally there is joint pain, most often in the knee.

Diagnosis and treatment. Lyme disease can be hard to diagnose. Early symptoms mimic the flu and other ailments or may be so minor that people ignore them. Available blood tests for Lyme disease yield many false results. More precise tests are still experimental.

If caught early, Lyme infection can be effectively treated with antibiotics. If left untreated, however, it can lead to arthritis, meningitis, facial paralysis, or heart trouble. If you have flulike symptoms and/or a localized round skin rash, and you think it possible that you've been bitten by a tick, inform your doctor immediately.

How to avoid infection. Avoid the ticks' habitats, especially in the summer. You are most likely to be bitten in wooded or grassy areas, especially along the Atlantic Coast from New England to Georgia (the disease, however, is spreading nationwide). If you do go into the woods, wear light-colored slacks and a long-sleeved shirt, and spray insect repellent containing diethyltoluamide (DEET) on shoes and pants legs (not on skin). Shower and check yourself for ticks right away. Check children, too—especially around the neck, ears, and in the hair. Pets that

go outdoors should wear a flea and tick collar; inspect animals after they've been out.

Removing a tick. Grip it with tweezers as close to your skin as possible. Gently but firmly pull the tick straight out, making sure that the head and all mouthparts are removed. If you don't have tweezers, cover your fingers with tissue before touching the tick. When you've removed it, drop it into a jar of alcohol to kill it. Wash your hands and disinfect the area of the bite with antiseptic.

No bigger than a pinhead, a deer tick infected with *Borrelia burgdorferi* bacteria is the main culprit in the spread of Lyme disease. Despite their name, deer ticks infest birds and animals other than deer. In fact, it's mice, not deer, that serve as the tick larvae's first host and source of infection.

The bull's-eye rash of Lyme disease may begin as a red dot at the site of a tick bite. The rash gradually expands into a ringlike reddish area several inches across and then fades. It's possible to have Lyme disease without ever developing the typical rash.

---

tact with animal feces or by picking up a parasite, bacteria, or virus in the course of handling a diseased animal. Young children (ages 1 to 3) who play in yards or sandboxes and ingest material contaminated by cat or dog excreta can develop a creeping

skin eruption called *visceral larva migrans*. Contact with the feces of infected cats may cause toxoplasmosis, an infection that is not usually a cause for alarm. However, if an expectant mother contracts toxoplasmosis early in her pregnancy, her baby may

suffer mental retardation, blindness, or other birth defects.

Keep sand in sandboxes fresh, and cover the boxes when children aren't playing in them to keep animals out. Don't allow toddlers to put sand or sandy fingers in their mouths. Pregnant women should not handle litter boxes and should wash their hands after touching a cat.

Children occasionally develop swollen lymph nodes and fever from superficial cat scratches or bites, but cat scratch fever, as it is known, is usually mild and goes away without treatment. However, if a cat scratch or bite is deep and the wound becomes infected, have it looked at by a physician.

Keep pets as free of mites, fleas, and ticks as possible, since they can migrate from a pet to family members. Mites and fleas cause itching and skin irritation, but are usually removed by bathing. Ticks, however, can cause Lyme disease or such illnesses as tularemia or Rocky Mountain spotted fever, which can be fatal if not treated. During the summertime tick season, check your children's skin and hair for ticks each night before they go to bed. (For ways to remove ticks, see *The Facts About Lyme Disease*, facing page.)

The key to avoiding contagion from pets is to make sure that they are healthy. Because a pet can carry a disease without seeming ill, have a veterinarian check its health before you take it into your home, and follow his or her recommendations for immunizations, feeding, worming, and general care. Don't adopt or let your child approach wild animals, such as raccoons, foxes, or skunks, since they often have rabies.

Good hygiene will protect your children too. Teach them to wash their hands after playing with an animal. Don't allow pets to sleep on children's beds at night. Keep a separate set of dishes that are used exclusively for the animals' food. Just a few sensible precautions will ensure that owning a pet is a happy experience for you and your children.

Can a child be harmed by playing on grass that's been treated with weed killer?

Some chemical herbicides have been associated with liver and kidney damage in animal studies. Others contain substances that may be carcinogens. If you use such products, read and follow package directions and warning labels carefully.

Babies and small children are at greater risk than adults because they tend to crawl around on the grass and ingest chemical residues. Keep young children (as well as pets) away from recently treated lawns until the chemicals have been dispersed by the elements. Better yet, find nonchemical ways to treat your lawn. You can keep weeds down by planting weed-resistant grass and not cutting the grass below 3 inches, which strengthens grass roots and denies many weeds the light they need to germinate. Weeds that are not near ornamental plants or shrubs can be killed with boiling salted water. Also, some large lawn-care firms now offer chemical-free service.

Are there any effective nonchemical alternatives for controlling garden pests?

If your garden is not large, simply handpicking the pests off your plants will keep their population down. Ladybugs will help eliminate mealybugs and other yard pests. Lacewings will demolish aphids, leafhoppers, and whiteflies. Praying mantises devour caterpillars. If you think that there are not enough of these "good" insects around, you can order them from garden centers.

Certain plants—nasturtiums, marigolds, rosemary, petunias,

and garlic—are repellent to certain pests. Try growing them throughout your garden.

If you are troubled by slugs or snails, dig holes near your plants and set dishes in them so that the rims are at ground level. Fill the dishes with beer to attract the slugs, which will fall in and drown.

Interspersing plant species sometimes confuses insects and makes it impossible for them to quickly demolish a row of their favorite crop. If you prefer to have the same crop in a single row or bed, putting up stakes and covering the bed with a tent of cheesecloth or plastic netting will keep out many pests.

What should I do if I touch poison ivy?

Poison ivy, poison sumac, and poison oak contain an oily resin called urushiol, which causes an allergic skin reaction in most people who touch them or who touch contaminated clothes or pets. (The smoke of a burning plant also carries the resin.)

To avoid contact in the first place, remember the old saying "Leaves of three, let them be." (Poison sumac, however, has paired leaves and clusters of greenish berries.)

Contact with poison ivy usually produces a red, itchy rash and tiny, oozing blisters. The rash peaks on the fifth day and disappears within a week or two.

Wash the affected area right away with strong soap and water. Wash contaminated clothing and pets too. Apply calamine lotion to the rash. Cover oozing blisters with sterile gauze pads moistened with a solution of 1 tablespoon of baking soda in a quart of water.

In some people, contact with poison ivy produces a severe reaction requiring medical attention and possibly treatment with prescription corticosteroid drugs.

What precautions can I take to avoid mishaps around my swimming pool?

You can minimize the risk of accident by never swimming alone and never leaving an infant or a small child alone, even in a baby pool. Infants have drowned in just a few inches of water.

Keep a rescue device—a ring buoy or a long, lightweight pole with a metal loop at the end—at poolside. Install a fence or wall around the perimeter of the area to prevent children from getting into your pool while an adult is not there. The barrier should not lend itself to easy hand-holds and footholds. Check that there are no nearby tree limbs or furniture that would enable children to climb over the wall.

Don't allow running or horseplay near the pool; explain to your children and their friends that the area around the pool is slippery and that a sudden fall could really hurt them. If you have a diving board, be sure it is securely anchored. The water under the diving board should be at least 6 feet deep. The American Red Cross recommends a depth of 9 feet.

If family members swim at night, be sure you have adequate lighting. Never allow electrical appliances to be used near water.

For adults, the greatest source of poolside danger is alcohol, which impairs motor coordination and judgment. Swim first and drink later (or not at all).

Are there health hazards that a craftsperson needs to be aware of?

Many crafts and hobbies, particularly in the fine arts, involve toxic or flammable chemicals. Some oil paint pigments still contain lead, solvents used in painting and printmaking give off toxic fumes, and clays used in pottery may contain silica and asbestos, for example. Chemicals used in photo processing can decompose and give off sulfur dioxide gas, which damages lung tissue and causes severe asthma.

To work at your hobby safely, follow these precautions:
☐ Choose the least toxic materials you can find. Replace solvent-based paints with water-based paints. Buy prepared clay and premixed dyes and glazes instead of the powdered form. (If you work with young children, use only nontoxic materials.)
☐ Read labels carefully. Recent federal legislation requires labeling of art materials with warnings about hazards, identification of any hazardous ingredients, and guidelines for safe use. Ask for the manufacturer's Material Safety Data Sheet.
☐ Set up your work area carefully; don't use normal living areas. Store your materials where children can't reach them, and don't decant toxic liquids into soda bottles or juice cans that someone might mistakenly pick up and drink.
☐ Take ventilation requirements seriously. Dilution ventilation—bringing in fresh air from one side of the room to dilute the contaminant and venting it with an exhaust fan at the opposite side of the room—will safely dissipate small amounts of many chemicals (the half cup of turpentine used in a day's painting, for example, or the chemicals used to develop black-and-white photographs in a darkroom). However, for larger quantities of toxic substances, you will need a special exhaust fan with a hood and filter to capture and vent the noxious fumes before they can mix with the general room air.
☐ Guard against fire by keeping limited supplies of flammable liquids, storing them safely (p.310), and not smoking or having open flames in the room. Install a smoke detector and a fire extinguisher in your workplace.
☐ Clean up carefully and dispose of hazardous materials safely. If you have a question, call the hazardous wastes department of your local government or the regional office of the Environmental Protection Agency.
☐ Wear appropriate protective clothing and gear—respirator, goggles, and gloves, for example.

I'm setting up a home workshop. What safety considerations should I keep in mind?

The careful organization that makes a workshop safe also can make it more efficient to use. Plan the space around the tasks you perform most often, keeping these guidelines in mind:
☐ Arrange tools out of the way, but within easy reach. If you have children, hanging cabinets with locking doors are better than pegboards for safe storage.
☐ Maintain your tools carefully; well-maintained tools are safer and more effective. Keep blades sharp. Read tool manuals, and clean and lubricate moving parts according to the manufacturer's recommendations.
☐ Choose a sturdy workbench that is freestanding, if possible, so that you can easily move around it and there is plenty of room for clamps.
☐ Surround stationary power tools with enough space to allow what you are working on to be maneuvered freely, unobstructed by nearby objects.
☐ Provide an appropriate electrical circuit for each power tool, using outlets with built-in fuses to protect power tool motors from overload. It's also advisable

to replace standard outlets in a workshop with ground fault circuit interrupters (p.309).

☐ Provide dust control for all power tools (sawdust and hot filings from a power grinder are serious fire hazards). Buy a wet-dry vacuum to collect dust and cooled filings.

☐ Create a fire-resistant area for storing flammable substances, where they will stay cool and dry and out of the reach of children.

☐ Install a fan to exhaust dangerous fumes outside.

☐ Put a smoke detector in the area and install an appropriate fire extinguisher.

☐ Buy—and use—safety goggles, earplugs, and dust masks.

How can I lower my risk of being in an automobile accident?

Begin by making sure that your car is in tip-top shape. Take it in for regular tune-ups. Keep your tires properly inflated and replace them when the treads become worn.

When you drive, observe basic safety rules. Above all, don't drink and drive (and don't ride in a car with someone who has been drinking). Use your seat belt and stay within legal speed limits. Before you start out on a long drive, make sure you have had enough sleep. Drivers falling asleep at the wheel cause 200,000 to 400,000 traffic accidents a year. Have your eyes examined regularly, particularly as you get older (see *Staying Sharp at the Wheel*, p.402).

Before traveling a new route, consult a map so that you know exactly where you will be going. On the road, signal early and enter other lanes smoothly. Yield in merging traffic.

Be a good defensive driver:

☐ Watch other drivers around you. Try to identify those who

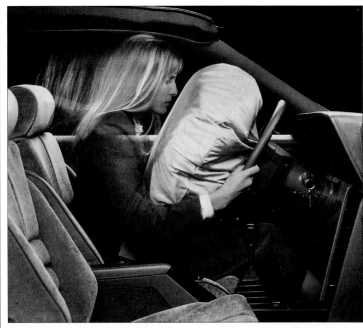

An air bag and buckled seat belts are a life-saving combination in a head-on crash.

will be slow to react in an emergency—people who are talking on car phones or eating with one hand while driving with the other, for example. Give them a wide berth.

☐ Beware of interchanges on crowded highways (the sites of more accidents than anywhere else). The most dangerous is a weave lane shared by entering and exiting traffic. To exit safely, signal early and wait for an entering car, if there is one, to reach the highway before easing into the exit behind it.

☐ Keep the quarter-mile of roadway (or 1 to 2 city blocks) ahead of you clearly in sight. Scan the scene constantly, checking the road surface, other vehicles around you, and in the city, pedestrian traffic. Be on the lookout for anything that may affect your path of travel.

☐ For safety (and time to stop), keep three car lengths between your car and the car ahead of you when you are going 30 miles per hour. Add two car lengths for each additional 10 mph of speed.

Do I need to use seat belts if my car is equipped with air bags?

Yes, you do. Air bags do not replace seat belts, but supplement them to give better protection in frontal and near-frontal collisions. Stored in the steering wheel assembly on the driver's side and in the dashboard on the passenger's side of the front seat, an air bag inflates instantly (in $1/20$ second) on impact and then begins to deflate, cushioning the jolt of the crash and keeping you from smashing into the steering wheel or dashboard. The inflating nitrogen gas, which escapes out the back of the bag, is harmless, although it is hot.

Since side or rear collisions don't cause air bags to inflate, seat belts are your only protection in such cases. Although federal regulations make passive restraints (defined as *either* air bags *or* automatic seat belts) mandatory in new cars, you need both for safety. Air bags used with both lap and shoulder belts are estimated to be 45 to 55 percent effective in reducing driver fatalities; lap/shoulder belts used alone, 40 to 50 percent; and air bags used alone, 20 to 40 percent.

I want to get a car seat to protect my child. What features should I look for?

Select a safety seat that suits your child's size and weight. Use an infant seat for a baby (from birth to 20 pounds), a convertible seat for a child who weighs less than 40 pounds, and a booster seat for a child weighing 40 to 70 pounds. Check the label to be sure that the seat meets federal standards set by the National Highway Traffic Safety Administration and the Federal Aviation Administration.

Before you buy it, try the seat in your car to make sure it fits properly. Seats for infants are designed to face toward the rear to prevent head and neck injuries (whiplash) as well as injuries by belts to fragile body parts. In general, children can face forward when they weigh more than 20 pounds.

Research suggests that one-third of all child seats aren't installed correctly, compromising their life-saving value. Follow the manufacturer's instructions carefully. Make sure the harness is fastened firmly over the child's shoulders. All but the last 20 percent of the seat should rest on the car seat. The car's safety belt should be routed through the seat correctly.

Aside from accidents, does flying pose other health risks?

If you are suffering from any kind of upper respiratory infection — whether it is a cold or a sinus flare-up — you may find the change in air pressure in a plane's cabin very painful, particularly during takeoffs and landings. If you can't postpone the trip, take a decongestant a half hour before boarding and if the flight is long, another one before landing. Chew gum or suck on a candy and swallow often to open painfully stopped ear canals.

Because differences in air pressure can cause or increase pain in dental cavities or gum abscesses, have such problems taken care of before you fly.

Although flight cabins are pressurized, the oxygen level in a plane is 80 percent of that at sea level. This may make breathing difficult for people with circulatory disorders or lung diseases like asthma and emphysema. If you have such a problem, your doctor can ask the airline to supply you with extra oxygen.

If you are allergic to tobacco smoke, you may have trouble finding smoke-free international flights. In the United States, all domestic flights lasting less than 6 hours are now smoke-free; longer flights still have smoking sections. Ask for a seat as far forward of the smoking section as possible.

Patients who have recently had surgery, a heart attack, or a stroke should not fly without their doctor's consent. Women with high-risk pregnancies should also consult their doctor before flying and check airlines for their policies on accepting pregnant passengers.

Airline personnel who are in the air for extended periods and frequent long-distance fliers are exposed to varying amounts of cosmic radiation, which has been linked to a higher risk of cancer and fetal damage resulting in retardation. Radiation exposure is believed to be greater for certain airline crews than for employees at nuclear power plants.

Some scientists are advising pregnant women to avoid long flights, especially from the 4th to the 15th week of pregnancy, the period when the fetus is most at risk of suffering retardation if exposed to radiation.

How can I best protect my child in an airplane?

Buy your child a ticket on the airplane (even if the youngster is less than 2 years old and could ride free in your lap). Bring along the child seat you use in your automobile and hook it up to the seat you have paid for. The Airline Passengers Association of North America, a consumer group, and the Association of Flight Attendants have both lobbied for legislation requiring the use in airplanes of the same child-restraint seats that have become mandatory in automobiles (such seats now carry a sticker of certification from both the National Highway Traffic Safety Administration and the Federal Aviation Administration).

Opponents don't argue safety; they are concerned about the prohibitive cost of flying for a family that must pay for an infant's seat. However, some airlines permit passengers to bring an infant car seat on board and attach it to an empty passenger seat, if one is available, without charge. If you are planning a trip with a child under 2, check with the airline about its policy.

What is a "sick" building?

A building is said to be sick when its air is contaminated and causes health problems for the people who live or work in it. In some cases, a specific pathogen is responsible for the spread of disease throughout a building: in 1976 in Philadelphia, for exam-

HEALTH AND SAFETY WATCHDOGS

The Environmental Protection Agency (EPA), created in 1970, is the federal agency responsible for safeguarding the U.S. environment. Among the EPA's areas of concern are toxic and solid waste sites, pesticides and other toxic substances, radiation hazards, threats to the nation's air and water supplies, and such international problems as acid rain and global warming.

The EPA sets standards for safe drinking water and clean air and regulates pesticide and other hazardous substance use, factory and car emissions, and waste disposal practices. It also offers information and advice to consumers through a series of 800-number telephone hotlines (see Appendix).

The Occupational Safety and Health Administration (OSHA), also created in 1970, is a Department of Labor agency that sets safety and health standards for workers in all industries. OSHA regulations and standards for specific industries are published in the *Federal Register*, available in most public libraries. OSHA also implements and enforces its standards through site inspections, citations, and fines. The National Institute for Occupational Safety and Health (NIOSH), an agency within the Department of Health and Human Services, conducts research on workplace hazards for OSHA.

---

ple, scientists traced an outbreak of deadly pneumonia to the air-conditioning system of a hotel. The lethal bacteria were bred in the system and then dispersed into the hotel air through cool air vents. The infection killed 29 people attending an American Legion convention in the hotel and is now known as Legionnaires' disease.

Bacteria and other microorganisms are only some of the pollutants that can contaminate the air in a large building (home pollutants are discussed on page 293). Asbestos from insulation and fire retardants can cause lung cancer. Formaldehyde from pressed-wood furniture, pesticides used by exterminators, tobacco smoke, and chemicals used in synthetic fibers and glues are all irritants that contribute to what is now known as sick building syndrome, a collection of symptoms that includes head-

ache, dizziness, nausea, stuffy or runny nose, dry respiratory mucous membranes, abnormal fatigue, and irritability.

Most sick buildings are tightly sealed, either to save fuel or because they were designed to be climate controlled and the windows cannot be opened. In another effort to save energy costs, too little fresh air may be circulated through a building to properly exhaust pollutants.

The key to a building's air quality is the design, operation, and maintenance of its ventilation system. If the fresh air intake is badly located, it can bring in car or truck exhausts or other pollutants. If ducts are blocked, air can't circulate. If filters aren't cleaned regularly, they may act as a breeding ground for mold or other microorganisms that will circulate through the building.

Remedies for sick building problems usually involve improv-

ing ventilation, removing the contaminant, or a combination of the two. Sometimes it's easy: a large hospital solved its pollution problem by screening the entrance of an air-intake pipe after it was found that pigeons had been nesting inside. In most cases, however, a consultant will have to identify the source of the pollution and offer solutions such as increasing fresh air circulation, cleaning ventilation ducts, sealing off the contaminants, or replacing furnishings made of synthetic materials with wood, metal, wool, or cotton versions.

My job involves handling toxic chemicals. How can I ensure my health and safety in the workplace?

First of all, make sure you have all the training you need to perform your work efficiently and safely. You should know and faithfully observe the correct procedures for handling the dangerous substance. Always wear the protective clothing and equipment needed for safe operation, such as respirators, goggles, and gloves. The Occupational Safety and Health Act, passed in 1970, requires employers to provide their workers with appropriate personal protective equipment and to see to it that the equipment is properly maintained. If you are unsure about what you should be wearing, check with your supervisor, a representative from your labor union, or the regional office of the U.S. Occupational Safety and Health Administration (see Appendix).

Since you are handling toxic chemicals, it is especially important to refrain from smoking on the job. Because smokers frequently put their hands to their mouths, they are at a higher risk of accidentally ingesting residues from the chemicals they have been handling. Also, toxic chemicals and cigarettes often interact, so that if you smoke and handle a chemical considered to be carcinogenic, you run a greater risk of contracting cancer than you would have from cigarettes or the chemical alone.

Try consistently to get enough rest at home so that you will be alert at work; avoid doing anything demanding a high degree of concentration if you are overtired. And of course, never use drugs or alcohol at the workplace; they can impair your performance and cause you to have an accident.

Does my working with toxic materials put the health of my wife and children at risk?

It's possible. Research is beginning to suggest that a father's exposure to toxic substances can directly affect his ability to sire children and impair the health of the children he does have. In Western Australia, for example, the Asbestos Disease Society studied the death certificates of children whose fathers worked in an asbestos mine from 1943 to 1966 and found evidence that enough asbestos fibers had been brought into the miners' homes to cause asbestos-related cancers among their children. In the United States, a National Cancer Institute study in 1979 found that children of men whose work involved high exposure to lead had three times more kidney tumors than children whose fathers did not receive such exposure.

If you work with toxic materials, be diligent about safety routines. Shower and change clothes before you leave work to avoid taking home fibers, fumes, or gases that may cling to your skin or work clothes. Never wash contaminated clothes at home.

Should a pregnant woman avoid certain kinds of work?

There is evidence that workplace exposure to certain toxic chemicals and materials can harm a growing fetus. Among these substances are ethylene oxide, used to sterilize surgical instruments; vinyl chloride, used in the manufacture of plastics; arsenic and its compounds, used in many industries; and the metals manganese, lead, and nickel.

The Supreme Court has ruled that women of childbearing age cannot be barred from jobs where toxic substances might harm a fetus. If you plan to become pregnant, find out about the chemicals and materials at your workplace. If you believe that you or your unborn child may be at risk, you can ask the company to transfer you to another area for the duration of your pregnancy. If no hazard-free areas exist, you may want to leave your job temporarily. If so, the Civil Rights Act, as amended in 1978, provides that women "disabled by pregnancy" must be treated in the same way as other temporarily disabled workers. That means you would be entitled to disability pay if you had to take a long maternity leave.

I've heard that photocopiers can be a health hazard. Is there anything to this?

Photocopiers are not a hazard for people who use them only occasionally. But people who work with them for most of the day can suffer ill effects if they do not follow proper procedures or if the machines are not located in a well-ventilated area and are not carefully maintained. Workers who handle the toners for machines have suffered skin rashes,

and others have complained of eyestrain from looking at the intensely bright light. A more serious potential health hazard is the ozone (p. 293) created by the action of the high-voltage electricity needed to make photocopies.

Almost all photocopiers give off some ozone, but the amount is usually less than the level considered hazardous by the Occupational Safety and Health Administration (more than 0.1 part per million). However, ozone levels can easily rise in enclosed spaces. An electrical or pungent odor coming from a copying machine is a sign that it is giving off too much ozone.

Many photocopiers come with an activated charcoal filter designed to break down ozone, but such filters are effective only if they are changed regularly, and many owner's manuals do not advise buyers that filters should be changed or how to change them. If they are not changed, the filters become clogged with dust and lose their effectiveness within a few weeks.

If you work with a copying machine routinely, take the following precautions:
□ Ask that photocopiers be located in open, well-ventilated areas.
□ Check that the machines are serviced and cleaned at regular intervals.
□ If you notice a pungent odor, report it at once so that the photocopier can be checked.
□ Find out whether the photocopier has an ozone filter and when it was last changed. If there is no filter, ask about the possibility of installing one.
□ Remember to use the document cover while you are working, to protect your eyes from the bright light.
□ If you handle toner, pour it slowly to avoid dispersing dust. Wear rubber gloves and a smock, and wash your hands

VDT SAFETY

For all its speed and efficiency, the modern computerized workplace can be a health hazard if you don't take preventive measures. Listed below are health problems that have been associated with work at a video display terminal (VDT) and ways to avoid them.

Eyestrain. Position the VDT about 2 ft. from your eyes. The entire display should be in sharp focus; brightness and contrast should be adjustable. If your work area is too bright, the screen will be difficult to read. But if you refer to papers as you work, you will need a lamp to light the text without causing glare on the screen. Glare is best cut by rearranging lights; otherwise, put a glare filter or hood on the screen. Periodically look away from the screen and focus on distant objects. Have your eyes checked regularly (p.136).

Neck and back pain. Make sure your screen, keyboard, and chair are at the right height for you. The top of the screen should be slightly below your horizontal line of sight; the viewing angle from your eyes down to the screen should be less than 25 degrees. Position a document holder right next to the screen. Sit up straight, arms and hands at a comfortable angle (see REPETITIVE STRAIN INJURY, below), feet flat on the floor. Use a comfortable, well-designed chair that shifts your weight slightly forward; a lumbar cushion may help relieve strain on the lower back. Get up from your chair and walk around periodically.

Reproductive disorders. A 1991 U.S. government study found that pregnant women who work with VDT's all day run no greater risk of miscarriage than women in other jobs. Scientists are still investigating possible links between birth defects and exposure to the electromagnetic radiation emitted by VDT's. To be on the safe side, workers are advised to sit at least 2 ft. away from their VDT screens and 4 ft. away from the back or sides of a colleague's VDT.

Repetitive strain injury (see below). Follow directions for avoiding neck and back pain. Adjust chair and keyboard heights so that your upper arms hang vertically, elbows bent at a 90° angle and wrists held straight, not bent up or down. Don't pound on the keyboard. Take a break at least once every 2 hrs.

when you are finished. Special cloths are available from office supply stores that attract and hold spilled toner more efficiently than paper towels do.

Repetitive strain injury (RSI) has had a lot of press coverage lately. What exactly is it?

You've read a lot about this occupational disorder because it is increasing faster than any other job-related illness. Known also as repetitive motion syndrome or occupational overuse syndrome, RSI is an impairment brought on by doing the same movements with arms and hands over and over again all day long.

RSI has been common for many years among violinists, typists, mechanics, and construction workers who use repetitive wrist movements in their jobs. Recently, however, high-speed keyboard technology has created RSI problems for a whole new set of workers who sit at computer terminals all day.

RSI affects different people differently. Some suffer tenosynovitis, an inflammation of the sheathing around tendons in the hand. Others may develop carpal tunnel syndrome, a condition in which the nerves that go through the wrist to the hand are pinched by swollen tissue.

Tenosynovitis caused by repetitive motion makes fingers

tender, painful, and hard to straighten (they hesitate and then pop out in a jerky motion). You may hear a cracking sound when your fingers move. Rest and anti-inflammatory drugs are the usual treatment, but sometimes steroids are prescribed.

Carpal tunnel syndrome causes a numbness or tingling sensation in the hand. Pain shoots from the wrist either up the arm or down into the hand. Discomfort may be worse at night and may even wake you up. Resting the wrist in a splint often relieves the pain, but persistent carpal tunnel syndrome is treated with steroid drugs or surgery.

Preventive measures for repetitive strain injury include sound work practices and adequate rest breaks (see *VDT Safety,* p.321), proper posture, and exercises to strengthen the wrist.

I sometimes have to work a night shift. Can this affect my health, and are there ways to adjust to night work?

Reasearch on the health effects of shift work is ongoing. Long-term studies indicate that shift workers have a higher incidence of heart attacks as well as accidents on the job than day workers do. In the short term, their health problems fall into two categories: fatigue and digestive disturbances. If you suffer insomnia during the day when you try to sleep, you'll have trouble staying alert on the job. If you eat at odd hours to which your body is not accustomed, gastrointestinal disturbances, including peptic ulcers, may result.

The human body's internal mechanisms are naturally geared to peak performance during daylight hours and tend to slow down at night. Someone who works at night for a protracted period of time may gradually adjust, but a day worker who works for a night or two and then returns to a normal routine is apt to experience the same symptoms as someone with jet lag (p.231).

Some people who work irregular hours compound their health problems by taking stimulants to keep themselves awake. Don't rely on caffeine or over-the-counter "pep" pills, which can make you jittery. Instead, re-orient your internal clock by keeping to a consistent eating and sleeping schedule, even on weekends. A 1990 study at Brigham and Women's Hospital in Boston has shown that workers adapt more easily to night hours if their workplace is brightly lit and if they darken their bedrooms with blackout shades while they sleep during the day. After a few days of working under bright lights and sleeping in a completely darkened room, you should be able to sleep soundly and feel more refreshed.

I work in a very noisy factory. What can I do to protect my hearing?

More than 9 million U.S. workers are exposed to dangerous noise levels at their jobs every day. The cumulative effect of such exposure over time can be a serious loss of hearing, even deafness. Although the Occupational Safety and Health Administration has set limits on noise levels in the workplace, companies that don't observe these standards are rarely cited.

Take initiatives to save your own hearing. Have a hearing test to establish your current hearing level. Most companies provide these tests as part of OSHA's hearing conservation program. If your employer does not, go to your own doctor or to a specialist he or she recommends. Continue to have your hearing checked at the intervals your doctor suggests so that you will be alerted to hearing problems early.

At work, always wear earplugs or other ear protectors. If you can make any changes on your own to reduce noise levels in your department (putting rubber pads under noisy machines, for example), do so. When you are not at work, you can give your ears a rest by avoiding loud noises (see *Living in a Noisy World,* p.300).

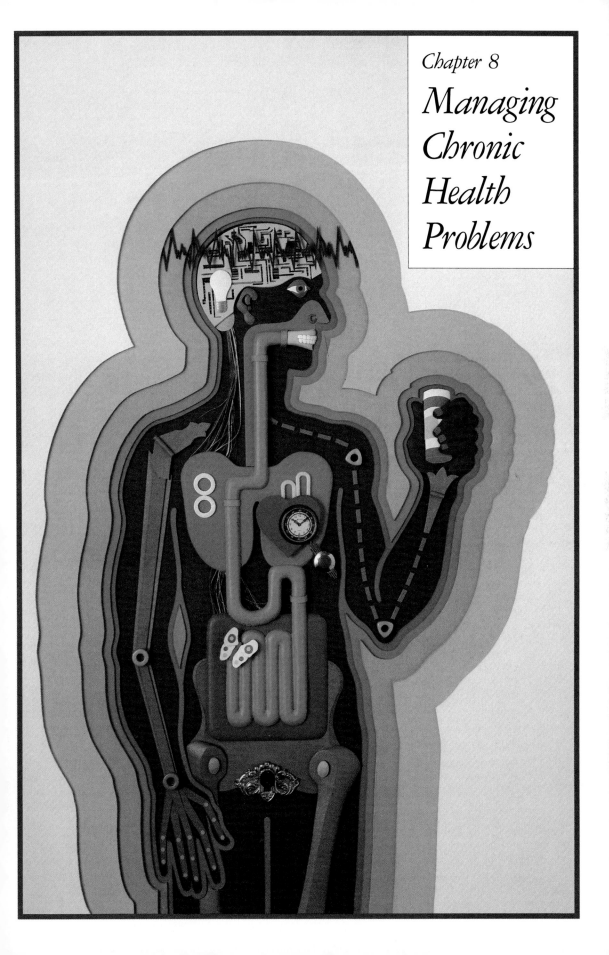

Chapter 8

*Managing
Chronic
Health
Problems*

"These Hands of Mine"

Before she was 18, Vicky P. had dropped out of high school, married, and had a baby. With few friends and fewer interests outside her family, Vicky would be the first to admit that her life in those days lacked direction. To make matters worse, shortly after the baby was born, Vicky developed rheumatoid arthritis, a debilitating joint disease that contorted her fingers and caused such severe pain in her shoulders and hands that she could not lift her baby.

Now in her early forties, Vicky has lost two fingers to the disease. Those that remain are gnarled, stiff, and painful; some have artificial joints. Yet her ongoing battle with arthritis has turned her life around. "It made me realize my talents and abilities," she says. "If I hadn't gotten arthritis, I wouldn't have the motivation I have today." After losing full use of her fingers, Vicky learned how to type. Today, she is an executive secretary at an insurance firm and, using two fingers on each hand, types 55 words a minute. She also sings in her church choir, leads public-speaking seminars, and has published two collections of poetry.

Pain is still very much a part of Vicky's daily life. She takes at least six aspirins a day, sometimes as many as 12. On days when the pain is really bad, her doctor prescribes stronger anti-inflammatory drugs, although she usually tries to get by on aspirin alone. Nothing, however, is as therapeutic for Vicky as her active lifestyle. The constant finger movements that her secretarial job entails help keep her fingers limber and lessen their pain (wrapping them in warm towels also helps). Her grandchildren are her joy; her poetry is her solace. As she wrote in one of her recent poems, "These hands of mine—these hands of mine Though crippled they're my own. I lift them up to show the world That through these hands I've grown."

A Dancer Fights Back

Richard T. was a young man on a fast track to fame and fortune. By the time he turned 30, Richard had already made a mark as a successful dancer and budding choreographer in Broadway musicals. Everything seemed to be going his way until just before his 35th birthday, when he began noticing a slight tremor in his hands. His body movements, too, were becoming stiff and cramped. At first Richard went about his business, trying to deny that anything was seriously wrong. But as his symptoms became more pronounced and debilitating, he was forced to face reality and see a doctor.

The diagnosis—Parkinson's disease—was a particularly devastating one for someone whose art and livelihood depended on smooth muscle coordination and graceful movement. With the curtain falling on his dance career, Richard responded with a fierce anger. At the height of his rage, he vowed to fight back and keep the disease from crippling his body.

Thirty years later, Richard is still active and still fighting. Medications are part of the story. To help control his symptoms, Richard takes three different antiparkinsonism drugs four times a day. But he attributes his success more to his determination and to his rigorous stretching program than to any drugs. Even before he gets out of bed in the morning, Richard stretches his muscles for 20 minutes to get rid of cramps. He spends 3 hours every day in a studio doing his complete body stretching routine. Finger exercises, such as practicing typing and picking up delicate objects, help maintain his manual dexterity.

Although his performing days are long past, Richard is still active in the theater as a director. He's also taken his message on the road, giving lectures and producing videotapes to encourage other people with Parkinson's disease to keep moving and keep fighting.

TEST YOUR HEALTH I.Q.

When Disease Won't Go Away

Most illnesses, fortunately, are short-lived; others recur again and again or simply never leave. Whether life-threatening or merely inconvenient, chronic conditions often force sufferers to make lifestyle adjustments. In some cases, the changes are temporary; in others, they're lifelong and dramatic. Either way, the key to living more comfortably with a chronic condition is understanding it. Can you tell which of the following statements about chronic diseases are true and which are common misconceptions?

1 A person is considered to have hypertension after a blood pressure reading of 150/100.

_____ True _____ False

2 Drugs are the best way to control high blood pressure.

_____ True _____ False

3 Angina sufferers nearly always go on to have heart attacks.

_____ True _____ False

4 Radiation from microwave ovens can damage pacemakers.

_____ True _____ False

5 Joint-replacement surgery is especially advisable for arthritis sufferers under age 50.

_____ True _____ False

6 Many children with asthma outgrow their symptoms in their teens.

_____ True _____ False

7 It's not a good idea to use decongestants on a long-term basis.

_____ True _____ False

8 Most diabetics must take daily doses of insulin.

_____ True _____ False

9 Smokers are twice as likely to get peptic ulcers as nonsmokers.

_____ True _____ False

10 Irritable bowel syndrome and spastic colon are different names for the same disease.

_____ True _____ False

11 A symptomless carrier of the hepatitis B virus cannot transmit the disease.

_____ True _____ False

12 Recipients of kidney and other organ transplants must continue taking immunosuppressant drugs for the rest of their lives.

_____ True _____ False

Answers
For more information on any of the quiz topics turn to the pages listed next to the answers.

1. False, p.326	5. False, p.336	9. True, p.346
2. False, p.327	6. True, p.338	10. True, p.347
3. False, p.328	7. True, p.342	11. False, p.349
4. False, p.331	8. False, p.343	12. True, p.353

What does it mean to say that a disease is chronic?

A chronic disease is any illness that a person must live with for a long time. Depending on the condition, the duration may vary from months to years to a lifetime. Most chronic illnesses are considered incurable, but the symptoms may come and go and there may be periods when the disease goes into remission. In contrast, an acute illness usually occurs suddenly, lasts a short time, and produces rapid changes (such as high fever or severe pain) in the afflicted person's condition from day to day.

The important thing to remember about a chronic disease is that it is likely to be permanent; the person who has it must learn how best to control it and cope with it in order to live as full and active a life as possible.

What are the most common chronic diseases?

High blood pressure (hypertension), heart disease, arthritis, asthma, chronic bronchitis, emphysema, sinusitis, and diabetes are among the most common chronic disorders. Many cancers are also common and chronic. Other chronic diseases are less common but still widespread, notably Parkinson's disease, multiple sclerosis, epilepsy, and lupus.

Several common chronic conditions that may not be thought of as diseases are nonetheless permanent or persistent. They are often disabling and may necessitate varying degrees of change in lifestyle. These include nearsightedness, blindness, deafness, varicose veins, migraine headaches, irritable bowel syndrome, and any paralysis or other crippling disability.

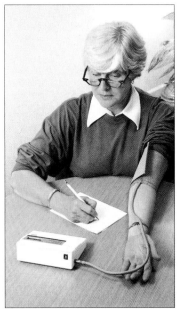

If you have hypertension, your doctor may advise you to track your blood pressure at home. Many different home blood pressure monitors are available; ask your doctor which type he recommends and how to use it. The digital model shown here allows you to record blood pressure without a stethoscope.

What is blood pressure?

Blood pressure is the force produced by the heart as it pushes blood through arteries and capillaries in the body. It normally goes up and down throughout the day in response to stress and exertion. Abnormally high blood pressure, or hypertension, occurs when the walls of the small arteries squeeze tight, leaving a reduced opening for the blood. To maintain the flow of blood through the body, the heart must pump harder.

Why the arteries constrict in some people and not in others is not fully understood. In 10 percent of people with high blood pressure, the condition is a symptom of some underlying, often correctable problem, such as a kidney or adrenal gland disorder. In the other 90 percent, however, the cause is unknown,

although there are a number of factors that increase a person's risk. These are age (blood pressure increases as you grow older); heredity (it tends to run in families); sex (men are more likely to get it); race (blacks have a 30 percent higher risk than whites); and obesity (up to half of obese people with high blood pressure can end it simply by losing excess weight). Smoking, heavy drinking, and stress may also be risk factors.

If blood pressure fluctuates normally, how is high blood pressure diagnosed?

Blood pressure is measured with a device called a sphygmomanometer, which consists of an inflatable rubber cuff attached to a pressure gauge (see *Screening Tests for Healthy Adults,* pp.124–125). Because blood pressure fluctuates with each heartbeat, the reading is given in two parts: the peak, or systolic, pressure, which is attained when the heart contracts; and the low, or diastolic pressure, attained when the heart relaxes between contractions. Both are measured in millimeters of mercury (mm Hg).

Hypertension is usually defined as a consistent systolic pressure of at least 140 mm Hg and a consistent diastolic pressure of at least 90 mm Hg. The key word, however, is *consistent*. The diagnosis is made only after the blood pressure is found to be elevated on three occasions at least several days apart.

What are the long-term risks of hypertension?

The heart of someone with high blood pressure works harder than it should. The extra strain on both the heart and arteries can lead to heart failure, heart attack, stroke, and atherosclerosis, or hardening of the arteries (see *The Facts About Atherosclerosis,* p. 329). Chronic hypertension can enlarge the heart, limiting its ability to function adequately. The brain, kidneys, and eyes can also be damaged by uncontrolled high blood pressure, which reduces the flow of blood to these vital organs. If the damage becomes severe enough, it can cause death.

Overall, about 1 million Americans die each year as a result of the effects of high blood pressure. As with cancer, however, many of these deaths could be prevented if the condition were detected and treated early. Once diagnosed, high blood pressure can almost always be treated.

Are drugs always necessary to control hypertension?

No, not at all. In fact, many of the recommendations for an overall healthy lifestyle given throughout this book will also help reduce blood pressure. Doctors usually prescribe drugs only after a patient has tried changes in lifestyle for 3 to 6 months without achieving a significant drop in blood pressure.

Stopping smoking, losing excess weight, limiting salt and alcohol intake, reducing stress, and getting regular aerobic exercise are the changes generally recommended for controlling hypertension. For more on keeping blood pressure within normal limits without drugs, see page 205.

My doctor prescribed a hypertension drug. Will I have to take it for the rest of my life?

Not necessarily. In some cases, the need for drug therapy can be reduced or even eliminated if you

---

THE LANGUAGE OF HEART DISEASE

Aneurysm. Bulge at weak point in wall of blood vessel or heart.

Angina (angina pectoris). Pain in chest, and sometimes shoulders and arms, caused by ATHEROSCLEROSIS in CORONARY ARTERIES (p. 328).

Aorta. The large main ARTERY leading from heart.

Arrhythmia. Heartbeat that is too fast, too slow, or erratic.

Arteries. Blood vessels that carry oxygen-rich blood from the heart.

Arteriosclerosis. "Hardening of the arteries," progressive thickening and loss of elasticity of walls of ARTERIES.

Atherosclerosis. Buildup of CHOLESTEROL and other fatty deposits (plaque) in the inner lining of ARTERIES, blocking normal flow of blood and encouraging clot formation; most serious form of ARTERIOSCLEROSIS (p. 329).

Blood pressure. The force exerted by flow of blood on blood vessels.

Cardiac arrest. Sudden stoppage of the heartbeat.

Cardiomyopathy. Heart muscle disease that weakens force with which heart contracts; may be caused by viral infections or degenerative changes.

Cardiovascular. Relating to the heart and blood vessels.

Cholesterol. A fatty substance that's an essential constituent of body cells; a higher-than-normal blood level increases risk of ATHEROSCLEROSIS.

Congestive heart failure. Inability of heart to pump enough blood to meet body's needs, causing fluid buildup in lungs, abdomen, and limbs (p. 332).

Coronary arteries. ARTERIES that branch from AORTA and supply blood to the heart itself; clogging of these arteries causes CORONARY HEART DISEASE.

Coronary heart disease. Damage to or malfunction of heart caused by narrowing or blockage of CORONARY ARTERIES. May manifest itself as ANGINA, ARRHYTHMIA, or MYOCARDIAL INFARCTION.

Coronary thrombosis. Obstruction of a CORONARY ARTERY by a thrombus (a clot that forms in an intact blood vessel).

Electrocardiogram (ECG, EKG). A graphic tracing of the heart's electrical activities, recorded by electrocardiograph machine (p. 124).

Embolism. Obstruction of blood vessel by an embolus (a blood clot, air bubble, or clump of material traveling in bloodstream).

Fibrillation. Irregular contractions of heart muscle fibers that cause heart to beat with an irregular, usually rapid rhythm.

Heart attack. Nonmedical term for MYOCARDIAL INFARCTION.

Hypertension. High BLOOD PRESSURE (see facing page).

Ischemia. Localized, usually temporary, deficiency of blood supply, often caused by a constricted or obstructed blood vessel.

Myocardial infarction (HEART ATTACK). Death of part of heart muscle due to sudden cutoff of its blood supply, usually as a result of a CORONARY THROMBOSIS. Underlying cause of most heart attacks is ATHEROSCLEROSIS that narrows the CORONARY ARTERIES and promotes clot formation.

Stroke. Damage to brain resulting from cutoff of blood supply due to blockage in a cerebral ARTERY or leakage of blood from a cerebral ARTERY.

Transient ischemic attack (TIA). Brief interruption of blood supply to part of brain, causing temporary impairment of movement, sensory perception, or speech; also called a ministroke, a TIA may foreshadow a full-scale STROKE.

lose weight and get enough regular exercise. But since there's usually no way to know in advance if that will be true for you, it's probably best to consider the medication a lifetime treatment. Incorporate it into your regular routine, and take it every day exactly as prescribed.

No matter what the reason, never stop taking a hypertension medication suddenly. Abrupt discontinuation can be extremely dangerous, producing higher blood pressure, heart palpitations, or even a heart attack. When your doctor stops a hypertension medication, readjusts your dosage, or substitutes another drug, it has to be done gradually over 1 or 2 weeks.

I've heard that drugs for high blood pressure can have unpleasant side effects. What can be done about them?

It is true that hypertension medications often produce side effects such as dry mouth, fatigue and drowsiness, dizziness or a tendency to faint when standing up suddenly, depression, and impotence. Take care to note any side effects you experience and report them to your doctor. The effects can usually be minimized by changing the dosage or switching to another drug.

What is angina and how does it differ from a heart attack?

Angina, also called angina pectoris ("spasm of the chest"), is a brief, recurring, unpleasant sensation in the center of the chest behind the breastbone. People who experience angina describe it variously as pain, heaviness, tightness, pressing, or squeezing in the chest. The feeling may spread to other body parts, such as the arms, neck, or jaws, and numbness may develop in the shoulders or arms.

Angina is usually a symptom of coronary heart disease, a condition in which clogged arteries reduce the supply of blood to the heart (see *The Language of Heart Disease,* p.327). During exercise or other stress, the heart can't get enough oxygen from its blood supply and the result is pain. A first-time attack of angina can be frightening and is often mistaken for a heart attack. The two events, however, are not the same. A heart attack is the result of a sudden, complete, and permanent cutoff of the blood supply to a part of the heart muscle. It almost always produces severe, prolonged pain and permanent damage (p.214). By contrast, the temporary shortage of blood to the heart that triggers angina causes no permanent heart damage. While some people with angina go on to have heart attacks, many don't. Still others develop angina after a heart attack as a symptom of progressive coronary heart disease.

How is angina treated?

The classic treatment for angina is nitroglycerine and other nitrate drugs, which dilate blood vessels. At the first hint of an attack, the patient slips a nitrate tablet under the tongue, where it dissolves and relieves the pain within seconds. Doctors advise some patients to take a tablet whenever they face an angina-provoking task, such as climbing stairs. Nitrates are now also given as skin ointments and long-lasting medicated skin patches.

Other drugs that counteract angina include a second group of blood-vessel dilators known as calcium-channel blockers. Also effective are beta-blockers such as propranolol, which slow the heart and reduce its need for oxygen. While all of these drugs relieve angina, none cure the underlying coronary heart disease, and a patient can expect to take them indefinitely.

Can coronary heart disease be reversed?

For years most researchers believed that coronary heart disease, the main cause of angina, could not be reversed; the best that medicine could do was to keep the disease from progressing. But based on newer studies by University of California and University of Washington researchers, some experts now believe that lifestyle changes together with medication can reverse coronary heart disease and eliminate, or at least reduce, angina. These changes include taking prescribed drugs along with stopping smoking, reducing stress, controlling blood pressure, and exercising regularly. Equally important is following a diet that lowers blood cholesterol and reduces weight. In another University of California study the participants who were most successful in reversing coronary heart disease were the ones who had reduced their fat consumption to well below the recommended 30 percent of calories, adopting a diet that was almost vegetarian. Before making such a radical change in diet, consult your doctor; make changes gradually. Even if you don't go to that extreme, adopting a generally healthy lifestyle can only help.

When is a coronary artery bypass operation necessary?

In coronary bypass surgery, a vein from the leg or another artery in the chest is used to create new blood pathways to the heart,

THE FACTS ABOUT ATHEROSCLEROSIS

What is it? Atherosclerosis—the most common form of arteriosclerosis, or hardening of the arteries—is a disease of the arterial walls. The walls' inner lining becomes thickened by deposits of cholesterol, fat, blood platelets, calcium, and other substances, known together as plaque. The buildup narrows the arteries, decreasing blood flow and increasing the chance that the blood will form clots. There are seldom any symptoms until the condition becomes advanced.

How does it affect the heart? Atherosclerosis is the underlying cause of coronary heart disease. When atherosclerosis narrows the arteries leading to the heart, that organ receives less oxygen and nutrients from the blood. Partial narrowing of the coronary arteries can cause the chest pain known as angina (facing page). If a coronary artery becomes completely blocked, the result is usually a heart attack. Blockage of an artery leading to the brain causes a stroke.

Who is most susceptible? Atherosclerosis is most apt to develop in people with any of these risk factors: high blood pressure, high blood cholesterol, smoking, diabetes, obesity, physical inactivity, heavy drinking, male sex, advanced age, and a family history of early heart attack.

Can atherosclerosis be prevented? The earlier in life you start paying attention to the correctable risk factors, the greater your chances of avoiding atherosclerosis and heart disease. Don't smoke. Control your weight. Keep to a low-fat diet. Use alcohol in moderation. Exercise regularly. Have your blood pressure checked regularly. If you have high blood pressure or diabetes, be meticulous about following all your doctor's instructions for controlling your condition.

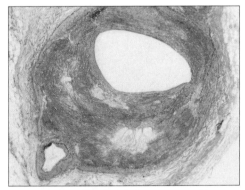

In a partially clogged artery, a hard mass of fatty tissue, known as atheroma, forms on the inner lining of the arterial walls, restricting blood flow through the artery.

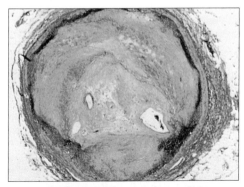

In a completely plugged artery, deposits fill the entire vessel, cutting off blood flow. If it's an artery to the heart or brain, the result may be a heart attack or stroke.

bypassing the blocked coronary arteries. It is the recommended treatment for people who have advanced coronary artery blockage. The procedure is definitely indicated in people who have angina and 75 percent blockage of the left main coronary artery, who have blockages in all three coronary arteries and have difficulty moving around, or who have persistent severe chest pain.

But whether coronary bypass surgery—now one of the most common major operations in the United States—should be performed on people who have clogged arteries but only mild angina is questionable. The landmark Coronary Artery Surgery Study, which followed 780 people with clogged arteries and angina for 10 years, found no difference in the lifespan of people who had

bypass surgery and those who were treated with only medication. The study did find that bypass surgery lengthened the lifespan of people whose hearts had been weakened by heart attacks, and another study showed that the operation improved a person's chances of surviving a heart attack. However, most experts today do not recommend bypass surgery to prevent heart

RECOVERING FROM A HEART ATTACK

During a heart attack, a blockage in a coronary artery cuts off blood to an area of the heart muscle. The affected area dies, while the surrounding heart muscle continues— far less efficiently—to pump blood. Immediate medical attention is crucial. Treatment with clot-thinning drugs (tissue plasminogen activator or streptokinase) within 4 hours of a heart attack can save a life (more than half of those who die from a heart attack do so within 1 or 2 hours) or reduce the amount of tissue damage. Proper treatment and rehabilitation will allow a healing scar to form and the heart to regain strength. Most patients can safely return to work within 2 months of the attack. Almost 40 percent of heart attack victims are still alive 10 years later.

Physical rehabilitation. The best post-attack therapy is gradual but steady physical activity. Patients now are encouraged to get out of bed within a few days of an attack and to start a supervised cardiovascular fitness program before leaving the hospital. Many hospitals and physicians' groups have set up therapy centers for heart patients; similar programs are offered by YMCA's and other community agencies (call your local chapter of the American Heart Association for a recommendation). Any rehabilitation class you join (with your doctor's approval) should be supervised by a doctor and should require a stress test (p.69) before accepting you.

Psychological rehabilitation. It is natural to be frightened by a heart attack. Some people become depressed afterward and find it hard to be optimistic about a future of curtailed activity. Patients and spouses who might benefit from affectionate contact fear even broaching the subject of sex after a heart attack. For general guidelines about resuming sexual activity after a heart attack, see page 333. Professional counseling or joining a self-help group for heart attack victims and their families may help restore your confidence and perspective. Ask the hospital or your doctor for names of such organizations.

Lifestyle adjustments. A heart attack is a sobering experience; it may encourage you to take seriously your doctor's recommendations about diet, exercise, losing weight, quitting smoking (p.201), and reducing stress (see *Learning to Relax*, pp.206–207).

Medical follow-up. Your doctor may prescribe small doses of aspirin (325 mg every other day) to avoid a recurrent heart attack (p.205). You may need other drugs to prevent angina pain, to restore a normal heart rhythm, to reduce fluid collection, or to lower your blood pressure. Follow doses exactly and report any side effects (your doctor may be able to change your medication). Go for checkups regularly and call your doctor if you have specific medical questions.

---

attacks in people with mild angina. Even for patients with severe arterial blockage and chest pain, surgery is recommended only when other methods of relieving the pain, such as drug therapy and lifestyle changes, have been tried unsuccessfully.

When the blockage is limited to just one or two segments of an artery, it may be possible to open the artery with a less invasive technique called balloon angioplasty. A catheter with a tiny balloon is inserted into the artery, and the balloon is inflated to stretch the artery walls and open up the narrowed portion. For increasing numbers of people with coronary heart disease, this procedure is becoming an alternative to bypass surgery.

What does a pacemaker do? When is it needed?

A pacemaker generates electrical impulses that stimulate the heart muscles to contract at a regular rate. The artificial device is surgically implanted in the chest or the abdomen when the heart's own natural pacemaker, an electrical generating center called the sinoatrial node, does not function properly or when the impulses that it sends to some parts of the heart are blocked. As a result of the malfunctioning, the heart may beat too fast, too slowly, or erratically (conditions called arrhythmia) or even stop altogether (cardiac arrest).

A typical pacemaker consists of a battery pack with a microelectronic circuit and a catheter that carries electrical wires to the heart. The device is usually preset to produce electrical impulses that stimulate a particular rate of heartbeats (generally 70 beats per minute). There are two types of pacemakers in common use today. A fixed-rate pacemaker, which produces impulses continuously, is implanted in patients whose natural signals have become very weak or irregular. A demand pacemaker monitors a patient's natural heartbeat and takes over temporarily if the heart slows down or misses a beat. A person who suffers from on-again, off-again arrhythmia is likely to receive a demand pacemaker.

For people who need them, pacemakers extend life. Studies show that the life expectancy of both children and adults who have pacemakers is frequently the same as that for healthy people of the same age.

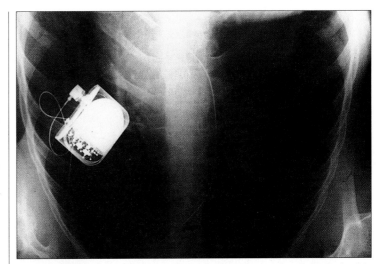

Most pacemakers control heartbeat with a single catheter connected to the heart's right ventricle (lower chamber). Some models, like the one in this chest X-ray, do the job more precisely with a second catheter to the right atrium (upper chamber).

My doctor says I may need a pacemaker. Is the surgery involved dangerous?

In most cases, implanting a pacemaker involves minor surgery, using local anesthesia. The procedure is not painful, either during or after the implantation. You may have slight soreness afterward, but it usually disappears within a few days.

Most pacemakers are implanted in the upper chest. To implant one, the surgeon makes an incision in a vein and threads the pacemaker's catheter through the vein into the right side of the heart. Then, just below the surface of the skin, the surgeon creates a small pocket to hold the pacemaker. Today's pacemakers are so tiny that the resulting bulge can hardly be noticed after the incision has healed.

During the first 2 days after receiving a pacemaker, the patient is carefully monitored with an electrocardiogram, and a chest X-ray is taken to make sure that the pacemaker is firmly in place. Strenuous activity should be avoided for about 2 weeks. After that, however, complete healing can be expected, and the patient can return to work and normal activity almost as soon as he wants.

A pacemaker may need its batteries replaced after several years, but the device itself usually lasts for 10 to 15 years before it needs to be replaced. Until then, the pacemaker must be checked periodically to make sure that it is working properly. This can be done with electrocardiograms in a doctor's office or even by telephone hookup to special pacemaker monitoring stations around the country.

Will receiving a pacemaker limit what I can do?

On the contrary, a pacemaker is likely to expand your range of activities, letting you undertake tasks that you may have avoided because of your heart problems. As a pacemaker recipient, just be sure to carry the device's name and type with you at all times, either on a medical identification bracelet or on a card in your wallet. Also carry your doctor's name and phone number and a list of any medications you take.

To make sure the pacemaker is performing correctly, you'll have to take your pulse at least once a day. You'll also need to be aware of other warning signs of a failing pacemaker: dizziness, fainting, heart palpitations, breathing difficulties, unexplained weight gain, and swelling of the ankles and legs.

Until the mid-1970's, people who wore pacemakers were warned to stay away from certain electronic devices, such as microwave ovens and electronic cash registers, which produce electromagnetic fields that could interfere with the pacemaker's functioning. Modern pacemakers are immune to interference from these common devices but can still be affected by sources of stronger electromagnetic fields, such as industrial engines, high tension wires, arc welders, and radio, television, and radar transmitters, including CB radios. Although frightening to the wearer, the effect of this interference is temporary and ends once you leave the scene. Another source of interference is the ultrasonic scaler

dentists use to remove plaque, so be sure your dentist knows about your pacemaker.

The security gates at airports don't affect pacemakers, but your pacemaker may set off the alarm; to avoid problems at the gate, carry a letter from your doctor when you travel.

What is heart failure? How does it differ from a heart attack?

In a heart attack, or myocardial infarction, part of the heart dies due to a cutoff of the blood supply to the affected area. Heart failure, on the other hand, means

RECOVERING FROM A STROKE

A stroke occurs when a blockage in a cerebral artery (a blood clot, an air bubble) or a hemorrhage cuts off the blood supply to a part of the brain. Without oxygen and glucose, brain tissue dies. In general, damage to the right side of the brain causes paralysis on the left side of the body, a loss of spatial perception, and forgetfulness. Damage to the brain's left side causes paralysis of the right side of the body, speech impairment, and difficulty understanding or remembering language.

Joint and muscle manipulation and other forms of passive physical therapy start immediately after the stroke to prevent bedsores, lung problems, thrombosis, and muscle atrophy. Special rehabilitation programs follow: physical therapists work on balance, spatial perception, and reeducating the patient's muscles; speech therapists deal with language difficulties; occupational therapists concentrate on daily living skills such as hygiene, feeding, and dressing.

Stroke victims frequently suffer depression, a frustrating barrier to rehabilitation for the patient and a cause of misunderstanding for family and friends who are trying to help. The patient's depression may well be caused by specific brain damage that occurred during the stroke; it isn't just a psychological reaction to the stroke, as people close to the patient may think.

Depression following stroke can often be successfully treated with antidepressant drugs that act chemically on the brain. However, family and friends can help by paying attention when the patient expresses feelings, by trying to find practical solutions to specific problems, and by offering encour-

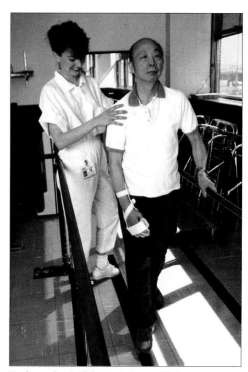

Under a physical therapist's watchful eye, a stroke patient tests his balance and gait by walking between parallel bars. Physical therapy is a critical part of the post-stroke rehabilitation process.

agement at each step toward recovery.

The goal of all therapy is to restore as much as possible the patient's independence and productivity. Some patients spontaneously recover their physical and mental functioning during the first 30 days after the stroke. Others make a nearly complete recovery with hard work and the support of family and friends; most patients, however, do suffer permanent limitations.

that the heart is unable to fully accomplish its main task—pumping enough blood to meet the needs of the body. Unlike a heart attack, heart failure is not immediately life-threatening, but it can eventually be fatal if not treated.

If the failure is in the heart's left side (which pumps oxygen-rich blood from the lungs to the body), it usually causes fluids to back up and accumulate in the lungs, resulting in difficulty breathing. If the failure is in the right side (which pumps oxygen-depleted blood from the body back to the lungs), fluids back up in body tissues. This can cause swelling of the ankles and legs and abdominal pain, as fluids swell the liver and crowd the intestines. Heart failure often affects both sides of the heart, causing both sets of symptoms. In this case, the condition is called congestive heart failure.

Heart failure can be caused by injury to the heart, most often stemming from a heart attack. It can also result from severe high blood pressure, badly clogged arteries, diabetes, inflammation of the lining of the heart muscle, rheumatic heart disease, and congenital heart abnormalities.

The usual treatment for heart failure is a reduction in physical activity, often including a period of bed rest. Diuretic drugs and a low-salt diet are generally prescribed to rid the body of excess fluids. A doctor may also order drugs to dilate the arteries, improve heart strength and rhythm, and treat other underlying conditions.

When is it safe to start having sex again after a heart attack?

Only your doctor can answer that question for you, but in general, if you are physically comfortable taking a short walk or climbing a

couple of flights of stairs, sex is probably safe. Most people feel this fit within 3 to 4 weeks of an attack. But depression, which sometimes follows a heart attack, diminishes a person's sexual desire and performance. Mild depression usually goes away on its own after a brief period; severe depression should be treated by a doctor. Many heart medications also lessen sexual interest and ability. Often a change in drug type or dosage will take care of the problem.

If you avoid sex just because you fear it might cause another heart attack, realize that such incidents are rare. Take a relaxed approach to lovemaking. Choose a time when you and your partner feel rested and free from stress, perhaps in the morning or after an afternoon nap. Try to defer sexual activity until 1 to 3 hours after a full meal and take any prescribed medication before engaging in sex. If you develop angina pains during intercourse, your doctor may recommend taking a nitroglycerine pill 15 to 30 minutes before having sex. Again, only your doctor can advise you on how much activity is safe during recovery.

If you find that your spouse is more apprehensive about making love than you are, be reassuring and communicate clearly what level of activity you find comfortable. Also, both of you may be more at ease if at first your partner assumes the more physically active role. Or you may want to try forms of lovemaking that require less exertion than full intercourse for a while.

Is cancer considered a chronic illness?

Although cancer is not usually included in lists of chronic diseases, many forms of cancer do fulfill the basic criterion for a

chronic condition: a health problem that persists for a long time. Certain cancers may go into remission for several months or even years, during which time patients may have no symptoms but must monitor their condition. Even when a cancer isn't in remission, however, patients may live with it for long periods of time. One in two people treated for cancer now has a normal life expectancy. This average does not include the easily cured basal cell and squamous skin cancers (p.372), which rarely result in a loss of life.

The word *chronic* is even used in the name of certain leukemias, such as chronic lymphocytic and chronic granulocytic leukemias. In this case the term is used to distinguish between the slow-growing leukemias and their acute counterparts, which may progress more rapidly.

A friend of mine has leukemia, but her disease is now in remission. Does this mean she's cured?

Not necessarily. Having a disease in remission is not the same as being cured but it is certainly the first step toward recovery. In a remission the symptoms and laboratory evidence of the disease have diminished or disappeared temporarily. The disappearance of all disease symptoms and signs is called a complete remission. The goal of treatment is to extend these periods of remission for as long as possible.

Unless the remission lasts for at least 4 years, however, most leukemia patients eventually experience a relapse of the disease, and treatment must be started anew. Leukemia patients who have remained in complete remission for 5 full years are considered recovered.

LIVING WITH CANCER

A diagnosis of cancer is no longer the automatic death sentence it was once considered to be. Today the cure rate is such that 50 percent of Americans with cancer are still alive 5 years after their original diagnoses. And a growing percentage have reached the 10-year mark and beyond.

New therapies are not only better at stopping some cancers, but they are also safer and less debilitating to patients. Surviving cancer involves four steps: diagnosis (confirming the disease and how far it has spread), treatment, rehabilitation, and follow-up. It takes a team of specialists to get you through all the steps, including social workers and hospital administrators who assist you in finding psychological and financial aid. The team is often led by an oncologist, or tumor specialist, recommended by your primary care doctor.

Although no two cancer treatments are exactly the same, most patients face some combination of surgery, radiation therapy, and chemotherapy. Cancer treatment can still be harsh. Agents powerful enough to kill cancer cells often destroy normal cells as well, causing side effects that may include nausea, vomiting, fatigue, impotence, difficulty swallowing, dry mouth, ulcers in the throat or mouth, dehydration, respiratory difficulties, hair loss, constipation, diarrhea, itchy skin, anemia, or infections. Fortunately, most of these side effects are temporary.

Like cancer treatments, pain control has improved. Some pain caused by the disease is alleviated by the treatment itself; other pain can be managed with analgesics such as aspirin, ibuprofen, and acetaminophen alone or in combination with codeine. In cases of severe pain, stronger opiates may be used. (There is little concern about a potential dependency when the drugs are used exclusively to relieve physical pain.)

Cancer surgery may cause disfigurement. Your rehabilitation may include reconstructive surgery or instruction in the use of a prosthesis if you have lost a body part to cancer.

Following are some general guidelines for dealing with cancer treatment.

Participate in your treatment. Your team of medical experts will interpret all the tests and tell you what they think and why, but only you should make final decisions about your care. Ask questions and be sure that you understand all your options and their risks. If you disagree with or don't trust your original oncologist, try to find another one quickly with whom you can comfortably discuss your care.

RECONSTRUCTIVE SURGERY

When cancer surgery involves certain parts of the body—the face or the breasts, for example—it can be disfiguring. To help alleviate a patient's fears about how he or she will look, a plastic surgeon is often consulted before the first operation. Just discussing the possibility of reconstructive surgery may be helpful in reassuring patients. In some cases, depending on the woman's age and condition, reconstructive breast surgery can be scheduled immediately after a mastectomy. Otherwise, the reconstruction may be done after a convalescence of several months.

The silicone implants used in many breast reconstructions may cause scarring and are suspected of increasing the risk of cancer and autoimmune disease. An alternative technique called pedicle flap surgery (shown right) is more difficult and time-consuming but creates a viable, living breast. In this operation, a flap of skin and other tissue is taken from the patient's abdomen to form the new breast mound (flaps can also be taken from the thighs and buttocks). Although the abdomen is left with a scar, the patient gets a free "tummy tuck" in the process. Such reconstructive surgery is expensive, but unlike cosmetic surgery, it is usually covered in part or completely by major medical insurance.

Which cancers have a high cure rate if they're detected early?

Skin, testicular, breast, uterine, cervical, prostate, and colon cancers are all fairly easily detected at an early stage by routine tests and exams. All have high survival rates (at least 70 percent) if they're detected and treated early. The tragedy is that many people who could be cured find out about their cancers only after the disease has spread. Once that happens, the chance for a cure is much less. For example, colon cancer that is treated early has a 5-year survival rate of 88 percent. After the disease has spread to nearby organs or lymph nodes, however, the rate drops to 58 percent, and by the time the disease has spread to more distant parts of the body, fewer than 7 percent of patients will live for 5 years.

Stick to your treatment. Whatever therapy you agree to, keep every appointment and take every pill exactly as prescribed.

Eat well. You may lose your appetite or find it hard to swallow, but you need nourishment to fight cancer. If necessary, eat smaller meals, but increase their protein and fat content. Drink soup, milkshakes, or milk instead of water. Enrich soups with powdered milk. Eat more dairy products.

Get enough rest. Fatigue is a normal side effect of the disease and the therapy. You may be able to keep a full work schedule if you get a nap in the afternoon and extra hours of sleep at night.

Exercise regularly. Exercise helps prevent stiffness, skin sores, constipation, breathing prob-lems, and other conditions related to inactivity. Ask your doctor to recommend an exercise plan. Try to take at least a short walk every day.

Don't give up intimacy. Ask your doctor what sexual limitations you can expect and encourage your partner to join in the discussion. Physical inti-macy is therapeutic and almost always possible.

Talk about it. Cancer patients need to talk openly with family and friends about what they are going through and how they feel about it. There are also support groups that can be found through the American Cancer Society (see Ap-pendix), the hospital, or your doctor. Some serve cancer patients in general; others serve people with a particular type of cancer. Support groups for families of cancer patients are also common.

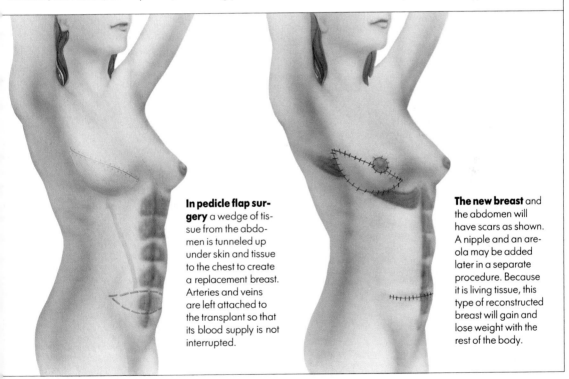

In pedicle flap sur-gery a wedge of tis-sue from the abdo-men is tunneled up under skin and tissue to the chest to create a replacement breast. Arteries and veins are left attached to the transplant so that its blood supply is not interrupted.

The new breast and the abdomen will have scars as shown. A nipple and an are-ola may be added later in a separate procedure. Because it is living tissue, this type of reconstructed breast will gain and lose weight with the rest of the body.

Early detection and treatment can save lives. For a schedule of recommended screening tests, see pages 124–125. For women, two screening tests are particu-larly important: a regular Pap smear, usually done as a part of a pelvic exam (p.252), and a mam-mogram every other year start-ing at the age of 40 and every year after 50. In addition, all women should examine their breasts once a month (p.203). These self-exams help a woman become familiar with the feel of her breasts so that she is more likely to notice any changes in them that may signal cancer.

For men, regular testicular self-exams (p.204) are recom-mended and, after the age of 40, an annual prostate exam (p.248). Both men and women with a family history or other factors in-dicating a higher-than-normal risk for certain cancers (p.204) may need more frequent exams.

JOINT REPLACEMENT SURGERY

Total hip and total knee replacement operations, greatly improved in recent years, offer pain relief and restored mobility to hundreds of thousands of American arthritis sufferers each year. Prosthetic devices—made of biocompatible metal and plastic—mimic the action of the natural hip and knee; they create stable, pain-free joints with a useful range of motion for more than 90 percent of patients. A recipient is able, after healing and physical therapy, to walk, climb stairs, swim, and possibly even ride a bicycle or play golf with an artificial hip or knee.

Loosening of the artificial joint components after 5 years or more is still the greatest problem. Most artificial joints are cemented to natural bone. If the bond gives way, the joint must be recemented in a second operation. Better cements and an alternative method of fusing artificial joints to bones without cement are being tested.

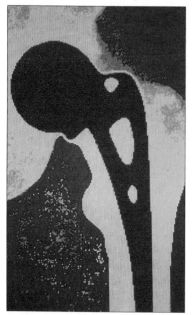

Joint replacement isn't recommended for everyone. People under 50, for example, may retain more use of their joints with less aggressive treatment. Because hips and knees are weight-bearing joints, obese people are not good candidates for replacements, nor are patients unwilling to exercise surrounding muscles.

A stemmed metal ball and plastic socket make up an artificial hip joint.

of cartilage and other joint tissue. In its mild form it is a natural and inevitable part of aging. Osteoarthritis most often affects joints that receive repeated stress or injury or that carry weight, usually the fingers, hips, knees, and spine. It not unusual for this form of arthritis to involve only one or two joints, without affecting other parts of the body.
☐ Rheumatoid arthritis is the most severe form of chronic inflammatory joint disease. It starts in one or more joints, inflaming and swelling the membrane surrounding the joint. The inflammation later spreads to the joint's cartilage and bone, and eventually may spread to other joints. Over time and without proper treatment, rheumatoid arthritis can cause joint deformity.
☐ Ankylosing spondylitis is an affliction of the spine that usually occurs in people between the ages of 20 and 40. Typically, the joints of the lower back become inflamed and the bones fuse together. After the inflammation recedes, the victim may have a permanently stiffened back.
☐ Gout is a form of arthritis caused by elevated levels of uric acid, a waste product normally removed by the kidneys. Uric acid crystals collect in a joint until they suddenly produce inflammation and intense pain. Gout occurs more often in men than women and usually affects only one joint at a time, often the big toe or another foot or hand joint.

Do the terms *arthritis* and *rheumatism* mean the same thing?

Not really. Rheumatism is an imprecise nonmedical term used to describe any disorder that causes pain and stiffness in muscles and joints, whether it involves only minor aches and twinges or a serious case of rheumatoid arthritis. Arthritis, by contrast, is a term used by doctors for more

than 100 different types of joint inflammation disease, all characterized by pain, swelling, stiffness, and redness. Depending on the type, arthritis may involve one joint or many and can vary widely in its severity. Described below are four major types of chronic arthritis in adults.
☐ Osteoarthritis, also called degenerative arthritis, is the most common type. This chronic condition is caused by the breakdown

How is osteoarthritis treated? How can I slow its course?

Osteoarthritis is the result of years of wear and tear on the joints. But even though bones and joints degenerate with age, much can be done to treat the symptoms and slow the development of osteoarthritis. An overall treatment program includes loss of excess weight, gentle exercise, heat and cold treatments, and avoidance of undue stress on the affected joints. Analgesics and corticosteroids can relieve pain, and nonsteroidal anti-inflammatory drugs can reduce joint inflammation. Aspirin, which both relieves pain and reduces inflammation, is a common treatment. Severe osteoarthritis may require surgery to correct deformity or relieve pain.

I've heard rheumatoid arthritis called an autoimmune disease. What does that mean?

The human immune system is designed to defend the body against invading bacteria, viruses, and other microorganisms by producing antibodies that recognize and destroy the intruders. In people with autoimmune disorders, these normal protective reactions are turned against the body's own cells and tissues.

Autoimmune disorders can be either organ-specific (directed against one particular organ, such as the pancreas, thyroid, or stomach) or non-organ-specific (widely spread throughout the body). Insulin-dependent (type I) diabetes, for instance, is considered an organ-specific disorder because antibodies attack only the pancreas, impairing its ability to produce insulin. Rheumatoid arthritis, on the other hand, is non-organ-specific because antibodies can attack almost any joint in the body.

My mother had rheumatoid arthritis. Does that increase my risk of developing it?

Having a parent with rheumatoid arthritis probably does increase your risk, but the odds that

---

FACT OR FALLACY ?

Arthritis is primarily a disease of older people

Fallacy. Arthritis can develop at any age. There are many different types of arthritis that can affect children, including a condition similar to rheumatoid arthritis in adults. The outlook for children and young people with arthritis, however, is usually better than it is for adults. The disease often goes into remission and in some cases disappears completely.

---

you have inherited a tendency toward the disease are still small. Researchers have found that more than half of the people with rheumatoid arthritis share a distinctive genetic marker on their white blood cells, while only about a quarter of the adult population at large have the marker. If one of your parents carries the marker, your chances of inheriting it and the tendency toward rheumatoid arthritis are greater than normal. However, most carriers of the rheumatoid arthritis marker don't get the disease; other, still unknown factors may have to be present to trigger its development.

My doctor says I have rheumatoid arthritis. What is the long-term outlook for me?

The outlook is very hopeful. Most people with rheumatoid arthritis can lead full productive lives, with a level of activity that is close to normal. The amount and severity of disability and deformity

---

usually associated with severe rheumatoid arthritis have been lessened by the treatment methods used today. These usually consist of cautious therapeutic exercises, warm compresses, cold packs, plenty of rest during flare-ups, and anti-inflammatory medications—aspirin and nonsteroidal anti-inflammatory drugs. Your doctor may also prescribe more powerful, so-called antirheumatic drugs, such as gold salts or penicillamine, which can halt or even reverse the course of severe rheumatoid arthritis. Corticosteroid drugs, which suppress the immune system, are reserved for cases that resist other medications. It's important to take your medications exactly as prescribed and to tell your doctor if any drug seems to be losing its effectiveness or is causing adverse side effects.

Successful management of your condition also depends on the proper mix of rest and exertion, which only you can control. You may need to build rest periods into your day. A regular exercise program may include gentle stretching and swimming in a heated pool as well as physical therapy. You'll learn through trial and error when to push yourself and when to take it easy. You'll also need to be aware of any changes in symptoms and to protect the affected joints from unnecessary stress. Devices such as buttonhooks, special door handles, and raised toilet seats can reduce stress on joints (see *Adapting a Home for Changing Needs,* pp.350–351).

A friend of mine has lupus. How serious a disease is this and how will it affect her life?

Lupus, or systemic lupus erythematosus (SLE), is another form of arthritis. It is a potentially serious chronic autoimmune disorder that causes inflammation of connective tissue in many organs of the body, most often in women of childbearing age. The cause of lupus is one of the great mysteries of medicine.

Lupus takes its name from a characteristic rash that extends across the cheeks and nose and is said to resemble the bite of a wolf (*lupus,* in Latin). Its symptoms are extremely varied and often mimic those of other diseases, such as rheumatoid arthritis, influenza, and anemia. They may include fever, fatigue, lack of appetite, weight loss, rashes, aches and pains, swollen glands, nausea and vomiting, headache, depression, bruising, hair loss, swelling, mouth ulcers, arthritis in two or more joints, anemia, chest pain, and seizures.

In most cases, the disease is mild, affecting only a few organs. In some people, however, the condition can be serious and disabling, affecting the skin, joints, kidneys, lungs, heart, nervous system, and blood. It is rarely fatal, but it can be life-threatening if the kidneys are involved. SLE is an unpredictable disease with symptoms that may come and go without apparent reason. Although people with lupus typically enjoy periods of remission, the disease almost always flares up again.

A much milder and more common form of the disease, called cutaneous or discoid lupus, is confined to the skin and characterized by persistent flushing of the cheeks or a patchy rash, usually in a circular pattern.

Has a cure for lupus been found yet?

No, not yet. But treatment of the symptoms has greatly improved over the last 20 years. Steroids and other drugs can slow or even stop the progress of the disease, and the kidney problems that are the source of most concern can usually be controlled. Many people with the most severe form of the disease live for 10 years or longer after diagnosis. And people with milder cases can expect a near-normal lifespan. As with other serious diseases, early detection and treatment are crucial to prevent severe and permanent damage to a person's internal organs.

What happens during an asthma attack?

The signs of an asthma attack are a tightness in the chest and difficulty breathing, usually accompanied by wheezing and coughing. In response to various triggers (see facing page), the lungs of people with asthma become swollen and inflamed. The airways in the lungs (bronchioles) narrow and fill with mucus, impeding the normal flow of air into and out of the lungs. Asthma attacks may last a few minutes or continue for hours. Their severity varies considerably from mild (the majority of cases) to life-threatening.

Is it true that children with asthma tend to outgrow the condition? Can you develop asthma later in life?

In many children with asthma, the symptoms will disappear during their teenage years, although attacks may recur later in life. Asthma in children is a common and serious condition that can affect their capacity to exercise and participate in sports and hurt their self-image as well.

It's also possible to develop asthma later in life. Allergic asthma, triggered by an allergen such as pollen or dust mites, usually develops before age 40. Non-allergic asthma, which has no obvious cause, usually starts after 40. Regardless of the sufferer's age or whether the condition is severe or mild, asthma should always be treated by a doctor.

What are the recommended treatments for asthma? Is it possible to prevent an attack?

Asthma attacks are treated with a variety of prescription drugs, taken by mouth or inhaled through a plastic inhaler. One type of asthma drug, the bronchodilators, relaxes and opens the airways. Other medications prescribed for asthma include cromolyn sodium, which makes the airways less sensitive to asthma triggers, and corticosteroids, which reduce inflammation and swelling in the airways.

If you use an inhaler to combat your asthma attacks, be sure you use it correctly; follow both your doctor's and the manufacturer's instructions. Don't overuse or underuse the medication. And pay careful attention to the expiration date on the inhaler.

Even though there is no cure for asthma, attacks can sometimes be prevented. If you are asthmatic, try to avoid, or at least reduce your exposure to, any asthma triggers that you are sensitive to. You can be tested to find out which allergens will trigger an attack. Keep in mind that aspirin is a trigger for some sufferers; consult your doctor before taking it or any cold medicine containing it.

Immunotherapy, or desensitization with allergy shots, can also help prevent asthma attacks in some people. Injections of an allergen are given in gradually increasing amounts in order to slowly build up the body's tolerance to the offending substance.

ASTHMA TRIGGERS

The particular allergens, activities, or conditions that irritate the bronchial tubes and bring on an asthma attack vary from person to person. Getting to know what affects you is an important first step toward controlling the condition. With this knowledge, you can either avoid a trigger altogether or use medications to prevent or control an attack when a trigger is unavoidable. Here are the most common asthma triggers.

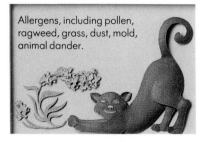
Allergens, including pollen, ragweed, grass, dust, mold, animal dander.

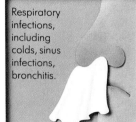
Respiratory infections, including colds, sinus infections, bronchitis.

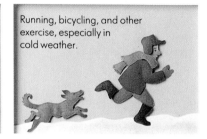
Running, bicycling, and other exercise, especially in cold weather.

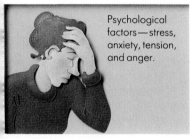
Psychological factors—stress, anxiety, tension, and anger.

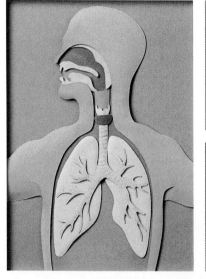

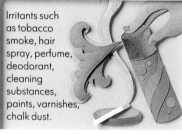
Irritants such as tobacco smoke, hair spray, perfume, deodorant, cleaning substances, paints, varnishes, chalk dust.

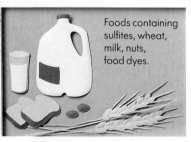
Foods containing sulfites, wheat, milk, nuts, food dyes.

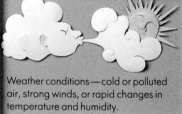
Weather conditions—cold or polluted air, strong winds, or rapid changes in temperature and humidity.

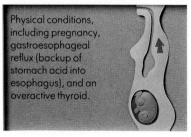
Physical conditions, including pregnancy, gastroesophageal reflux (backup of stomach acid into esophagus), and an overactive thyroid.

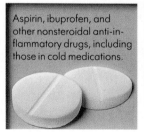
Aspirin, ibuprofen, and other nonsteroidal anti-inflammatory drugs, including those in cold medications.

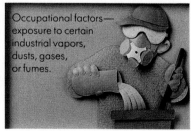
Occupational factors—exposure to certain industrial vapors, dusts, gases, or fumes.

I had a bout of bronchitis after a cold. How does this differ from chronic bronchitis?

It is not uncommon to develop acute, or temporary, bronchitis after a severe cold. Acute bronchitis is an inflammation of the bronchial tubes that branch into the lungs. Although viruses and bacteria are responsible for most cases, acute bronchitis can also be caused by heavy smoking, dust, or air pollution. Symptoms include coughing, excess mucus production, and sometimes chest pain and low-grade fever. The condition usually lasts for a few days or a few weeks at most.

Chronic bronchitis is diagnosed when a mucus-producing cough is present for at least 3 months of the year, 2 years in a row, with no other disease that could explain it. The symptoms of chronic bronchitis—coughing and shortness of breath—re-semble those of asthma (p.338), but they persist whereas asthma symptoms typically come and go, and vary in intensity. Heavy smoking is the major cause of chronic bronchitis.

What can be done for chronic bronchitis?

Treatment for chronic bronchitis is designed to reduce irritation in the nose, sinuses, throat, mouth, and airways and to encourage the elimination of mucus. Broncho-dilators may be prescribed to relax and open the airways. In some cases, antibiotics may also be given to treat or prevent bac-terial infection.

In addition, there is much that people with chronic bronchitis can do for themselves. First of all, they shouldn't smoke. Giving up cigarettes will almost always prevent bronchitis from pro-gressing. Other sources of lung irritation, such as secondhand smoke, polluted air, and dusty working conditions, should also be eliminated (p.297). Bron-chitis sufferers can help maintain their resistance to infection by eating nutritious foods, exercis-ing regularly, and maintaining an overall healthy lifestyle. Running a humidifier or inhaling steam can help loosen mucus, allowing it to be coughed up.

Is there a link between chronic bronchitis and emphysema?

Yes, indeed. Chronic bronchitis and emphysema are distinct dis-eases, but both are caused over-whelmingly by cigarette smoking, and many people who have one disease also have the other. The conditions occur together with enough frequency that the com-bination is known medically as chronic obstructive lung disease.

While bronchitis is congestion of the bronchiole tubes, in em-physema, the tiny air sacs in the lungs (called alveoli) that absorb oxygen and expel carbon dioxide are badly damaged or destroyed, making it very difficult to breathe. The lungs also lose the flexibility that normally helps keep the air-ways open. As the condition progresses, it becomes impossi-ble for a person to exhale fully.

Is emphysema curable?

No, which is one of the main rea-sons not to smoke. Once the lung tissue has been damaged by emphysema, it cannot be re-paired, although proper treat-ment can control the disease and prevent it from progressing. Treatment consists primarily of inhaling bronchodilators to open the bronchial passages and ease breathing. Of course, a per-son with emphysema has to swear off smoking for life. Other-wise the lungs will continue to deteriorate, putting a serious strain on the heart and making it necessary to have home oxygen equipment to aid breathing.

Why do I seem to get sinusitis after every cold? Can I avoid it?

Sinusitis is an inflammation of the membranes of the sinuses, the air-filled cavities in the bones around the nose, eyes, and cheeks. It often develops after a cold when mucus doesn't drain properly from the sinuses and an infection spreads from the nose into the sinuses. As mucus col-lects in the sinuses, it swells the membranes, causing headache, facial pain, and sometimes fever. Some people also lose their abili-ty to smell. Unfortunately, once you have sinusitis, the sinus membranes become extra-sus-ceptible to repeated infections.

As a result, there is a good chance that sinusitis will recur whenever you catch a cold or have an allergy attack.

Even though it is often a com-plication of a cold, sinusitis is usually not caused by a cold virus but rather by a secondary bacte-rial infection. Treatment includes antibiotics to fight the infection along with oral and nasal decon-gestants to reduce inflammation and drain the sinuses. When sinusitis is the result of an aller-gy, antihistamines may tempo-rarily reduce swelling and let you breathe a bit easier. But both de-congestants and antihistamines should be taken with care. Used too often, decongestants can have a "rebound" effect, which causes nasal passages to become even more congested. Long-term antihistamine use can dry up sinuses, making the mucus even thicker and harder to expel.

For patients with severe, re-current sinusitis, a new type of surgery, in which a thin fiberoptic scope is used to scrape away tis-sue blocking the sinuses, offers relief without the incisions and blood loss that conventional sinus surgery involves.

Home treatments include us-ing a vaporizer to promote drain-age, drinking warm liquids, and taking hot steamy showers.

What is an allergy? What substances are people allergic to?

An allergy is an exaggerated reaction by the body to some-thing that is completely innocu-ous to most people. The function of the human immune system is to defend the body against dan-gerous foreign substances. In people with allergies, however, this defense mechanism becomes hypersensitive; it not only pro-duces disease-fighting antibodies to attack harmful foreign sub-

SEASONAL ALLERGIES: WHEN AND WHERE

If you suffer from hay fever (seasonal allergic rhinitis), you can blame your runny nose and itchy eyes on plants that seasonally flood the air with microscopic pollens. Depending on your own particular sensitivities, you may be allergic to pollen from deciduous trees, grasses, weeds (especially ragweed, sagebrush, and pigweed), or a combination of sources. As the chart below shows, peak allergy seasons vary by region of the country and by type of pollen.

Mold spores also cause seasonal allergies but are less easily mapped. Mold thrives in warm, moist conditions, and spores abound after summer rains. They are present all year in the South but are rare in the nation's dry regions.

Map regions: Rockies and Great Plains; Northeast; Midwest; Southwest; Southeast; Central and Southern California; Northwest and Northern California

Legend: TREES, GRASSES, WEEDS

Chart — peak allergy seasons by region (months Jan. through Dec.):

Region	Jan.	Feb.	Mar.	Apr.	May	June	July	Aug.	Sept.	Oct.	Nov.	Dec.
Northeast												
Midwest												
Rockies and Great Plains												
Northwest and Northern California												
Central and Southern California												
Southwest												
Southeast												

stances (known as antigens) but forms antibodies against substances that are normally harmless. These otherwise benign or even beneficial substances are called allergens. Depending on the type, an allergic reaction can affect the skin, the respiratory or digestive systems, or some other part of the body. The result can be inflammation, irritation, runny nose, watery eyes, itching, hives, wheezing, coughing, shortness of breath, sneezing, and many other reactions.

A first encounter with an allergen causes no outward reaction in an allergic person. Instead, that first exposure sensitizes the person by causing the immune system to form antibodies that will recognize the allergen. Then, on subsequent exposures to the allergen, these antibodies provoke an allergic response. Common allergens are pollens, mold spores, animal dander (flakes of dead skin), animal saliva and urine (on feathers and hair), house-dust mites (p.299),

wool, various chemicals, certain drugs, and venom from insect stings. Food allergens include dairy products, strawberries, eggs, shellfish, and cereals.

How can I find out what's causing my allergies?

The most obvious way to determine what you are allergic to is by observation. If you have a rough idea of the kinds of things you might be allergic to, after a

LIVING WITH ALLERGIES

More than 35 million Americans have an allergic condition. The most common include asthma, allergic rhinitis (hay fever), and allergic reactions to foods, dust, mold, chemicals, animals, and insects. No matter what form your allergy takes, there is much that can be done to alleviate discomfort.

Medications. Several effective medications are available. Consult your doctor if they cause any unpleasant side effects.
☐ Antihistamines relieve or prevent the symptoms of allergic rhinitis by blocking histamine, the substance produced by the body during an allergic reaction. If an antihistamine makes you too drowsy or loses its effectiveness after a while, as often happens, switch to another type. Or ask your doctor about prescription antihistamines, which may not have these problems.
☐ Decongestants in tablets or nose-drop form relieve nasal and sinus congestion by narrowing blood vessels. Limit use of either type to a few days; otherwise increased congestion may occur when you stop. Oral decongestants raise blood pressure; avoid them if you have hypertension or heart problems.
☐ Bronchodilators are inhaled directly into the lungs to open the air passages and provide immediate relief from coughing, wheezing, and shortness of breath. You can also use them preventively before an allergy-triggering activity. Check with your doctor first if you have hypertension or heart problems.

Lifestyle changes. Besides avoiding your specific allergens whenever possible, try these overall suggestions:
☐ Stay inside as much as you can on dry, windy days and in the mornings when pollen and mold counts are highest.
☐ Avoid chemical irritants (perfume, household cleaners, chlorinated pool water) that can increase your sensitivity to inhaled allergens. Cold weather also affects some people's sensitivity.
☐ Reduce dust, especially in your bedroom. Try keeping floors and walls as bare as possible and other surfaces free of clutter. Wash bedding once a week; vacuum mattresses regularly. For more on controlling dust allergies, see page 299.
☐ Run your air conditioner. It cuts down on airborne allergens, and it keeps the air dry, preventing the formation of mold.

while you may begin to notice that you get an allergic reaction every time you come in contact with a certain substance or eat a particular kind of food.

Laboratory tests may also be able to reveal the cause of an allergic reaction. Although the science of allergy testing is not yet foolproof, doctors are often able to zero in on the offending substance by using either skin tests or blood tests. In skin testing, tiny amounts of suspected allergens are applied to the skin. If you are allergic to a certain substance, your skin will become irritated or develop a welt. The most reliable skin tests are those for pollen, dust, molds, and other airborne allergens; those for food allergens are considered much more questionable. Even when skin tests are relatively accurate, however, they can be painful, and they are not reliable at all for children under 3 years old, since the immune systems of young children are not yet mature enough to show a measurable response to an allergen.

A blood test called the radioallergosorbent test (RAST) is less painful and uncomfortable than skin tests, but more expensive and often less sensitive. The RAST procedure tests a person's blood for the presence of antibodies that react with specific allergens. Typically, the blood is examined for antibodies to 20 to 30 different substances that cause allergic reactions.

I began suffering from hay fever in my mid-thirties. Is this unusual?

No, not at all. In fact, it is not unusual for people to develop their first symptoms of hay fever (or any other allergic disease) after age 60 or 70.

The term *hay fever,* incidentally, is a misnomer. Hay fever is caused by pollens and molds, not hay, and there is rarely any fever involved. The correct medical term for the allergic condition called hay fever is allergic rhinitis. It is usually treated by limiting contact with the allergen and taking antihistamines when needed.

A friend of mine has had diabetes since childhood. How does her condition differ from diabetes that starts later in life?

Both types of diabetes involve the pancreas, one of whose functions is to produce the hormone insulin, which the body needs to process glucose (sugar), its chief source of energy. Without sufficient insulin, blood glucose levels rise, causing the classic symptoms of diabetes—excessive urination, hunger, and constant thirst. The type of diabetes that usually starts in childhood is called insulin-dependent, juvenile-onset, or type I diabetes. In this case, the pancreas has lost all or most of its ability to make insulin, and affected individuals need daily injections of the hormone to stay alive. Insulin-dependent diabetes appears suddenly, usually at an early age, and progresses quickly. Only about 10 percent of all people with diabetes have this form of the disease.

The other 90 percent of people with diabetes have type II, or non-insulin-dependent, diabetes. In this case, the pancreas does produce insulin, but either the amount is insufficient to meet the body's needs or the amount is sufficient, but the body is unable to use it effectively. Non-insulin-dependent diabetes occurs mainly in adults over age 40 who are overweight. The onset is usually gradual and often symptomless (untreated type I diabetes always produces symptoms). Some people with non-insulin-dependent diabetes may need oral medications or injections of insulin to help control their blood glucose levels, but many can control this type of diabetes through diet and exercise alone.

No matter what the type, it's important that diabetes be monitored and treated carefully. Left untreated, diabetes can severely impair health and lead to heart or kidney disease, stroke, blindness, gangrene, and even death. With proper treatment and diligent self-monitoring, however, a diabetic can expect to lead a full and satisfying life. The life expectancy of a type I insulin-dependent diabetic whose condi-

tion is well monitored is about the same as for a nondiabetic. However, it's slightly shorter for type II non-insulin-dependent diabetics, who often have some preexisting cardiovascular and kidney problems.

I'm 35 years old and have recently been diagnosed with type II diabetes. How will this affect my life? What is my outlook?

First of all, be happy that you know about your condition and can start to do something about it. Of the estimated 11 million Americans with non-insulin-dependent diabetes, about half are unaware of their condition, because the early symptoms are so mild and slow to develop.

If you are careful about controlling your weight and blood glucose levels through proper diet and regular exercise, you may not need any other treatment. Your doctor will show you how to regulate your food intake with carefully planned and spaced meals and how to keep track of your blood glucose levels. (see *Diary of a Type II Diabetic*, p. 344). Glucose monitoring (p. 213) should become a regular part of your daily routine, just like brushing your teeth. A few type II diabetics have to take oral diabetes drugs or insulin injections to keep glucose levels within a normal range and to prevent serious complications.

Diabetes is a chronic condition that takes effort on your part. It is a daily responsibility, both to keep informed and to watch what you eat. Diabetes is not something you can wish away or pretend does not exist. But if you adhere closely to the lifestyle your doctor recommends and take any medication regularly, your outlook is good.

Remember that you are not alone. Millions of other people in this country and around the world also have diabetes. Sometimes it helps to talk with other diabetics or with counselors who specialize in diabetes. Check with your doctor, hospital, or local affiliate of the American Diabetes Association, which can supply useful information and put you in touch with support groups and other helpful programs.

As a diabetic, will I ever be able to have a piece of candy or cake?

Yes, but you have to be sensible about it. It is a myth that people with diabetes have to avoid all sweets. In general, you should avoid concentrated sugar, because it is absorbed quickly into the bloodstream, causing blood glucose levels to rise. As long as your overall diet is sound, eating small amounts of sugary foods on special occasions should be no problem. Both the American Diabetes Association and the American Dietetic Association include limited quantities of such sweets as cookies, ice milk, and sherbet in their exchange lists (p. 344) for people with diabetes.

My daughter has type I diabetes. Can she have a normal pregnancy?

Yes, although she will need to take certain precautions. Ideally, proper control should start well before a diabetic woman becomes pregnant. Whether she is insulin-dependent (type I) or non-insulin-dependent (type II), a diabetic woman should have normal blood glucose levels for at least 2 months before conception and any diabetic complications (cardiovascular, kidney, or eye problems) should be under control. During pregnancy, a woman

DIARY OF A TYPE II DIABETIC

The key to controlling type II diabetes–and often avoiding medication–is keeping your blood glucose levels as near to normal nondiabetic levels as possible through diet and exercise. Monitoring your blood glucose two or three times a day at least 2 days a week is also important.

An essential guide for any diabetic is a food exchange list, available from your doctor or the American Diabetes Association (see Appendix). Such a list indicates which foods you can eat, which you can substitute for others, and proper portion sizes. You'll find keeping a written record helpful both for analyzing your diabetes-control regimen and for planning ahead.

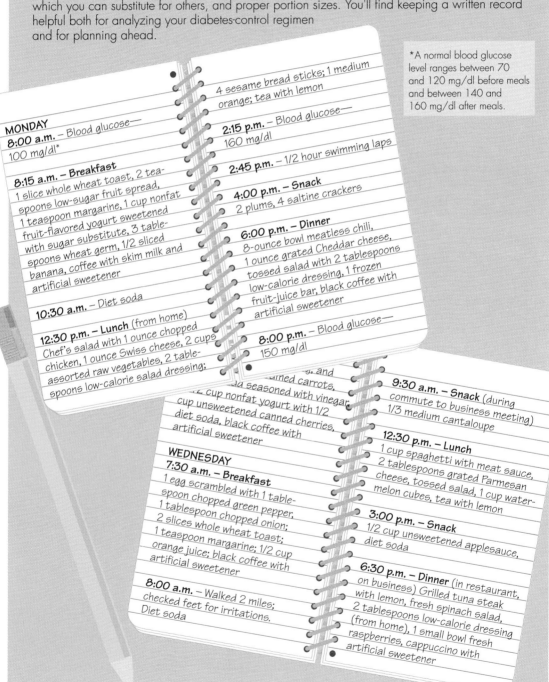

*A normal blood glucose level ranges between 70 and 120 mg/dl before meals and between 140 and 160 mg/dl after meals.

MONDAY
8:00 a.m. – Blood glucose— 100 mg/dl*

8:15 a.m. – Breakfast
1 slice whole wheat toast, 2 teaspoons low-sugar fruit spread, 1 teaspoon margarine, 1 cup nonfat fruit-flavored yogurt sweetened with sugar substitute, 3 tablespoons wheat germ, 1/2 sliced banana, coffee with skim milk and artificial sweetener

10:30 a.m. – Diet soda

12:30 p.m. – Lunch (from home)
Chef's salad with 1 ounce chopped chicken, 1 ounce Swiss cheese, 2 cups assorted raw vegetables, 2 tablespoons low-calorie salad dressing;

4 sesame bread sticks; 1 medium orange; tea with lemon

2:15 p.m. – Blood glucose— 160 mg/dl

2:45 p.m. – 1/2 hour swimming laps

4:00 p.m. – Snack
2 plums, 4 saltine crackers

6:00 p.m. – Dinner
8-ounce bowl meatless chili, 1 ounce grated Cheddar cheese, tossed salad with 2 tablespoons low-calorie dressing, 1 frozen fruit-juice bar, black coffee with artificial sweetener

8:00 p.m. – Blood glucose— 150 mg/dl

...ng, and ...anned carrots, ...a seasoned with vinegar ...2 cup nonfat yogurt with 1/2 cup unsweetened canned cherries, diet soda, black coffee with artificial sweetener

WEDNESDAY
7:30 a.m. – Breakfast
1 egg scrambled with 1 tablespoon chopped green pepper, 1 tablespoon chopped onion; 2 slices whole wheat toast; 1 teaspoon margarine; 1/2 cup orange juice; black coffee with artificial sweetener

8:00 a.m. – Walked 2 miles; checked feet for irritations. Diet soda

9:30 a.m. – Snack (during commute to business meeting)
1/3 medium cantaloupe

12:30 p.m. – Lunch
1 cup spaghetti with meat sauce, 2 tablespoons grated Parmesan cheese, tossed salad, 1 cup watermelon cubes, tea with lemon

3:00 p.m. – Snack
1/2 cup unsweetened applesauce, diet soda

6:30 p.m. – Dinner (in restaurant, on business) Grilled tuna steak with lemon, fresh spinach salad, 2 tablespoons low-calorie dressing (from home), 1 small bowl fresh raspberries, cappuccino with artificial sweetener

with diabetes has a higher-than-normal risk of developing complications. She must be vigilant about controlling her blood glucose not only for her own sake but because poor maternal blood glucose levels can produce jaundice or hypoglycemia (low blood glucose) in the baby or cause the child to be abnormally large or stillborn. A woman who develops gestational (pregnancy-related) diabetes must be equally careful.

A diabetic woman's chances for a healthy pregnancy and baby are also improved if she selects an obstetrician who is experienced in treating women with diabetes and is affiliated with a hospital with an obstetrical center that specializes in high-risk cases. Most of these centers also offer programs to help diabetic women achieve control of their condition before becoming pregnant and clinics that provide close monitoring of mother and child during pregnancy.

A concern of many diabetics who are parents or are planning a family is that their children will develop the disease. Both types of diabetes tend to run in families. But those who are predisposed to type I diabetes are less likely to actually develop the disease than those with a family history of type II diabetes. A child of a parent with type II diabetes has a 10 to 15 percent chance of developing the disease. Even so, you can help minimize your children's risk by instilling in them healthy habits regarding weight control and regular exercise.

How important is exercise in managing my diabetes?

There's evidence that middle-aged men who exercise regularly lower their risk of developing type II diabetes. For those who already have diabetes, exercise is extremely beneficial. It keeps you in shape and promotes weight loss, an especially important goal for individuals with weight-related type II diabetes. Exercise also increases metabolism, which helps bring down blood glucose levels, and it enhances the body's use of insulin, making diabetes drugs and insulin injections more effective. The role exercise plays in reducing blood pressure, lowering blood fats, and establishing healthy cholesterol levels is especially important for diabetics, who have a high risk of heart disease.

If you have the more common non-insulin-dependent diabetes and both your condition and any diabetic complications are well under control, you can undertake the same activities as a nondiabetic person in similar physical condition, provided your doctor agrees. If you are an insulin-dependent diabetic, though, you do have to be careful. If you are not properly prepared—by being in good physical condition and by eating something beforehand—exercise that is too strenuous or that lasts too long can cause a risky drop in your blood glucose. Ask your doctor to help you find the types and amount of exercise that are best for you.

Is hypoglycemia a real disorder?

Hypoglycemia—abnormally low levels of glucose in the blood—is a real, but often misunderstood, disorder. Almost all true cases of hypoglycemia occur in people with diabetes, usually insulin-dependent diabetes. When a type I diabetic injects too much insulin, doesn't eat enough or skips a meal, or exercises too long or vigorously, the resulting oversupply of insulin in the blood may cause a sudden decline in blood levels of glucose, which is essential to brain function. If the glucose level remains very low for extended periods of time, the brain can be irrevocably damaged.

The symptoms of hypoglycemia include sweating, dizziness, racing pulse, weakness, confusion, shaking, headache, hunger, tingling around the mouth, jerky movements, and skin pallor. In extreme cases, the victim passes out and, if not treated, may die.

The treatment for hypoglycemia is a quick jolt of sugar—orange juice, soda, raisins, glucose tablets, or even a sugar cube. Since hypoglycemia is always a possibility for people with insulin-dependent diabetes, they should keep some form of sugar with them at all times.

If an attack of hypoglycemia results in loss of consciousness, injections of glucagon, a hormone sold as a prescription drug, will raise the blood glucose level and rouse the victim in about 15 to 20 minutes or less. A person with insulin-dependent diabetes should keep glucagon handy and be sure that a relative or friend, both at home and at work, knows how to inject it.

What are peptic ulcers, and why do they form?

Peptic ulcers are sores that form in the lining of the upper gastrointestinal tract—the stomach, the duodenum (the first part of the small intestine), and less commonly, the esophagus. The word *peptic* is derived from pepsin, an enzyme secreted by the stomach lining, which, along with hydrochloric acid, helps break down food. When peptic ulcers form in the stomach, they are called gastric ulcers. When they form in the duodenum, they are called duodenal ulcers.

The same gastric juices that help digest food would eat away at the lining of the stomach and duodenum were it not for a protective layer of mucus secreted by the lining. Ulcers form when the balance between corrosive elements (gastric juices) and protective elements (mucous layer and mucus-producing cells) is upset. In some people, the gastrointestinal lining secretes too much acid, but more commonly, the lining produces too little mucus or irritants such as alcohol or aspirin weaken the mucous layer, leaving it vulnerable to damage by even normal amounts of gastric juices.

Many people think that stress causes ulcers, but that is not necessarily true. Stress may make it harder to cope with an ulcer or may make an existing ulcer worse, but there is no conclusive evidence that stress can actually generate an ulcer.

Although ulcers can be symptomless, most people with ulcers complain of a gnawing or burning pain in the abdomen, sometimes accompanied by loss of appetite, weight loss, belching, a bloated feeling, nausea, or vomiting. The surest way to diagnose an ulcer is with endoscopy or a barium X-ray (see *Diagnostic Tests,* pp. 126–127).

Possible complications of an ulcer include bleeding, which can be serious, and perforation of the tract wall, which is a medical emergency. A small number of gastric ulcers become malignant and must be removed surgically.

Are some people more likely to develop peptic ulcers than others?

Yes. Smokers are twice as likely to get ulcers as nonsmokers. Smoking also slows the healing process and increases the likelihood that an ulcer will recur.

Arthritis sufferers and others who regularly take aspirin or nonsteroidal anti-inflammatory drugs, such as ibuprofen, form another risk group. These drugs irritate the stomach lining and reduce its ability to produce protective mucus.

Heredity also plays a role. People with close relatives who have ulcers are three times more likely to develop an ulcer than the general population.

Although the incidence of ulcers in women has been increasing recently, ulcers are still more common in men. Duodenal ulcers usually develop in young adults, age 20 to 40; gastric ulcers, in people over 40. Ulcers are rare in children and teenagers.

My husband has developed an ulcer. Is he doomed to a life of eating bland food?

No, not at all. The thinking about food and ulcers has changed completely in recent years. Your husband should avoid drinking alcohol, coffee, and tea, which irritate the stomach, and above all, if he smokes, he should stop now. Otherwise, for most people with ulcers, a special diet is not necessary. In fact, that old staple of ulcer diets, milk, is now thought to stimulate, rather than neutralize, acid secretion. Even spicy or acidic foods are no longer thought to aggravate ulcers. Of course, certain foods will upset anyone's digestion, whether or not there's an ulcer present. It's up to your husband to determine which foods don't agree with him.

What are the standard treatments for ulcers?

Antacids neutralize excess stomach acid, providing temporary relief of ulcer pain and promoting healing. Many different types of antacids are available without a prescription (p. 215).

When antacids fail to control symptoms, ulcer-healing drugs may be prescribed. Cimetidine and ranitidine reduce acid secretion; sucralfate forms a protective coating over the ulcer.

For the small percentage of people whose ulcers do not respond to treatment with either antacids or medication, surgery may be needed.

What is inflammatory bowel disease?

The term refers to a group of chronic diseases that cause inflammation in the intestines. The main types of inflammatory bowel disease are ulcerative colitis and Crohn's disease. The former causes inflammation and ulceration in the large intestine (the colon), including the rectum. Crohn's disease can cause inflammation and thickening in any part of the bowel, but affects mainly the terminal ileum (the end of the small intestine at the point where it joins the colon). When it affects the ileum, Crohn's disease is also known as ileitis.

Ulcerative colitis and Crohn's disease have similar symptoms—frequent diarrhea, abdominal pain, rectal bleeding, pain in the joints, and fever. The symptoms may come and go, and people with either disease may experience long periods of remission. Possible complications in other parts of the body include eye inflammation, arthritis, and skin disorders. Both conditions are associated with higher rates of cancer. Diagnosis is usually based on endoscopic examination of the bowel, barium X-rays (see *Diagnostic Tests,* pp. 126–127), and biopsy (p. 144).

An estimated 1 to 2 million Americans have inflammatory bowel disease. People under 30 are most often affected, although the disease occurs in men and women of all ages. When children contract ulcerative colitis or Crohn's disease, the symptoms are apt to be more widespread and severe than in adults.

No one knows exactly why, but inflammatory bowel disease is more common in Jewish people than in Gentiles, and occurs in whites more often than in other racial groups. The cause of inflammatory bowel disease has not been identified, but emotional distress is not thought to be a factor. The most likely current theory is that a virus, bacteria, or some other outside agent interacts with the immune system to switch on the inflammatory process.

How successful is drug therapy in controlling Crohn's disease? Is surgery ever necessary?

Although there is still no cure for Crohn's disease, several anti-inflammatory drugs can effectively control abdominal cramps and diarrhea and sometimes prevent recurrences. The most frequently prescribed drugs are corticosteroids and sulfasalazine.

Crohn's disease may also be treated with immunosuppressive drugs, such as azathioprine and 6-mercaptopurine, while antibiotics are used to fight related infections. All these medications can have unpleasant side effects, such as nausea, headache, dizziness, acne, weight gain, and anemia. It is important for people with Crohn's disease to work closely with their doctors to monitor their drug reactions so that any adjustments that are needed can be made.

If medication does not control the symptoms, or if a person develops an intestinal obstruction or other complication, surgery will be necessary. Generally, the diseased part of the intestine is

removed and the two ends of the healthy intestine are reattached. Unfortunately, surgery is not a cure for Crohn's disease; the condition tends to recur near the area of the intestine that was removed.

What is the outlook for a patient suffering with ulcerative colitis?

It's generally good. People can often manage ulcerative colitis just by avoiding certain types of foods—such as milk and other dairy products or very spicy foods—that seem to set off intestinal disturbances. For most other patients, a corticosteroid drug or sulfasalazine effectively controls the disease.

Fewer than 25 percent of people with ulcerative colitis ever have symptoms severe enough to require hospitalization. However, if the disease can't be controlled with medication, if the colon becomes very swollen, or if malignancies are suspected, a colectomy (surgical removal of the colon) may be necessary. Sometimes the rectum can be joined to the upper intestine to allow normal evacuation. Most cases, however, require the removal of the entire colon and rectum, followed by an ileostomy, in which an artificial outlet for body wastes is created in the abdomen. The procedure is similar to a colostomy (p.348), but involves the small intestine rather than the colon. Colon removal brings about a marked improvement in the health of ulcerative colitis patients, although those who've had an ileostomy require time and support to adjust to a new lifestyle.

It is important to remember that neither ulcerative colitis nor Crohn's disease need interfere with leading a normal life. Despite the limitations people with either form of inflammatory bowel dis-

ease experience from time to time, most are active, productive, and otherwise healthy.

What is irritable bowel syndrome, and how does it differ from inflammatory bowel disease?

Irritable bowel syndrome is a chronic condition that causes changes in the way the colon contracts. Certain parts of the bowel contract too quickly, and others too slowly, causing a "spastic" movement that accounts for the condition's other names, spastic colon and spastic colitis. Symptoms include constipation alternating with diarrhea, and abdominal cramps and bloating. Because it involves muscle disturbances rather than inflammation or tissue damage, irritable bowel syndrome is a much less serious condition than inflammatory bowel disease.

Doctors term irritable bowel syndrome a functional disorder rather than an organic disease because no signs of disease show up on X-rays or other diagnostic tests. Diagnosis of irritable bowel syndrome is usually made only after X-rays, endoscopy (see *Diagnostic Tests*, pp.126–127), and fecal analysis have ruled out cancer, inflammatory bowel disease, and other possible causes for the patient's symptoms.

There is no link between irritable bowel syndrome and inflammatory bowel disease—that is, irritable bowel syndrome will not progress to become ulcerative colitis or Crohn's disease, nor will it lead to cancer.

The causes of irritable bowel syndrome are not clear, although stress and other psychological factors are thought to play a role. Treatment may include antispasmodic drugs to reduce intestinal spasm, antidiarrheal drugs to

TYPES OF OSTOMY

When bowel blockage, inflammation, or cancer requires the removal of all or part of the colon (large intestine), a new opening may have to be created to permit the elimination of digestive waste. The procedure is known as an ostomy; the two most common types are shown below.

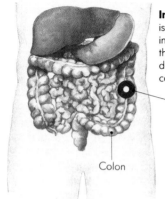

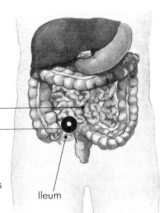

In a colostomy, part of the colon is brought through an opening in the abdomen. The location of the opening, or stoma, varies depending on the part of the colon that has been removed.

Stoma

Colon

Small intestine

Stoma

In an ileostomy, a portion of the ileum (the end of the small intestine) is brought through an opening in the abdomen. This is usually done when the entire colon must be removed.

Ileum

relieve prolonged diarrhea, and for some patients, a high-fiber diet. No sure cure for irritable bowel syndrome exists; various treatments may have to be tried before the right one is found.

If you have irritable bowel syndrome, you are not alone. Overall, the condition accounts for about one-half of all visits to doctors for digestive complaints.

My husband needs a colostomy. Can he lead a normal life after this procedure?

He certainly can, but first make sure you both understand what a colostomy is and why it is being recommended. In this procedure, a part of the colon, or large intestine, is passed through an incision in the abdomen and formed into a new, surgically created opening called a stoma. Body wastes are then eliminated directly through the stoma into a special pouch called an appliance. A permanent colostomy is required when all or part of the rectum or anus as well as part of

the colon must be removed (because of cancer, for example), making normal defecation impossible. Fewer than 15 percent of people with colorectal cancer, however, need a colostomy. Moreover, some colostomies are temporary—that is, a person recovering from intestinal surgery may need to evacuate into an external bag for a few months, after which time a second operation is performed to close the temporary colostomy.

Assuming your husband does require a permanent colostomy, you and he have every reason to be optimistic. Your husband would be joining people from all walks of life who continue to be just as active and outgoing as they were before their surgery.

As with anything new, living with a colostomy takes some getting used to. The look, size, shape, and location of the stoma vary from person to person, but in general, stomas are strong and resilient. They cannot be injured during normal everyday events, such as showering or bumping into something.

There are two types of colostomy appliances in common use—more expensive disposable pouches, which are discarded after a few days, and reusable pouches, which can be cleaned and used repeatedly, provided good hygiene is observed.

Today's appliances are made of sturdy materials and fit very securely; they can also be deodorized with drops or powders. While it is natural to worry about odor or leakage, such problems are much less likely to occur than they were in the past.

People who have had a colostomy do not require a special diet, although they may be advised to increase fiber intake as an aid to both digestion and elimination. To prevent problems with intestinal gas, the intake of high-fiber foods should be increased gradually and foods that tend to produce a lot of flatulence (p. 33) should be avoided.

Many women and men with colostomies are able to remain just as sexually active as they were before their surgery. Sexual counseling is available for those who do experience emotional or other problems. In addition there are support groups throughout the country that give people with colostomies a chance to compare notes and observe how well others in the same situation are functioning. For more information on living with a colostomy, contact the United Ostomy Association (see Appendix).

How does cirrhosis differ from hepatitis?

Cirrhosis is a form of chronic liver damage that sometimes develops as a complication of hepatitis but is more often caused by alcohol abuse, especially when combined with poor nutrition. (Cirrhosis can also be caused by various other diseases of the liver and digestive tract as well as by congestive heart failure [p.332], cystic fibrosis, some inherited metabolic disorders, and in rare cases, by prolonged exposure to certain drugs or toxic chemicals.) Unlike hepatitis, cirrhosis is not contagious, but it is a more serious disorder, with a higher incidence of fatality. Over time, cirrhosis damages normal liver cells. As these cells die, they are replaced by scar tissue. The result is that the liver can no longer perform its vital role in aiding digestion, monitoring blood glucose levels, storing nutrients, and filtering wastes from the blood. People with cirrhosis often develop fluid buildup in the legs, and some acquire a yellowish cast to the skin, resembling jaundice. Confusion and coma occur in the late stages of advanced cirrhosis.

The progress of cirrhosis can be slowed by avoiding alcohol in cases related to alcohol consumption or by treating other underlying causes. In some cases, a liver transplant offers the only possibility of a cure.

THE FACTS ABOUT HEPATITIS

What is it? Hepatitis is an inflammation of the liver that in some cases may lead to liver scarring (cirrhosis) or liver cancer; it is considered chronic if it lasts for 6 months or more. Most frequently caused by one of several hepatitis viruses, the disease can also develop as a result of other viruses that attack the liver (mononucleosis, for example), alcohol or drug abuse, exposure to certain chemicals (such as dry cleaning fluids), or damage caused by an autoimmune reaction (p.337).

How do the hepatitis viruses differ? There are five identified hepatitis viruses. Hepatitis A, common in developing countries, is spread by direct contact with an infected person's feces or indirect fecal contamination of food, water, shellfish, hands, and utensils. Hepatitis B, formerly called serum hepatitis, is the most serious form of the disease; it's spread from mother to child at birth or shortly afterward or through sexual contact, blood transfusion, kidney dialysis, or contaminated needles. Hepatitis C, formerly called non-A, non-B hepatitis, and hepatitis D, which exists only in conjunction with hepatitis B, are spread via infected blood or contaminated needles. Hepatitis E is similar to hepatitis A and spread in the same ways, but it's found primarily in the Indian Ocean area.

What are the symptoms? Fatigue, mild fever, loss of appetite, nausea, and aching joints are common signs of hepatitis. Some patients develop dark urine, jaundice, abdominal swelling, and even coma. Others have no symptoms. It's possible for a person with symptomless hepatitis B, C, or D to transmit the disease. Diagnosis is usually made by means of blood tests; in some cases a liver biopsy may be used to confirm diagnosis.

How is it treated? Most people with hepatitis A, B, D, and E recover completely with rest, abstinence from alcohol, and good nutrition; mild flare-ups may recur over a period of several months. About 5 percent of hepatitis B patients and up to 50 percent of hepatitis C patients develop chronic liver disease. Some of these cases respond well to treatment with alpha interferon. In severe cases, a liver transplant may be the only option.

How is it prevented? Adequate sanitation and personal hygiene prevent the spread of hepatitis A and E. (If you're traveling to developing countries, see your doctor about taking immune globulin; drink only bottled water and eat well-cooked food.)

Health-care workers and others who risk exposure to the hepatitis B virus can be protected by one of several vaccines. Blood tests can identify hepatitis carriers, and such screening is now routine for high-risk mothers. Babies of mothers infected with the B virus are given a preventive vaccine at birth.

Blood screening has largely eliminated the risk of getting hepatitis B from a tranfusion and is reducing the risk for hepatitis C.

Adapting Your Home for Changing Needs

Maintaining independence and self-esteem despite a debilitating disease or trauma is much easier if you can manage some basic remodeling around the house. You may need a contractor for big jobs like lowering kitchen cabinets or covering stairs with ramps, but many safety and convenience products can be installed by a handyman. Today, hundreds of products are available to make life — and everyday chores — easier and more comfortable for people with impaired mobility or dexterity. (See Appendix for product sources.)

A phone with outsize numbers and pushbuttons facilitates dialing.

This versatile faucet moves up and down, as well as from side to side, making it easier to fill tall pots.

An outdoor entryway light, equipped with a timer or a dark-sensitive bulb that goes on at dusk, makes the approach to the house brighter and safer and lets you see to unlock the door.

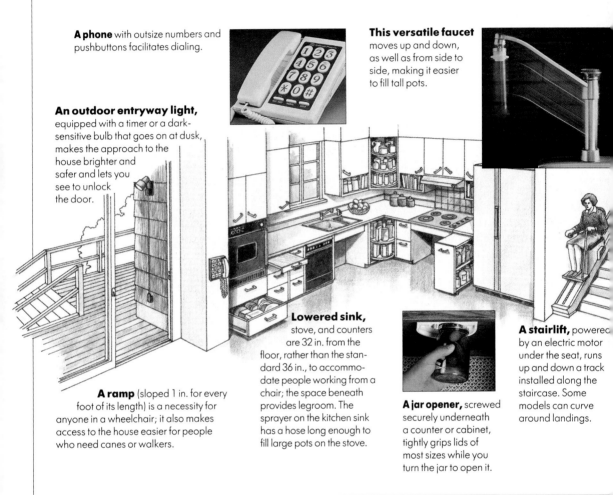

Lowered sink, stove, and counters are 32 in. from the floor, rather than the standard 36 in., to accommodate people working from a chair; the space beneath provides legroom. The sprayer on the kitchen sink has a hose long enough to fill large pots on the stove.

A ramp (sloped 1 in. for every foot of its length) is a necessity for anyone in a wheelchair; it also makes access to the house easier for people who need canes or walkers.

A jar opener, screwed securely underneath a counter or cabinet, tightly grips lids of most sizes while you turn the jar to open it.

A stairlift, powered by an electric motor under the seat, runs up and down a track installed along the staircase. Some models can curve around landings.

Gadgets That Make Life Easier

Put on socks or stockings without having to bend down with this molded stretcher, which holds the hose top open while you slide your foot in.

A buttonhook makes dressing less frustrating for those with stiff fingers; a hook on the other end is for pulling up zippers.

Long-handled brush is angled to allow a person with restricted arm movement to manage a coif successfully.

Globe-shaped pencil holder takes pressure off painful arthritic joints as you write. The holder can also be clamped around a toothbrush.

Loop scissors cut with a squeezing motion that is easier on arthritic hands than the pinching required by conventional scissors.

Extension gripper has a claw that grasps objects securely as you bring them toward you. A lug hooks soft items; a magnet pulls in metal objects.

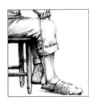
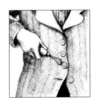

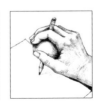

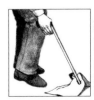

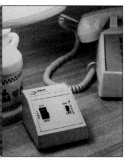

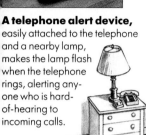

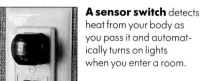

A sensor switch detects heat from your body as you pass it and automatically turns on lights when you enter a room.

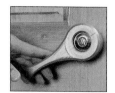

A lever handle, which fits over any standard knob, makes opening doors easier for stiff arthritic hands.

A telephone alert device, easily attached to the telephone and a nearby lamp, makes the lamp flash when the telephone rings, alerting anyone who is hard-of-hearing to incoming calls.

Lowered closet rod and shelf can be reached from a wheelchair.

An over-bed table has casters for mobility and an adjustable top that can be raised and tilted.

Offset hinges swing a door out and away from the door frame to allow a wheelchair access through the opening.

A hospital bed can be raised to 30 in. (nursing height) or lowered to 19 in. (wheelchair level). A pushbutton control also adjusts the positions of the bed's head and foot.

Wall grab bar has a zigzag shape and scored inner surface for better gripping at several different heights.

Wheelchair-accessible shower has a barrier-free entry, a hand-held shower head, a water-mixing valve that controls water temperature with a single knob, grab bars, and a wheelchair-level seat.

A single-lever faucet handle makes it easy to regulate water temperature and flow.

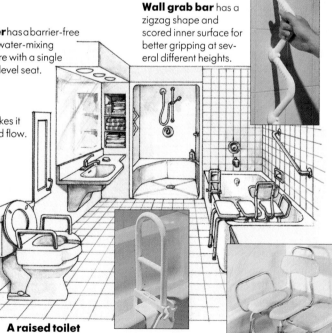

Special eating utensils, such as thick-handled flatware, knives with curved blades, lipped plates, and non-tip, double-handled cups, are designed to make holding them more comfortable and using them less difficult for people with limited or impaired manual dexterity. You may have to try different styles before you find the best ones for your situation.

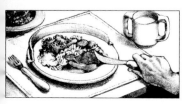

A raised toilet seat clamps on to a standard toilet bowl. Padded arms offer extra support.

A tub grab bar, which clamps over the edge, allows you to get safely into and out of your bath.

A tub seat, adjustable for height, lets you bathe comfortably while sitting down.

What is chronic kidney failure, and what causes it?

Chronic kidney failure is the gradual and progressive loss of the kidneys' three vital functions: removing wastes and excess fluid from the body; maintaining the body's natural balance of water, salt, potassium, and acid; and regulating blood pressure.

Unlike acute kidney failure, in which a sudden shutdown of kidney functions produces alarming symptoms such as swelling, breathlessness, and dramatic weight gain within a matter of days, chronic kidney failure develops gradually over many years. Symptoms such as loss of appetite, nausea, weakness, and frequent urination may not become apparent until the kid-

neys have lost a good portion of their ability to function. If left to progress untreated, chronic kidney failure eventually results in coma and death.

A number of factors can cause kidneys to fail. These include infections, inflammation, obstructions, high blood pressure (which is both a cause and a result of chronic kidney failure), diabetes, polycystic kidney disease (an

---

THE FACTS ABOUT DIALYSIS

For a person whose kidneys fail to filter waste products and excess fluid from the blood, dialysis is a life-saving alternative. There are two main types of dialysis. In hemodialysis, the patient's blood is filtered by an artificial kidney machine. In peritoneal dialysis, the filtering process takes place in the patient's own body. Either procedure can be done in a hospital, a special clinic, or at home, depending on the patient's medical condition, personal desires, and financial situation. Patients must continue dialysis for the rest of their lives or until they receive a kidney transplant.

Hemodialysis. Before the first treatment, a special plastic shunt is implanted between an artery and a vein in the patient's arm or leg to allow regular access to the bloodstream for quick removal and return of the blood. The machine is made up of two parts—one for the blood and one for the solution (dialysate) used to clean the blood. An artificial membrane separates the two compartments. This design allows the blood's components—primarily red and white blood cells and protein—to remain in one compartment, while smaller particles of waste products are filtered through the membrane into the dialysate. Treatments usually last 3 to 4 hours and are needed three times a week.

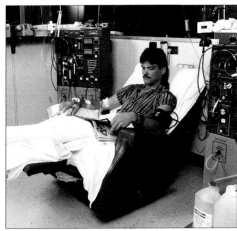

In hemodialysis, an artificial kidney machine substitutes for a patient's real kidneys, filtering waste products and excess liquid from his blood.

Peritoneal dialysis. Before the first dialysis, a soft plastic catheter is surgically implanted in the patient's lower abdomen. In peritoneal dialysis, the lining of the patient's own abdominal cavity (the peritoneum) serves as a filtering membrane. The dialysate (cleansing fluid) is drained by gravity from a soft plastic bag into the abdominal cavity and left there for 4 to 5 hours. During that time, waste products and excess water from the blood vessels lining the cavity seep through the

peritoneum and mix with the dialysate, which is then drained back into the bag and discarded. The procedure is usually performed at home by the patient as many as four times a day. While the liquid is in the abdominal cavity, the patient can unhook the bag and go about normal activities. The procedure can also be done by a machine that cycles dialysate in and out of the cavity several times during the night while the patient sleeps.

inherited disorder in which many cysts form on the kidneys), and excessive, long-term use of painkillers or of certain illegal drugs, such as heroin. A diagnosis is usually based on kidney function tests, which measure levels of urea and other waste products in the blood. Contrast X-ray imaging, ultrasound scanning, radionuclide scanning (see *Diagnostic Tests,* pp.126–127), and biopsy (p.144) may be used to detect the underlying cause of kidney failure.

Can chronic kidney failure be slowed down or halted? Is it possible to avoid dialysis or a kidney transplant?

The progression of chronic kidney failure due to diabetes or high blood pressure can be slowed through a combination of diet, medication, and exercise aimed at controlling blood glucose or blood pressure.

Although much has yet to be learned about the relationship between diet and kidney disease, there is some evidence that a low-protein diet is beneficial. Striking the right protein balance, however, can be tricky: too much protein can overload the kidneys; too little results in poor nutrition and will impair general health. Always consult your doctor before making any drastic changes in your diet.

Once chronic kidney failure reaches an advanced stage, however, dialysis (the artificial cleansing of the blood) or, when possible, a kidney transplant is the usual form of treatment.

How successful are kidney transplants?

The outlook for a kidney transplant patient is quite good, especially if the donated organ comes from a living relative. (Unless something goes wrong with the remaining kidney, which rarely happens, there is no risk to a donor's health in living with only one kidney.) But even when the kidney comes from the cadaver of someone who is unrelated to the recipient, the success rate of kidney transplants is much greater than that of heart or liver transplants.

Although it's possible for a patient with chronic kidney failure to lead a relatively normal life with dialysis, the treatment of choice is a kidney transplant. This is a serious operation, whose primary danger is that the recipient's immune system will recognize the donated organ as foreign tissue and reject it. To guard against this possibility, transplant recipients must take immunosuppressant drugs (medications that lower the body's ability to fight foreign invaders— either cold viruses or transplanted organs) for the rest of their lives. Unfortunately these drugs can produce serious complications and they don't always work effectively. If, despite treatment with immunosuppressant drugs, the donated kidney is rejected, the patient returns to dialysis. Another kidney transplant may be possible if the patient is otherwise in good health. Researchers are working on new techniques that in the future may allow kidneys and other organs to be transplanted successfully without the recipient having to take immunosuppressant drugs.

My younger sister has been diagnosed as having epilepsy. What causes her seizures?

Epilepsy is a physical condition marked by sudden, brief changes in the way the brain functions. Seizures result when normal electrical signals in the brain misfire. An uncontrolled surge of electrical energy may occur spontaneously, or it may be set off by some outside factor, such as a flash of light. Seizures last for a short time, from just a second to a minute or two.

There are two main types of seizure—generalized and partial. In a generalized seizure, the epileptic loses consciousness as the whole body stiffens and then twitches and jerks. In a partial seizure, which affects a more limited area of the brain, the victim may remain conscious during the episode. A partial seizure, however, can turn into a generalized one. (A type of generalized seizure, absence seizures are momentary losses of consciousness that usually occur in children. During these blank periods, which may recur hundreds of times a day, the epileptic appears to be daydreaming or inattentive.)

Epilepsy can develop at any age but is most likely to begin in childhood or adolescence. The condition may develop for no apparent reason, or it may result directly from a head injury, brain disorder, drug abuse, or lead poisoning. It sometimes develops as a complication of such diseases as meningitis, encephalitis, or severe measles.

Is it possible to tell when my sister is about to have a seizure? What should I do to help her when one starts?

It is seldom possible to know that a seizure is imminent. Sometimes just before a seizure an epileptic will experience a strange sensation—a feeling of fear, sickness, or irritability, or an odd smell or taste. This so-called aura results from an increase in the brain's electrical activity. However, seizures are rare for most epileptics today, thanks to modern medications. If your sister does have one, keep calm and reassure others. Clear the surrounding area of anything hard or sharp, and put something soft under her head. Loosen tight clothing, jewelry, or anything around her neck that may make breathing difficult. Keep the airway open by turning your sister gently on her side. Don't restrain her or put anything in her mouth.

Stay with your sister until the seizure is over, and be calm and reassuring as consciousness returns. If a seizure occurs away from home, help your sister to get home safely as she may seem confused or disoriented.

How is epilepsy treated?

For most people, drug therapy alone will prevent seizures. A variety of anticonvulsant drugs are used to control different types of seizures. These drugs may produce unwanted side effects, such as drowsiness and lack of concentration, and it may take some trial and error before the most effective drug or combination of drugs is found. Women with epilepsy who wish to have children may be advised to change their medication before becoming pregnant to reduce the risk of birth defects.

If a person remains seizure-free for an extended period, the doctor may consider discontinuing drug therapy. But epileptics should never stop taking a prescribed medication suddenly on their own. An abrupt withdrawal of the drug may bring on seizures and other problems.

In rare cases, surgery is used to treat epilepsy if drugs have been unsuccessful or if only one, well-defined part of the brain is thought to be affected.

THE FACTS ABOUT PARKINSON'S DISEASE

What is it? Parkinson's disease is a chronic brain disorder that affects muscle control and movement. The first sign, which may become apparent in the fifth or sixth decade of life, is often a slight tremor in a resting hand, arm, or leg. In time, the tremor affects both arms and legs and the head. Other symptoms include stiffness, weakness, difficulty in initiating movement or changing position, a stooped posture, a shuffling gait, diminished blinking, a frozen facial expression, dribbling, and difficulty in swallowing. Speech may become slow and hesitant, and in the later stages of the disease, intellect may be affected. Depression is common among Parkinson's disease patients.

What causes it? Parkinson's results from damage to or degeneration of the substantia nigra—a layer of gray matter deep within the brain containing nerve cells that produce dopamine, a neurotransmitter (p.161). Smooth muscle movement depends on a balance between dopamine and another neurotransmitter, acetylcholine. When dopamine is lacking, the balance is disrupted and the symptoms of Parkinson's begin to appear.

Why the substantia nigra deteriorates is unknown. Exposure to environmental toxins, such as pesticides and chemical fertilizers, is thought to play a role. Certain drugs, especially antipsychotics (p.171), produce the symptoms of Parkinson's as a side effect.

The disease is not contagious, nor does it seem to be inherited. Men are more likely to develop it than women.

How is it treated? There is still no cure for Parkinson's disease, but its symptoms can be alleviated by a combination of drugs and physiotherapy designed to maintain and improve mobility. Antiparkinsonism drugs fall into two main groups. Anticholinergics block the effect of acetylcholine to compensate for the dopamine deficiency. Levodopa and other dopamine-boosting drugs raise the level of dopamine activity in the brain. Although they can be remarkably effective in relieving symptoms, antiparkinsonism drugs produce side effects in many people and their effectiveness declines over time. Drug therapy for Parkinson's disease requires careful monitoring and experimentation on the part of the doctor to determine the most effective drug(s) and dosage(s) for any given stage of the disease, while minimizing side effects.

A still experimental treatment involves transplanting dopamine-producing tissue from a patient's adrenal glands into the brain.

What is the outlook? Parkinson's isn't fatal, and drugs have greatly improved the quality of life for many patients. In time, however, the disease becomes harder to control and routine tasks become more difficult. Home aids (see *Adapting a Home for Changing Needs,* pp.350–351), self-help groups (see Appendix), psychotherapy, and family support can help patients cope with the psychological and practical problems the disease poses.

How does MS affect the human body?

Multiple sclerosis (MS) is a disease of the central nervous system that destroys myelin, the protective covering around nerve fibers in the brain, spinal cord, and elsewhere in the body. Although the cause of MS is unknown, the main suspects are a slow-developing virus, an autoimmune reaction, or a combination of the two. The disease occurs more often in colder areas than in the tropics and is twice as common in women as in men. It primarily strikes young adults, with the first attack often occurring between the ages of 20 and 40. Onset is rare in children and older adults. Genetic factors also play a role, since relatives of people with MS have a higher risk of developing the disease than the rest of the population.

In a healthy body, myelin acts as a nerve fiber insulator, helping to maintain the flow of electrochemical impulses that keep the different parts of the body in constant communication with each other. In people with MS, the myelin is destroyed and gradually replaced with hard scar tissue that distorts or even blocks nerve signals. As a result, depending on which parts of the brain, spinal cord, or other nerve tissue are affected, the disorder can cause such symptoms as numbness, tingling, weakness, fatigue, loss of coordination and balance, double vision, slurred speech, tremors and shaking, impaired bladder control, sexual problems, and paralysis. Although not a mental illness, MS sometimes interferes with memory and decision making.

MS symptoms vary from person to person. In some people they are mild and cause very few problems. Others experience flare-ups between periods of remission. Although MS is usually considered a chronic condition, in rare cases it causes a single flare-up and no more. MS is rarely life-threatening, but unfortunately, many MS sufferers must learn to cope with progressive disabilities.

What is the treatment for MS? Are there ways to prolong a remission?

Although there is as yet no cure for multiple sclerosis, much can be done to help people who have the disorder to remain active, independent, and productive.

Treatment with corticosteroid drugs or adrenocorticotropic hormone (ACTH) can sometimes shorten or reduce the severity of an MS attack. Other medications may be prescribed to alleviate specific symptoms, such as tremors or shaking.

Physical therapy can strengthen and relax muscles and help patients maintain function following severe attacks. Some people may need braces to help them move about. Rather than being a mark of disability, braces and other such devices should be regarded as the means by which people with MS achieve and maintain their independence.

Researchers are working hard to improve treatments for the disease and to help prolong remissions. In the meantime, people with MS are advised to guard against infections and try to maintain optimum health by eating well, scheduling regular rest periods, and avoiding overwork, excessive fatigue, and stress. Although it's important for people with MS to remain active, becoming overheated can exacerbate symptoms. For this reason, doctors often advise their MS patients to take up swimming, which provides a good workout without overheating the body.

Is chronic fatigue syndrome a real disorder? If so, is there a treatment for it?

There is a growing recognition that this somewhat controversial condition—once dismissed as a figment of the patient's imagination—is real and very disabling. Since there's still no laboratory test for chronic fatigue syndrome, the illness is defined by its symptoms: overwhelming fatigue that has persisted for at least 6 months, accompanied by at least six of the following symptoms—severe headaches, joint or muscle pains, muscle weakness, nausea and vomiting, abdominal cramps, confusion, irritability, inability to concentrate, depression, and sleep problems. The disease seems to strike many more women than men and more adults than children.

The causes of chronic fatigue syndrome are unclear. Some researchers believe that one or more viruses may be involved, or that something happens to switch on the body's ready-alert defenses, throwing the immune system into a chronic state of overactivity. According to other theories, chronic fatigue is a result of muscle breakdown or of a magnesium deficiency.

Whatever the cause, chronic fatigue syndrome does not appear to be contagious. Over time most people with the syndrome get better, although it may take several years for a person to feel completely normal again.

Researchers are still working to find a cure for chronic fatigue syndrome. Meanwhile, people who suffer from it are advised to stay in the best possible condition by eating a balanced diet and getting plenty of rest. In addition, they can help themselves by keeping informed about the latest research and by joining with fellow sufferers for emotional support and encouragement. (For the names of support groups, see Appendix.)

I've suffered from migraines for years. What causes these terrible headaches?

The causes of migraines are still a mystery. The severe, throbbing pain of a migraine is thought to be due at least in part to dilation of blood vessels in the head. As the blood vessels expand, they trigger the release of pain-inducing chemicals. The scalp's nerve endings become irritated, and the head throbs with pain.

Migraines tend to run in families. Some researchers think that people who are susceptible to migraines may inherit a defect in the way the brain handles the neurotransmitter serotinin (p. 161), a chemical messenger that can influence the way a person perceives pain.

Of the two basic types of migraine, the relatively rare classical migraine is often preceded by warning signs, such as flashing lights, blurred vision, and sometimes partial blindness that clears up in about 20 minutes. A common migraine does not telegraph its arrival as clearly, if at all.

The factors that trigger migraines vary with the individual. Some of the most common triggers are anxiety, stress, tension, fatigue, bright or flashing lights, and extremes of temperature. In women, oral contraceptives and changing hormone levels during menstruation or ovulation may cause migraines. Certain foods can act as triggers, especially those containing a chemical called tyramine that constricts the arteries. The chief food offenders are alcoholic beverages (especially red wine), chocolate, cheese, citrus fruits, nuts, and caffeine.

Have there been any recent advances in the treatment or prevention of migraines?

Some very effective options are now available. These include drug therapy, biofeedback, stress reduction, exercise, and control of triggering factors.

Mild migraine attacks can sometimes be averted with aspirin or acetaminophen. There is also some evidence that taking an aspirin every other day can prevent migraines. But do not embark on aspirin therapy without consulting your doctor.

If mild painkillers don't work, your doctor may prescribe a drug called ergotamine tartrate, which, if taken early in the course of an attack, helps shrink dilated arteries in the brain and has proven very effective in relieving migraines. Unfortunately, ergotamine can cause serious side effects and should be taken only occasionally. If used regularly, ergotamine can even increase the frequency of attacks.

Other drugs, such as the beta-blocker propranolol, may be prescribed to avert more frequent attacks of migraine. But because such drugs can also cause serious side effects, they should be taken only under careful medical supervision.

Biofeedback (p. 207) is a technique that can help you gain control over such basic biological functions as muscle tension and temperature. By learning to raise the temperature in your hand, for example, you may be able to direct the flow of blood away from the head, thus constricting painful swollen arteries.

Since stress can trigger migraine attacks, sufferers should try to get enough sleep, exercise regularly, and practice relaxation techniques (see *Learning to Relax*, pp. 206–207).

A small percentage of people may be able to prevent migraines by identifying and eliminating the foods that trigger their attacks.

Can a disorder in one part of the body cause pain to be felt somewhere else? If so, how does this happen?

Oddly enough, it is possible to feel pain in a part of your body other than the part that is actually causing the pain. For example, you may feel a pain in your hip that stems from arthritis in the knee. Or you may feel a pain in your right shoulder that really signals an inflammation of the diaphragm in your chest or a liver problem. Perhaps the most familiar example of this phenomenon, known as referred pain, is a heart attack or angina that is felt as a pain in the left arm.

Most cases of referred pain are due to the convergence in the spinal cord of nerves from two different areas of the body. The brain attributes impulses from one area as coming from the other, obscuring the location of the pain's true source.

I've been told that chronic pain can occur mysteriously without any sign of injury or disease. Is this true?

Yes. Some people suffer free-floating pain that has no discoverable source. In some cases, pain persists after the illness or injury that caused the pain in the first place has been resolved. In other cases, no known physical cause precedes the onset of pain.

People with pain that has a source, no matter how bad the ache, at least know why they are hurting. But the suffering of people with free-floating pain is compounded by uncertainty and

THE FACTS ABOUT CHRONIC BACK PAIN

What causes it? At some point in their lives, most people suffer back pain. The most common back problems are usually the result of poor posture, overweight, weak abdominal and back muscles (which support the spine), or strain (often from lifting a heavy load incorrectly). To deal with this type of back pain, see *Relief for an Aching Back,* pp.218–219. More serious and persistent back pain arises from a trauma, congenital spinal defects, tumors, or one or more of the conditions described below.

When should I consult a doctor? If severe back pain isn't relieved by rest and home therapy within a few days, if back pain immobilizes you for more than 2 days, if pain shoots down the back of either leg, or if back pain is accompanied by other symptoms such as high fever, dizziness, or abdominal pain, see your doctor as soon as possible.

Osteoarthritis (p.336) in the joints between vertebrae can cause pain and stiffness anywhere along the back or in several different spots simultaneously.

Sore muscles or ligaments, usually caused by poor posture, tension, recent exercise or other exertion, or infection, can be felt anywhere in the back.

Herniated disc, also known as prolapsed or slipped disc, is most likely to occur in the spine's lumbar region. Discs—the shock absorbers between vertebrae—can wear down and protrude enough to put pressure on a spinal nerve.

Spinal stenosis is a narrowing of the spinal canal often caused by bony growths that alter the contours of vertebrae.

Ankylosing spondylitis is an inflammation of the joints between vertebrae or between spine and pelvis, which can lead to fusion and a severe loss of movement.

Facet joint displacement is a locking of two vertebrae out of alignment at the facet joint, which connects pairs of vertebrae and enables the spine to move. Irritation within the joint itself or pressure on a nerve causes pain.

Sciatica, pain that follows the sciatic nerve from the buttocks to the foot, is caused by pressure on the nerve from a slipped disc, tumor, or bone infection.

Coccyx pain occurs at the spine's base, often after the coccyx (tailbone) hits a hard surface in a fall.

How is chronic back pain treated? The first line of defense is usually rest (on your back on a firm surface with a pillow under your knees), moderate applications of ice or heat, and analgesics. Your doctor may prescribe anti-inflammatory drugs or a muscle relaxant; he or she may also recommend that you be put in traction, wear a back or neck brace, or undergo physical therapy.

When is surgery necessary? Spinal tumors and herniated discs that put pressure on spinal nerves can be removed surgically. Fusing two or more vertebrae together may stabilize an unsteady spinal joint. Surgery is rarely recommended, however, before extensive nonsurgical treatment and testing. Back surgery is risky. Consult a qualified surgeon, then seek a second opinion.

fear. Such people often go from doctor to doctor, searching in vain for a diagnosis. Their pain may bring on serious psychological problems, compounded by dependence on alcohol or drugs. However, intensive medical and psychiatric care can help control this type of chronic pain.

What are the latest advances in pain management?

Some of the most interesting research involves endorphins, the body's own natural pain relievers. For example, exercise has been found to stimulate the production of these soothing proteins. Inactivity not only shuts down the production of endorphins, but can also lead to muscle deterioration. As a result, pain specialists are now prescribing a planned program of exercise for their patients with chronic pain.

Some people with chronic pain have found relief through a therapy called transcutaneous electrical nerve stimulation (TENS). Brief pulses of electricity are applied to the nerves just under the skin near the pain site. Exactly how this works or why it works on some patients but not others remains unclear. It may be that TENS triggers the production of endorphins or blocks pain signals from reaching the brain. Recent studies, however, are casting doubt on the efficacy of TENS as a pain reliever.

Researchers are also learning how to harness the power of the placebo effect. It has been known for some time that a sugar pill or other inactive placebo can often make a sick person feel better. Somehow, the power of suggestion or the patient's own optimism or belief in his or her physician sets in motion a cycle of healing. It is now believed that the placebo effect may have a neurochemical component that allows certain people to tap into the supply of endorphins in their brains.

Depending on the source of a pain, physicians may also prescribe various types of drug therapy, ranging from mild painkillers such as aspirin and acetaminophen to powerful prescription drugs such as codeine, morphine, propoxyphene (Darvon), and meperidine (Demerol).

Psychological methods of pain relief include psychotherapy, behavior modification, hypnosis, relaxation and meditation, and biofeedback (see *Learning to Relax,* pp. 206–207).

In cases of extreme chronic pain, surgery may be an option. The procedure usually involves cutting several nerves leading from the pain site to the spinal chord and brain. This leaves the previously painful area with no sensation whatsoever, a cure that may be worse than the ill.

The best sources of information about the management of chronic pain are your family physician and the many pain clinics located throughout the United States (for further information contact the American Chronic Pain Association, Inc., or the National Chronic Pain Outreach Association; see Appendix). Unfortunately, charlatans and phony pain-relieving gimmicks abound in the field of pain management. Reputable pain clinics usually employ a team of medical specialists who can tailor diagnosis and treatment to fit the individual patient's needs.

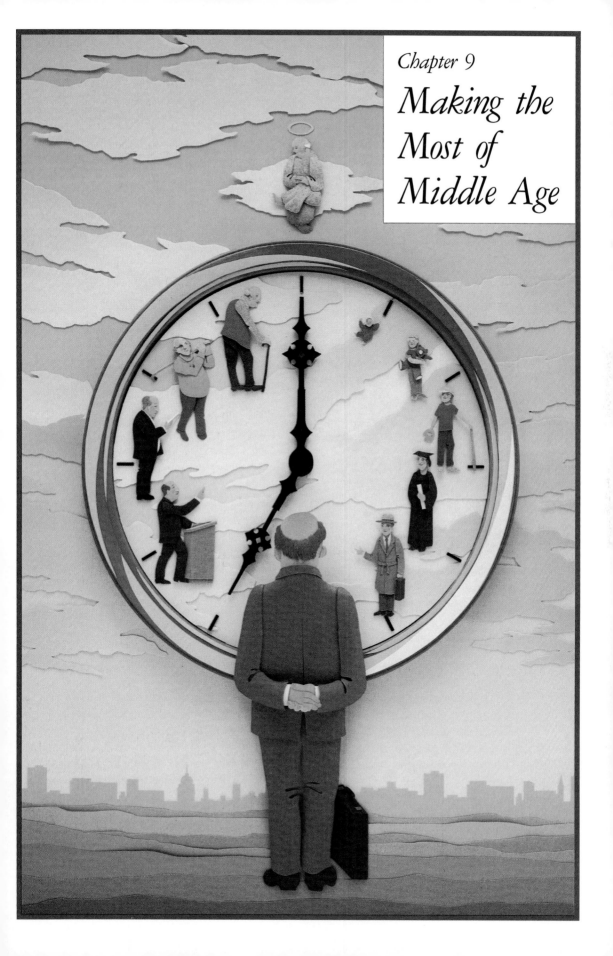

Chapter 9

*Making the
Most of
Middle Age*

Caring for a Sick Parent

When Jean R.'s widowed mother developed Alzheimer's disease at age 68, life for Jean, a homemaker in her mid-forties, changed abruptly. Faced with a rapid decline in her mother's mental functioning, Jean decided to bring her mother home and care for her herself.

Jean's children felt displaced in their own home and were ashamed to have friends over because of their grandmother's unpredictable behavior. Jean's husband, while supportive, missed the intimacy he had shared with his wife, and began to spend more time at work. Exhausted and overextended, Jean wondered how long her own health would hold out.

Concerned about her family's well-being, Jean decided to reassess her situation. By now, her mother no longer recognized her and needed almost constant attention. After a great deal of deliberation, Jean made the difficult decision to place her mother in a nursing home. Knowing that her mother was well cared for by professionals, Jean began to reclaim her life and rebuild her relationships with her family.

Baldness Averted

Despite coming from a long line of prematurely bald men, David D., a successful 41-year-old lawyer, had retained his hair for most of his thirties. By the time he turned 40, however, there was no denying his receding hairline and ever more visible crown. To David, his thinning hair and growing paunch were clear and distressing signs of waning youth.

One day, after seeing him attempt to hide his bald spot, David's wife reminded him that he had a doctor's appointment in a week and suggested that he discuss his hair loss.

When David mentioned his concern about going bald, his doctor referred him to a local dermatologist who had had success treating balding patients with minoxidil, an antihypertension drug that often stimulates hair growth. The fact that David was healthy and had only recently begun to lose hair made him a good candidate for minoxidil. After 10 months of treatment with minoxidil ointment, David's crown is no longer visible. His new hair has improved not only his looks but his self-confidence too. It even inspired David to do something about that paunch.

A Midlife Turnaround

Eleanor K.'s forties had been tumultuous. She divorced her alcoholic husband, went to work, put three children through school, and began studying for an advanced degree at night. Armed with her new degree, Eleanor landed a well-paying job and felt that things were finally coming together for her.

As she neared 50, however, Eleanor suddenly wasn't so sure. Her children finished college and moved out, leaving her alone and lonely in a large house. She embarked on a promising relationship with a divorced man, but let her insecurities get in the way and cause a breakup. To make matters worse, Eleanor's menopause was proving difficult. She was having hot flashes day and night and often complained of dizziness and palpitations. Listless and irritable, Eleanor went to her gynecologist for help.

After a complete physical and a discussion of the pros and cons of hormone replacement therapy, Eleanor and her doctor decided to give it a try. Almost at once, the hormone treatments relieved Eleanor's hot flashes and other physical symptoms. Within months she felt better in other ways too. With her spirits much improved, she was socializing more and meeting new people. After a difficult transition, life really was begining anew for Eleanor at 50.

TEST YOUR HEALTH I.Q.

Facing Up to the Passage of Time

Change is a fact of life at any stage, but especially so in the middle years. New responsibilities emerge, such as paying for children's college education, taking care of declining parents, and planning for retirement. New concerns arise, such as reducing the health risks that an aging body is subject to. For some, the midlife transition is confusing and traumatic. For most, it's a time to reevaluate the present and plan for a better future.

Many myths surround the middle years. See if you can tell fact from fallacy by choosing the phrase or phrases that most accurately complete the following statements.

1 Middle age begins when a person _____ .

- **A.** reaches age 40
- **B.** becomes a grandparent
- **C.** has grown children
- **D.** feels middle-aged

2 _____ may play a major role in the aging process.

- **A.** Free radicals
- **B.** A built-in genetic program
- **C.** A death hormone

3 Weighing slightly more at 40 than you did at 20 _____ .

- **A.** is detrimental to health
- **B.** may be beneficial in some cases
- **C.** results in part from a natural slowing of metabolism

4 _____ have a higher risk of developing glaucoma than others.

- **A.** Very fair-skinned people
- **B.** Diabetics
- **C.** People with a family history of glaucoma
- **D.** Blacks

5 The medical term for an eye tuck operation is _____ .

- **A.** genioplasty
- **B.** otoplasty
- **C.** blepharoplasty

6 A possible cause of liver spots is _____ .

- **A.** overproduction of bile in the liver
- **B.** a diet too high in fat
- **C.** years of overexposure to the sun
- **D.** insufficient exposure to the sun

7 The hair of _____ tends to turn gray earliest.

- **A.** Asians
- **B.** whites
- **C.** blacks
- **D.** Native Americans

8 A postmenopausal woman should wait _____ after her last period before she can safely stop using contraceptives.

- **A.** 6 months
- **B.** 1 to 2 years
- **C.** 3 to 4 years

9 Divorce is most likely to occur among couples in the _____ age range.

- **A.** 15- to 24-year
- **B.** 25- to 34-year
- **C.** 35- to 44-year
- **D.** 45- to 53-year

Answers

For more information on any of the quiz topics turn to the pages listed next to the answers.

1. D, p.362	4. B,C,D, p.369	7. B, p.373
2. A,B,C, p.363	5. C, p.370	8. B, p.375
3. B,C, p.364	6. C, p.371	9. A, p.378

When does middle age begin and what are its signs?

When midlife begins is a matter of some debate today as better diets and healthier habits help people live and feel younger longer. Most of us think of midlife as the years from about 40 to 65, but being middle-aged has less to do with chronology than with changes in relationships, attitudes, and experiences. At 45, some contemporary men and women are already grandparents, others are putting children through college, and still others are raising preschoolers. How you feel about your age and the changes that midlife brings really determines when middle age starts for you.

The harbingers of midlife are subtle at first. Many people admit to being middle-aged when they can no longer deny the presence of fine wrinkles and gray hairs or when they notice that it takes longer to recover from sessions of strenuous exercise. The acquisition of reading glasses, a thickening waistline, and the appearance of brown spots on hands underscore the passage of time.

Middle age often brings with it new or at least different responsibilities and significant changes in lifestyle and tastes. This is a time of maximum earning power for some, and of sometimes wrenching career decisions and changes for others. Men often begin to focus more on the pleasures of the hearth, while women, particularly those with grown children, get bolder in their career ambitions.

It's also the time many people start thinking of retirement and the need to plan for it. As your children venture out on their own, your parents may start demanding more of your time and help. Cultural tastes may change. (One sign of impending middle age is said to be the failure to recognize the latest pop music.)

In midlife, people tend to become more introspective. They begin to think more about their own mortality and how to make the most of the time that they have left. In a process that psychologist Erik Erikson termed *generativity*, concern shifts in the middle years from the self to family, society, and future generations. At work you may enjoy becoming a mentor, or you may volunteer for more responsibilities in the community.

The transition to midlife was once viewed as potentially traumatic, a time of crisis in which men embarked on affairs to prove their continuing virility and women became depressed and felt useless in their newly emptied nests. Today, however, that notion is giving way to a much more positive view of middle age as a time of fulfillment, both per-

---

DEFINING MIDLIFE

The very notion of middle age is a relatively recent one—not surprising considering the fact that until the 20th century it was uncommon for people to reach what we now consider the middle years. The average age at death was only 18 for prehistoric men and women, in the twenties for ancient Greeks and Romans, and about 30 throughout the medieval period. Such figures, however, are somewhat misleading in that they take into account the extremely high infant and maternal mortality rates that were the norm until this century. People who survived infancy could, and sometimes did, live to a ripe old age, but even as recently as 1900, only 4 percent of the U.S. population was over 65.

In 1900 the average life expectancy in the United States was 47 years. By 1950 that figure had risen to 66 years, thanks mainly to dramatic declines in infant and maternal mortality. Since then, the availability of vaccines and antibiotics and other medical advances have helped slow the death rate, with the result that today the average American can expect to live into his or her seventies.

Although youth and old age have been studied extensively, research into middle age as a distinct stage of life is relatively recent and incomplete. This situation is changing, however, as the post-World War II baby boomers swell the ranks of the middle-aged. In a major effort to close the gap in knowledge about midlife, the Chicago-based MacArthur Foundation launched a multi-million-dollar research project in 1989. By the time the study is completed (it's expected to last at least 7 years), researchers hope to have a clearer picture of the medical, social, and psychological factors that allow people to navigate midlife successfully.

sonal and professional. Wiser and more experienced than they were in their youth, many people flower in middle age.

How and why do we age?

Scientists have developed many theories to explain aging, but no one really knows how and why it happens. According to one theory, our cells contain a built-in genetic program, a DNA clock that sets the pace of aging and determines the outer limit of an individual's life span. Another view holds that the body contains a fixed amount of energy that gradually dissipates over time and is finally used up. Some scientists blame aging on the vicissitudes of daily living (cells are damaged by the foods you eat, the air you breathe, and the wear and tear you put your body through) or on the gradual deterioration of the immune system, which makes the body more susceptible to infection and disease.

One school of thought emphasizes the role of free radicals (molecules with free, unpaired electrons) in the aging process. Free radicals exist normally in the body, but are also produced by tobacco smoke, sun, burned foods, and certain drugs. In the presence of oxygen, free radicals trigger a chain reaction that causes cells to deteriorate in much the same way as exposure to salt air causes metal to rust.

Still another theory suggests that a gland, possibly the pituitary, secrets a death hormone, which triggers the aging process and eventually ends life.

Intriguing new research seems to support the idea that human cells contain the seeds of their own destruction. Scientists in the United States and Japan have succeeded in growing certain cells indefinitely in a laboratory culture. Investigating these so-called immortal cells, the scientists found that all of them lacked a specific human chromosome. When the missing chromosome was introduced into the cells, they began to age.

Research on aging continues on many fronts. Although it may not produce a unified theory that will help doctors prolong human life (aging may be too complex for that), the work is likely to help doctors better understand and treat diseases associated with aging such as Alzheimer's (p. 410) and atherosclerosis (p. 329).

What can I do to slow the aging process?

Good genes, good luck, and an absence of disease help determine to a great extent how kind the aging process will be to you. (For more on the pace of aging, see page 386.) There are, however, important steps you can take to maintain your vitality, youthful appearance, and good health as long as possible.

☐ If you smoke, stop (p. 201). In addition to being disastrous for your health, smoking promotes wrinkling of the skin.

☐ Excessive exposure to the sun can lead to skin cancer and premature wrinkling. Try to limit your exposure, and when you do go out in the sun, be sure to protect yourself adequately with sunscreen (pp. 218–219).

☐ Eat a balanced diet and try to maintain a steady weight. Losing and gaining weight repeatedly weakens the elasticity of the skin, causing sags and wrinkles.

☐ To replenish the natural moisture lost by aging skin, drink six to eight glasses of liquid each day. Don't rely on coffee, tea, cola, or alcoholic drinks exclusively for your liquid intake; these beverages act as diuretics, draining water from the system.

☐ If you drink alcohol, do so in moderation.

☐ Stay physically active. A regular exercise program approved by your doctor will not only make you feel more energetic but may help you look younger and live longer too.

☐ Stay mentally active. If you take a lively interest in the world around you and keep yourself intellectually challenged, your mental agility and capacity for learning will continue to grow.

☐ Remember that wrinkles and gray hair are not the end of the world. Perhaps the best way to deal with aging is to accept gracefully the changes life brings you at different stages.

How does the transition to midlife differ for men and women?

Men at midlife tend to follow more predictable patterns than women—possibly because men at midlife have been the focus of more studies and possibly because men define themselves almost exclusively in terms of their careers. A man's vulnerability at midlife usually involves his sense of where he stands at work. If his own particular dreams have not been achieved, a man may be distressed to see younger men and women winning more recognition on the job. Socialized to be tough and independent, however, he may have trouble expressing his feelings. Emotionally isolated men can have a hard time making the transitions they need to make at this stage of life.

On a brighter note, a man who has concentrated his energies on climbing a career ladder may now find that he is at or near the top of his potential. The achievement of personal goals and the development of interpersonal relationships can now take higher priority in his life.

Although women face major losses at midlife—grown children leave home, menopause ends their years of fertility, their parents' health may fail—most seize this opportunity to pursue their own interests. Midlife can be a liberating time for women; particularly for those who are mothers, it can be a time to reconnect with delayed ambitions.

For women who have postponed having a family, entering midlife means confronting their biological clocks and realizing that their childbearing years are coming to a close. Many such women make having a child their number-one priority.

What can I do to ease the transition into midlife and make the most of it?

Acknowledge the fact that your life is changing. Give yourself time to accept the transition you're going through and to contemplate the significance of your experience at midlife. What's missing in your world? What unfulfilled dream can you go back and recapture? What's good about your life? What aspects do you wish to develop further? At midlife, most people are becoming less concerned with others' opinions and more secure in their own point of view. Allow the wisdom you've accumulated over the years to guide you.

The losses of midlife are undeniable. In a culture obsessed with physical beauty, men and women alike mourn the fading of youth. The risks for developing heart disease and other illnesses increase. Women in midlife are more likely to develop breast cancer (pp. 202–204) and to undergo hysterectomies (p. 253). Men in midlife can develop prostate troubles (p. 248). New emotional burdens may include

---

FACT OR FALLACY?

Most people undergo some sort of midlife crisis

Fallacy. Midlife is a turning point for many people but this transition assumes the dimensions of a crisis for only a few. At about age 40, many people take a long, hard look at themselves. No longer young, they can evaluate the achievements and errors of their early years. Not yet old, they still have time to make changes.

Most people change gradually, responding to events, taking advantage of opportunities, and allowing their inner feelings to guide them. Some people, however, make hard decisions in their twenties and never question them. At midlife, such people often discover that a bit of soul-searching is in order. A person who delays acceptance of some crucial reality—waiting until the children are grown to acknowledge the failure of a marriage, for instance—may indeed experience the sort of midlife identity crisis the media love to chronicle.

---

caring for aging parents, dealing with teenage children, or letting go of children who have grown up and are ready to leave home.

Midlife's gains may be more subtle than its losses, but they can be deeply satisfying. People in their middle years are often more self-assured and comfortable with themselves—and more

---

generous toward others—than they were in youth. Psychologist Erik Erikson wrote in the 1950's that altruism, or a concern for the general good, is the hallmark of psychological growth. Although such growth can occur at any age, it seems to be a particular characteristic of middle age.

Several recent studies assessing midlife emotional development in Americans suggest that many adults do change priorities in their forties and fifties and become more caring and compassionate, particularly if their careers and marriages are successful. This altruism can take the form of coaching a Little League team, helping a younger colleague, or simply deepening relationships within the family.

It's much easier now to put on weight and harder to take it off than it once was. Is this usual? Do I need to change my diet?

As you age, your metabolism slows and you need fewer calories to maintain the same weight. You may also be less active than in the past. If you eat as much as ever and exercise less, you'll inevitably gain weight. After 30, it's not unusual for people to gradually gain as much as 20 pounds; some weight charts reflect this tendency (see *Determining Your Ideal Weight,* p. 57). In the absence of such conditions as hypertension and diabetes, weighing a bit more at 40 than your ideal weight at 20 may be beneficial, especially for women. A few extra pounds may ease some of the effects of menopause and help prevent osteoporosis.

In an effort to regain a youthful appearance, some middle-aged people go to the opposite extreme, becoming too thin. Excessive dieting can lead to nutritional defi-

THE SANDWICH GENERATION

If you find yourself in middle age caring for failing parents while still raising school-age youngsters, not to mention holding down a job and and trying to maintain a marriage, welcome to the sandwich generation. Adding to the generational squeeze in a growing number of U.S. households are the so-called boomerang kids, adult children in their twenties or older who return to the nest, unable to make it on their own thanks to low starting salaries and high living costs.

Survival tactics. Don't let guilt make you accept responsibilities you cannot handle, and don't jump into a custodial role when it's not required. Fostering an adult child's dependency isn't productive parenting. And just because a person is old doesn't mean she cannot take care of herself. Before an aging parent or adult child comes to live with you, discuss expectations and what each generation will contribute to household finances and chores.

The cost of elder care can strain a family's budget to the breaking point. Work out a long-range financial plan with your parents while they are still in good health. Consult a professional financial planner who specializes in retirement and geriatric issues.

Reaching out. If you're responsible for the care of a frail parent, share the responsibility with the whole family. If you have siblings, devise a plan for a fair division of labor and expenses. Community services for the aged can be very helpful; contact your local agency on the aging for information. Day care for physically or mentally impaired elderly individuals is available in many areas. Or maybe all your parent requires is a chance to socialize at a senior citizens center. Find home-care help through family or friends if possible. If you use an agency, interview candidates and check references carefully. If a dependent parent lives far away, consider hiring a geriatric care manager to arrange for housekeeping, schedule doctor's appointments, pay bills, and coordinate other aspects of your parent's care. For more information, contact the National Association of Private Geriatric Care Managers (see Appendix).

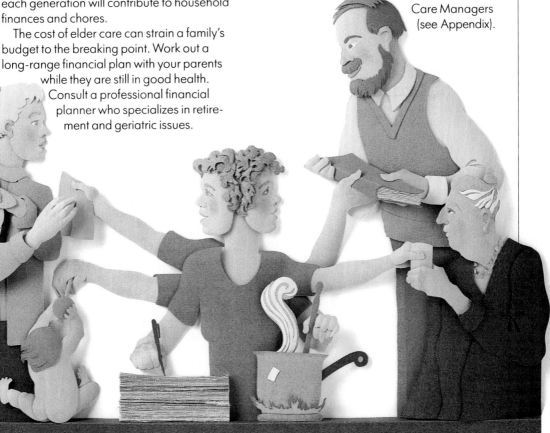

ciencies, and being underweight increases your risk of developing osteoporosis in later life.

The most sensible way to temper your body's natural tendency toward weight gain is to establish healthier eating habits and engage in regular exercise. Eat more whole grains, fruits, and vegetables and fewer sweets, fats, and cholesterol-rich foods. Take smaller portions of meat, especially fatty red meats. Pay attention to how well your diet is balanced and concentrate on nutrition and health rather than weight. Pass up empty calories such as those found in alcohol and sugar, for example, which have no nutritional value.

Yo-yo dieting—quickly losing and regaining weight—is the worst thing you can do. Weight lost too fast depletes muscle tissue as well as fat. Aging skin, which loses its elasticity, can't accommodate a sudden weight loss without wrinkling. And feast-or-famine eating patterns undermine good nutritional habits.

I've exercised regularly for years. Should I start slowing down now that I'm in my forties?

As long as you're healthy and have developed a regular exercise routine, there's no reason to slow down now. Although peak performance capacity does diminish with age, proper conditioning can improve aerobic capacity and muscle tone at all stages of life. When you work out aerobically, pay attention to your pulse rate to make sure you stay within your training zone (see *The Facts About Aerobics,* p. 71) and take sensible precautions to avoid injury (see *Sports Injuries,* p. 108).

People who develop regular exercise routines as young adults and maintain the regimen throughout life may be able to postpone

some of the effects of aging. In fact, doctors now believe that many of the adverse changes in body function long associated with the aging process may be the result of a sedentary lifestyle. Regular exercise strengthens the cardiovascular system, reduces the risk of a stroke, and may retard the development of such diseases as arthritis and diabetes. Exercise helps to lower cholesterol levels and counters midlife problems of weight gain and muscle stiffness.

Even if you haven't been exercising regularly, it's not too late to start now and reap the benefits. If you are thinking of embarking on an exercise program, consult your doctor and don't overdo it at first (see *Before You Start,* p. 73).

How should I change my health maintenance schedule during my middle years?

Taking good care of yourself at midlife is the best way to stay fit and to prepare for a vital old age. In the absence of a chronic condition or a suspected medical problem, it is probably enough to see your doctor for a physical exam (p. 122) every 2 to 5 years before age 60; every 2 years between 60 and 65. For a suggested screening test schedule, see *Screening Tests for Healthy Adults,* pp. 124–125.

However, if you have a family history of diabetes, cancer, or heart disease, make sure that your doctor is aware of this so that he or she can recommend an appropriate schedule of tests and checkups. For example, a woman at risk for breast cancer (see *Common Cancers: Assessing Your Risk,* p. 204) may be advised to have a breast exam and a mammogram more often than a woman with no risk factors.

If you wear glasses, you are probably accustomed to having your eyes examined regularly (p. 136). Even if you have never had vision problems before, as you enter middle age you may experience increasing difficulty reading small print, sewing, or performing other activities that require close-range focusing. A visit to an ophthalmologist or an optometrist will determine whether your vision needs correction. At the same time you should be screened for glaucoma.

Many people visit the dentist once or twice a year for routine cleaning and examination. If this has not been your habit, now is the time to start (see *A Dental Exam,* p. 137). Middle-aged teeth and gums are particularly vulnerable to periodontal disease (p. 138), which can lead to tooth loss. Scrupulous home care (p. 227) and regular cleanings and checkups at the dentist's office can prevent these problems.

What other kinds of dental problems can I expect in middle age?

Despite all your own and your dentist's best efforts, it's quite possible to lose teeth to periodontal disease or infections in middle age. Dentists prefer to save natural teeth whenever possible through periodontal therapy or root canal work (see *Glossary of Dental Terms and Procedures,* pp. 138–139), but sometimes there is no choice but to pull a tooth. To fill its place in the mouth, the dentist has several choices: a removable bridge, a fixed bridge, or an implant. A bridge is attached to the adjacent teeth on each side of the missing tooth or teeth. It either snaps into and out of position with metal clasps or is permanently cemented in place.

An alternative to bridges and

A LIVING WILL

Middle age is a time for looking ahead and planning for the future. If you haven't done it yet, drawing up a living will is an important part of this process. Modern medical technology, miraculous as it may be in reversing traumas, can also keep people alive who are irreversibly incapacitated and cannot speak for themselves. If you don't want this to happen to you, take steps now to make your wishes clear by means of a living will.

To be legally binding, however, your living will must conform to your state's regulations. The national organization Choice in Dying (see Appendix) provides living will and medical power of attorney forms for each state. It is not necessary to have a lawyer draw up a living will, but in some states you may need one to create a medical power of attorney (see below).

You make a general statement about not wanting your life to be prolonged if you are severely incapacitated or terminally ill.

Living Will Declaration

To My Family, Doctors, and All Those Concerned with My Care

I, _____, being of sound mind, make this statement as a directive to be followed if I become unable to participate in decisions regarding my medical care. If I should be in an incurable or irreversible mental or physical condition with no reasonable expectation of recovery, I direct my attending physician to withhold or withdraw treatment that merely prolongs my dying. I further direct that treatment be limited to measures to keep me comfortable and to relieve pain.

These directions express my legal right to refuse treatment. Therefore I expect my family, doctors, and everyone concerned with my care to regard themselves as legally and morally bound to act in accord with my wishes, and in so doing to be free of any legal liability for having followed my directions.

I especially do not want: _____

Other instructions/comments: _____

Proxy Designation Clause: Should I become unable to communicate my instructions as stated above, I designate the following person to act on my behalf:

If the person I have named above is unable to act on my behalf, I authorize the following person to do so:

Name _____
Address _____

Name _____
Address _____

Signed: _____
Witness: _____
Address: _____

Keep the signed original with your personal pa[...] at hom[...]
Review your Declaration from time to time; initial a[...] date[...]

You reiterate your right to refuse treatment and ask those involved to respect your wishes by honoring them.

You can spell out procedures you don't want used on you — cardiac resuscitation, a respirator, or intravenous feeding, for example.

Even if you refuse artificial life support systems, you may want to ask for pain medication and nursing care to ease your death.

Living wills can't clearly address every possible medical situation. Sometimes these wills are contested by hospitals concerned about both ethics and liability. To leave no doubt, you may name a proxy in your living will to speak for you when you are dying and cannot make decisions yourself. For more-encompassing protection you should also draw up a medical power of attorney, naming a health-care agent who will have the authority to make decisions about your treatment should you become totally incapacitated without having a terminal condition.

Sign and date the living will according to your state's witnessing requirements. Then distribute copies to your proxy and health-care agent (who may be the same person), family members, doctors, and lawyer. Discuss your wishes so that they are clearly understood by all concerned.

dentures (p.395) for people who can't or don't want to use them, a dental implant is a support for artificial teeth that is surgically attached to the jawbone. There are two basic types of implants. An endosteal implant is a peg, blade, or screw made of titanium or other biocompatible materials that is embedded directly into the jawbone to provide an anchor for a single crown or a bridge of artificial teeth. A subperiosteal implant is used when the jawbone has deteriorated so much that an implant cannot be inserted in it. Instead, an individually designed metal framework is fitted over the remaining bone beneath the gums. Posts projecting from the framework serve to anchor artificial teeth. This type of implant may be used to replace a few teeth or all of them.

Implants are expensive, and they are not for everyone. On the other hand, implants look and feel natural, and unlike bridges, they don't disturb the teeth on either side. If you are considering dental implants, see a dentist who has had training in implantation procedures.

Is some hearing loss to be expected during the middle years?

By the age of 50, most people do experience some hearing loss, especially in the upper frequencies (you'll have more trouble hearing a woman's or a child's high voice than a man's deep baritone). Hearing loss usually occurs so slowly that most people don't notice it at first. If you suspect that your hearing has diminished, get tested and discuss the situation with your doctor. You may be able to slow the decline by reducing the amount of noise around you (p.300). Or you may be suffering from a reversible problem such

as otosclerosis, a condition in which abnormal bone growth prevents sound vibrations from entering the inner ear. Surgery can usually correct otosclerosis.

What vision changes should I expect in my middle years?

Around age 45, most people begin to have trouble reading fine print or threading a needle. Presbyopia, a term coined from Greek roots meaning "old eye," is probably the reason you find yourself squinting and holding a sewing needle at arm's length. What's happening is that the lens of your eye is adjusting less readily as you switch your gaze from far to near. In a gradual process that becomes noticeable in midlife, an accumulation of fibers in the lens reduces its elasticity, making close-range work frustratingly difficult to see.

The simple solution to middle-age presbyopia is reading glasses that magnify close work. You may be able to use inexpensive ones bought at the drugstore (p.225). If you already wear corrective lenses, your ophthalmologist may suggest bifocals; for more on bifocals and how to get used to them, see page 225.

Besides becoming far-sighted, are there other eye problems that I should be aware of?

Since night vision tends to deteriorate with age, you may gradually notice that you cannot see as well as you used to when you drive a car at night (the lights of other cars may begin to bother you as well).

You may also start noticing floaters, semitransparent specks, hairs, or strings in your field of vision. Harmless by themselves, floaters are shadows cast on the

retina by microscopic structures in the vitreous humor, or jellylike fluid, in your eyes. As you age, it's natural for the vitreous humor to shrink and pull away from the retina, often making you see floaters quite vividly.

In some people, however, the vitreous humor is so strongly attached to the retina that as it shrinks, the vitreous tears the retina or detaches it from the underlying tissue. Signs of a possible retinal detachment include seeing a flurry of floaters, often accompanied by dramatic flashing lights, or experiencing an abrupt eclipse, as if a curtain were being drawn across the eye.

Nearsighted, or myopic, people are especially prone to retinal detachment in middle age because the shape of their eyeballs—elongated from front to back—stretches and thins the retina. Trauma such as being hit in the eye by a flying ball can detach the retina at any age.

If you even suspect a retinal problem, see an ophthalmologist without delay. Only immediate medical attention can prevent lasting vision impairment. When a tear or hole in the retina is still small, laser or cryopexy (freezing) treatment under local anesthesia will usually seal it. Surgery for extensive detachment requires general anesthesia. In this case, the retina may be reattached by freezing or by the application of a silicone band. The success rate of retinal surgery has improved dramatically in recent years to between 80 and 90 percent.

In middle age, your risk of developing such vision-threatening conditions as cataracts, glaucoma, and macular degeneration also rises. Cataracts (p.399) are a clouding of the lens of the eye, which blocks out light and blurs vision. The usual treatment for cataracts is surgery, which

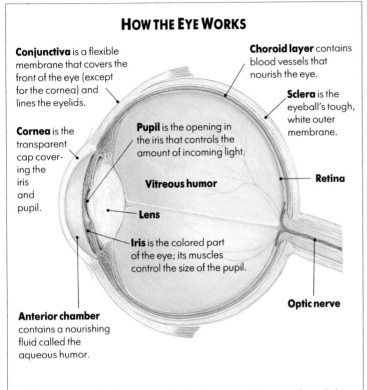

HOW THE EYE WORKS

Conjunctiva is a flexible membrane that covers the front of the eye (except for the cornea) and lines the eyelids.

Choroid layer contains blood vessels that nourish the eye.

Sclera is the eyeball's tough, white outer membrane.

Cornea is the transparent cap covering the iris and pupil.

Pupil is the opening in the iris that controls the amount of incoming light.

Vitreous humor

Retina

Lens

Iris is the colored part of the eye; its muscles control the size of the pupil.

Optic nerve

Anterior chamber contains a nourishing fluid called the aqueous humor.

Light rays entering the eyes are bent by the cornea, then pass through the pupil to the lens, which focuses the light through the jellylike vitreous humor onto the retina. Retinal cells convert light into nerve impulses, which travel via the optic nerve to the brain's visual cortex, where they're interpreted.

has proven highly successful in improving vision.

Glaucoma is a buildup of pressure inside the eyeball that can damage the optic nerve and cause blindness (see *The Facts About Glaucoma*, p.398). Blacks, diabetics, and people with a family history of glaucoma are most likely to develop the disorder. Open-angle glaucoma, the most common form, is effectively treated with eyedrops—if it's detected early. A glaucoma test (p.136) is recommended for everyone at about age 35 and annually thereafter for those with a risk factor for the disease.

Macular degeneration (p.396) is a progressive deterioration of the macula, or central part of the retina, which may lead to loss of central vision. Although usually associated with the elderly, macular degeneration can affect middle-aged eyes as well. For a simple home test to detect macular degeneration, see page 397.

Why does skin wrinkle as we age? Is there any surefire way to get rid of wrinkles?

Wrinkling is an inevitable part of the aging process. The skin consists of two layers—the epidermis, a thin protective outer layer made up partly of dead cells, and the dermis, or true skin, which contains water, elastic fibers, collagen (the fibrous protein that holds body cells and tissues together), blood vessels, nerve fibers, sweat glands, oil glands, hair follicles,

lymph vessels, and muscle cells. A fatty layer lies under the dermis. As we grow older, the fatty layer thins out, natural stores of collagen deteriorate, and the oil and sweat glands slow down. Losing its plumpness and elasticity, the skin sags. Stripped of its natural moisturizers, it dries out and begins to wrinkle.

Some people have a genetic tendency to wrinkle earlier than others—the fair-skinned Irish, English, and Scandinavians, who are more subject to sunburn—also wrinkle sooner than dark-skinned peoples.

Wrinkles can't be wished away with a magic potion, but they can be postponed. To keep your skin looking younger longer, follow the advice for slowing the aging process given on page 363. In addition, wash your face with gentle cleansers and warm, not hot, water, avoid astringent toners, and use moisturizing creams or light oil-based lotion to protect your skin from the wind and cold when you go out.

Although the facial expressions that accompany emotions—from surprise, joy, and laughter to frowns, tears, and anger—do etch lines in faces over time, most people appreciate the character such lines give their own and other people's faces.

However, if your fine lines disturb you, there are a few home treatments that may make them less noticeable. A facial mask will tighten and smooth your skin temporarily. Using a moisturizer (even the least expensive brand) on your face every day helps the skin look and feel better.

Other treatments require a visit to the doctor's office. Tretinoin, a prescription salve derived from vitamin A and sold commercially as Retin-A, is believed by some experts to smooth fine wrinkles and to revitalize skin (pp.220–221). A der-

TYPES OF COSMETIC SURGERY

At some point in their lives, a great many people make the decision to "do something" about the sags and wrinkles that age brings or about a feature they're not happy with. Described here are some of the most common cosmetic surgery procedures. The pros and cons of cosmetic surgery in general are discussed at right.

Breast lift (mastopexy)	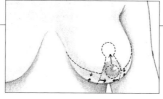 Breast reduction	Raises sagging breasts through skin tucks and repositioning of nipples higher on the breasts.
Breast reshaping (mammoplasty)		In reduction mammoplasty, breast size is reduced by removing excess tissue and moving nipple higher on breast. In augmentation mammoplasty, implants are inserted in breasts to enlarge them. Silicone implants may harden; some types have been linked with increased cancer risk.
Chemical peel (chemosurgery)	Caustic chemicals strip away top layers of facial skin, smoothing fine wrinkles but leaving skin very vulnerable to sunburn.	
Chin augmentation (genioplasty)	Adds size and contour to a receding chin by moving lower jawbone forward and wiring it in place or by implanting a prosthesis. Chin augmentation	
Dermabrasion	Skin is scraped with a diamond stone or wire brush to smooth fine wrinkles or acne scars; healing skin is sensitive to the sun.	
Ear surgery (otoplasty)	Resets prominent ears closer to the head by removing skin at the back of the ear and reshaping cartilage to create a more prominent fold in the central portion of the ear.	
Eye tuck (blepharoplasty)	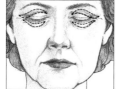 Eye tuck Face lift	Reduces pouches under the eyes, wrinkled skin folds in the upper eyelids, or both through surgical removal of excess skin and associated fatty deposits. Postoperative black eyes usually heal within a week.
Face lift (rhytidectomy)	Smooths and tightens skin of the face and neck through surgical removal of excess skin and fatty tissue.	
Forehead lift	Improves drooping eyebrows and decreases wrinkles on the forehead and at the top of the nose through surgical removal of forehead muscle and skin.	
Hair transplant	Plugs of hair-bearing scalp are removed from areas of heavy growth and grafted onto bald areas. Results vary. Even when transplants succeed, treated areas can become bald again.	
Liposuction	Fat deposits on hips, buttocks, arms, or thighs are suctioned out through a tube. This is not a weight-reduction technique, nor does it smooth out dimpling in fat-expanded skin (cellulite). Liposuction	
Nose surgery (rhinoplasty)	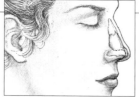 Nose surgery	Reduces the nose's overall size, reshapes its tip, or recontours it in some other fashion by trimming, cutting, or manipulating bone, cartilage, and skin.
Tummy tuck (abdominoplasty)	Removes excess wrinkled skin and associated fat from the abdomen and tightens the muscles of the abdomen wall to create a firm, flat tummy.	

COSMETIC SURGERY PROS AND CONS

Every year hundreds of thousands of American men and women undergo cosmetic, or esthetic, surgery designed to enhance appearance. (Reconstructive surgery is used to correct disease- or accident-associated disfigurement or congenital malformations.) Some patients want to improve their facial features by altering the size of a nose, pinning back ears, or augmenting a chin. Other patients choose to resculpt their bodies—lifting breasts or slimming thighs. Older patients may seek to minimize signs of aging with face lifts, eye tucks, or hair transplants.

Cosmetic surgery should never be undertaken lightly. Removing fat deposits through liposuction, for example, is major surgery that often involves general anesthesia, 2 or 3 days in the hospital, bruising, and pain. Even a so-called minor procedure like an eye tuck, performed with a local anesthetic in a doctor's office or clinic, can have complications. Healing after cosmetic surgery may require 2 to 3 weeks or more—time when you may not want to be seen by any but your closest friends. The cost of cosmetic surgery is high ($1,000 and up) and often must be paid in advance. Such fees are not usually covered by health insurance policies, nor do they qualify as a health expense deduction on your federal income tax.

Certain cosmetic surgery procedures may also entail risks beyond infection and surgical complications. In some women, for example, the scar tissue that forms after surgery wraps tightly around a silicone breast implant, causing hardness and discomfort. This can occur shortly after the operation—or years later. There are still many unanswered questions about the possible long-term cancer risks associated with breast implants.

Although successful cosmetic surgery can bring about remarkable changes in appearance, it isn't magic. It can't make a 60-year-old man or woman young again; it can't solve the social, sexual, or career problems of an insecure 30-year-old. The best candidates for cosmetic surgery are people who have specific cosmetic goals ("I just want to get rid of the bags under my eyes") and are realistic about the improvements they can expect.

matologist can also inject animal collagen under the skin to fill out superficial wrinkles. Relatively painless, the procedure must be repeated at least every 9 months in order to maintain the effect. (Some people are allergic to animal collagen, which is why pretreatment testing is necessary.) For more drastic ways of dealing with wrinkles, see *Types of Cosmetic Surgery,* left.

How do I choose a qualified plastic surgeon?

If, after weighing the risks and benefits, you decide to undergo cosmetic surgery, consult your own doctor first. Be sure that no health problems, such as heart disease, uncontrolled hypertension, or glaucoma, make plastic surgery unusually risky for you. Ask your doctor for a reference and ask for recommendations from friends who have had cosmetic surgery.

Pick a surgeon who devotes his practice to plastic surgery and is certified by the American Board of Plastic Surgery. You can call the American Society of Plastic and Reconstructive Surgeons for a list of qualified doctors (see Appendix). There are other legitimate professional societies, but some serve only to bolster the credentials of less qualified doctors. For other ways to check a doctor's qualifications, see page 119.

Look for a doctor who is on the staff of a major hospital and who has privileges to perform the procedure you are considering at that hospital. Even if you are treated in his office, the hospital accreditation is reassuring.

When interviewing plastic surgeons, beware of anyone who promises too much. No one can guarantee 100 percent success or make you appear 20 years

younger. Dramatic before-and-after pictures are also suspect. No surgeon can guarantee how well any particular patient will respond to a procedure, so photographs of others' results are misleading. Also be suspicious of a doctor who doesn't discuss risks with you. Ask how many times the doctor has done the procedure you want (you don't want to be among the first).

Three-quarters of all cosmetic surgery is performed as an outpatient procedure in a doctor's office or an ambulatory clinic. If you are scheduled for outpatient surgery, make sure that the clinic is accredited.

I'm noticing many more brown spots on my skin. Should I be concerned?

Liver spots, or age spots, are small, flat, light brown to black patches that often appear on the back of hands or on the faces of people in their middle years. The spots look like oversize freckles and are no cause for alarm. Despite the name, they have nothing to do with the liver; they may result from years of overexposure to the sun, but no one knows what really causes them.

If their appearance bothers you, cover them up with makeup or fade them with bleaching creams. Be precise when you use these creams; if you apply them carelessly, white spots, or "halos," can form around the spots. Also be aware that bleached skin may turn blotchy when exposed to the sun.

How do I know if I have a skin cancer, and what do I do about it?

Skin cancer is so prevalent in our sun-worshiping society (more than 500,000 new cases a year in the United States) and cure rates are so high (90 to 95 percent if the cancer is caught early) that it is worth having any suspicious spot on your skin looked at by a doctor. You should give your skin a monthly check, using a full-length mirror and a hand mirror to see your back. Any new growths, moles, sores, or discolorations, and any changes in existing ones should be evaluated by your dermatologist.

Slightly raised yellow, brown, or black spots with a waxy, crusted surface are most likely harmless seborrheic keratoses. These wartlike spots, which appear to be "stuck on" or loosely attached to the skin, occur most often on the back and chest, and sometimes on the face and neck. If you want to have them removed for cosmetic reasons, your dermatologist can perform the procedure in his office.

Other blemishes may signal skin cancer, of which there are three main types:
☐ Basal cell carcinoma is the most common. It starts as a fleshy bump, usually on the head, neck, or hands. Left alone, the bump bleeds, crusts over, and then bleeds again. Untreated, a basal cell carcinoma slowly continues to grow, destroying the tissue directly beneath it, but not spreading to other parts of the body.

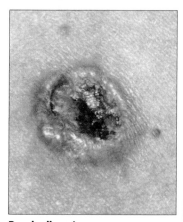

Basal cell carcinoma

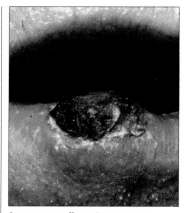

Squamous cell carcinoma

☐ Squamous cell carcinoma usually develops on the face, particularly around the mouth, or on the rims of the ears. This type of skin cancer begins as a bump or a red, scaly patch and grows more quickly than a basal cell carcinoma. Squamous cell carcinoma can metastasize, or spread to other parts of the body.

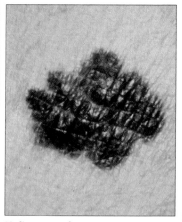

Malignant melanoma

☐ Malignant melanoma is the most dangerous form of skin cancer because it is the quickest to spread throughout the body. Although it accounts for only 5 percent of skin cancer cases, it is responsible for 75 percent of deaths from skin cancer. Malignant melanoma often starts in or near a mole (which is why changes in existing moles need

to be checked), but a melanoma can also suddenly appear anywhere else on the skin. The American Cancer Society has devised an ABCDE system for identifying malignant melanoma: A is for asymmetry (the two halves of the sore don't match); B is for border irregularity (the edges are ragged or blurred); C is for color (shades of tan, black, and brown may be mixed with red, white, and blue); D is for diameter (the growth is larger than the size of a pencil eraser or it appears to be getting bigger); E is for elevation (the growth protrudes from the skin).

Depending on the type of cancer and whether or not it has spread, skin cancer can be removed by surgery, electrodesiccation (drying up the tumor with a high-frequency electric current), cryosurgery (freezing), or radiation therapy. Early detection makes removal of the cancer easier; surgery is usually performed in the doctor's office with a local anesthetic.

What causes varicose veins, and what can I do to alleviate the discomfort they produce?

Varicose veins are twisted and swollen veins that are visible beneath the skin of the legs. Normally, valves in veins prevent blood that is being pumped back to the heart from draining downward with the pull of gravity. When a valve becomes stretched or weakened and can't close properly, blood pools in these veins, causing them to swell, sometimes painfully.

A tendency to develop varicose veins runs in families, with women being more susceptible than men. In some people, inadequate nutrition, physical inactivity, and poor muscle tone can contribute to the problem, but age also plays a part. Most people start to notice varicose veins in their thirties. Women often develop them during pregnancy due to weight gain or an increase in blood volume, or because the growing uterus impedes blood flow through the pelvic veins.

If varicose veins cause discomfort, try wearing support hose, which are available in a variety of colors and styles in many stores. Or your doctor can give you a prescription for more substantial medical support hose. Don't cut off circulation by crossing your legs at the knees or by wearing constricting garters or elastic-topped stockings. Try not to stand or sit in a single position for long periods of time. Elevate your legs whenever possible. Walking and other forms of exercise help. Keep your weight down and don't smoke.

More painful or disfiguring varicose veins can be treated with sclerotherapy, a procedure in which an irritant solution is injected directly into the vein, causing it to harden and shrivel away. Thanks to the availability of very fine needles, sclerotherapy can also be used to treat spider veins, the small feathery, red or bluish varicose veins that appear on the legs and occasionally on the face.

Varicose veins that are very painful, ulcerated, or prone to bleeding may have to be stripped, or removed surgically.

Why does hair turn gray and begin to thin out as we age?

Hair doesn't really turn gray; it simply loses its color. As the years pass, the production of pigment in the hair roots gradually slows down and eventually stops. Strands of unpigmented hair are actually white but look gray when mixed in with darker-colored hair. Race and heredity play a role in determining when your hair will gray. Caucasians begin to go gray earliest (in their mid-thirties) and blacks latest (in their mid-forties). And if either of your parents turned gray prematurely, there is a good chance that you will too.

As your hair loses color, it also changes texture. It dries out (good news for oily-haired people) and individual hair shafts lose thickness. As you grow older, the 50 to 120 hairs you normally lose each day are no longer replaced with long, thick strands, but rather with thinner, finer hairs. By the time they're in their sixties, many people have baby-fine hair. This change in texture accounts in part for the impression that hair thins out with time. In addition, the number of hair follicles in your scalp begins to diminish, and those that remain grow out more slowly. Youthful hair normally grows as much as half an inch a month, but that rate slows in midlife.

For hair to look and feel noticeably thinner, you must lose about 40 percent of it. Most men suffering from common male pattern baldness (progressive hair loss at the temples and crown) easily meet that quota by middle age. But the timing and extent of male pattern are dictated mainly by heredity; some men start going bald in their twenties or younger. (For more on male pattern baldness and possible remedies for it, see page 222.) A woman, on the other hand, isn't likely to notice thinning hair until after the hormonal changes of menopause.

The hair thinning that some women experience during pregnancy or that men and women suffer after a severe illness is a temporary condition. Once the body recovers, hair begins growing again at a normal rate.

Some women weaken their hair—and precipitate its loss—by constantly coloring and perming it and by pulling it back into ponytails, chignons, and other tight, sleek styles.

Does intelligence decline during midlife?

Not at all. Mental powers can actually improve with age, depending on how active people are intellectually, how motivated they are to use their minds, and how hard they try.

The idea that intelligence declines with age is an old one based on giving older adults the kinds of intelligence tests young people take. Reaction time, computational speed, and short-term memory may decline as the years go by, but other skills—vocabulary, general knowledge, arithmetic ability, communication techniques—often improve.

While it may take longer for older people to react and to solve problems, they have the advantage of experience. With age, thinking becomes more pragmatic, more subjective, and emotionally richer. Older people learn and remember information that they wish to learn, ferreting out what is important to them.

People who remain open to learning new things in their middle and later years often find that intellectual stimulation keeps them feeling young and vital. In fact, researchers suspect that there is a close connection between the mind and the immune system; staying mentally active could actually help you live longer.

Normal, healthy people should be able to continue learning and improving their intellectual skills well into old age. When intelligence does decline in middle age or in the later years, the cause in most cases is organic. Some medications, such as cer-

IMPROVING YOUR MEMORY

Forgetting things is always aggravating, but as you grow older forgetfulness can become unsettling, even frightening. When you misplace your house keys, can't remember where you parked the car, or suddenly draw a blank on the name of the movie you saw on Saturday night, you find yourself interpreting these lapses as signs of aging. In fact, they are, but this benign forgetfulness is not so sinister as you think. Long-term memory—bringing to mind your important experiences and knowledge—remains sharp long into old age for most people. It is short-term recall—the name of the movie, where you parked the car—that first starts letting you down.

Categories of memory. How many separate memory tracks exist in the brain is controversial, but most psychologists do agree on three general categories of memory: episodic (memories of specific events), semantic (retention of knowledge and facts), and implicit (things you remember automatically like how to speak your native language or how to ride a bicycle). Episodic memory declines with age, researchers say, but the process is gradual. Substantial problems don't occur for most people until they're in their seventies.

Honing memory. Motivation aids memory. Most people, for example, have no trouble remembering to deposit their paychecks. Routine helps too. Always put your purse, wallet, or keys in the same place and jot down appointments on the same calendar, which you check regularly. There are also a number of exercises that help keep your memory sharp. Called mnemonic devices, these memory tricks are familiar to most people from the child's rhyme, "Thirty days hath September..." that spells out the vagaries of the calendar. Following are some easy tactics to help you jog your memory.

☐ Pay attention to what you want to remember. If you don't listen carefully when people are introduced, you won't recall their names.

☐ Associate names with visual images, the more outrageous the better (they will stay in your mind longer). If you meet a man named Gene, for example, you might think of blue jeans. Let's say that Gene is tall; think of a long pair of blue jeans. The next time you meet him, you will notice his height and that should trigger the image of extra-long denim pants, which will help you come up with the name Gene. If a name doesn't conjure an image, try rhyming it with a word that does. Use the same technique to associate images with numbers you have to remember.

☐ Link a series of things you want to remember with familiar places. This loci (Latin for "places") method goes back to ancient Greece. To memorize the segments of a speech, for instance, associate each element with a room in your house. Start at the front door with the introduction and walk into the foyer for the first idea. Place the second idea in the living room, and so forth. When you rise to deliver your talk, take the walk mentally.

---

tain types of tranquilizers and antiparkinsonism drugs, can interfere with intellectual function. Abnormal blood chemistry, malnutrition, cardiopulmonary disease, and sight or hearing problems can also be responsible for apparent intellectual deterioration. A sharp, sudden decline in intellect may be caused by a stroke or some other physical disorder, but such a loss of cognitive powers is by no means a normal part of the aging process.

Is it true that you need less sleep as you get older?

No, your need for a certain number of hours of sleep a day remains about the same throughout adulthood. However, a good night's sleep may seem harder to come by as you get older because the nature of your sleep pattern changes.

There are two types of sleep: REM (rapid eye movement) and

NREM (nonrapid eye movement). During REM sleep your eyes move rapidly and you dream. For most adults REM sleep constitutes about a fifth of a night's sleep. The rest of the time is divided among four stages of NREM sleep, which get progressively deeper. Stage IV sleep is the deepest and most difficult to wake up from (it is also in Stage IV sleep that you talk in your sleep or sleepwalk).

As you age, your REM sleep

stays consistent, but your NREM sleep patterns change. Starting sometime after age 30, you begin to reach the deepest sleep states less often and for briefer periods each night. By 40, some people no longer reach Stage IV sleep at all. The result is that the slightest noise or disturbance may wake you, you are aware of waking up and going back to sleep throughout the night, and you wake up feeling less refreshed than you once did. (The same thing happens to young people, but less often, and they tend not to remember it the next day.) Some people adapt by using their wakeful time in the middle of the night to read or listen to music, and then go back to bed.

Another effect of changed sleeping cycles may be that you feel like going to bed earlier at night and getting up earlier in the morning than you used to.

By the time you reach 60, even more of a night's sleep is spent in the lighter stages (one study tallied 150 awakenings a night for subjects 60 and older). And as hard as it is to get a full night's sleep, you will have no trouble dozing in the daytime.

Not all sleeplessness is a result of changing patterns. The same things that kept you awake when you were younger—anxiety, for example, or too much caffeine or alcohol—are even more likely to interfere with sleep in middle age. Luckily, the same remedies (see *Falling Asleep*, p. 208) work at any age.

What kinds of birth control are best for women at midlife? When can I safely stop using birth control?

Birth control pills increase the risk of heart attack for women over 35 who smoke, but for healthy women who don't smoke

there is no reason to abandon oral contraceptives. IUD's can trigger or exacerbate the heavy menstrual flow some women experience preceding menopause. But if an IUD does not cause you to bleed excessively, and if you have only one sexual partner (which reduces the risk of developing pelvic inflammatory disease), an IUD is a good, convenient choice for you.

Barrier methods of birth control—diaphragms, condoms, sponges, and foam—are the best choices for women who can't use oral contraceptives or IUD's. If used correctly, latex condoms also offer protection against AIDS and other sexually communicable diseases (p. 243).

Midlife is a particularly dangerous time to use the natural methods of birth control since premenopausal changes often cause irregular ovulation. Sterilization of one partner is an option for midlife couples who anticipate a decade or more of fertility (p. 247). For more on the pros and cons of the various methods of contraception, see *Preventing Pregnancy*, p. 246.

A woman can safely stop using birth control after menopause when her doctor confirms that she is no longer ovulating—usually 1 to 2 years after her last menstrual period.

We are thinking about having a "midlife" baby. What pitfalls should we be aware of?

The availability of sophisticated fertility counseling and genetic testing—as well as new techniques for transferring fertilized eggs into the wombs of older women with ovarian failure— makes the possibility of having a healthy baby later in life a safer and more realistic ambition these days than ever before.

But a baby is more than a charming idea; it is a dependent being that takes years of tender care to raise. Are you ready to rock a colicky infant who is up all night? To teach a 6-year-old how to roller-skate? To go through menopause before your daughter goes through adolescence? To finance college when you're already living on retirement income?

If these prospects don't dissuade you, you may find that the patience you've developed and the wisdom you've accumulated over the years will make you a better parent than you ever could have been (or were) in your twenties or thirties.

Here are a few things to ponder before you make your decision. If this baby will be your first child, consider how profoundly his arrival will change your life. Are you perhaps too set in your ways after so many childless years? Are you really able to accept the restrictions on your independence that a baby will inevitably bring?

If you already have older children, are you prepared for how they will view an addition to the family? Adolescents and even young adults can feel threatened when parental attention suddenly changes focus.

Think about how old you will be when the child reaches milestones such as the start of first grade, the first prom date, graduation from college, and marriage. How might this child feel about having parents so much older than his friends' parents at parent-child events?

If you can face all these questions with equanimity and a sense of humor, chances are you will get a great deal of joy out of raising a midlife child. And the child will benefit immeasurably from having loving parents who really want him.

I'm 45 and have noticed that my periods are not as regular as they once were. Is this the start of menopause? What signs and changes should I expect now?

Menopause technically means the end of menstruation, but the natural changes in a woman's body that cause menopause can take place over many years. This transitional period between the childbearing years, marked by monthly menstrual cycles, and the later years when fertility ends and menstrual cycles stop is referred to clinically as the climacteric and popularly as the change of life.

The hormones estrogen and progesterone drive the female reproductive cycle. During a woman's childbearing years, her ovaries produce enough of these hormones each month to cause the lining of the uterus to thicken and nourish a fertilized egg; if there is no fertilization, the hormone levels drop, the lining of the uterus breaks down, and menstruation occurs. After age 35, the ovaries gradually begin to produce less of these hormones. At about age 40, the decline in hormone production becomes more pronounced and menopause nears. The ovaries eventually stop releasing eggs and producing progesterone but continue to produce small amounts of estrogen.

Your irregular periods are indeed a typical sign of changing hormone levels, which affect different women in different ways, just as menstruation does. Monthly bleeding may become heavier or lighter and cycles may become shorter or longer. You may miss a period or two and then begin menstruating regularly again. Or you may simply stop menstruating after a normal

FACT OR FALLACY?

Men go through a menopause of their own

Fallacy. Since men don't menstruate, they can't experience menopause (the end of menstruation) as women do. However, a small minority of men (about 5 percent) go through what is called the male climacteric at midlife or later. Victims suffer a sudden drop in testosterone levels that makes them feel tired and irritable and often dulls their sexual appetites. Some become impotent and require hormone therapy. Normally a man's testosterone levels peak in his teens and then decline gradually. While sperm count begins to diminish after age 40, men remain fertile into their eighties and nineties.

period with no irregularities at all.

The change, or climacteric, is complete only after a woman has stopped menstruating altogether and her body has adjusted to the changes in estrogen and progesterone production—a process that can take as long as 5 years after the final menstrual period.

Menopause can occur at any time between ages 45 and 55, with 50 the average age among American women. Premenopausal women who undergo a hysterectomy that includes the removal of both ovaries experience a sudden estrogen level drop and what is known as an artificial, or surgical, menopause.

Along with changes in the menstrual pattern, menopausal

women may experience hot flashes and/or vaginal dryness. Moodiness, depression, and other emotional reactions to menopause do occur, but not as often as cultural myths would have you believe. Your general health and state of mind determine to a great extent how easily you'll undergo change of life. If you are happy and have been taking care of yourself, you are unlikely to suffer any particular distress related to menopause.

Fears about menopause persist, however, despite the fact that few women actually suffer debilitating symptoms. Many women who have been through menopause report new surges of energy and a heightened sense of well-being in a new stage of life.

What causes a hot flash?

Hot flashes are among the most common and most disturbing symptoms of menopause. Sudden waves of heat are sometimes accompanied by feelings of anxiety, heart palpitations, dizziness, and headache. During a hot flash, women typically feel a rush of warmth either throughout the upper body or all over. As surface blood vessels expand and the flow of blood to the skin increases, a flushing sensation is felt and red splotches may appear on the face, chest, neck, back, shoulders, and upper arms. Perspiration and a cold clammy feeling often follow as the body tries to readjust.

Not every woman experiences hot flashes during the climacteric and those who do may experience them only intermittently. In some cases, hot flashes cease within a year of the final menstrual period; in other cases, the problem continues for several years. Each episode usually lasts from a few seconds to a few minutes, but in severe cases, a hot flash may last as long as 15 minutes or more. Some women have hot flashes once a week; others, several times a day. While they are more likely to occur at night, hot flashes can be embarrassing when they happen during a business meeting or at a formal social event. In most cases, a woman's sudden temperature change is not noticeable to the people around her.

Exactly what causes hot flashes is not known, but they are probably connected to the drop in estrogen levels a woman experiences prior to menopause. Such hormonal changes appear to stimulate the hypothalamus, the part of the brain that regulates body temperature. Some researchers speculate that the hypothalamus releases extra norepinephrine, a chemical that tells the body that it is overheating. The body responds by dilating blood vessels and sweating.

What are the pros and cons of hormone replacement therapy?

From the mid-1960's to the mid-1970's, doctors routinely prescribed estrogen pills to replace the hormones a woman's body no longer produces in sufficient quantities after menopause. In the mid-1970's research studies began to question the safety and effectiveness of estrogen replacement therapy. Estrogen therapy was found to increase a woman's risk of developing breast cancer, ovarian cancer, uterine cancer, gallbladder disease, and uterine fibroids.

Today, estrogen is usually combined with progestin (a synthetic form of the hormone progesterone) in doses designed to replicate the hormone levels that occur naturally during the menstrual cycle. The combina-

tion, which is thought to be safer than estrogen alone, is prescribed by many doctors for premenopausal women who have had their ovaries removed and for women who suffer severe menopausal side effects. Doctors may also prescribe hormone therapy to prevent or to treat osteoporosis (see *The Facts About Osteoporosis,* pp.378–379).

Assessing the risks and benefits of hormone therapy, however, is no easy matter. It's fairly well established that estrogen therapy increases a woman's risk of developing cancer, especially breast and endometrial cancer. On the other hand, there is no question that hormone therapy helps to prevent osteoporosis and to relieve such menopausal symptoms as hot flashes and vaginal dryness. In 1991 a major study sponsored by the National Institutes of Health concluded that estrogen significantly reduces a woman's risk of heart disease. Since postmenopausal women are far more likely to die from heart disease than from cancer, the benefits of estrogen therapy seem to outweigh its risks. However, the NIH study focused only on women (most of them white) with no history of cancer or heart disease, and it did not examine the effects of combining estrogen with progestins. A new, more broadly based NIH-sponsored study is expected to provide a clearer picture of the risks and benefits of hormone-replacement therapy.

In the meantime, you must weigh the pros and cons carefully before beginning hormone therapy. Make sure that your doctor is aware of your family and medical history and discusses the risks with you. Consider trying less controversial remedies for menopausal problems (see next question) before agreeing to hormone therapy.

The National Women's Health Network, a Washington-based research group, recommends the use of hormone therapy only for premenopausal women who have had their ovaries removed, for women who experience extreme menopausal discomfort, and for women who are at high risk of fractures from osteoporosis. The Network does not regard estrogen as a valid treatment for preventing cardiovascular disease.

What can I do on my own to reduce the discomforts and risks of menopause?

Keep a record of when you have hot flashes; you may see patterns that will help you predict and be prepared for these experiences. Try dressing in layers so that you can remove, say, a sweater or jacket during a hot flash. In a meeting or social gathering, situate yourself (when possible) so that you can step outside to cool off unobserved. A cold drink also brings relief, as does taking a cool shower, if circumstances permit.

Healthy eating is always a smart preventive measure. Caffeine, alcohol, and spicy foods can exacerbate hot flashes; try cutting them out of your diet. Some women say that vitamin E helps reduce the number and severity of hot flashes.

Many women report that they are more likely to experience menopausal symptoms in times of stress. If you can't avoid tension-provoking situations, use meditation or exercise to help yourself relax and cope (see *Learning to Relax,* pp.206–207).

Also, talk about what you are going through with your family and friends; it will give you perspective—and maybe a sense of humor—about the effects of this very natural process.

How will menopause affect my sex life?

No longer concerned about getting pregnant, many women report increased sexual pleasure after menopause. Others report no change in their sexuality.

For some women, however, the physiological changes that accompany menopause do create problems. A drop in estrogen production affects the vaginal walls: they become drier and less elastic and, in some cases, intercourse becomes quite painful. Hormone replacement therapy (p.377) is one way of treating menopause-related vaginal changes. Applying moisturizing gels regularly and lubricants just before intercourse also helps.

Men at midlife may develop sexual problems too, and ongoing relationships can suffer when one or both partners experience difficulties with sex. Partners who are willing to talk honestly about their sexual problems and to try new techniques to improve the situation are likely to work things out together. Regular sexual activity, with a partner or through masturbation, will help maintain vaginal elasticity and lubrication. Staying physically fit and emotionally grounded also helps to keep sexual experience satisfying at any age.

Are there other physical changes or problems a woman should watch out for at midlife?

Women become more vulnerable to a number of health problems as they grow older; these are some of the most common ones:
☐ Heart disease. Six times more women die of heart attacks than of breast cancer. After menopause women are more likely to suffer heart attack and stroke than they were before,

possibly as a result of estrogen loss (p.205). The risks of developing cardiovascular disease continue to increase with age and are higher for black women than for white women—19 percent higher for coronary heart disease and 79 percent higher for stroke.
☐ High blood pressure. The risk of high blood pressure also increases as women age. More than half of all women over age 55 have high blood pressure; women over 65 are more likely to develop the condition than men of that age.
☐ Lung cancer. More women today are dying of lung cancer than of breast cancer, primarily because those women who do smoke are smoking more heavily than women did in the past. Quitting smoking (p. 201) reduces your chances of developing not only lung cancer, but also such life-threatening conditions as emphysema and heart disease.
☐ Osteoporosis. See *The Facts About Osteoporosis*, facing page.
☐ Breast cancer. The risk of breast cancer, the most common cancer in women, continues to increase with age.
☐ Vaginal bleeding. Premenopausal women who experience prolonged, heavy bleeding between menstrual periods and postmenopausal women who have any vaginal bleeding should check with their doctors immediately. Such episodes can be symptomatic of a range of health problems from benign fibroid tumors (p.252) to more serious uterine cancer.

Is divorce more likely to occur during midlife? Does divorce affect women and men differently?

Recent divorce rates for women are highest among 15- to 19-year-olds and for men, among

BONE MAINTENANCE

In the fight against osteoporosis, prevention is far more effective than any treatment now available. According to the National Osteoporosis Foundation (see Appendix), building up bone mass before age 35 can do more to delay the onset of osteoporosis in later life than any other preventive measure. To build up bone mass your body needs plenty of calcium, particularly during adolescence, when bones are growing rapidly, and during pregnancy and breast-feeding, when a woman is in effect feeding two.

Although the recommended dietary allowance for calcium is 800 mg per day for adults over 24, the National Osteoporosis Foundation suggests that adult men and premenopausal women consume 1,000 mg of calcium per day; postmenopausal women not on hormone therapy should increase their daily calcium intake to 1,500 mg.

For optimum calcium absorption, your body also needs vitamin D, which you either manufacture yourself after exposure to the sun or get from egg yolks, saltwater fish, and fortified milk.

The body absorbs calcium most efficiently from food sources—milk, cheese, yogurt, oysters, sardines (with bones), salmon (with bones), broccoli, collard and turnip greens. An 8-oz glass of skim milk contains 302 mg of calcium; a cup of cooked fresh collard greens, 357 mg.

If you can't get enough calcium from your diet, however, consider drinking calcium-fortified juice or taking a calcium supplement. Calcium comes in many forms, some more effective than others, so read labels carefully. Calcium carbonate supplements are a good choice. Some antacid pills consist mostly of calcium carbonate and are available in sodium-free versions (another advantage of calcium carbonate antacids is their low price). Calcium citrate, calcium lactate, and calcium gluconate all contain a lower percentage of calcium than calcium carbonate. Avoid bone meal or dolomite, which may contain lead or other toxic metals.

Regular weight-bearing exercise (weight training, low-impact aerobics, and jogging) strengthens bones and builds bone mass in young people and may help decrease or defer bone loss in older people.

THE FACTS ABOUT OSTEOPOROSIS

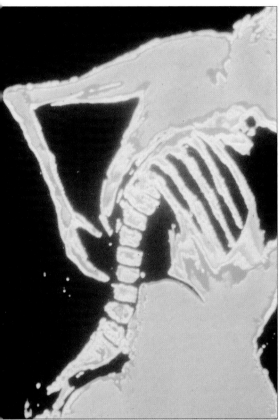

What is it? Osteoporosis ("porous bone") is a condition that decreases bone mass and makes bones—particularly vertebrae, wrists, and hips—fragile and easy to break.

What are its symptoms? Osteoporosis often progresses without causing any symptoms. The earliest signs—an aching back, a broken wrist, or a fractured hip—usually appear first when a person is in her sixties or seventies. Later, tiny fractures of the vertebrae may cause the spine to bend, decreasing height and producing a hunched-back posture. Elderly victims of osteoporosis are susceptible to broken hips, which prove fatal to 12 to 20 percent of those who suffer them.

What causes it? No one knows exactly. From childhood until you reach your mid-thirties, the density of your bones increases. The process then gradually reverses and you begin to experience a natural decrease in bone mass that continues throughout the rest of your life. Osteoporosis accelerates the rate of decrease. Most experts believe that the sharp decline in estrogen production that occurs after menopause hastens the loss of bone in middle-aged women. In fact, women, who generally have less bone mass than men to begin with, develop osteoporosis much earlier and six to eight times more often than men. Caucasian and Asian women are more at risk than black women.

Other osteoporosis risk factors include age (the longer you live, the more bone mass you are likely to lose), a diet chronically deficient in calcium, a sedentary lifestyle, an early (before age 45) menopause (surgical or natural), a family history of the condition, smoking, and excessive alcohol consumption.

How is it treated? A diet rich in calcium and vitamin D and exercise to strengthen bones and muscles are essential. For some postmenopausal women, hormone replacement therapy (p.377) may be recommended. Severe, progressive osteoporosis is sometimes treated with the hormone calcitonin, which regulates calcium levels in the body and slows the loss of bone density.

A "dowager's hump," a classic sign of osteoporosis, is evident in the X-ray above. In adults, most bones consist of hard, dense bone on the outside and a layer of soft, spongy bone on the inside. The latter contains marrow, which produces blood cells. Collagen (a protein) gives bone elasticity, while calcium gives it hardness. The bone thinning that characterizes osteoporosis is caused mainly by a loss of collagen and calcium that affects hard and spongy bone alike. Relatively dense spongy bone (right, top) contrasts markedly with the same type of bone affected by osteoporosis (right, bottom).

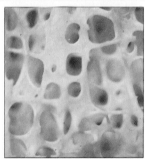

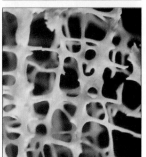

20- to 24-year-olds. The same statistics show more than a third of divorces taking place before a couple's fifth anniversary.

Ironically, most studies indicate that marital satisfaction starts out high and steadily declines during the busy middle years when child rearing and other responsibilities leave little time for couples to nurture their partnerships. Many people stay married even when they are unhappy, fearing the alternatives and hoping that their marriage will improve in the future.

The misconception that midlife divorces are epidemic may be based on the visibility of such divorces. People take notice when couples who have been together for years split up. And as the years go by, the total number of people who have been divorced (and have not remarried) increases so that the accumulation of divorced people is much greater among the middle-aged than among young adults.

Divorce is hard on everyone. Financially, women—especially older women who have not held jobs—have a harder time than men do. A woman who has spent years supporting her husband's career development may suddenly find herself alone, without job skills, and faced with the responsibility of raising her children.

Women past 40 have limited prospects for remarriage. (An unattached man in his forties, by contrast, is often hotly pursued.) Women, however, usually have stronger relationships with family and friends to help them through tough times, and thus tend to manage better emotionally as single people than men do.

Although men may fare better financially after a divorce, they can find themselves socially isolated, estranged even from their own children. Youngsters often rally around their mother,

the partner they see as needing more support. Many men who've been married for decades are at a loss when it comes to cooking, running a home, or taking care of themselves; in fact, statistics indicate that men between 45 and 64 who live without a spouse are twice as likely as married men to die within 10 years.

My youngest child is moving out of the house soon, and I feel great about it. Is this unusual? Shouldn't I be experiencing empty nest syndrome?

You are not unusual. Study after study confirms that most contemporary parents find the transition to an empty nest a happy time. The syndrome that equates children leaving home with the end of a parent's useful life usually afflicts women who have devoted years of their lives exclusively to raising children. Fewer and fewer women fit that description these days. And even many full-time mothers report a mixture of emotions as their children grow up and gain independence. The prospects of more personal freedom, more time and energy to devote to postponed ambitions, help to compensate for any losses felt.

Mothers and fathers who have maintained careers and other outside interests throughout their child-rearing years are likely to have positive feelings about launching their children into the world. Most parents share a sense of accomplishment and relief when their parental responsibilities have been fulfilled. This transition can lead to renewed intimacy and satisfaction in the couple's relationship and to the formation of deep and loving friendships with newly independent children.

We've recently become the grandparents of a beautiful baby boy. I should feel ecstatic, but I actually have mixed feelings about being a grandparent. How do I get over this?

Some young grandparents wholeheartedly welcome the change in their status, but for those middle-aged people who equate becoming grandparents with growing old, the new arrival is often received with mixed emotions. Becoming a grandparent at an especially young age usually means that your children are having children early, and your concern about the wisdom of their decisions may dampen the joy you feel at the arrival of a baby.

You may fear that you will be called into duty as baby-sitters and spend more hours than you would like changing diapers and rocking a squalling infant. If you are concerned about being exploited, discuss this frankly with your children. Offer to baby-sit one evening a week, if you wish, but don't do more than you want to do.

Then relax and enjoy the baby. As grandparents you have special roles in the child's life. You are his link with another generation. Not on the firing line 24 hours a day, you can take the time to explain and persuade instead of simply saying no to a request. You can have the fun of teaching some of your favorite skills to your grandson and the satisfaction of providing perspective to upsetting events in his life. You can afford to just listen when he needs to talk.

Don't let foolish vanities spoil your fun. Being identified as a grandmother or a grandfather doesn't make you old and unattractive any more than a few gray hairs or a few wrinkles will.

PLANNING FOR RETIREMENT

Everyone knows (and hates to be reminded) that it's never too early to start planning and saving for retirement. Once you hit midlife, however, the issue really can't be avoided. Whether you intend to stay employed indefinitely or expect to retire early, you need to know if you will have enough money to live comfortably and still be able to pay for medical emergencies and other contingencies. Your mental and physical well-being as you grow older become more and more dependent on the financial security you've structured for yourself in middle age.

Assess your current finances. The first step in serious financial planning is to figure out how much money you have and how much you are spending. Add up your assets: bank accounts, stocks and bonds, retirement funds, home, automobile, and other valuables. Determine your monthly income and expenses for 6 months and take an average; this should give you a good idea of where you stand now.

Set goals. Once the status quo is clear, think about future goals. What do you want for your retirement? To have enough money to live where you are or in smaller quarters elsewhere? To be able to travel? To help your children buy a house? Estimating the amount of money you will need to achieve your goals is the next step. Financial experts say that the average person can live in retirement on 70 percent of pre-retirement income. Use that figure or be more precise, determining your actual personal needs. You can make firm estimates on some expenses; others, such as medical costs, are unpredictable and you'll need a contingency fund to cover them.

Make a realistic plan. You may be shocked at the discrepancy between your savings and the amount of money you'll need to live even modestly after retirement. Social Security will provide a minimal income base, and pension plans add on to that for many people. If you don't have pension coverage, you can save a considerable amount of money each year tax-deferred through an IRA, Keogh, or other self-employment pension plan.

Get professional help. An independent financial planner (one who makes a living consulting, not selling financial products) can help you get an overview of your finances and suggest ways to meet your goals through diversified investments appropriate to your situation. A professional can also give you a clear perspective on cutting your current budget. You may be carrying too much insurance, for example, or there may be a better, tax-advantaged way to help out your parents financially. Such practical, unbiased advice is not only worth the cost, but should be sought out every few years as your needs and circumstances change.

. . . AND MAKING OUT A WILL

Drawing up a will is a critical part of midlife planning. A will explains in legally binding terms how you wish to dispose of your property after death. If you die intestate (without a will), a probate court will distribute your assets according to state laws, a lengthy process that may cost your estate not only the state-appointed executor's fees, but also inheritance taxes that could have been avoided with the help of a lawyer and a will.

Hire a lawyer who specializes in estate planning to draw up your will and advise you on tax law and ways to preserve the greatest part of your estate for your heirs.

A will should designate who will administer your estate (the executor of the will), who will be your heirs, and what each heir will inherit. Because you don't know how much your estate will be worth at the time of your death, it's best to divide it proportionately among heirs (50 percent to a spouse and 25 percent to each child, for example) instead of in fixed dollar amounts.

After a friend died of a heart attack at age 47, I've been brooding about his death and the possibility of my own. Is this unusual at midlife?

An increased awareness of your own mortality is not unusual at midlife. It is a natural part of adult development. So many major and minor losses confront you now. Your body is aging, your children may be leaving home, and your parents may be failing.

A parent's death reminds you that your turn will come; a contemporary's death tells you it could happen at any minute. There is no stronger catalyst for facing your own life's limits. Some psychologists suggest that men are more shocked by mortality than women, but coming to terms with it is certainly a universal crisis that all adults must work through in midlife.

When confronted with the death of a contemporary, many people find themselves temporarily obsessed with their fears of death. Fortunately, this obsession passes. After the rituals of a friend's death are over, middle-aged people appear to be no more obsessed with death than members of any other age group are. While your morbid preoccupation is undoubtedly temporary, the way that a recognition of mortality affects your experience of life may well be permanent. Accepting the idea of your own death opens you up to a richer, deeper appreciation of life. Knowing that the time you have is limited, you are more likely to use it well. People change their values and life goals after profound confrontations with death. And they may suddenly become more appreciative of their own health. If your friend's death was related to smoking, his funeral may provide the stimulus for you to stop. In such instances, the awareness of limits is paradoxically liberating.

I'm still working, but my recently retired husband seems to be at loose ends. How can I get him interested in other pursuits?

Men, especially those who have been highly involved in their careers, often find the transition to retirement difficult. For years, work provided a sense of identity, status, and self-esteem, and all that is missing now. The structure work gave to daily life is also gone. Your continuing enjoyment of your career may be contributing to your husband's sense of superfluousness. You can help him by suggesting activities and by being supportive of his efforts, but it is up to him to redirect his own life.

Some people begin second careers after retirement. If your husband has an avocation, he may wish to pursue it more seriously now. Starting a business at home is one option. Obtaining part-time employment or consulting work can revive your husband's feelings of usefulness and self-esteem, as well as his social life. In the first months of retirement, he may miss work camaraderie more than he realizes.

Volunteering is a time-honored way to explore new interests. Several organizations help match retirees with people and programs that can use their skills (p. 420).

An adult education course at a local college may interest your husband. Studies show that people who remain mentally active stay healthy longer. Your husband may have educational ambitions worth reviving; more and more people are pursuing college degrees or graduate work in midlife. Universities and community colleges commonly offer dozens of extension courses. And learning doesn't have to take place within the walls of accredited institutions. A museum lecture series, a Bible class, or a book club will also provide intellectual stimulation. For other ideas and resources for staying active after retirement, see page 420.

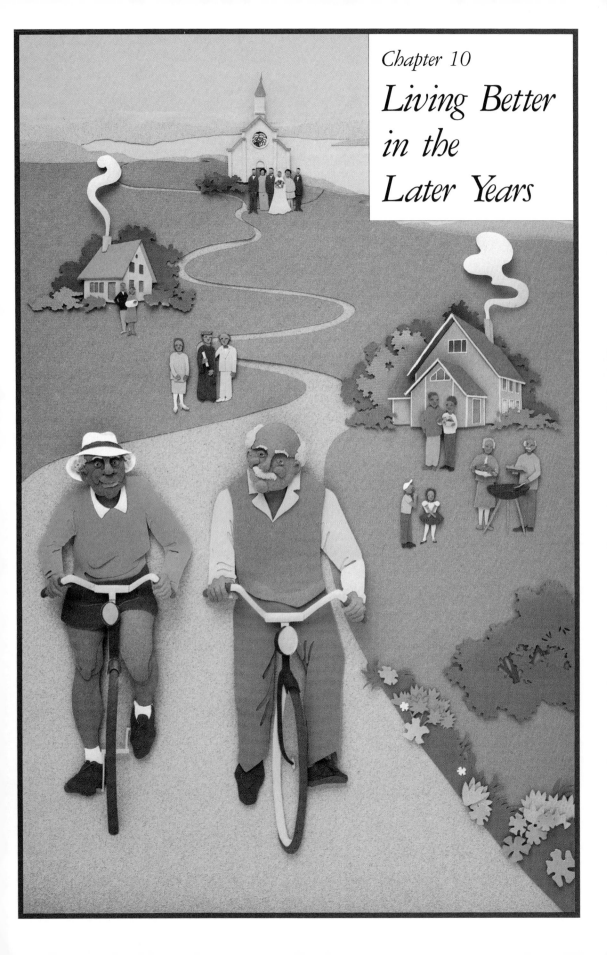

Chapter 10

*Living Better
in the
Later Years*

Intergenerational Living

ileen E. and her husband, both professors at a small New England college, decided to stay in their off-campus house after retirement rather than move to a sunnier climate. Throughout her sixties and most of her seventies, Eileen remained strong and capable of handling household tasks that her older, frailer husband could not. When he died, Eileen made up her mind not to move.

As her 80th birthday neared, however, Eileen began to feel less secure living by herself. Running the house was not as easy as it used to be, and inflation was squeezing her budget.

Chance and a housing crisis at the college came to Eileen's rescue. One of her former students, who had become the college registrar, asked her whether she'd be interested in taking in a student lodger. Although fearful that a stranger in her home would be intrusive, Eileen agreed to give it a try. Her first student was a young man who negotiated a lower rent in exchange for doing regular chores. Eileen soon came to find the student's company refreshing, his help a relief, and the extra money a decided boon. At 85, Eileen is still living happily at home with the help of her student lodgers.

Saving a Good Eye

acular degeneration is the most common cause of vision loss among the elderly, and by the time Nancy M. was 75, the dry form of the disease had dimmed her left eye. Although she knew there was no cure for this type of macular degeneration, Nancy was not discouraged. She saw well enough with her right eye to lead an active social life and indulge her fondness for bingo.

One day, while playing her favorite game, Nancy noticed that the lines on her bingo card looked wavy and that the numbers were hard to read. Terrified at the idea of losing her re-

maining sight, Nancy dropped her card and abruptly left the bingo hall to call her eye doctor for an appointment.

The doctor confirmed that Nancy had macular degeneration in her right eye, but it was the wet form of the disease, which is treatable with lasers if caught early. Nancy underwent the 30-minute procedure in the doctor's office and within 3 weeks was back playing bingo. Aware that wet macular degeneration can recur, Nancy sees her eye doctor regularly and does her own vision check at home with an Amsler grid, a chart not unlike a bingo card.

Loss, Recovery, and Renewal

oel M. at 68 was a vigorous man accustomed to being in control. A devoted husband and proud father and grandfather, Joel still commanded the respect of the town he had served as police chief for many years. The day his wife died in a car crash, however, Joel's world fell apart. Hobbled by grief, he lost interest even in his family and withdrew further and further into himself.

At his son's urging, Joel began attending meetings of a local support group for the bereaved. Slowly Joel realized that he wasn't

alone, that there were others who understood his feelings, and that together they could help each other recover from their loss.

Joel also found that he could still have very strong feelings for a woman. In his group was a widow with grown children of her own. A tentative first date over a cup of coffee led to many other dates; 6 months later the couple became engaged. Seeing their parents' happiness, both sets of children put aside whatever reservations they had about their parent's new relationship and gladly welcomed the marriage.

Toward a Healthy Old Age

Stereotypes about older people abound in a society that is still largely youth oriented. Fortunately, as the ranks of the elderly increase, a more accurate picture of the potential and problems of old age is emerging. This chapter will guide you through the changes you can expect as you get older and the actions you can take to turn your later years into your prime years. But first, test your knowledge of the aging process by identifying which of the following statements are fact and which are fiction.

1 **Men between the ages of 65 and 70 begin to lose bone mass at the same rate as women do.**

_____ True _____ False

2 **Despite medical advances, human life expectancy has remained constant since the mid-19th century.**

_____ True _____ False

3 **Once a person passes 70, the health benefits of giving up smoking, losing weight, or starting an exercise program are minimal.**

_____ True _____ False

4 **The overuse of laxatives can result in constipation.**

_____ True _____ False

5 **Older people need to increase their drug dosages because gradually, over time, their bodies build up a tolerance to most medications.**

_____ True _____ False

6 **New techniques for filling and reconstructing teeth are making dentures obsolete.**

_____ True _____ False

7 **Cataract surgery is one of the most successful operations performed today.**

_____ True _____ False

8 **A woman's risk of developing breast cancer declines as she gets older.**

_____ True _____ False

9 **There is little doctors can do to treat incontinence among the elderly.**

_____ True _____ False

10 **Sleeping patterns change with age.**

_____ True _____ False

11 **A stiff and shuffling gait can be the result of a sedentary lifestyle.**

_____ True _____ False

12 **Depression is much more common among the elderly than among younger people.**

_____ True _____ False

Answers
For more information on any of the quiz topics turn to the pages listed next to the answers.

1. True, p.386
2. False, p.387
3. False, p.388
4. True, p.390
5. False, p.393
6. False p.395
7. True, p.399
8. False, p.404
9. False, p.406
10. True, p.407
11. True, p.409
12. False, p.412

I've noticed that some of my friends in their mid- to late seventies are leading healthy, active lives while others are declining rapidly. What causes the difference?

That people age at different rates is plain to see; why that happens is less clear. Genes, environment, lifestyle, and attitude all play a role in determining the pace of aging.

Susceptibility to a number of diseases, such as heart disease and certain cancers, may run in families. But such a familial predisposition to a disease does not necessarily mean you'll develop it. Preventive health care (p.200), eating well, staying mentally and physically active, managing stress (see *Learning to Relax*, pp.206–207), quitting smoking, and reducing your exposure to sunlight and environmental toxins can greatly increase the odds in your favor.

It's quite likely that your active friends are more outgoing and optimistic than those who are declining. No matter what your age, but especially as you grow older, attitude plays a critical part in maintaining good health. Recent studies have shown a link between people's self-assessment of their health and their mortality, even when physical exams and objective lab reports contradict the self-assessment. In one study, older people who believed they were in poor health were shown to be seven times more likely to die during the next 12 years. While you can't wish yourself to good health, your beliefs about your state of health can become a self-fulfilling prophecy, causing you to act in ways that will make the self-assessment come true. In other words, have a positive attitude and you'll take good care of

yourself; have a negative attitude and you may neglect your health.

For more on the aging process and what you can do to slow it, see page 363.

I was once 6 feet 2 inches tall; now I'm barely 6 feet. What happened?

Some loss of stature is a normal part of aging. Curvature of the spine, compression of the spinal discs, loss of elasticity in the joints, and a flattening of the arches of the feet often begin in midlife and gradually become more pronounced, so that by age 70 or so the body may have shrunk several centimeters.

A more substantial reduction in height, such as you describe, could mean that you are losing bone mass, a sign of osteoporosis. Although osteoporosis is often regarded as a woman's disease, men aren't immune. As their male hormone levels decline with the passing years, men between the ages of 65 and 70 begin to lose bone mass at the same rate that women do. After age 75, nearly half of all men and women have some degree of osteoporosis.

In a 3-year study of 77 healthy men ages 30 to 87, researchers at Oregon Health Sciences University found 50 percent more spinal bone loss than they had anticipated. Among the factors responsible for loss of bone mass in elderly men (as in women) are inactivity, poor diet, cigarette smoking, and heavy alcohol use; steroids that are prescribed to treat some diseases can also lead to the breakdown of bone.

For more on osteoporosis, its causes and prevention, see *The Facts About Osteoporosis*, pp.378–379. To protect your spine, watch your posture and keep your back and abdomen strong through exercise (see *Relief for an Aching Back*, pp.218–219).

What other physical changes can I expect as I enter my seventies?

Many of the physical changes that are associated with normal aging begin in a person's thirties and progress gradually over decades. Although people don't necessarily age faster in their later years, the effects of the aging process are cumulative, and thus signs of it become more noticeable the older you get. As the years go by, you will experience at least some of the physical changes listed below, but their effects and impact on quality of life vary dramatically from one individual to another.

☐ As pigmented hairs fall out and are replaced by white strands, hair appears grayer (p.373).

☐ Skin becomes drier and less elastic. Wound healing is slower, and the skin is more easily damaged by the sun.

☐ Eyesight and hearing may be less acute; the senses of taste and smell may diminish.

☐ Reflexes and reaction times become somewhat slower.

☐ There may be lapses in short-term memory, even though long-term memory remains clear.

☐ The brain shrinks, losing about 10 percent of its weight as it ages. As a result of nerve cell loss, the ability to memorize and learn new skills is reduced.

☐ Internal organs—heart, lungs, liver, kidneys—operate less efficiently, losing function at the rate of about 1 percent a year from the age of 30 on and becoming less resistant to disease.

☐ Muscles shrink and body fat increases, although these changes can be minimized by regular exercise.

☐ A slightly irregular pulse rate and a mild increase in blood pressure are not unusual.

☐ Secretion of digestive juices lessens, and constipation may

THE GRAYING OF AMERICA

The number of people over 65 in the United States has nearly doubled since 1960 and thanks to aging "baby boomers" will double again by the year 2050. Unlike the stereotype of the sedentary retiree, today's senior generation is fitter and more independent than ever. Only 5 percent of Americans age 65 or older live in nursing homes. Many are still actively engaged in careers or community service. And although retirement income is often one-half to two-thirds of working income, the elderly also wield more economic power than ever before, a trend that has not gone unnoticed by businesses and advertisers.

But an aging population raises serious questions for society as a whole, not the least of which is how to pay for the medical care and support services that keep the elderly going. Today's older people are often called upon to bear without adequate resources the physical, emotional, and financial burdens of caring for themselves or their spouses through serious illnesses. A burgeoning older population will place added strains on a

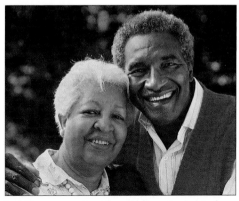

health-care system that is already short of geriatricians (p.392) and care givers.

As their numbers increase, however, older people are organizing to focus attention on their special concerns. Thanks in part to this new political clout, the mandatory retirement age was abolished in the United States in all but a few professions, and health-care reform and other issues of vital importance to the elderly are being pushed to the forefront of the nation's agenda.

---

occur with greater frequency.
☐ Metabolism in general slows down in the later years.
☐ After menopause, women may develop incontinence (p.405) as pelvic muscles weaken and the uterine ligaments no longer offer the same support to the bladder. Older men may develop incontinence or have difficulty urinating.
☐ Sexual hormone levels decline, although this does not necessarily lead to loss of sexual interest or ability. When sexual activity declines with age the reason is not always physiological.
☐ Sleep patterns usually change (p.407); older people may sleep less, at different hours, or more lightly than before.

It's important to be aware of the difference between the natural effects of aging and symptoms of disease (see *Recognizing Illness,* p.392). Many researchers today believe that the debilitating effects of aging have been overstated. They note that such conditions as atherosclerosis, once considered an inevitable part of aging, are often preventable; and a significant decline in mental faculties is now recognized as a sign of disease, not a normal consequence of getting older.

Has modern medicine really increased human life expectancy?

Dramatically so. Since the mid-19th century, human life expectancy has nearly doubled, from age 40 to about 75. If advances in medicine and in our standard of living continue, Americans born in the year 2050 can expect to live to be 80. Although the maximum human life span seems to be about 120 years, very few people reach that mark. Some scientists speculate that the middle eighties are probably the ceiling for human life expectancy, even if cures are found for heart disease and cancer.

Why aren't there more centenarians? No one really knows. According to one school of thought, a person's life span is programmed in the cells from birth; other experts place more importance on the role of stress and environmental factors in limiting longevity. Diet is another critical factor in determining how long an individual will live. (Researchers have found that rats limited to 40 percent of their normal caloric intake live more than twice as long as their counterparts who eat whatever they want.) Emotional pain—loneliness or depression—appears to depress the immune system and age people prematurely. In areas where strong kinship and community ties flourish, people often live to be much older than the general population.

Of course, the advantages of living to a ripe old age must be balanced against quality of life considerations. As medical science conquers killer diseases, our society will have to pay increasing attention to such issues as poverty among the elderly, the quality of nursing home care, and other emotional and social needs of the aged (see *The Graying of America*, p.387).

A friend of mine smokes, has several drinks a day, and does not seem to pay very much attention to his diet. Yet he's well over 80 and is thriving. How can this be?

A partial explanation can be found in heredity; the genes of people like your friend may make them less vulnerable to certain diseases or less likely to gain extra weight than other people.

Other aspects of your friend's lifestyle may compensate, to a certain degree, for his harmful health habits. He may take long walks every day, for example, to work off those extra calories he consumes.

There will always be people who beat the odds, but statistically they are rare, and exceptional cases like your friend should not inspire you to play Russian roulette with your health. Rather than concentrating on the exceptions that prove the rule, your best bet is to do all you can to create a healthy environment for yourself and adopt good health habits that work for you.

I'm 68 years old. Is it still worthwhile for me to make lifestyle changes?

It's never too late to change. In 1988 and 1989, a group of sedentary nursing home patients from the Boston area, ages 86 to 96, were introduced to weight lifting. After training for about 2 months, most of these elderly bodybuilders at least tripled the strength of their leg muscles. Two of them gave up their canes, and one woman regained her ability to get up from a chair without using her arms.

Surprisingly, statistics show that older people have more success breaking bad habits and making good ones than younger people do. If you don't succumb to negative thinking ("The damage is already done"), your maturity, and the perspective and patience that often comes with it, can work to your advantage. If you need reasons for making changes, here are a few.
☐ When people stop smoking, regardless of how long or how much they've smoked, the body begins to heal rapidly. It is never too late to reduce your risk of heart disease and cancer (see *If You Quit Smoking Today*, p.200).
☐ Improving your diet can enhance the quality of your life almost immediately. You can conquer minor medical problems like constipation and fatigue, and control more serious ones, such as diabetes or high cholesterol.
☐ Some older people begin to drink excessively in reaction to illness or loneliness (p.413). With counseling, however, late-onset alcoholics can discover better ways to cope, and they often find it easier to stop drinking than younger people do.

When you have decided which lifestyle changes will be of most benefit to you, here are two ways to make them work.
☐ Introduce change gradually. Radical changes are more likely to lead to relapse than to success.
☐ Make changes you can integrate into your life. Temporary change works only temporarily. (The nursing home bodybuilders lost about one-third of their newly acquired muscle tone when they stopped working out for 4 weeks.) There is no reason to try to become an Olympic athlete in your seventies. Instead, aim for more modest results that will last a lifetime.

Food doesn't taste the same to me anymore, and I'm eating less. Is this normal?

Sensations of taste and smell sometimes deteriorate with age, although exactly how this happens—and how commonly—is unclear. It was once thought that the number of taste buds decreases with age, but this is no longer accepted as true. Today doctors are more likely to investigate a variety of possible causes for taste loss, including infections, disease, and poor dental hygiene (the last can produce a constant bad taste in the mouth that interferes with the enjoyment of food). Some drugs can also affect the taste of food.

As anyone who's had a bad cold knows, taste and smell are closely related; if your sense of smell is diminished, which is often the case among the elderly, food tastes bland. Sinus inflammations, nasal polyps and other blockages of the nasal passages, damage to the receptor cells in the nasal cavities, viral infections, and head injuries can all cause olfactory loss. The loss is usually permanent, although in some cases, the sense of smell returns when the underlying cause, such as chronic sinus disease or a polyp, is treated. A "scratch-and-sniff" test can help a doctor identify the cause of olfactory impairment and, if possible, devise a treatment plan.

A reduced appetite is not the most serious consequence of olfactory loss. People who can't smell a gas leak or a pot burning are in real danger. If your sense of smell is impaired, be sure to install smoke detectors throughout your house and test them regularly (p.310); consider installing an industrial-grade gas detector, near the ceiling for natural gas, near the floor for propane.

You can compensate for diminished taste sensations by giving more attention to the texture of your food. Crunchy vegetables, for example, are more interesting than soft ones. When you prepare your favorite dishes, experiment with seasonings and garnishes. Even if you're on a salt-, sugar-, or fat-restricted diet, you needn't resign yourself to unappetizing meals—fresh herbs like dill and tarragon, garlic, spices, and lemon juice can add a delightful new flavor to almost any recipe.

I've read about older people who aren't poor yet still suffer from malnutrition. Why does this happen?

There are many reasons why a person may neglect his or her nutrition, even when money is not an issue. Today's older generation grew up at a time when knowledge about nutrition was less advanced than it is now and nutritional awareness less widespread. Many elderly people live alone and have a hard time adjusting to solitary dining. Nursing home residents are often served meals they don't choose at hours when they're not ready to eat them and, not surprisingly, find the food unappetizing.

People whose diets are restricted for health reasons may have difficulty adjusting to new foods and so may lose their appetite. People with missing teeth or ill-fitting dentures have trouble chewing and may choose foods because they are soft rather than for their nutritional content. Medical conditions such as stroke, arthritis, or Parkinson's disease can make cutting food, lifting it to the mouth, and chewing difficult. Some prescription drugs cause such side effects as nausea and indigestion, which make eating an unpleasant chore.

Adult children, friends, and neighbors who are concerned about an older person's nutrition and well-being can help by regularly inviting him or her over for dinner or dropping off a home-cooked casserole. Whenever possible, nursing homes should encourage residents to get out of bed and take meals with others in the dining room. Socializing stimulates appetite by making meals a more pleasant occasion.

Because poor nutrition impairs general health, anyone whose medical problems interfere with nutritional needs should make a point of talking to a doctor or registered dietitian. A doctor may be able to change or adjust prescriptions for drugs that diminish appetite. A dietitian can help plan varied, well-balanced meals that take into account restricted diets, physical handicaps, or digestive problems.

Since my husband died 2 years ago, I've stopped cooking formal meals for myself. My daughter says that I'm endangering my health? Is she right?

You are describing a common but unfortunate phenomenon. Widows who once enjoyed preparing nutritious meals for their families may sip tea and nibble at toast or crackers, unwilling to make a meal for one. Widowers who may never have shopped for food or cooked for themselves when their wives were living are often reluctant to learn.

If you're in the habit of eating several healthy snacks during the day, your daughter need not worry. As long as your diet is balanced on a daily basis, you don't have to meet all your nutritional needs at one sitting. But if your eating habits are causing you to lose weight or lack energy or are otherwise endangering your health, your daughter is quite right to be concerned.

Instead of cooking formal meals for yourself, try experimenting with new ways of cooking. Meals don't have to consist of several courses in order to be good for you. In response not only to the needs of single diners but also to help working mothers who make up a great part of the labor force today, there is now an entire subspecialty of cookbooks dedicated to making quick-and-easy one-dish dinners and simplified menus geared to flavor and good health.

Cooking your favorite dishes in quantity and freezing small portions is another way to ensure appetizing meals with minimal bother. Sign up for Meals on Wheels, if you qualify, to give yourself a break from cooking.

If sitting down alone makes you less likely to enjoy your meals, try treating yourself like a guest. Setting an attractive table can make mealtime more of a special occasion.

You don't always have to dine alone, either. Make a point of inviting your daughter or close friends over for a meal. Make a regular arrangement with a good friend to take turns cooking and serving meals.

A friend of mine claims that vitamins help keep her young. Should I start taking vitamin supplements now that I'm over 65?

A vitamin supplement does not convert a poor diet into a good one. If you are in good health, the best way to meet your nutritional requirements is by eating a well-balanced diet. The components of such a diet (see *Foods for a Healthy Diet,* p.24) will deliver vitamins and minerals to your body much more efficiently than supplements do. However, because the body's ability to absorb calcium and synthesize vitamin D (which aids calcium absorption) declines with age, many doctors recommend that otherwise healthy older men and women take a calcium supplement to protect against osteoporosis (see *The Facts About Osteoporosis,* p.379); drinking a cup of milk every day or sitting in the sun for 10 minutes twice a week can meet most people's requirements for vitamin D.

By itself, the aging process does not necessarily increase a person's need for most nutrients; in fact, the number of calories required to maintain a healthy weight declines with age as metabolism slows and activity levels tend to fall off. However, illness, injury, the process of recuperation, certain medications, and a poor diet may cause nutritional deficits. Thus, older people who eat very little, who have chronic health problems, or who take prescription drugs regularly may benefit from a vitamin supplement. A multiple vitamin containing the full Recommended Dietary Allowance (RDA) for vitamins and minerals (p.12) will suffice in most cases.

For more on vitamin and mineral supplements, see pages 40–42.

I'm having more and more difficulty chewing my food. How can I modify my diet to make eating easier?

It's important to chew food thoroughly to aid digestion and avoid choking. To make eating easier for yourself, try putting foods through a processor or a blender. If you do go on a soft foods diet, however, make sure you don't decrease your intake of fiber (pp.31–32). Soft and chewable sources of fiber include wild or brown rice, legumes (beans, peas, and lentils), squash, cooked leafy green vegetables, and hot or cold whole-grain breakfast cereals, such as oatmeal and shredded wheat.

Chewing food becomes harder for people with missing teeth; the wider the gap, the more difficult chewing becomes. If this is your problem, the best solution is to have the missing teeth replaced with a fixed or removable bridge, implants (pp.366–368), or a set of dentures. If you decide on dentures, make sure they fit well (pp.395–396) and remember that people who wear dentures, even well-fitting ones, must chew food longer than people with natural teeth do.

My husband has all his own teeth and chews his food thoroughly, but he still has trouble swallowing. Why is this?

Your husband's saliva glands may be malfunctioning. Several commonly prescribed drugs, such as antidepressants, antihistamines, antihypertensives, diuretics, analgesics, and antiparkinsonism drugs, can interfere with saliva production; so can radiation treatments for the head and neck, bacterial infections, and a weakened immune system.

Dry mouth is not a normal result of aging, nor is it the only cause of swallowing difficulties (others include muscular and neurological disorders and strokes). Your husband should see a doctor to find out what's wrong and what remedies are available. If a drug is the problem, for example, an alternative prescription may be the solution. Meanwhile, your husband should drink plenty of water with his meals.

I often suffer from constipation. Should I take a daily laxative?

Older people report problems with constipation five times more often than younger people do, but such reports are often unfounded. Most of us have been taught that anything less than a daily bowel movement means constipation. In fact, normal bowel functioning varies with individuals, and there is no reason to think you are constipated unless the normal pattern of your bowel movements has changed.

Among the most common causes of constipation in the elderly are a sedentary lifestyle, inadequate diet, and insufficient fluid intake. Antacids containing large amounts of aluminum and some prescription drugs, such as codeine, can also cause constipation. The next time you see your doctor, bring a list of every drug you take (including over-the-counter medications) and find out if any of them could be constipating you.

Ironically, overuse of laxatives is a frequent cause of constipation (see *The Facts About Regularity,* p.216). Most doctors will advise their patients to take a dietary approach to constipation before prescribing any other remedy. Try taking a brisk daily walk, drinking lots of fluids, and adding more fiber to your diet.

Can I reverse osteoporosis by beginning an exercise program now?

Exercise can't reverse the bone loss of osteoporosis once it has occurred. If begun early in life and practiced consistently, exercise may help prevent osteoporosis—but there's no guarantee.

This does not mean, however, that exercise at this stage in your life is worthless. In combination with other therapies—namely, a calcium-rich diet and estrogen replacement, when appropriate—exercise can help to preserve bone density (see *The Facts About Osteoporosis*, p.379). In addition, by strengthening muscles that protect brittle bones and vulnerable joints, exercise lowers your risk of injury.

Anyone who has been sedentary for years should begin a program of exercise slowly and gradually (see *Before You Start*, p.73). Consult your doctor first. Then choose a weight-bearing exercise (p.103) that you enjoy and will be able to perform regularly. Some good bets are weight training, walking, jogging, low-impact aerobics, and tennis. Non-weight-bearing exercises, such as swimming and bicycling, have less effect on bone loss, but will help you maintain flexibility and balance. By keeping limber, you guard against falls, which are a danger for people with easily broken bones (p.403).

My grandchildren are amazed that their 70-plus grandmother jogs and plays tennis. Is there any reason not to exercise as long as I can?

Let's hope that your grandchildren learn a thing or two from you. Maintaining a sensible, lifelong exercise program is among the very best things you can do

for yourself as you get older. Research shows that weakened muscles, brittle bones, and creaky joints—once considered inevitable aspects of aging—are more likely to be the preventable consequences of a sedentary lifestyle. (For more on the benefits of exercising later in life, see page 72.)

Staying physically active throughout life is more important than early athletic achievement, studies show. Some older people are reluctant to exercise because they are afraid they will fall and hurt themselves or even that exercise will give them a heart attack. But it is people who lead sedentary lives who may be more vulnerable to injury and disease. The regular exercise you now

get will help you maintain your agility and balance and remain steadier on your feet.

Injuries do occur when people exercise too strenuously, too abruptly, or for too long a period. Always listen to your body, and rest when you begin to feel tired or out of breath.

I'm now dependent on a wheelchair to get around. How can I stay as fit as possible?

It's important to use your muscles whether or not you are in a wheelchair, because unused muscles will shrink and become very weak. A physical therapist can help you adapt a variety of exercises to suit your needs.

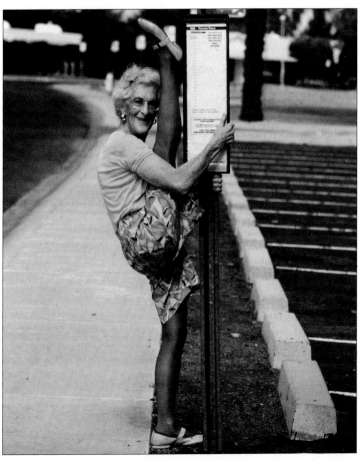

Limber great-grandmother Foofie Harlan, 76, stretches at an Arizona bus stop.

Stretches for the arms, legs, and back, and even sit-ups, can be performed from a wheelchair or an armchair (see *Exercises for the Disabled*, p. 75). By slouching down and leaning forward, you can tone your abdominal muscles. Hand-held elastic bands, passed under feet or thighs, can provide resistance for muscle-strengthening movements. Weight training—with free weights or with weight machines—is especially beneficial.

No matter what your physical limitations may be, regular exercise will help you gain strength and muscle tone and improve your cardiovascular functioning.

Now that I'm past 70, do I need to see my doctor more often?

After age 65 you should see your doctor for a thorough physical examination (p. 122) more often than before—probably every year. Women over 50 should have a gynecological exam (p. 252) every year as well. Regular checkups give your doctor a baseline to work with. He or she should keep detailed, accurate records and be familiar with your general condition when you are healthy so that any change from the norm—for example, a sudden weight loss, a rise in blood pressure, or a change in an EKG—can be noted and its cause investigated.

Your annual checkup will probably include more screening tests than you may have had when you were younger (see *Screening Tests for Healthy Adults*, pp. 124–125). It also provides an opportunity to review your medications and to discuss your lifestyle in general. Your doctor will want to know about your diet, whether you exercise regularly, and how well your social network functions to support you. Think

these things through before your visit, and answer in detail (for more on doctor-patient communication, see pages 120–121). If you schedule your physical in the fall, you can get your annual flu shot at the same time (p. 128). (You should have received a one-time pneumococcal vaccine at age 65 to protect against pneumonia; if you didn't, discuss this with your doctor at your next visit.)

In addition to seeing your primary care physician every year or so, you should continue having your eyes and teeth examined on a regular basis (pp. 136 and 395). It's also a good idea to have your hearing tested regularly. Your primary care physician can do a basic screening for hearing problems as part of your regular physical examination.

RECOGNIZING ILLNESS

Older people are rarely hypochondriacs. In fact, several studies confirm they are more likely to tolerate pain and ignore signs of disease than to report superficial problems to a doctor. Some older people have simply been brought up to be stoic about discomfort. Others may assume that their physical problems, however unpleasant or unusual, are attributable to old age and can't be helped. It may be difficult to distinguish a temporary ache or pain from a sign of illness, but certain symptoms are definitely not caused by aging and warrant immediate medical attention. If you experience any of the problems listed here, see your doctor without delay.

☐ Shortness of breath that occurs while you are resting or during the night.
☐ Heart palpitations (irregular heartbeats) not associated with strenuous exercise.
☐ Persistent or recurrent pain anywhere in the body.
☐ Constant fatigue, even when you've had plenty of rest.
☐ Double vision.
☐ Persistent or loud ringing in the ears.
☐ Sudden unexplained weight loss.
☐ Persistent thirst.
☐ Persistent low-back pain.
☐ Loss of power in an arm or a leg.
☐ Sudden change in bowel habits.
☐ Bleeding from any source.

My primary physician has always been an internist. Should I switch to a geriatric specialist at this stage of my life?

If your internist has been treating you for a long time and to your satisfaction, there's no compelling reason to change now. The particular specialty of your primary care physician is generally less important than his or her manner (does the doctor listen to your concerns and treat you with respect?), general skill, and ability to distinguish between signs of illness and normal aspects of aging. However, there are some advantages to switching to a geriatric specialist (geriatrician), especially if you are not in good health. A geriatrician is trained in the care and treatment of the aging and has relatively more experience working with them. A geriatrician is usually skilled in rehabilitation and will probably have a wider network of appropriate contacts for referrals than other specialists.

Elderly people often show different symptoms of disease than younger people do. Conditions sometimes overlap and mask one another. A geriatrician is trained to differentiate. He or she is also apt to be sensitive to visual impairment, hearing problems, and other aspects of aging that may hinder communication between doctor and patient.

Whether you stay with your internist or switch to a geriatrician, it's important to have a single primary care physician. Many older people are referred to specialists for specific conditions. As a result, they may see two, three, or more physicians who treat them and prescribe medications for them. Other care givers— nurses, dentists, physical therapists, social workers—may also be part of a health-care team. By coordinating and monitoring all aspects of your health care, a primary care physician will help you avoid treatments that duplicate or conflict with each other. (For advice on choosing a primary care physician, see page 118.)

Should drug dosages change as one ages?

They should be reduced in most cases. Because the body's sensitivity to drugs increases with age, older people can suffer serious side effects from drugs at dosages that would be harmless to younger people.

Because the kidneys and liver function less efficiently with age, the elderly metabolize and excrete drugs more slowly than the young. As a person gets older,

total body fat increases and total body water decreases. This means that fat-soluble drugs tend to build up and have a longer-lasting effect in an older body, while water-soluble drugs become more concentrated in the blood.

Older people are often particularly sensitive to psychoactive drugs—sleeping pills, tranquilizers, antidepressants, and stimulants—which act on the central nervous system. Unfortunately, overdoses of these drugs among the elderly often go unrecognized; even doctors misinterpret symptoms—dizziness, fatigue, confusion, memory losses—as part of the natural aging process, rather than as side effects of overmedication. According to the Public Citizen Health Research Group, 61,000 older adults develop drug-induced parkinsonism every year; 32,000 people fracture their hips in drug-induced falls; 163,000 suffer memory loss or impaired thinking due to drugs they are taking; and 243,000 are hospitalized for treatment of adverse drug reactions.

During a recent visit to my sister, I was alarmed at the number of pills she takes in the course of a day. Could she be overmedicating herself?

It's quite possible. As people get older, they are more likely to develop diseases and to have ongoing health problems for which medicines are prescribed, often by several doctors who may not be aware of what their colleagues are doing. If your sister does not have a single physician coordinating her treatments, she runs the risk of taking medications that duplicate each other's function or, even worse, that interact adversely. The use of over-the-counter medications often compounds the problem.

Many older people also hold on to old prescriptions and medicate themselves in attempts to save money on doctor's visits or because trips to the pharmacy have become too difficult. Others fill prescriptions but have trouble following the doctor's directions for taking them.

Talk to your sister about the medications she's taking. Encourage her to discuss the issue with the physician she sees most often to find out if any of the pills she takes are not necessary or potentially harmful.

What precautions should I take to avoid overmedication?

Take an active interest in your own health care, but don't act as your own doctor when it comes to pill-taking. Find a doctor you trust, and talk to him or her about the drugs you are using. Speak up whenever you don't understand the need for or how to take a drug. Ask your doctor to write down instructions for taking a new drug or to give you an instructional leaflet. (For questions to ask about a new drug, see page 151.) If you have doubts about a medication, ask your doctor if there is a nondrug treatment you can try first. The fewer drugs you take, the less likely you are to overmedicate.

If your doctor doesn't schedule a periodic review of your drugs, ask for one. Take an inventory of your medicine cabinet and draw up a list of all the drugs—prescription and over-the-counter medications, including vitamins— you take. Show the list to your doctor or better yet, put all the drugs in a bag and bring them into the doctor's office with you. Together with the doctor, make decisions about which drugs you should keep taking and which you might do without.

A WEEKLY MEDICATION DIARY

One way to remind yourself when and how to take your medicines is to keep a diary, or check-off chart, like the one shown here. (For other suggestions, see p.229.) Draw up the checkoff chart on index cards or on the pages of a notebook. Under the days of the week, write in the times you should take each drug every day. Whenever you take a medication, draw a line through the time of day. On a separate index card or notebook page, list each drug you take (both prescription and over-the-counter), what it looks like, what it's for, and all directions and cautions. Review this list periodically with your doctor; update it whenever he or she prescribes a new drug.

The Medicines I Take

Drug	Description	Use	Directions & Cautions
Digoxin	Small white tablet	For heart	0.25 mg once a day. Take at the same time every day.
Lasix	White tablet	Fluid in heart	40 mg twice a day. Causes frequent need to urinate.
Dilantin	White capsule with orange band	Seizures	100 mg 3 times a day. No alcohol.

Drug Checkoff Chart

Drug/directions	Sun.	Mon.	Tues.	Wed.	Thurs.	Fri.	Sat.
Digoxin. 0.25 mg once a day	8	8	8	8	8	8	8
Lasix. 40 mg twice a day	8 6	8 6	8 6	8 6	8 6	8 6	8 6
Dilantin. 100 mg 3 times a day	8 4 10	8 4 10	8 4 10	8 4 10	8 4 10	8 4 10	8 4 10

I seem to catch every cold and bug that passes my way. Is this usual as one gets older?

Unfortunately, it's not uncommon. Researchers believe that as people age, changes in their immune systems may make them more vulnerable to disease. However, the exact nature of those changes and their impact on general health is still not clear. Distinguishing between the normal effects of aging and changes due to disease is especially difficult in the case of the immune system.

It's quite clear, however, that people over 65 are likelier to catch the flu and suffer more severe consequences from it than younger people. Older people who suffer from chronic respiratory conditions are especially vulnerable to colds and infections, as is anyone being treated for cancer or other diseases with immunosuppressive drugs. Implanting such devices as pacemakers, heart valves, and prosthetic joints increases the patient's risk of infection, as do other types of surgery. Malnutrition, loss of independence, social isolation, and depression also lower resistance to disease.

To protect yourself against pneumonia and the flu, make sure you get a one-time pneumococcal immunization at age 65 (p.128) and a flu shot in the autumn of every year (p.129). For ways to ward off colds and better cope with those you do get, see pages 209–213.

My son mentioned the other day that he thought I was neglecting my teeth. How frequently should I be seeing a dentist?

Maintaining sound gums and teeth through proper home care and regular dental examinations is good not only for your appearance and morale, but for your overall health. Many dentists suggest having your teeth examined every 6 months (see *A Dental Exam*, p.137), but you may need to see your dentist more or less often depending on the condition of your mouth and on the efficiency of your home dental care (see *Caring for Your Teeth*, p.227). The important thing, especially as you get older, is to work out a schedule with your dentist and to stick to it. At this stage in life, plaque builds up more quickly on tooth surfaces and around gums, increasing your risk of developing periodontal disease and suffering tooth loss. As gums recede and expose the roots of teeth, cavities tend to develop on the root surface. This problem is made worse by a decline in saliva production that is quite common among older people (p.390). (Saliva functions as a natural dental rinse, diluting and neutralizing the acid in plaque that eats away at tooth enamel.)

My arthritis makes dental hygiene difficult. Is there an easier way to clean teeth, and is it all right to use toothpicks as a substitute for dental floss?

Devices to help people with arthritis or other physical problems brush and floss more easily are available at drugstores and through catalogs featuring aids for the handicapped (see Appendix). If it's difficult to hold a toothbrush, you can purchase special wide-handled models or modify an ordinary toothbrush by affixing a sponge around the handle or inserting the handle into a rubber ball. Wrapping adhesive tape around the handle can also make gripping easier. Some people find that an electric toothbrush is easier to manipulate than a regular one.

Drugstores carry special floss holders that make flossing somewhat easier. The American Dental Association does not recommend toothpicks as a substitute for dental floss because picks do not clean below the gum line and can damage sensitive gum tissue. Interdental cleaners, also available at drugstores, are a more effective substitute. If all else fails, rinsing thoroughly after every meal with water or a mouthwash will help dislodge food and is certainly better than doing nothing at all.

With the new techniques for filling and reconstructing teeth, is it true that dentures are fast becoming obsolete?

Not quite yet. For a variety of reasons more than 29 million Americans over age 65 have lost all their teeth, most often to gum disease. Luckily, modern dentures, which are held in place with suction or adhesives, are less clumsy than those of a generation ago. Since techniques for making and fitting dentures have improved significantly, no one need suffer uncomfortable dentures beyond the first few weeks of wear.

It does take time, however, to get used to the sensation of wearing dentures and for the muscles of the cheeks and lips to adjust to them. Eating may be awkward at first. And your dentist may have to check the fit of your dentures several times before you feel that they are as comfortable as they should be.

Precise fit is very important because you want to wear your dentures all day long without having to think about them. If they are uncomfortable, you will be self-conscious and miserable. And if you don't use your dentures regularly, your mouth will start to reshape itself, ensuring that the dentures won't fit properly when you put them in the next time.

If a new set of dentures continues to be painful after several weeks of wear, consult your dentist. The problem may be projecting bone or tooth chips, which the dentist can remove.

My dentures don't seem to fit in my mouth as well as they once did, and they are beginning to bother me. What could be causing this?

It's not unusual for dentures to become uncomfortable after months or years of wear. Once you've lost most or all of your teeth, the shape of your mouth is likely to change. Changes in the gums and in the bones supporting them can make your dentures feel uncomfortable after a time.

In general, it's a good idea to schedule regular dental appointments to have your dentures checked and refitted, if necessary. Poorly fitting dentures can irritate your gums, tongue, and cheeks, causing infections and other problems. Eventually, the ridges of irritated gums can shrink to such a degree that it becomes impossible to fit them with a new set of dentures.

If your dentures are no longer comfortable, don't try to fix them yourself because you might dam-

CARING FOR YOUR DENTURES

Whether they're made of porcelain or acrylic, false teeth collect plaque just like natural teeth and should be cleaned daily. First, take dentures out of your mouth and rinse them to remove food particles. Then, using a soft brush specially designed for dentures (or a soft regular toothbrush), brush thoroughly but gently with baking soda, hand soap, a mild dishwashing liquid, or a special denture-cleaning paste (check with your dentist about the best choice for your particular dentures). Be careful around metal clasps; you don't want to change their shape. To remove tartar, soak your dentures in a solution of 1 tablespoon white vinegar to 8 ounces of water.

Handle your dentures carefully. They'll crack or bend easily if dropped on a porcelain basin, so keep a towel under them as you work or fill the basin with water.

Even if you have dentures, it's important to keep your mouth clean. While the dentures are out, brush your gums, your tongue, and the roof of your mouth with a soft-bristled toothbrush and toothpaste to remove food debris and bacteria and to stimulate circula-

tion. If you wear a partial denture, take good care of your remaining teeth (see *Caring for Your Teeth,* p.227). When you brush and floss each day, pay particular attention to the teeth where denture clasps are connected—plaque collects in these places.

Dentists often recommend that you wear new dentures 24 hours a day for a few days to get used to them. After that, you should take them out at night to give your mouth a rest. Since dentures need to be kept moist to hold their shape, place them in a container of cool water or of denture-cleaning solution (ask your dentist for advice). If your dentures have metal parts, don't soak them longer than the recommended time in cleaning solution, or the metal may discolor. Never put dentures in hot water; heat can warp them.

To keep your mouth healthy and to check for beginning signs of oral cancer and other diseases, continue regular dental check-ups. If the fit of your dentures changes, see your dentist right away; ill-fitting dentures can cause serious gum irritation and even serious bone loss.

---

age them. If necessary, use a denture adhesive to secure them until you can see your dentist. If you continue to have trouble with fit, ask your dentist about implants (pp.366–367).

My husband complains that straight lines look crooked to him. What's happening to his sight?

Have your husband see an ophthalmologist for a complete eye exam (p.136) as soon as possible. The symptom you describe is a sign of age-related macular degeneration (ARMD), the most common cause of vision loss in older people. Basically, macular degeneration occurs when age takes its toll on the macula, the part of the retina responsible for

sharp central vision and color (see *How the Eye Works,* p.369). The condition is painless and can progress undetected for some time. It usually affects both eyes, either simultaneously or one after the other. In addition to age, risk factors for the more common "dry" form of macular degeneration include family history, being female, and having blue eyes; overexposure to sunlight is also thought to play a role. In dry macular degeneration, the cells of the macula waste away, leading to a decrease in image sharpness and gradual loss of central vision. When the patient peers out of the corner of his eyes, vision may seem fine, but when he turns to look at something directly, it may appear blurred or grainy.

In the less common, but more ominous "wet" type of macular degeneration, abnormal blood vessels growing under the macula leak, causing dark spots at the center of vision and making straight lines appear wavy. Wet degeneration may result in sudden, severe loss of central vision.

Since dry macular degeneration can develop into the wet type, early detection and regular follow-up exams are crucial. An ophthalmologist can check for visual distortion with an Amsler grid (facing page) and examine the condition of the retina with a slit-lamp microscope (p.136) and a fluorescein angiogram (the latter is obtained by injecting into the bloodstream a dye that highlights the retina and then photographing the retina with a special camera to detect leaking blood vessels). Early-stage wet macular degeneration can often be treated with lasers. Unfortunately, there's no treatment for dry macular degeneration.

To protect his eyes from sunlight, your husband should use special sunglasses that block all or most UVA and UVB rays (p.220), and have his regular glasses coated with a UV filter. He should check his vision daily with an Amsler grid, and notify his ophthalmologist promptly if he notices vision changes.

Macular degeneration can cause permanent vision damage, but because side vision is unaffected, it rarely leads to total blindness. Today, fortunately, there is a wide array of products designed to help people with limited vision, including magnifiers, easy-to-read watches and timers, telephone attachments, and "talking" books and calculators. For more information on such aids, contact the American Foundation for the Blind or the National Association for the Visually Handicapped (see Appendix).

What is diabetic retinopathy?

People with diabetes (pp.342–345) are subject to a number of serious complications, including retinopathy, or damage to the retina. Complications are more likely to occur if diabetes has not been well controlled, but they can also affect patients who have been diligent about monitoring and treating their disease. It is estimated that over 75 percent of people who have had diabetes for more than 30 years experience some retinal damage.

Diabetes can weaken blood vessels throughout the body, but because the capillaries that nourish the retina are so tiny and delicate, they are especially vul-

A HOME EYE TEST

The grid shown below was designed by the Swiss ophthalmologist Marc Amsler to screen patients for macular degeneration. To test your own eyes, put the grid in good reading light at the distance you normally hold a book. If you wear reading glasses, use them for the test. Cover one eye and focus on the dot in the middle of the grid with the other eye. You should be able to see the dot and the entire grid clearly and without distortion or blurring (the lines should look parallel and straight, and no part of any line should be missing). Repeat the test on the other eye. If the grid doesn't appear intact with either eye, see your eye doctor and describe the test results. Early diagnosis and treatment can often forestall serious vision problems.

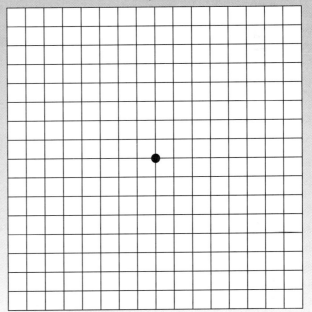

What grid distortion may mean. Wavy lines (below, left) anywhere on the grid may indicate wet macular degeneration. A blank spot (below, right) is a sign of dry macular degeneration. Not everyone's symptoms are the same—seeing graininess or dark spots may also signal retinal problems.

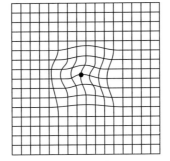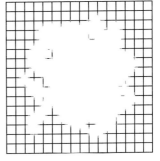

THE FACTS ABOUT GLAUCOMA

What is it? In a normal eye, a fluid called the aqueous humor constantly bathes the lens and iris (see *How the Eye Works,* p.369). As new fluid is produced, excess fluid drains out of the eye into the bloodstream through a complex drainage system. In glaucoma, the drainage channels become blocked, causing fluid to build up in the eye. The resulting increase in intraocular pressure eventually damages the optic nerve. Left untreated, glaucoma can severely reduce peripheral vision and lead to blindness.

The most common type of glaucoma is chronic open-angle glaucoma, in which the drainage channels are blocked gradually, causing a slow rise in eye pressure. In acute closed-angle glaucoma, the blockage and rise in pressure occur suddenly and painfully.

Glaucoma can also be caused by disease or injury to the eye. In rare cases, a child may be born with congenital glaucoma.

Who is most at risk? Glaucoma affects some 2 million Americans. Blacks, diabetics, and people with a family history of glaucoma are at higher risk of developing the disease than the rest of the population. One of the most common major eye disorders in people over 65, glaucoma rarely strikes before age 40.

What are the symptoms? Progressive and painless, chronic glaucoma often damages the optic nerve without the patient being aware of it. If there is an early symptom, it's usually a subtle loss of peripheral vision.

In an attack of acute glaucoma, vision blurs, usually in one eye. Halos may appear around lights. The eye may become hard, red, and painful enough to cause nausea and vomiting.

Diagnosis and treatment. The basic test for glaucoma is a measurement of the pressure within the eye with a tonometer (see *Examining Your Eyes,* p.136). An ophthalmologist will also test peripheral vision and examine the back of the eye for optic nerve damage.

Starting at age 35, have your eyes tested for glaucoma every year if you are at risk for the disease; every 2 to 5 years if you're not.

If caught early, chronic glaucoma is easily controlled with drugs that relieve pressure in the eye. (These drugs come in the form of eyedrops or pills, and are taken singly or in combination.) After years of treatment, some patients develop a tolerance for one drug and must switch to another. When drugs fail, laser surgery becomes necessary to open up drainage channels or create artificial ones.

Acute glaucoma requires emergency treatment to reduce intraocular pressure with eyedrops, pills, or intravenous fluids. Once the pressure is brought down, an operation called an iridectomy may be performed. Using lasers or a scalpel, the surgeon creates a tiny opening in the iris to allow the aqueous humor to drain more easily.

SEEING THROUGH PROBLEM EYES

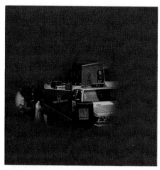

Glaucoma in its early stages may cause a gradual peripheral vision loss.

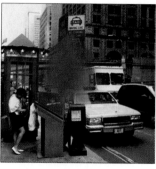

Macular degeneration may blur, distort, or destroy central vision.

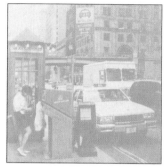

Cataract, a loss of transparency in the eye's lens, clouds vision.

nerable. As the capillaries deteriorate in the nonproliferative form of the disease, they can bulge and leak, leaving fluid deposits in the retina. Depending on where the leaks occur and how extensive they are, the patient may experience slight to moderate vision loss or none at all. Diffuse leakage throughout the macula can cause it to swell and lead to moderate to severe vision loss. Eventually, capillaries may close altogether, creating oxygen-starved patches of retina.

About 5 percent of patients with nonproliferative retinopathy develop the advanced, or proliferative, form of the disease, in which weak new blood vessels form to replace the closed-off capillaries. These abnormal blood vessels can hemorrhage within the retina or into the vitreous humor, seriously obscuring vision. Although the blood is sometimes reabsorbed, scars may form on the retina that can lead to retinal detachment, a medical emergency requiring immediate treatment (p.368).

Some diabetics notice visual disturbances in the early stage of retinopathy; others experience no vision loss until the disease has progressed significantly. Regular ophthalmological screening, including examination with a slit-lamp microscope (p.136) and flourescein angiography (p.396), can provide the early diagnosis, which along with controlling the underlying diabetes, can help prevent or postpone vision loss.

Laser surgery is the treatment of choice for retinopathy. Lasers may be used to reduce swelling, destroy closed vessels, and seal weak ones. The procedure is performed under a local anesthetic (in the form of eyedrops) and takes about half an hour. Severe cases, in which bleeding has greatly clouded the vitreous, may require a more complicated operation, called a vitrectomy, in which the vitreous is removed and replaced with an artificial solution.

I've been told that I have cataracts, but I'm hesitant about having my eyes operated on. Is surgery the only treatment for cataracts?

A cataract is a gradual clouding of the lens of the eye that affects most older people to some degree. Its cause in the elderly is unknown. (Cataracts in younger people may be due to diabetes, Down's syndrome, exposure to radiation, use of cortisone drugs, or maternal infection early in pregnancy.) The condition is painless and often goes unnoticed in its early stages. The main symptom is a progressive loss of visual acuity and increasingly blurry vision.

Not all cataracts require surgery. Some develop so slowly that a person may go through life without needing an operation. Whether or when you decide to have your cataracts removed will depend in part on the degree to which they interfere with daily activities, such as working, driving a car, going to the movies, or watching TV.

Depending on the size and location of your cataracts, there are alternative treatments that may help you avoid or postpone surgery. Prescription glasses can sometimes compensate for minor vision loss. If you have small cataracts near the back of your lenses, eyedrops can widen your pupils to allow more light to enter your eyes.

To make living with cataracts more comfortable, avoid direct sunlight by wearing a hat and proper sunglasses (p.220) outdoors. Utilize the sun visor in your car to cut glare while you drive. Avoid direct light indoors.

To cut glare from a printed page, some people with cataracts find it helpful to cover the page they are reading with a sheet of a dull black paper in which a slit has been cut. They read a few lines at a time through the slit and move the paper up and down as needed. When you watch television, make sure there is no light source between you and the television screen.

On the other hand, a cataract doesn't have to be "ripe," or completely opaque, before it can be removed. Doctors tend to recommend surgery when sight is impaired to such an extent that daily functions are compromised.

How successful is cataract surgery? How is it done?

Advances in medical technology have made cataract surgery one of the most successful operations doctors perform these days. In about 95 percent of cases, vision is markedly improved. Of course even minor surgery carries some risk, especially for people who have serious heart or lung disease, or severe hypertension; no responsible doctor would fail to determine whether you are a good candidate for surgery before proceeding with it. In addition, a cataract patient must be able to lie quietly during the operation; an uncontrollable cough, for example, could compromise the safety of the procedure.

Before cataract surgery is performed, careful measurements of the length and curvature of the affected eye are taken to enable the surgeon to select an implant that will most closely restore the patient's normal vision. The operation itself takes about an hour and is performed in a hospital on an outpatient basis or in an ophthalmologist's operating suite. The patient is given local or general anesthesia, and drops are applied to the eye to widen the pupil and expose the lens. Using a fine diamond-tipped instrument, the surgeon makes a small incision around the outer edge of the cornea. Next, a clear gel is injected between the cornea and the lens to maintain the space between them and allow removal of the lens. An artificial lens is slipped into the natural lens capsule and is held in place with plastic hooks. The incision is sewn up with a very thin suture thread. To prevent infection, the patient is given antibiotics immediately after the operation.

In most cases, the replacement lens restores normal vision, although some people will need to wear glasses too. If a permanent plastic implant is not advisable because of the presence of eye disease or because a patient is very young (it is not known whether implants last indefinitely), removable contact lenses or, rarely, special glasses may have to be worn instead.

Most people recuperating from cataract surgery experience nothing more than a few days of mild discomfort. The incision heals completely in about a month, and glasses, if they are needed, can be fitted in about 10 weeks.

My husband seems to have difficulty hearing women's voices, but not men's. Is this common? What's happening to his hearing?

Your husband may have age-related hearing loss, or presbycusis. Common among older people, presbycusis is usually caused by gradual wear and tear on the receptor cells of the inner ear and is often the result of a lifetime's exposure to loud noises (for ways to noiseproof your environment, see *Living in a*

Noisy World, p. 300). Men are more likely than women to suffer hearing loss, probably because more of them traditionally worked in noisy places. As women increasingly move into different kinds of occupations, more of them will no doubt experience hearing losses.

Changes in hearing are usually noticed much later in life than changes in vision. The first sign of age-related hearing loss is often difficulty hearing high-pitched sounds, like a woman's voice or the sound of certain musical instruments. Words tend to sound mumbled, certain consonants may be hard to hear and understand, and listening in a crowd becomes especially difficult. A person with presbycusis may also become very sensitive to loud noises. Even raising your voice to make yourself understood can be quite uncomfortable for your husband.

There is no cure for age-related hearing loss although a well-fitting hearing aid (facing page) can usually make listening easier and more enjoyable.

Another possible form of hearing loss among older people is conductive hearing loss, in which a blockage or impairment of the structures of the outer and middle ears prevents sound vibrations from reaching the inner ear. The underlying problem may be a buildup of wax in the ear canal (p. 226), a punctured eardrum, or an ear infection. To people with this type of hearing loss, voices and other sounds may seem muffled, but their own voices sound amplified. Conductive hearing loss is often correctable with medications or surgery.

Hearing may also be affected by poor circulation that diminishes blood supply to the ears, as well as by certain antibiotics and antihypertensive drugs and by large doses of aspirin.

I am having trouble convincing my husband that his hearing is not what it used to be. What can I do?

Ask him (gently) to try a few tests. Have him sit down, cross his feet, and rub his shoes together. Can he hear the sound the rubbing makes? Can he hear the television or radio when it is set at a sound level pleasant to your ears? Can he hear water dripping from a faucet? Can he listen to telephone conversations equally well with both ears? If he has difficulty with these hearing checks, your husband may have a mild hearing loss. The next step is a visit to the doctor to determine the cause of the loss and whether it's treatable.

In the meantime, you can help your husband cope by speaking in a slightly louder than usual tone, at your normal rate of speech, if it does not seem too rapid for him. Don't mumble and don't shout. Shouting is patronizing, it can distort sounds, and for people with presbycusis, can be very uncomfortable.

For your own sake as well as your husband's, keep background noise to a minimum. Avoid running noisy household appliances simultaneously or while you are speaking. Turn down the television or radio and wait until your neighbor stops mowing his lawn before starting a conversation. If your husband does not catch something you have said, rephrase it in short, simple sentences. Give clues to help key him into a conversation. For instance, "Since we're talking about the economy, dear, how well do you think the governor is managing?" If you want to ask him a question, call him by name first. "Robert, would you like to go for a drive?" is better than "Shall we go for a drive?"

BUYING AND CARING FOR A HEARING AID

If your hearing is troubling you, see your doctor. He or she may refer you to a specialist in hearing disorders (an otolaryngologist or an otologist) or suggest that you see an audiologist, a professional (though not a physician) with a graduate degree in evaluating hearing. Using a series of tests, the doctor or audiologist can assess the extent and type of your hearing loss (see facing page) and prescribe a hearing aid, if necessary. Hearing aids are sold by audiologists or by hearing aid dealers (the latter are licensed in most states to test hearing and sell aids).

The most commonly used hearing aid is the in-the-ear aid, which lies flush with the outer part of the ear; it's useful in all but the most severe cases of hearing loss. The in-the-canal aid fits entirely within the ear canal; it's used for mild to moderate hearing loss. The behind-the-ear aid is suitable for almost all degrees of hearing loss; because of its size, it's the easiest to handle.

Hearing aids aren't cheap. Prices vary depending on the type and brand of hearing aid, on the number of special features it has, and on the dealer—it pays to comparison-shop. There's usually a 30-day trial period after purchase, during which time the dealer should adjust the device and make sure you're using it properly. If you're not satisfied, be sure to go back to the dealer.

Getting used to a hearing aid takes time. You must learn to insert and remove it and to adjust the volume. Distinguishing sounds will be tricky at first. Practice at home a few hours a day and be patient. The first week is usually the hardest. Feedback (a high-pitched whistling from sound that has been reamplified) can occur when a hearing aid has not been inserted or fitted properly. Your hearing aid dealer can help you solve this problem.

To care for your hearing aid, keep it away from high temperatures and harsh chemicals, including hair spray. When you take it out at night, turn it off, disengage the batteries to extend their life, and wipe the exterior with a dry cloth. Keep your ears free of earwax (p.226).

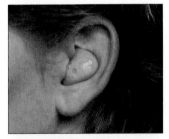

In-the-ear hearing aid

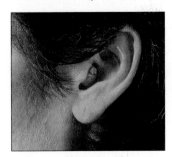

In-the-canal hearing aid

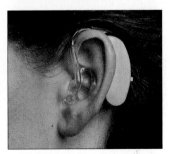

Behind-the-ear hearing aid

My mother complains of dizzy spells. What could be causing them?

It depends on the type of dizziness. Most doctors distinguish between light-headedness, in which the person feels faint or woozy, and vertigo, in which the person feels that she's spinning or that the room she's in is spinning around her.

A mild sense of unsteadiness or light-headedness may mean that your mother is tired, anxious, or depressed. Dizzy spells can also result from one of several different medical conditions, including anemia, hypoglycemia (p.345), hypotension (low blood pressure), and other cardiovascular problems.

Vertigo, on the other hand, is often related to disorders of the inner ear, where the balance centers are located. A viral infection in the ear, for example, can cause vertigo and impair hearing if not treated promptly. Vertigo can also occur in cases of agoraphobia (p.168) or as a side effect of certain medications.

Persistent attacks of severe vertigo may be a sign of Ménière's disease, a condition caused by an increase in the amount of fluid in the canals of the inner ear that control balance. In an attack of Ménière's, vertigo may be accompanied by nausea, vomiting, sweating, and in the affected ear, deafness, tinnitus (ringing or buzzing), and pressure or pain. Ménière's disease can be treated with drugs or, if necessary, surgically.

If your mother experiences brief, severe attacks of vertigo when she moves her head in a certain way or changes position, she may have what is known as positional vertigo, a benign condition that usually subsides with time. Attacks can be prevented by identifying and avoiding positions that trigger them.

Dizziness is a common problem among the elderly that can result in falls or in a disabling fear of walking. Although many cases are mild and clear up on their own, dizziness can be a sign of a serious underlying problem, including stroke, transient ischemic attacks (facing page), and in rare cases, a brain tumor.

Have your mother see her doctor for an ear exam and perhaps other diagnostic tests to determine the cause of her dizziness. Dizziness due to disorders of the inner ear is often treated with antihistamine or antiemetic drugs. Among the latter, dimenhydrinate (Dramamine) provides effective relief for the nausea associated with inner ear disorders; it is also used to treat motion sickness and many forms of vertigo. The drug can cause drowsiness, however, and your mother should not drive or drink alcohol if she takes it.

I sometimes get dizzy when I get up from a chair. Is this a cause for concern?

The annoying experience you describe is not unusual among the elderly (as well as among younger people with chronically low blood pressure). Up to 30 percent of older people suffer from postural hypotension, a condition in which blood pressure drops significantly when a person rises or sits up suddenly. Some people with hypotension never have symptoms, but those who do are often afraid that they will faint or fall when they get up from a chair or from bed.

Prolonged bed rest can lead to postural hypotension, while some commonly prescribed drugs can exacerbate the condition or even cause it. Among these drugs are certain antihypertensives, sedatives, diuretics, antidepressants,

and antipsychotic drugs, nitroglycerin preparations, a widely prescribed antiparkinsonism drug (Sinemet), and some drugs used to treat heart-rhythm disturbances. If you think that a medication you are taking is making you dizzy, ask your doctor about it.

Some practical precautions can help you to minimize the effects of postural hypotension.

☐ When you get out of bed in the morning, sit up for a few moments before rising to your feet.

☐ Avoid sitting or standing for prolonged periods.

☐ When you sit, elevate your legs on a footstool or some other support whenever possible. When you're lying down, use pillows to keep your legs raised at or above the level of your heart.

☐ Always stand up slowly, especially if you have been sitting for a very long time.

☐ Support stockings can help prevent blood from pooling in the lower legs. Avoid tight knee-high stockings or any constricting elastic, such as garters, that could impede circulation.

☐ Pointing your feet, then flexing them upward toward the knees several times before you stand up, will help raise your blood pressure and pulse rate.

☐ Drinking coffee after meals and sprinkling salt on your food can keep your blood pressure up, if this is not contraindicated by other medical problems.

Notify your doctor if your dizziness persists or if you have fainting spells.

KEEPING SHARP AT THE WHEEL

Age alone doesn't define a driver's competence. But the changes that occur in vision, hearing, reaction time, and physical flexibility as you grow older can make driving more difficult. Responsible older drivers recognize and acknowledge these changes in themselves when they happen, learn to compensate for the deficiencies when they can, and stop driving when they can't. Listed below are ways you can make up for some of the effects of aging and still be a safe driver.

☐ When you buy a car, pick a midsize model (such cars have better visibility than compacts and are easier to maneuver than large cars). Choose power steering and brakes for easy, fast response. If you drive at night, avoid fully tinted windshields.

☐ On an expressway keep pace with the traffic around you. If you must drive more slowly, use the right-hand lane. Avoid expressways at rush hour when quicker reactions are needed.

☐ Exercise to keep your body flexible so that you can observe the road from all angles and maneuver the car more easily.

☐ Avoid driving at dusk and daybreak, when light is tricky.

☐ Don't drive at night if you have problems with night vision.

☐ Have your eyes checked regularly. If you wear glasses, keep your prescription up-to-date and pick frames that won't interfere with your peripheral vision.

☐ Have your hearing checked regularly and, if you need a hearing aid, wear it when you drive.

☐ Before a long trip get plenty of sleep and take rest stops as needed along the way.

Why are falls such a danger for older people? What are the principal causes?

Falls are the most common type of accident—and the leading cause of accidental death—for people over age 65. Falls become more dangerous as people age because their bones break more easily, sometimes resulting in permanent impairment. In addition, the lengthy bed rest necessitated by a bad fall can lead to weakened muscles, pneumonia, and other complications.

Most falls result from a combination of physical frailty and an environmental hazard. And it isn't always the most enfeebled among the elderly who have the greatest risk of falling, but rather those who have yet to acknowledge and adapt to their physical limitations. More than half of all reported falls involve previously diagnosed infirmities such as weakening eyesight or hearing, diminished muscle control (sometimes after a stroke), an unsteady gait, arthritis, and dizziness or fainting. When they walk, older people tend not to pick their feet up as high as they used to, which makes them more apt to trip. Mental impairment, alcohol abuse, and the side effects of prescription drugs are other factors often involved in falling accidents.

What can I do to minimize my risk of falling?

Have your vision and hearing checked regularly. Keep your ears free of earwax, which can interfere with equilibrium. Go over all prescriptions with your doctor; make sure that you are taking the right dosages and that none of the medications impair your mental functioning or sense of balance. Exercise great care if you drink alcohol, since even small amounts can impair judgment and slow reflexes.

Don't wear poorly fitting or worn shoes. Check your home for danger spots; accident-proof your surroundings as much as possible (see *Adapting a Home for Changing Needs,* pp. 350–351).

Even after a minor fall, fear of falling causes some people to curtail physical activities. This is usually the worst policy for you or anyone caring for you to adopt. Make a point of staying in good physical shape. A program of regular exercise—anything from stretches to low-impact aerobics—will improve your balance and range of motion. Most falls are preventable. Physical fitness and attention to simple measures can keep you on your feet and out of the hospital.

After a few minutes of vacuum cleaning, I sometimes develop chest pains. Could I have a heart problem?

It's possible. If insufficient oxygen is reaching the heart muscle (usually because of narrowed coronary arteries), your heart can't accommodate sudden physical exertion and the result may be the chest pains known as angina (p. 328). Angina is not the same as a heart attack, but rather a warning sign of developing coronary disease.

Angina is a likely explanation for your symptoms, but there are others, including stomach, esophagus, gallbladder, lung, muscle, or bone problems.

Whatever may be causing your chest pain, don't try to diagnose it yourself. See your doctor for an evaluation and treatment. Many people ignore chest pains because they are afraid of getting bad news. This is a serious mistake. In the case of heart attack, delay—or denial—can be fatal.

About 60 percent of heart attack deaths occur within an hour of the onset of symptoms. If in doubt, seek medical attention right away.

Does hypertension affect older people differently?

Some increase in blood pressure (and with it an increase in heart attack and stroke risk) often occurs as people age. In many cases, this increase affects primarily the systolic pressure, the first figure in a blood pressure reading (p. 326). Until recently, isolated systolic hypertension was thought to be a natural part of the aging process, a way for the body to compensate for the effects of hardening arteries. And because antihypertensive drugs can produce serious side effects (p. 328), especially among the elderly, doctors sometimes resisted treating isolated systolic hypertension with drugs.

Although diet and lifestyle changes (p. 205) remain key elements of any hypertension treatment plan, a recent study indicates that treating isolated systolic hypertension with a low dose of an inexpensive diuretic drug (chlorthalidone) significantly reduces stroke risk in older people, even in patients over 80.

What is a transient ischemic attack?

A common problem in people over age 65, a transient ischemic attack (TIA) is a temporary interruption of blood supply to the brain that results in strokelike symptoms lasting no more than a day, often only seconds or minutes (see *Recovering From a Stroke,* p. 332). TIA's are usually caused by an embolism in a cerebral artery or by a narrowing of a cerebral artery due to atherosclerosis (see *The Language of*

Heart Disease, p.327). Although symptoms may be imperceptible or no more alarming than a momentary episode of dizziness or numbness, TIA's are dangerous in that they are often the prelude to a full-blown stroke.

A suspected TIA should be brought to your doctor's attention without delay. He or she can perform diagnostic tests to rule out other causes of your symptoms and to look for evidence of atherosclerosis. Treatment, often with aspirin (p.205) or anticoagulant drugs, is aimed at preventing a major stroke. Patients with more than 70 percent blockage of one of the internal carotid arteries, the main arteries to the brain, may be candidates for carotid endarterectomy, a stroke preventive operation in which the inner layer and attached fatty deposits are removed from the artery.

Although I've never smoked, I've developed a persistent cough. How serious is this?

A cough is one of the body's most ingenious defenses. Coughing keeps potentially dangerous organisms and foreign bodies out of the lungs, helping to prevent infections and blockages. Most coughs are triggered by irritation of the airways caused by dust, smoke, or mucus dripping from the back of the nose.

A minor cough often accompanies a cold, allergy, or a bout of influenza and lasts about as long as the underlying viral infection does. A persistent cough, however, can be a sign of a serious pulmonary condition, such as bronchitis (p.339), emphysema (p.340), and even lung cancer.

Coughing is also a sign of pneumonia, an inflammation of the lungs usually caused by infection with bacteria or viruses. In cases of bacterial pneumonia,

coughing produces phlegm and is typically accompanied by fever, chills, and acute chest pains. In addition to fever, aches, and other flulike symptoms, viral pneumonia produces a persistent dry cough that may interrupt sleep. A common complication of the flu among the elderly, pneumonia is a leading cause of death for people over 65. This is why a one-time pneumococcal vaccine (p.128) and a yearly flu shot are so important once you reach that age.

A cough that brings up bloody phlegm and is accompanied by weight loss and a low-grade fever may indicate tuberculosis. Although this disease is not common in the general population, it is increasing among older people, especially those who are malnourished or who abuse alcohol.

The first line of treatment for a cough is to drink plenty of fluids and get lots of rest. To relieve nighttime discomfort, eat a little honey or suck on hard candy or cough drops. For a discussion of the pros and cons of cough medicines, see page 214.

Any cough that doesn't go away within a week or so may signal a condition more significant than a cold or minor allergy. If your cough persists or is severe, brings up greenish or bloody phlegm, or is accompanied by pain or breathing difficulty, see your doctor without delay.

I'm well over 70. Do I still need to do breast self-examinations on a regular basis?

Regular self-examination is more important than ever as you get older. American women now face a 1 in 9 chance of developing breast cancer, and the risk is even higher for older women. More than 80,000 breast cancer cases are reported every year in women over age 65.

It cannot be said too often or too emphatically that a good prognosis for breast cancer depends on early detection. Examine your breasts every month at a time that you can easily remember, such as the first day of the month (see *The Breast Self-Exam,* p.203). In addition, be sure your doctor examines your breasts during your annual physical, and have a mammogram every year to help detect disease before it progresses.

Keeping to a regular self-examination schedule helps you to stay familiar with the shape and texture of your breasts, so that you are more likely to notice any small lumps that develop. If you do notice a change, inform your doctor right away.

Should you develop cancer, remember that the guidelines for living with the disease (pp.334–335) are valid no matter how old you are. Do not let age or embarrassment stand in the way of protecting your health. Stay informed about your condition and treatment options. If you are unsure of a recommended treatment, get a second opinion.

My doctor says I need to have some polyps removed from my colon. Does this mean I have an increased risk of colon cancer?

It depends on the type of polyp. Polyps are small mushroomlike growths, which often develop in the colon (large intestine), especially in older people. An estimated two out of three Americans over 60 have some kind of abnormal growth or lesion in their colons. Some polyps (called pseudopolyps or inflammatory polyps) result from injury or inflammation of the intestinal lining, often after a severe bout of colitis (pp.346–347); these growths are not thought to pose a significant health risk.

Although benign, adenomatous polyps are usually considered to be precancerous—that is, they have the potential to become malignant—and your doctor may advise removing them. The procedure, called a polypectomy, is a relatively uncomplicated one, in which a specially equipped fiber-optic tube, or endoscope (see *Diagnostic Tests,* pp. 126–127), is inserted into the colon to excise the polyps. When polyps are particularly large or firmly attached to the wall of the colon, intestinal surgery through an abdominal incision may be needed.

Most doctors believe that the larger a polyp is, the greater the risk that it will become cancerous, and many advise removing all but the tiniest polyps as a preventive measure. Surgery to remove precancerous growths is elective, which means that you can decide whether or not you want to have it done. If you are otherwise healthy and your doctor feels you are a good candidate for surgery, it's probably a good idea to go ahead with it.

I developed diabetes in my forties, but that was 20 years ago. What changes in treatment will be necessary as I get older?

If you've had diabetes for years, you know that losing weight—even a little weight—helps control diabetes and that diet and exercise are the best ways to keep your weight down and control your blood glucose (sugar) level (pp. 342–345). But as you get older, especially if you live alone, it may seem more difficult to maintain a healthy diet. You may also be getting less exercise: in the later years many people fall into a sedentary lifestyle,

and exercise—even if it's just a daily walk—can seem like a chore when you're not feeling well.

For these reasons, diet and exercise alone may no longer control your diabetes, and your doctor will prescribe medication. Hypoglycemic pills, which help the pancreas make more insulin, are usually the first choice. If these drugs eventually stop working, your doctor may start you on insulin injections.

You are undoubtedly aware that stroke, kidney failure, heart disease, and visual impairment can occur as complications of long-term diabetes. If you maintain regular contact with your doctor and follow your treatment plan faithfully, you should be able to avoid or at least control many diabetic complications.

Diabetic neuropathy (nerve damage) may eventually produce a tingling, aching, or burning sensation in your legs and feet, or induce numbness. Numbness is a hazard because it can prevent you from noticing injuries on your legs and feet before they become infected. Untreated infections can ulcerate and, in the worst cases, result in the amputation of a foot or leg. Be diligent about bathing your feet and inspecting them daily for blisters, cuts, or bruises. Get professional help for any ingrown toenails, corns, or bunions rather than trying to treat them yourself. Exercise caution around hot water, heating pads, or electric blankets, which can burn you without your knowing it.

Older people sometimes have multiple health problems and take several medications. Keep your primary care physician up-to-date about every drug you are taking, prescription or over-the-counter (p. 393). If you're given a special diet for another condition and you think that it conflicts with your diabetic diet, mention

this to your doctor too. It's usually a simple matter to work other nutritional requirements into your diabetic meal plan.

Frankly, the worst part of growing old for me has been the loss of bladder control. What are the causes of this embarrassing problem?

There are several different types of incontinence with many different causes. Although incontinence is often age-related, it is not an inevitable part of aging, and it is treatable.

In stress incontinence, urine leaks out when a person coughs, sneezes, laughs, exercises, or moves in a way that puts pressure on the bladder. This type of incontinence is common in women of all ages.

Urge incontinence is the inability to hold urine long enough to reach a toilet; it is associated with such conditions as stroke, Alzheimer's disease, Parkinson's disease, and multiple sclerosis, but can occur in otherwise healthy elderly people too.

Overflow incontinence is the leakage of small amounts of urine from a bladder that is constantly full. A common cause in older men is an enlarged prostate (p. 248) that blocks the flow of urine. Overflow incontinence is also associated with diabetes.

Other possible causes of incontinence include urinary tract infections (pp. 248–249), bladder stones, damage to the urethra, a dropped bladder or uterus, weak pelvic muscles, prostate cancer (p. 248), stress, and anxiety. Incontinence can also occur as a side effect of diuretics, sedatives, antidepressants, and other medications. And in addition to all the other problems it causes, smoking has been linked to loss of bladder control.

Aside from using adult diapers, how else can I control incontinence?

Adult diapers and incontinence pads are widely available now and can be very useful. But they are by no means your only option. Because incontinence can be caused by so many things, your first step should be to have your doctor determine why you are incontinent. Before your visit, keep a diary for a week or two that notes when you have made it to the toilet, the times and circumstances when you have had an accident (were you hurrying? coughing? laughing?), and whether only a few drops or a stream of urine was voided. This information will help your doctor make an accurate diagnosis and begin appropriate treatment. Here are some frequently recommended therapies.

☐ Eliminate alcohol, caffeine, sugar, spicy foods, and acidic fruits and juices from your diet for a few weeks. These foods are known to irritate the bladder.

☐ Behavior modification techniques, including bladder retraining and biofeedback (see *Learning to Relax,* pp. 206–207), are frequently helpful.

☐ Kegel exercises to strengthen the muscles of the pelvic floor (p. 238) can relieve mild to moderate stress incontinence (p. 405). New tampon-shaped graduated weights are available that add resistance to these exercises.

☐ Drugs that soothe bladder spasms by blocking the release of certain chemicals in the nervous system may be prescribed to treat urge incontinence.

☐ In some medical centers, collagen injections are being used, as an alternative to surgery, to repair a damaged urethra or lift a dropped bladder.

☐ Several surgical procedures have been devised to relieve incontinence. Although surgery is usually attempted only after noninvasive therapies have failed, it is often very effective.

For more on controlling incontinence, contact Help for Incontinent People (see Appendix).

I'm 75 years old, and my skin is getting very dry and scaly. Is this a normal part of aging?

A certain degree of wrinkling, drying, and loss of elasticity is the natural result of hormonal changes and long-term wear and tear from the sun, wind, cold, and other environmental assaults. If you are troubled by dry skin, these home remedies may help.

☐ Check that the air in your home is sufficiently humid.

☐ Keep detergents, rubbing alcohol, bleaches, and other drying substances away from your skin.

☐ Limit bathing to once a day, and use only mild soap.

☐ Apply a moisturizer or emollient such as petrolatum to dry areas immediately after your bath, while your skin is still moist.

CARING FOR A BEDRIDDEN PATIENT

To minimize the sense of dependency that illness fosters, allow a bedridden patient to brush his teeth, comb his hair, and do as much on his own as possible. Unless they're seriously ill or incapacitated, most convalescents prefer to feed themselves. When you bring in a meal, make sure the patient is propped up enough to ensure safe swallowing. If you must spoon-feed the patient, chat during the meal, but don't expect replies all the time. Leave enough time between bites for chewing and swallowing. The aids for the bedridden mentioned below are available from specialty stores and catalogs (see Appendix).

Preventing bedsores. A serious threat to anyone confined to bed, bedsores, or pressure sores, most often develop where bones are near the skin—at the hips, elbows, knees, ankles, and heels. Bedsores first appear as reddened areas on the skin, which soon darken and ulcerate. Without prompt medical attention, bedsores can become infected, and such infections can be life-threatening. Frail older people with thin skin are at particular risk.

To prevent bedsores, change the patient's position at least every 2 hours. Roll the body gently, smoothing sheets taut underneath. Keep the patient's skin clean and dry (this is especially important if the patient is incontinent) and lubricate it with a body lotion. An inexpensive foam rubber egg-crate mattress pad will help alleviate pressure. You can also use noncompressible pillows and special sheepskin protectors to cushion vulnerable parts of the body.

Using a bedpan. Be sensitive to the patient's need for privacy. Accompany a mobile patient to the bathroom when necessary. A less mobile patient may be helped onto a portable toilet placed next to the bed. You'll need a bedpan for a patient who cannot leave the bed.

Before using a bedpan, wash it with hot water (to warm it) and dry it. With one hand, help the patient raise the buttocks while you slip the pan underneath. Be ready to remove the bedpan promptly when the patient is through without seeming to hurry the process. Don't leave the bedpan in place longer than necessary; the resulting pressure can lead to the formation of bedsores.

If a patient is incontinent, use waterproof pads across the bed that you can change quickly and easily (see CHANGING THE BED, facing page). Wash the patient gently, pat dry, and apply a moisturizing cream and a layer of petroleum jelly.

No one knows your skin better than you do. If you think that the dryness and scaliness you are experiencing is unusually severe, it is time to consult your doctor. Especially in the later years, the condition of your skin can provide important clues to the state of your general health. An underactive thyroid, for instance, can cause skin to look older than it should and feel thick, dry, and cool to the touch. (Brittle nails and hair loss on the outer eyebrows are among other signs of hypothyroidism.) If you experience any of these symptoms, see your doctor. Untreated hypothyroidism can raise cholesterol levels and lead to weight gain, anemia, fatigue, memory loss, depression, and other serious complications. Fortunately, hypothyroidism is easy to control with a synthetic form of the thyroid hormone thyroxine.

Itchiness that has no obvious cause can be a sign of kidney or liver disorders, leukemia, diabetes, or an allergy to one or more of your medications. The appearance of scaly spots or raised, coarse-textured growths may be signs of skin cancer (pp.371–372). Monitor your skin carefully and report unusual changes promptly to your doctor.

I've noticed that my sleep patterns have been changing lately. Is this abnormal?

It is not at all unusual. Although some people in their later years feel they need to sleep more or fewer hours than they once did, most older people get the same amount of sleep as ever but on a changed schedule (pp.374–375). They are apt to be more wakeful at night and make up the missed sleep with daytime naps.

Falling asleep can be easier than ever as you age; it is sustaining sleep that gets difficult. If you go to sleep at 9:30 or 10 P.M., you may nod right off, but then wake up at 3 or 4 A.M. You toss and turn until the sun comes up and then get out of bed feeling tired. Sleep researchers suspect that people with this pattern may actually have been well rested by 4 A.M. and that it's the extra hours spent tossing in bed that makes them groggy. One solution is to alter the body's circadian rhythms (the internal clock that tells each of us when to rest and when to wake) by taking a short nap midway through the evening, then staying up until 1 A.M. That way, you get the amount of sleep you need while waking up at a more conventional time. For more home remedies for insomnia, see *Falling Asleep,* p.208.

Are sleeping pills advisable at my age?

Try to do without them, if possible. Elderly people represent only 12 percent of the U.S. population, but between 35 and 40

Bathing. To bathe a bedridden patient, you will need two large towels (one to keep the bed dry, the other to cover the patient); a wash basin; two sets of wash cloths and towels (one to clean the genital area, the other for the rest of the body; don't forget to change the water after washing the genital area). Use mild soap and warm water for washing, and pat the skin dry (don't rub the skin). Start at the head and work down, uncovering only the part of the body that you are working on. Shampoo the patient's hair with a dry shampoo, or use an inflatable basin designed for washing hair in bed. Basins like the one featured here are available from specialty suppliers (see Appendix).

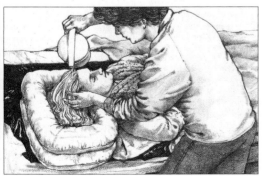

Changing the bed. Two people can change a bed with the patient still in it. Make sure the room is warm; keep the patient covered throughout. Remove the spread, all but one blanket, top sheet, and pillows. Roll the patient to one side of the bed. While your helper supports the patient as shown, untuck and roll the used bottom sheet toward the middle of the bed, then tuck in a clean bottom sheet and unfold it toward the middle of the bed. Roll the patient over the ridge of sheets to the other side of the bed. With the helper still supporting the patient, remove the used sheet; unroll and tuck in the other half of the clean bottom sheet. Change pillowcases and top sheet; replace blankets and spread.

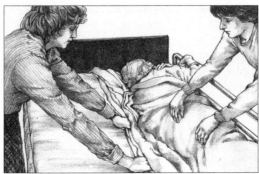

BEATING THE WEATHER

As you grow older, your body becomes less adept at adjusting to temperature changes. In the elderly, continued exposure to cool temperatures—even as mild as 60°F—can trigger hypothermia, a dangerous lowering of body temperature that requires emergency room treatment. At the other extreme, heat exhaustion or heatstroke can also be life-threatening. Never ignore symptoms like fatigue, faintness, dizziness, or nausea during a spell of hot weather.

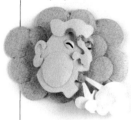

Commonsense cold weather precautions:

☐ Dress warmly before going outdoors, and always wear a hat (your body loses 20 percent of its heat through your head).

☐ Wrap up especially well against brisk winds, which increase the chill on cold days.

☐ Beware of getting caught in a storm. If a sudden downpour leaves you with damp clothing and wet feet, warm yourself and put on dry clothes immediately.

☐ When it's very cold outside, stay home or, at the very least, don't travel alone.

☐ At home, keep the thermostat set at a minimum of 65°F—higher when you're sick—and dress warmly.

☐ Since body temperature drops while you sleep, use plenty of covers in bed. A down quilt is a good investment, and so is a woolen nightcap if your bedroom is chilly at night.

☐ If you take tranquilizers or antidepressants, dress more warmly. These and some other medications lower your perception of how cold you are. Check with your doctor about any drugs that you are taking.

☐ Keep up your physical activity and eat regular, nutritious meals during the day.

☐ Drink warm fluids—tea, cocoa, or soup— between meals but avoid alcohol, which keeps your body from retaining heat.

Commonsense hot weather precautions:

☐ Take it easy when the temperature goes into the nineties, and don't try to accomplish too much or to do even routine tasks as quickly as you would in milder weather.

☐ Wear loose-fitting clothes made of cool, porous fabrics, such as cotton or linen.

☐ Drink plenty of liquids—water or fruit juice—throughout the day.

☐ Stay out of the sun, especially around midday when it is hottest.

☐ On especially hot, humid days, stay indoors and don't do heavy work. Cool off with lukewarm showers and baths or stay in an air-conditioned room.

---

percent of prescriptions for sedatives and hypnotic tranquilizers are written for people over 60. Sleeping pills are highly addictive and can interact dangerously with other medications (of course, you should never mix sleeping pills with alcohol). Also, since older people metabolize drugs more slowly (p.393), the drowsiness brought on by a sleeping pill often carries over into the following day, increasing the risk of falls and other accidents.

In many cases, sleeping pills mask rather than solve the real problems that lie behind sleepless nights. Many older people suffer from a variety of physical and psychosocial problems that affect their need and appetite for sleep. Anxiety and depression keep some people (young and old alike) awake at night (p.169). Alzheimer's and other neurological diseases interfere with sleep patterns; so do respiratory conditions, cardiovascular disease, and pain. If you have many sleepless nights, consult your doctor rather than automatically reaching for a sleeping pill.

Sometimes painful leg cramps wake me up in the middle of the night. What should I do when this happens?

Nocturnal leg cramps aren't dangerous, but they can disrupt sleep and be extremely painful. Researchers have ruled out bad circulation as the cause but have not yet determined what brings on these sharp, sudden cramps.

As a preventive measure try this gentle stretching exercise: Stand facing a wall from a distance of 2 or 3 feet and place your outstretched hands flat on the wall. Keeping your legs straight and your heels on the floor, lean slowly forward until you feel a pulling sensation in your calves. Your calves should feel stretched but not painful. Hold the stretch for 10 seconds, straighten up and relax for 5 seconds, then stretch again. Repeat three times daily. If you get a cramp in bed, try sharply flexing your foot and ankle toward your knee, in opposition to the cramp. Some people find relief by taking an over-the-counter quinine preparation (ask your pharmacist) or by drinking tonic water.

If you are awakened at night by twitching leg movements, you may have a condition unrelated to cramps known as "restless legs." People with this problem, which can occur day or night, say their legs feel on pins and needles or as if a current were passing through them. Muscle-relaxing drugs, including oxycodone and carbamazepine, may be prescribed to ease the jerky movements of restless legs.

My husband used to enjoy his after-dinner walks, but now after a few minutes he says his legs are hurting him. What could be wrong?

The problem could be intermittent claudication, the medical term for cramplike pains that occur in one or both legs after exercise. (The word *claudication* comes from the Latin *claudicare*, "to limp.") Usually caused by a restriction in the blood supply to the calves, the condition is a common consequence of atherosclerosis (see *The Facts About Atherosclerosis*, p.329) or diabetes (pp.342–345); risk factors include smoking, a sedentary lifestyle, and a high-fat diet. Because

intermittent claudication can be a sign of a serious underlying problem, your husband should see his doctor. People with intermittent claudication are advised to stop smoking, cut down on fatty foods, lose weight, and build up their exercise routines gradually. Your husband's doctor may also prescribe drugs to improve circulation to his legs.

My grandmother's walk has become increasingly stiff and shuffling. Is this just a sign that she is getting older or a symptom of disease?

It could be either. A stiff gait can be a sign of Parkinson's disease, although a slight hand or arm tremor is a more usual early symptom (see *The Facts About Parkinson's Disease*, p.354). Arthritis, Huntington's chorea, Lou Gehrig's disease, a tumor in the brain, and multiple sclerosis can all produce a shuffling gait. So can certain medications prescribed to control agitation and other nervous conditions. If your grandmother feels a numbness or weakness in one leg, she may have had a transient ischemic attack (for the causes and treatment of TIA's, see page 403).

If your grandmother's physician rules out disease as a cause, her stiff and shuffling gait is probably the result of a sedentary lifestyle. Her muscles may be weakening and her joints stiffening because she does not use them enough. Ask her if her feet give her any trouble. Suggest that she try a daily walk (in well-fitting shoes) and some gentle exercise (see *Firming and Toning Exercises*, pp.88–89). Or ask a physical therapist to design an exercise program that your grandmother can easily incorporate into her daily routine.

What is the difference between "normal" memory loss and dementia?

The memory lapses that begin to plague people in their middle years (see *Improving Your Memory*, p.374) don't become any less annoying or less frequent as you get older. Especially when under pressure, an older person is indeed likely to have some memory problems, but given an opportunity to relax, the mind will usually come up with the missing information. Fatigue, grief, sensory loss, lack of concentration, or attempting to remember too much can all cause the temporary memory lapses that doctors refer to as age-associated memory impairment. Luckily, the techniques for sharpening memory described on page 374 work at any age.

Far from being a normal part of the aging process, memory loss that is severe, progressive, and disabling is one of the symptoms of dementia, a generalized decline in all areas of mental function usually due to brain disease. Other common symptoms of dementia include poor judgment, confusion, anxiety, delusions, paranoia, depression, and other personality or behavioral changes. Memory loss that begins to interfere with normal activities should be evaluated by a doctor and never dismissed as an inevitable part of growing old.

Is dementia reversible? What diseases other than Alzheimer's can cause dementia?

Unfortunately, most cases of dementia are irreversible. Alzheimer's disease is the most common cause of irreversible dementia, accounting for about 70 percent of cases. Multi-infarct

THE FACTS ABOUT ALZHEIMER'S DISEASE

What it it? Alzheimer's disease is a progressive degeneration of nerve cells in the brain that results in dementia (impaired memory, thinking, judgment, and behavior). The disease causes the brains of its victims to atrophy and to develop abnormalities, such as tangles of fibers and clusters of degenerating nerve endings, in areas that play an important role in memory and other intellectual functions. Unfortunately, these abnormalities become evident only in autopsy.

Named for Alois Alzheimer, the German physician who first described it in 1907, Alzheimer's disease affects some 4 million people in the United States and is the leading cause of dementia in people over age 65.

What causes it? No one really knows. Theories suggest genetic predisposition, viruses, toxic elements in the environment (particularly aluminum), deterioration of the body's immune system, or a combination of these factors.

What are the symptoms? Early symptoms may be barely perceptible, but gradually the patient shows increasing signs of dementia. Although Alzheimer's manifests itself differently in different people, there are three main phases. In the first, patients may be aware of their own memory and concentration problems. Normal tasks such as driving, reading, balancing a checkbook, or socializing become harder. In the second phase, memory loss becomes more severe, and patients have more trouble with speech and orientation. Anxiety and paranoia increase; erratic mood and personality changes occur. In the third phase, patients become so confused and agitated that they can no longer care for themselves in even the most basic way. The disease may take years to run its course, but once the patient becomes incapacitated and bedridden, life expectancy is not long.

How is it diagnosed? Short of an autopsy after death, there is no single definitive diagnostic test for Alzheimer's disease. When symptoms are noticed, the patient should undergo complete physical, psychiatric, and neurological examinations by physicians experienced in the diagnosis of dementing disorders. (A family physician can refer the patient to suitable specialists.)

To determine whether a patient is suffering from dementia and whether the condition is due to a treatable illness rather than to Alzheimer's, the exams should include a medical history, psychiatric and neurological tests, blood and urine analyses, chest X-ray, electroencephalogram, CT scans, and electrocardiogram (see *Diagnostic Tests,* pp.126–127).

Identification of distinctive Alzheimer's disease proteins in a patient's spinal fluid and a new computer-enhanced X-ray technique may soon allow doctors to make more accurate diagnoses of Alzheimer's.

How is it treated? There is still no cure. Symptoms of the disease, such as anxiety, depression, psychotic thinking, sleeplessness, and behavioral disturbances, may be treated with drugs, but medications to slow or reverse the progression of Alzheimer's remain experimental and controversial.

Even if there is no cure, it's very important for an Alzheimer's patient to be under the care of an experienced physician. Other key elements in the management of Alzheimer's include proper nutrition, guided exercise and physical therapy, and the maintenance of a daily routine and social contacts. There is much that family and friends can do to help an Alzheimer's patient (see facing page).

The vast majority of Alzheimer's patients are cared for at home by members of their families. The Alzheimer's Association (see Appendix), a national voluntary organization, provides information for care givers and sponsors support groups for families of people with the disease. Many communities have day-care programs for Alzheimer's patients, and some have respite services to give relief to care-giving families. For patients in the later stages of Alzheimer's disease, care in an institution may be advisable (more than 50 percent of all nursing home patients have Alzheimer's or a related disorder).

dementia, which is the result of a series of small strokes, accounts for another 10 percent of cases. The remaining irreversible dementias are caused by a combination of Alzheimer's and cerebrovascular disease or by such conditions as advanced Parkinson's disease, AIDS, and other viral and genetic disorders.

While Alzheimer's disease usually causes a slow, steady decline in mental ability, multi-infarct dementia starts rapidly and then follows an uneven course. Severe bouts of confusion may be separated by periods of normal reasoning. Multi-infarct dementia occurs most often in men and is often associated with diabetes and hypertension. Sometimes, treating these conditions can slow or even arrest the progression of multi-infarct dementia.

Reversible dementia may be due to physical or psychological factors. The former include diabetes, hypothyroidism, cerebral infection and certain brain tumors, nutritional deficiencies, and drug reactions. Among the psychological causes are stress, alcoholism or other substance abuse, depression, and psychosis. In these cases, dementia is a secondary symptom; treatment of the underlying condition may reverse the dementia.

How can family and friends cope with someone who suffers from dementia? Does the type of dementia make a difference?

Although the prognosis for reversible dementia patients is more optimistic than for those with Alzheimer's or multi-infarct dementia, the care for anyone suffering from dementia is similar. Your aim is to keep the patient safe and comfortable and to lessen, in any way you can, the fear and confusion that the disease produces. Remember, the progress of Alzheimer's disease is usually slow. The victim in the early stages realizes something is wrong and can become extremely frustrated by what the disease is doing.

Stress—from changes in routine or from a physical illness such as an infection or fever—can bring on more severe manifestations of dementia. Removing the stress—returning the patient to familiar surroundings or lowering the fever—can restore a more normal state.

There are several kinds of help a friend can offer. First, try to think of interesting ways for the patient to pass an afternoon. Arrange for old friends to visit, for example. Or encourage the patient to pursue old interests (was she a gardener? did he like going to baseball games?) or help to develop new ones like taking a daily walk or learning to dance.

Second, try to provide cues for orienting the patient. People with dementia are easily upset when they don't know what time it is or where they are, especially if they wake up during the night. A clock with a bright digital readout of the hour and a nightlight, for example, take care of that particular problem. Use your ingenuity to solve others.

Third, remind the patient about upcoming events just before they happen and keep providing cues during the event. People suffering from dementia can become confused when confronted by a visiting friend or relative whose name they can't remember. Tactful reintroductions help ease the situation.

Finally, be sure the patient's vision and hearing are regularly checked. Poor eyesight or hearing robs the patient of sensory information, which simply adds to the confusion of daily life.

My mother is neglecting her hygiene. How do I deal with this?

It isn't easy. Your mother may or may not realize how her hygiene has deteriorated. She may welcome your help or she may become defensive. Either way, talk to her in a straightforward manner. Avoid platitudes. Don't compare her to others who are managing better than she is. Assure her that you're there to help.

Try to determine what's causing your mother to neglect herself. Has some event altered her life? Is she in mourning? Is she no longer able to participate in her favorite activities? Has her living situation changed recently? The response to such unwanted life changes is often depression, which can make people apathetic and bored by rituals—such as personal hygiene habits—that once pleased them. If you think your mother is depressed, encourage her to see her doctor or a counselor. (For more on the signs and treatment of depression, see pages 169–172.)

If your mother's hygiene continues to deteriorate, don't put off a visit to the doctor. Since her problems may be due to changes in mental functioning brought about by an underlying disease, it's essential that the condition be properly diagnosed.

If your mother's hygiene is poor because she is too weak to take proper care of herself, try to arrange assistance for her. If she has dementia, however, she may not remember how to bathe or take a shower. You can help by running the bath, arranging the towels, slippers, and robe for her, helping her in and out of the tub if necessary, and making sure soap and sponge are easily accessible. Similarly, limit clothes selection to choices that won't overwhelm your mother.

My grandmother often seems very down. Is depression common among older people?

Old age can be a time of great fulfillment and satisfaction, and statistically, depression is less common in the later years than in middle age. However, the elderly do face special hardships that can result in depression. The deaths of spouses, other relatives, and friends come more often now. Retirement brings freedom but often a lot of empty time. When health problems make it difficult to get out and do things, the days can pass slowly— and sometimes painfully. Loss of control over one's affairs and over one's body is not easy to take. In this society, which places such value on youth and vitality, the elderly can be made to feel useless and forgotten.

Unlike younger people who suffer from depression, older depressed patients do not always report feeling "down." They are more likely to make repeated trips to their doctor to report various physical problems. They may suffer from delusions not only about their health (that they have cancer or some other life-threatening disease) but about money too (that they are impoverished). An older depressed person may also lose interest in food and grooming, have difficulty concentrating, feel less energetic, develop sleep disturbances, and refuse contact with the outside world by not answering the door or telephone.

The good news is that the elderly are remarkably resilient and that depression is a highly treatable illness (pp. 169–172). Try to convince your grandmother to see her doctor for an evaluation and treatment, if necessary. Since depression can have many physical causes and

COPING WITH THE LOSS OF A SPOUSE

Every year close to a million American husbands and wives are widowed (a woman is more than twice as likely as a man to lose a spouse). When you lose a spouse, you lose not only the person closest to you—with whom you have shared your thoughts and everyday rituals—but a central part of your identity as one half of a couple. It's no wonder, then, that it takes most widows and widowers a long time to recuperate, and that bereaved spouses face a higher risk of dying than husbands and wives who still have each other.

The recovery process. The first step toward recovery is to allow yourself to grieve (p. 174). Express your feelings openly among loving family and friends. Talk to your clergyman or rabbi. Some widows and widowers go through a period of "enshrining" the lost spouse, maintaining the house exactly as it was, speaking only in reverential terms of the dead person, and surrounding themselves with memorial photographs. This isn't healthy. You need to refocus your attention on yourself and on remaking your life. As soon as you can after your spouse's death, ask a friend to help you go through your husband's—or wife's—belongings. Save a few mementos, give away useful clothing and equipment, and dispose of the rest.

Returning to a full life. It's a good sign when you can acknowledge that you are lonely; it means that you are facing up to your feelings and soon will be ready to overcome your pain. Everyone needs companionship. Reestablishing a social life is a positive first step. Going out will not only help take your mind off your sadness but will get you reinvolved in the world around you. At first, you may feel guilty or disloyal even thinking about rebuilding a full life, but seeing people and doing things will soon become natural again.

Specific techniques for gradually working yourself out of bereavement will also keep you too busy to brood. Avoid oversleeping. Don't automatically turn on the television. Take care of your health: eat well, exercise regularly, and don't use alcohol to ease your pain. Start again the familiar activities that you enjoy. Play golf. Go out shopping and to lunch with a good friend. Invite adult children to supper or take a grandchild to an art exhibit or a baseball game. After a while, you will be ready to expand your horizons. Join a swim club or a hiking group. Volunteer at a homeless shelter or become active in a local environmental organization. Visit a friend who lives in another part of the country. Plan an ambitious vacation, an adventurous trip you've secretly always wanted to take. A good travel agent can suggest all kinds of exciting and unusual trips. Eventually, as you heal, you may find that a few hours of solitude will no longer make you feel lonely. In fact, you may learn to cherish time to yourself—to read, listen to music, or work on hobbies.

consequences and in the elderly may mimic dementia (p.409), it's especially important that your grandmother's condition be properly diagnosed.

In addition to suggesting a trip to the doctor, what else can I do to help my depressed grandmother?

You can do a lot to brighten her life just by visiting often. Make plans to take her out shopping, to exhibits or concerts. If she likes to play cards or go to the movies, help her organize a group of like-minded friends for regular card games or afternoon trips to the theater.

But don't help out too much. Researchers have found that one reason some elderly people seem to slip into depression is because the people who care for them don't allow them enough independence. Many studies have shown that elderly people are more likely to flourish when they are able to take control of their lives (p.156). Encourage your grandmother to figure out what she really wants to do and to fulfill her dreams as creatively as possible. If she does, she will enjoy greater self-esteem and go a long way toward recovering from her depression.

I've always enjoyed a cocktail before dinner and a glass of wine with my meal. Is there any reason to give up drinking now?

Moderate drinking is usually harmless, relaxing, and may even be beneficial to your health. Some studies show that light drinkers live longer than either heavy drinkers or teetotalers. So there is no reason to give up alcohol completely unless you

are very overweight; have a medical problem such as diabetes, ulcers, or high blood pressure; or have a family history of alcoholism that makes drinking inadvisable. If you do drink, however, there are certain age-related health considerations you should be aware of.

☐ As people grow older, their tolerance for alcohol decreases. Age-related metabolic and physical changes cause older people to become intoxicated faster and stay drunk longer than they did when they were younger.

☐ The way liquor makes a person feel may also change with age. Some older people become irritable or hostile rather than euphoric after a drink or two.

☐ Drinking affects physical coordination and reaction times more quickly in the later years. Falls, automobile accidents, and other injuries are some of the undesirable consequences.

☐ Drinking heavily with a meal increases the chances that you will choke on your food, especially if you wear dentures.

☐ If an older person suffers from any memory impairment, alcohol may worsen the condition.

☐ Excessive drinking has a negative impact on nutrition at any age, but substituting the empty calories of alcohol for needed nutrients is especially dangerous for the elderly.

☐ Older people, who constitute less than 13 percent of the population, take more than 30 percent of all prescription medicines, a large portion of which are sleeping pills and tranquilizers. Mixing these drugs with alcohol can be lethal. Always ask your doctor about the effect of alcohol on any medication you are taking, and never assume that it's safe to take an over-the-counter medicine with a drink; you could have a serious adverse reaction, for example, to an antihistamine or to aspirin.

My mother is 68, and for the first time in her life she has taken to drinking heavily. Can one become an alcoholic in later life?

Older people become alcoholics at about the same rate as middle-aged and younger people do. It has been estimated that up to 10 percent of our over-60 population—about 4 million Americans—are problem drinkers. Of the people 65 and over enrolled in the Mayo Clinic's alcoholism treatment program in Rochester, Minnesota, more than 40 percent said they had developed symptoms after age 60.

Older people who drink excessively are often responding to the stresses of aging—loneliness, bereavement, physical pain, boredom after retirement. And unfortunately, alcoholism in the elderly often goes untreated because the signs of problem drinking, such as memory loss, repeated falls, and loss of appetite, are mistakenly regarded as the frailties of old age. In addition, inappropriate social stigmas against alcoholics, especially women alcoholics, sometimes prevent family members from acknowledging the problem and prevent the woman who drinks from seeking help.

You are to be commended for squarely facing up to your mother's drinking problem. Al-Anon support groups exist to advise relatives of alcoholics, and it may be that you and other family members or trusted friends can convince your mother to seek help (see *The Facts About 12-Step Programs*, p.164). Another national self-help group, Women for Sobriety, specializes in the problems of women alcoholics; and Golden Years support groups now operate in some communities (see Appendix).

LIVING ALTERNATIVES FOR THE LATER YEARS

The majority of elderly people want to live out their lives in the their own homes. Many retirees, however, either can't afford the cost or don't want the responsibility of maintaining the house in which they raised their children or spent their working years. Affluent older people have many choices, but even for retirees on tight budgets, creative housing alternatives are being pioneered. Here's a sampling of today's retirement housing options.

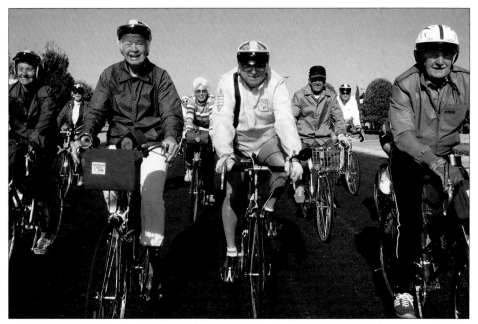

Retirement community. The bike club of Sun City West, Arizona, typifies the energetic lifestyle encouraged at Sun City complexes and other active retirement communities. Begun in 1960, the original Sun City, also in Arizona, was the first community designed exclusively for the elderly in the United States. With their busy sports facilities and recreation centers, Sun City and its offshoots represent the high end of the retirement community spectrum. More affordable options, ranging from high-rise apartments to modest houses clustered around a community center, have been built by commercial developers as well as by nonprofit groups, such as unions, educational institutions, and religious organizations. Some retirement communities, like the Sun Cities, offer medical and nursing care; others do not.

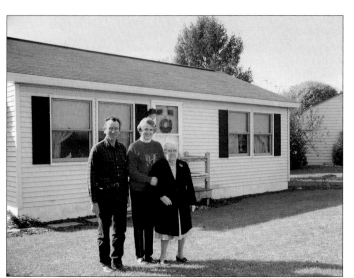

Elder cottage housing opportunity (ECHO). An independent house on her daughter and son-in-law's property allows a 93-year-old widow to live independently but safely. Living among her own things and keeping her own schedule, she can quickly summon her family if she needs help (her daughter's house is visible at the right of the photograph). The prefabricated ECHO house can be taken down when no longer needed.

Based on an Australian concept, ECHO housing allows the generations to mix easily without infringing on each other's privacy. If an elderly parent becomes ill, children—and grandchildren—are close at hand to provide nursing help and meals.

In some parts of the United States, families wanting to build an ECHO house may run afoul of local zoning regulations. Several states, however, have passed laws to allow ECHO houses and in-law apartments.

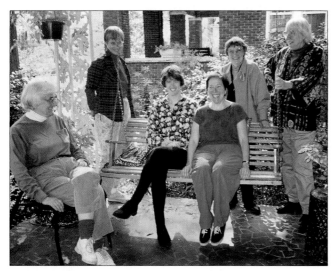

Cooperative living. Long interested in cooperative living, Elizabeth Freeman (seated at far left) purchased a small apartment house in Durham, North Carolina, and turned it into the Molly Hare Cooperative, now home to six women, most of them over age 50. Each member bought in at a modest price and pays a monthly fee based on the size of her apartment. The residents of the Molly Hare Cooperative consider themselves friends and neighbors, sharing chores and, if they choose, meals and other social activities, as well as a safe, convenient, and affordable living space.

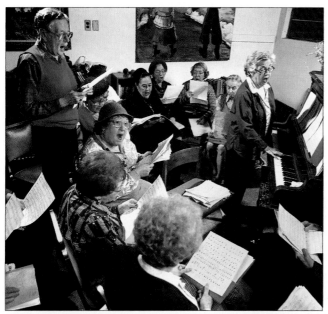

Naturally occurring retirement community (NORC). This term refers to apartment buildings and other housing complexes not originally intended for the elderly, but which evolve into retirement communities as their residents grow older. At Penn South, 10 high-rise co-op apartment buildings in New York City built by the state housing division and the International Ladies Garment Workers Union, more than two-thirds of the residents are 65 or older. A consortium of nonprofit agencies provides social and health services. (Not all NORC's offer such services.) Penn South residents also voluntarily take care of each other when necessary and join in recreational and educational activities, such as the choir rehearsal shown above.

CHOOSING A NURSING HOME

When the time comes to find a nursing home for a loved one, ask your doctor, friends, and local social service agency for recommendations (see Appendix for other sources of information). Try to involve the future resident in the search.

Whether it is run by a proprietor, a nonprofit organization, or the government, a good facility offers professional care in a clean, safe, attractive environment that encourages visits from friends and relatives. The business office should be knowledgeable and helpful about exploring a resident's financial entitlements.

Theoretically, homes that qualify for Medicare or Medicaid payments must comply with federal law on the rights of nursing home residents, but abuses do occur. When visiting a nursing home, look for the home's and the director's state licenses (both should be current and on display); ask to see an up-to-date inspection report and Medicare certification.

The best way to evaluate a home is to visit it often and at different times of day. Speak with residents. Visit residents' rooms, common lounges, the dining room at mealtimes, and outdoor recreation areas. Observe the staff. Are they pleasant with residents and attentive to their needs?

Use this checklist to evaluate homes you are considering.
☐ Is the nursing home located where friends and relatives can visit easily?
☐ Is a doctor on call 24 hours a day? Is there an affiliation with a good, accredited hospital?
☐ Are there planned activities?
☐ Do residents receive transportation to outside activities?
☐ Is a resident's privacy respected by doctors, nurses, and aides?
☐ Is the food nutritious and tasty, and are meals pleasant?
☐ Does the staff help to create a homey environment?

My father is becoming increasingly suspicious in his old age. Is paranoia common among the elderly? Is there anything I can do about it?

While elderly people are often accused of being paranoid, they are no more likely to have paranoid delusions than anyone else. Paranoia, a mental disorder in which people believe they are being conspired against, persecuted, spied upon, or otherwise badly treated, most commonly strikes people between the ages of 35 and 45.

In some communities, older people grow more suspicious for the perfectly valid reason that they have heard of cases of people robbing or cheating the elderly. Other people have a hard time giving up control when younger family members take over their household and financial responsibilities. Has your father recently given up driving or moved in with one of his children? Such changes could leave him feeling angry and helpless.

Sometimes it is easier for someone with memory lapses or visual problems to conclude that a possession has been removed rather than acknowledge that he can't find it. And someone who doesn't hear well may hear his name spoken and think that people are discussing him behind his back. If your father is hard of hearing, help him to find a good hearing aid (p.401). If his

RECORDING YOUR PERSONAL HISTORY

Everyone has stories to tell. Whether they are formal memoirs or funny anecdotes swapped around the dinner table, these personal narratives link the past to the present and hand down family traditions—and perhaps a few myths—to the next generation.

The value of reviewing your life. In the past, some psychologists took a negative view of reminiscing, seeing it as an unhealthy escape from the present. That attitude is changing. Recent studies suggest that reminiscing helps older people to maintain self-esteem and a sense of identity. What you gain by reminiscing and writing a personal history is a sense of perspective on your life. Remembering and re-creating its main events help to put your story into a meaningful framework.

To write or to tape. Stories that are told and retold invariably get distorted. Writing down—or taping—your personal history freezes those important moments in time and keeps them fresh and clear for each new family member. Most personal histories are written, but tape recordings are increasingly common. Writing gives you a chance to edit and polish your storytelling as you go, but talking into a tape recorder adds the personal flavor of your voice, your accent, and your inflections. If you are a gifted storyteller, you may be depriving the family if you don't use a tape recorder.

Make it a family project. If compiling your personal history alone seems overwhelming, involve relatives. The process can draw generations in a family closer together. Because the young are often eager to know where they came from, a grandchild, niece, or nephew may be the perfect collaborator. Collect your source material by letting all of your family and family friends know that you are looking for memorabilia. Old diaries are best, but letters, photographs, scrapbooks, school yearbooks, and official records such as school report cards and marriage licenses can fill in important pieces.

Outside help. The American Association of Retired Persons (see Appendix) offers instructional materials to help people reminisce in a constructive way. While working on a personal history, many people feel a greater sense of perspective if they can relate their lives to a family tree. For assistance with genealogical research, you can contact the National Archives in Washington, D.C., or visit your library. Many how-to books on tracing families are available.

I'll always remember the time we first arrived in this country. It was in the Fall and never seen such colors!

eyesight is failing, make sure his glasses correct his vision as well as possible. If he spends too much of his time alone, your father may feel uncomfortable in the company of other people. What may seem like a suspicious attitude to you may just be loneliness and social awkwardness, and anything you can do to lessen his isolation will help him.

My grandfather is always talking about the "good old days." Is all this reminiscing healthy?

Reminiscence is a healthy source of pleasure for older people. After all, when you've lived a long and eventful life, it's fun to savor the extraordinary (and ordinary) moments. Just as it is natural for you to make plans for the future and visualize your horizons expanding, it is natural for your grandfather to look back and enjoy his fondest memories. Remembering triumphs, tragedies, and lessons learned may help him to cope with the difficulties of his later years and to put things into perspective.

Most older people wish to have their experiences admired and appreciated. Younger family members can help elders nurture and share precious memories by asking questions and listening attentively. That is how families pass down wisdom and traditions from generation to generation.

If you are concerned that your grandfather is too preoccupied with the past, help fill up the present. Give him a diary in which he can record his current thoughts and feelings. Keep him apprised of family news and spend time with him at family gatherings. If your grandfather is telling the same stories over and over again, divert him by expressing interest in another aspect of

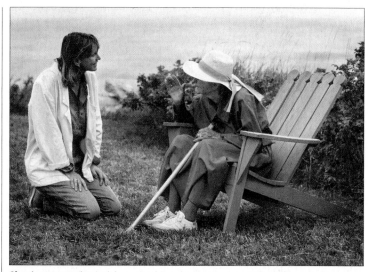

Sharing memories with her granddaughter animates a lively nonagenarian.

his life. Be patient; rather than becoming annoyed with him, try to learn from his experiences.

I've been dating a widow my own age and we're considering moving in together, but my children are giving me a hard time about it. How can I tell them that my personal life is not their affair?

In the interests of mutual understanding, consider some of the reasons that children might behave in the way you describe. If your friend is from a different background or poorer or less educated than you, your heirs may be worried that she is after your money. If she has a health problem, the family may think that you will get stuck nursing her through a serious illness. Are your friend's interests very different from yours or your children's? Your children may focus on such differences because they fear that her influence on you is eclipsing theirs. And whether it's rational or not, many children feel that a father is being disloyal to their mother by even considering living with another woman.

Occasionally, family members see signs of real trouble ahead that a person in love doesn't see.

While your children are offering unsolicited advice to you, you can probably remember times not long ago when they scorned your advice. Remind them that, like them, you are capable of making your own decisions and that you should not be expected to settle for a life of loneliness. Family criticism usually simmers down once a decision has been made. If you actually do move in with the widow, your children should begin to accept that reality. If you marry her, they are even more likely to welcome her into the family, if your unconventional living arrangements were bothering them. Meanwhile, don't be apologetic but keep the lines of communication open.

I've just had an offer of marriage, but at 70, I think I'm just too old for it. My friends say this is nonsense. Who's right?

Too old for what? Do worries about being sexually active at your age hold you back? Our society's Victorian attitudes toward sex among the elderly can make older people feel shy about expressing their desires. This is unfortunate, because being touched, cuddled, and caressed is a basic human need that remains consistent from infancy onward and does not diminish as one grows older.

The social considerations involved in any new marriage can be intimidating. You may be leaving your home and old friends and establishing a new social network. When two people who have accumulated investments and property over the years wed, the financial and legal ramifications can be complex. If one or both of you have grown children, you will have to decide what you now wish to leave them and what you will want your new spouse to inherit when you die; you'll also want to update your will (p.381) and the list of beneficiaries on your insurance policy.

Do you feel too old to cope with all these changes? Take things slowly and make decisions one at a time. You and your partner should frankly disclose your financial situations. Where you will live should be deter-

mined jointly. If each of you owns a home, consider the tax advantages of selling one or both of them while you're still single; federal tax laws allow an important exemption for homeowners over 55, but if one of you takes the exemption while single, neither of you is entitled to another exemption after you are married.

It is natural for you to value your friends' opinions, but what really matters is what *you* think and feel about an impending marriage and, most importantly, the person you will be sharing your life with. You and your partner are the only ones qualified to judge the wisdom of committing yourselves to this relationship.

I'm going out with a man whom I find very compatible, but he seems reticent about starting a physical relationship. What can I do to move things along?

It may be that your friend has accepted social taboos against sex in the later years and believes he should do without it. Or his religious upbringing may have taught

him that lovemaking outside the bonds of matrimony is wrong.

Some older men, perhaps experiencing episodes of impotence for the first time, think that they are losing their sexual powers and stop having sex to avoid embarrassment and disappointment (p.238). Other men become preoccupied with their health and begin to fear, mistakenly, that sex could trigger a stroke or a heart attack (p.333). Medical problems—disease, disability, the side effects of a drug, or alcohol—can also suppress sexual response.

However, unless illness or the death of a partner intervenes, there is no reason that sexuality and its expression cannot last as long as you live. Although a man's sexual response very gradually slows down during the later years and he may need more time to achieve an erection, positions for intercourse can be chosen to facilitate sex for older couples. If the woman is on top or the partners lie side by side, both partners are apt to be more comfortable.

Respect your friend's reticence; some people are naturally reserved and approach sex tentatively. His slow pace may mean that he is serious about you and doesn't want to let any impulsive action threaten his chances for a long-term relationship. Without rushing or pressuring him, you can undoubtedly think of subtle ways to let him know you think he is attractive.

I'm 75, love my job, and see no reason to quit. My family, however, is pestering me to do so. Should I listen to them?

The average age at retirement in the United States has been dropping for decades, but as people live longer (and remain healthy

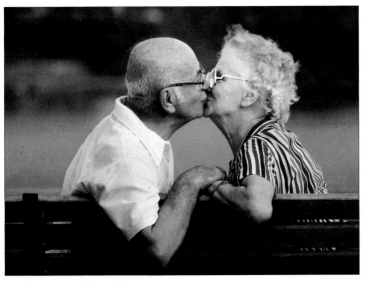

Kisses and other expressions of affection are healthy—and fun—at any age.

MEDICAL MONEY MATTERS

The rising cost of health care in the United States poses a financial threat to many people living on retirement incomes. Since Medicare does not pay all the costs of a major illness, supplemental health insurance policies have been developed to help cover the Medicare gap (see *The Facts About Medicare*, p.149). Here are basic facts about supplemental health insurance, as well as ways to control the mounting costs of medications.

Medigap insurance. Designed to pay for certain medical expenses not covered by Medicare, medigap policies have been a source of confusion and, in some cases, fraud. A federal law standardizing medigap insurance went into effect in 1992. The hundreds of medigap policies once available have been reduced to 10. The core medigap policy must cover:

☐ The patient's copayments (see *The Language of Medical Insurance,* p.148) for days 61 through 150 of a hospital stay and all costs from day 151 on, for a total of 365 free hospital days over a lifetime.

☐ The patient's 20 percent copayment for Medicare-approved doctors' fees.

☐ Blood costs not covered by Medicare.

The nine other medigap policies, not all of which are available in every state, offer limited coverage for such services as medical emergency care abroad, preventive health care, home recovery care after an illness, and partial reimbursement for prescription drugs. The broader the coverage, the costlier the policy.

Long-term-care policies. After a hospitalization of at least 3 days, Medicare pays all covered services for the first 20 days in a skilled-care nursing facility and provides partial coverage for the next 80 days. But neither Medicare nor medigap policies pay for long-term custodial care at home or in a nursing home. Long-term-care policies partially fill this gap, paying a fixed amount per day for care in a nursing home or for custodial care at home. Contact the Health Insurance Association of America (see Appendix) for a list of companies that offer long-term-care policies.

Cutting medication costs. Although prescription drug prices skyrocketed in the 1980's, there are ways to pay less.

☐ Use fewer drugs; ask your doctor if there are alternative treatments for your condition, such as exercise, diet, or physical therapy.

☐ Ask your doctor whether a cheaper generic drug (p.152) or even an over-the-counter drug might work as well as your name-brand prescription drug.

☐ Comparison-shop among pharmacies.

☐ Buy your medications by mail through the pharmacy service sponsored by the American Association of Retired Persons (see Appendix) or other reputable mail-order organizations.

☐ Buy drugs you must take regularly in bulk; discounts are highest for larger quantities.

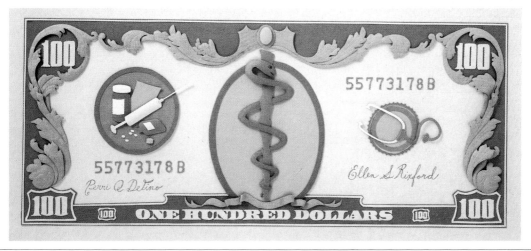

and energetic longer), more workers like yourself will want to remain at their jobs. Those people who were most ambitious and successful, and who enjoyed their work the most, are also most likely to be uncomfortable spending their mornings playing golf and their afternoons puttering around the house.

If you want to keep working at 75, the law is on your side. A federal bill passed in 1986 prohibits most employers from forcing people to retire at a specified age, and many states have similar laws against mandatory retirement. Starting in the year 2000, the legal retirement age at which you can collect full Social Security benefits will go up.

Retirement is a very personal decision. If you are happy at your job and have a rewarding life outside the office, and if your family does not complain that they don't spend enough time with you, there is no reason to retire. On the other hand, if you are spending all your time at the office and neglecting your family and other interests, perhaps you should begin thinking about the issue. Some companies are recognizing the need for diversity when it comes to retirement age. They help employees plan everything from investments to part-time jobs to prepare them for this major life transition; employees are learning that retirement can be rewarding and doesn't mean that they are finished and useless.

The idea of retiring frightens me. Working hard keeps me sharp. How can I keep busy without my job?

Retirement can be the time to fulfill long-held ambitions—seeing the world, learning to play the piano, or "giving back" to the community through volunteer work. As you suspect, elderly people don't keep their minds alert and their bodies in shape by watching the world go by from a rocking chair; they keep healthy by staying active and taking on new challenges for themselves or in their community.

Many organizations offer opportunities for service, travel, or study—often at discounted prices—to retirees. Some national groups are listed below (see Appendix for their addresses and phone numbers); check your phone book for the names and numbers of local organizations for retirees.

☐ The American Association of Retired Persons (AARP) provides many valuable services (including discounts on medications and travel) to members age 50 and older and acts as a clearinghouse for information on issues relevant to older citizens. AARP members, who pay a nominal yearly fee, receive a monthly newsletter and the bi-monthly magazine *Modern Maturity*.

☐ ACTION, the federal domestic volunteer agency (which includes Foster Grandparent Program, Retired Senior Volunteer Program, Senior Companion Program, and VISTA), helps match older volunteers with programs that will put their skills and experience to best use.

☐ Elderhostel offers a worldwide network of noncredit courses at reasonable fees on college and university campuses for students over the age of 60.

☐ Outward Bound programs designed specifically for older people challenge participants to sharpen their coping skills in wilderness and urban environments.

☐ SCORE (Service Corps of Retired Executives) matches senior volunteers who have business expertise with would-be or struggling entrepreneurs.

I've been thinking of going back to college and finally getting my degree, but at 68 aren't I too old?

Absolutely not. As long as you are in good health, there is no reason why you shouldn't return to school, enjoy the experience, and excel in your courses. Some older people find that it takes them longer to absorb new information than it did in college. They may also require a study environment that's relatively free of noise and other distractions. However, research studies have shown that normal decline in memory, reasoning, and I.Q.'s in healthy elderly people is so minor as to be inconsequential. In fact, studying may actually help improve mental agility. When research animals were forced to negotiate a maze in order to survive, they grew new connections between their brain cells. Animals deprived of mental exercise lost these connections.

Some researchers believe that sociability and flexibility are key factors in maintaining and improving mental skills in later life. Asked to evaluate senior citizens auditing classes at Wichita State University in Kansas, 75 percent of the teachers polled said that their older students were at least as quick as younger ones, and 64 percent said the older students seemed more motivated. Older students reported that while they felt they benefited most from their classes, what they most enjoyed was the contact with people on campus.

Colleges and universities across the country have special programs that address the needs of older students; some offer credit for life experiences. And many states have adopted laws waiving tuition for seniors at state-supported institutions.

I worry about how my affairs would be handled if I became incapacitated. Where can I go for advice?

Facing the difficult prospect that you may outlive your ability to make solid financial and health-care decisions is one of the smartest and bravest things you can do to protect your family and yourself. The most important thing to do is to write a will or to be sure that the one you have still reflects your wishes (p.381). Next, you can draw up a living will, specifying what artificial life supports you wish to be used under particular circumstances (p.367). You can also appoint someone to exercise medical power of attorney for you. This person will make decisions based on your health-care wishes if you become incapacitated.

Durable power of attorney gives someone you name decision-making power over your financial assets, including your property, bank accounts, and income, in case of your incompetence. If you worry that your relatives live too far away or are too closely involved to be impartial, designate a banker, lawyer, or friend whom you already know you can trust. While choosing someone to have power of attorney now may make you feel anxious, the alternative is to wait and let a court appoint someone (who

DYING WITH DIGNITY: HOSPICE CARE

The central fact of life is the inevitability of death, and a critical part of the aging process is coming to terms with this reality and preparing for it. Dying in a hospital, however, can be unnecessarily impersonal and unpleasant for both the dying and their families. Hospitals, after all, are designed to save lives, not necessarily to ease death. To some observers, using technology to prolong the lives of terminally ill patients robs the dying of their autonomy. The hospice movement (named for the lodgings used by travelers in the Middle Ages) offers a humane alternative.

The basic tenet of hospice care is that the dying should be able to make their own choices about how they want to spend their final days. Hospice care emphasizes nurturing, spiritual serenity, and preparation for dying. The goal is neither to hasten nor to delay death, but rather to allow an individual to die when the time comes with the support and comfort of family and friends and without the intervention of high-technology medicine.

The first modern hospice was founded in London in 1967 by Dr. Cicely Saunders. Listening to what terminally ill patients had to say about the kind of care they wanted, Dr. Saunders designed a program and a facility to meet their needs. Since then, the hospice movement has spread worldwide. In the United States alone, there are now more than 1,700 hospice programs (the first was started in 1974 by doctors, nurses, and clergy in New Haven, Connecticut).

The organization of hospice programs may vary, but most share these common features:
☐ The patient, in consultation with family and hospice staff, makes all care decisions.
☐ A team consisting of a doctor, nurses, social workers, trained volunteers, and a chaplain, along with family and friends, coordinates services for the patient and makes sure that help is available around the clock.
☐ Care is given in the patient's home or in a homelike environment in a hospital or nursing home where family and friends (and even cherished pets) are welcome.
☐ Pain management allows the patient to be as comfortable and as alert as possible.
☐ Care encompasses the physical, psychological, social, and spiritual needs of the terminally ill and their families. If the patient is at home, family members are taught nursing skills. If the family faces financial or emotional problems, the social worker will make appropriate referrals. Bereavement counseling continues for the family after the death.

Medicare, Medicaid, and many health insurers cover hospice programs that meet their guidelines. Hospice care tends to be less expensive than hospitalization, especially if the patient remains at home. For more information about hospice programs in your area, contact the National Hospice Organization (see Appendix).

may not have been your own choice) after you no longer have a voice in the decision.

Setting up a revocable living trust or transferring property to children while you're still healthy is another way to make sure your assets go where you intend them to go and to protect your estate from undue taxation. If your financial situation is complicated, it is a good idea to let your bank work with your lawyer or a financial planner to tailor trusts, savings, and investment plans for your specific needs.

I'm in good health and spirits now, but I want to make sure my affairs are in order when I die. What should I include in my plans?

Getting your affairs in order now is a great kindness to the people you love, because it relieves them of the burden of making decisions while they are in mourning. Find a suitable place—a fire-proof strongbox, for instance—to hold your important papers and let a family member or trusted friend know exactly where these records are. Among the essential papers you'll want to assemble are your will, insurance policies, deeds and mortgages, statements of all bank accounts, copies of income tax returns for the previous 3 years, veteran's discharge papers, birth and marriage certificates, and your living will and organ donor card (if you have them).

If the conduct of your funeral is important to you, leave written instructions about it. Many people today plan their own funeral services, specifying what they should contain and where they should be held. If you would like to be cremated, be sure to state this. If there is a special place where you wish to be buried, it's wise to buy a cemetery plot while you're still living, because later on the location you want may no longer be available. If funeral costs will be a concern, you can consult a memorial society; memorial societies are nonprofit organizations that can help you identify the most repu-table funeral directors and the most reasonably priced arrangements in your community (see Appendix). Taking care of these responsibilities can prevent disagreements or even friction among family members, who may have differing opinions about what you would have wished.

As part of your preparations, you may wish to review your life, either sharing your thoughts with those who are close to you or writing them down (see *Writing Your Personal History,* p.416). When possible, take steps to heal old wounds and to pay back any financial or emotional debts. The people best equipped to face death are those who view their lives as meaningful and who feel they have fulfilled their goals. The presence of loving relationships in your life and your religious faith or other philosophical beliefs will help you face the end of life calmly and courageously. And knowing that your loved ones will find your affairs in order will give you great peace of mind.

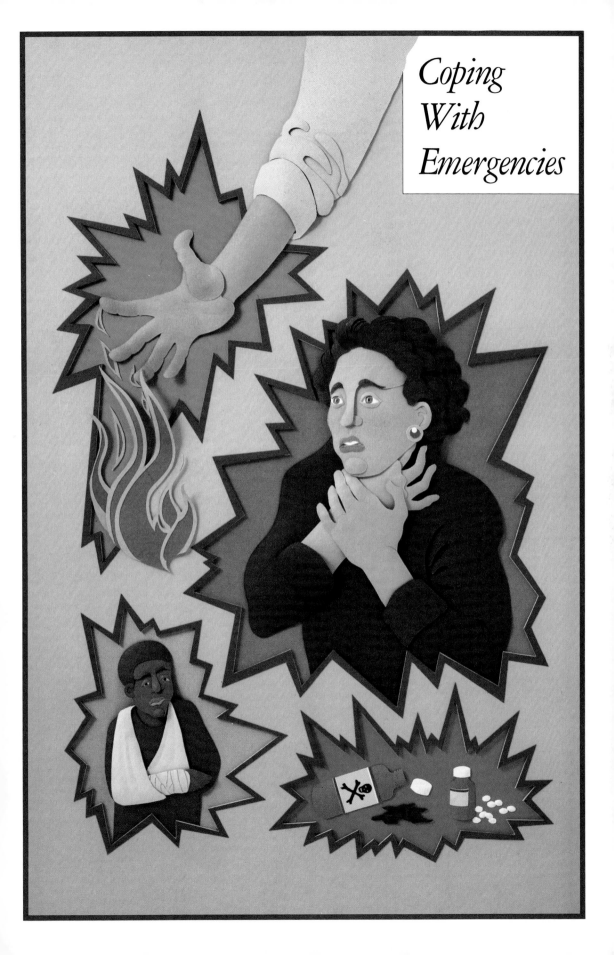

*Coping
With
Emergencies*

WHEN EMERGENCY STRIKES

F amiliarize yourself with this section and learn the basics of first aid before you have to face an emergency. Knowing what to do ahead of time wards off the sense of helplessness and panic that hinders your ability to cope. A victim may also respond positively to your confidence.

Preparations

☐ Take an artificial respiration and a cardiopulmonary resuscitation (CPR) course. These first-aid techniques can save lives. Ask the nearest American Red Cross or American Heart Association chapter where and when courses are offered (they usually last 4 to 8 hours).

☐ Keep an updated list of emergency numbers close by your telephone. Include your local hospital emergency medical service, fire and police departments, poison control center, and your doctor's office and home. Find out the emergency number in your area; 911 applies to many, but not all, communities.

☐ Learn the shortest route to the hospital, so that you can get there quickly in an emergency.

☐ Periodically update your medicine chest (p.229).

☐ Install smoke alarms and fire extinguishers (p.310) in your home; test them often.

General Rules

☐ There are three major medical emergencies that call for immediate action: when a victim stops breathing (pp.426–428), when you can't detect a heartbeat or a pulse (p.428), and when bleeding is severe (pp.432–433). If you believe that a patient's condition is serious, call—or ask someone else to call—for the local emergency medical service. Apply appropriate emergency measures while waiting.

☐ Check the victim for a medical I.D. bracelet or pendant, which will indicate an existing condition such as epilepsy or diabetes.

☐ Loosen the victim's clothes, cutting them open if necessary, but keep the patient covered to lessen the chance of shock.

☐ Do not give an emergency patient anything to eat or drink unless you are dealing with a diabetic crisis (p.436) or heatstroke (p.444).

☐ Do not move a victim unless safety demands it.

☐ Be prepared to tell a doctor or emergency medical service technician what has happened, what the victim's injuries or symptoms are, when the accident occurred or the symptoms first began, what a poison victim might have swallowed and when, where you and the victim are, and the number of the telephone closest to your location.

☐ Ask what more you can do to help.

THE RECOVERY POSITION

When a person is unconscious or has sustained a serious injury, it's imperative to place him or her in the recovery position as soon as possible. This position is designed to keep anything—the tongue, blood, saliva, or vomit—from blocking the windpipe and choking the victim. If the victim is bleeding profusely or isn't breathing, call for help and begin emergency first aid right away to stanch bleeding (p.433) or restore breathing (p.427). Once bleeding is under control or breathing has stabilized, place the victim in the recovery position and tend to any other wounds. *However, if the person has sustained a neck or back injury, do not move him or her at all.*

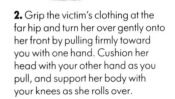

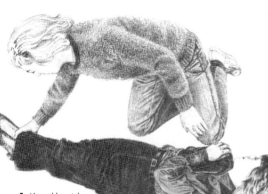

1. Kneel beside the victim and turn her head toward you. Tuck the near arm under the body, keeping it straight. Put the other arm across the chest as shown, and then lift the far ankle over the near ankle.

2. Grip the victim's clothing at the far hip and turn her over gently onto her front by pulling firmly toward you with one hand. Cushion her head with your other hand as you pull, and support her body with your knees as she rolls over.

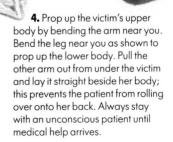

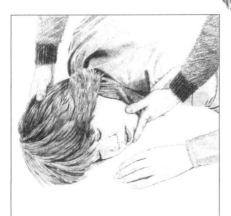

4. Prop up the victim's upper body by bending the arm near you. Bend the leg near you as shown to prop up the lower body. Pull the other arm out from under the victim and lay it straight beside her body; this prevents the patient from rolling over onto her back. Always stay with an unconscious patient until medical help arrives.

3. Tilt the victim's chin back to straighten the throat. This will keep the airway open, preventing the tongue from slipping back into the throat and allowing the victim to go on breathing freely.

Abdominal pain

Mild stomach upsets and digestive problems are not emergencies, but if the pain is severe and persistent—and possibly accompanied by nausea, cramping, or fever—call your doctor or go to a hospital emergency room.

APPENDICITIS

A dull pain in the abdomen may be the first sign of appendicitis. The pain is caused by inflammation of the appendix, a short tube, closed at one end, that projects from the junction of the small and large intestines.

Appendicitis can occur if the end of the appendix that connects to the large intestine is blocked by fragments of hard waste matter, or if the appendix becomes kinked. As a result, infection sets in and the walls of the appendix become inflamed and swollen.

If the condition is acute, the pain increases until the appendix finally bursts, spreading the infection through the area immediately around it or throughout the abdominal cavity (the latter condition is called peritonitis). A burst appendix is a surgical emergency, requiring immediate treatment. For this reason, a doctor should be seen as early as possible if appendicitis is suspected.

The symptoms of appendicitis can take between 4 and 48 hours to develop. And because they are extremely variable, the condition can be very difficult to diagnose. Arrange to see a doctor without delay if the pain gets worse, becomes continuous, keeps the sufferer awake, or lasts longer than 4 hours.

The warning signs
☐ Constant, dull pain. At first the pain may be felt near the navel, but sometimes it is in the lower right side of the abdomen.
☐ After a few hours, constant severe aching may be felt in the lower right side of the abdomen.
☐ The lower right side of the abdomen is tender to the touch. The pain becomes more severe if the sufferer moves, and it may interfere with sleep.
☐ The sufferer may vomit. Often there is constipation, although the bowels may move normally or even be loose.
☐ The victim exhibits a complete lack of appetite and generally feels nauseated.
☐ Walking or passing urine may be painful.
☐ Body temperature generally rises to 102°F in adults and can register even higher in children. In some cases, however, there is little or no increase in body temperature.

What you should do
Get the patient to a hospital right away. In the meantime, don't give the patient any medication, food, or liquid of any kind and don't administer an enema.

GALL AND KIDNEY STONES
When gallstones enter the bile duct and when kidney stones pass through the ureter, both can cause unexpected and excruciating pain. In the case of gallstones, pain is felt in the upper right side of the abdomen, between the shoulder blades, or in the right shoulder; pain from kidney stones, which is sharp and intermittent, starts in the side and moves toward the groin. People with either kind of stones may experience nausea and vomiting.

What you should do
Get the patient to a hospital right away. (Surgery may not be necessary unless an infection develops or a stone blocks passage to the kidney or obstructs the bile duct.) Don't give the patient a painkiller, a laxative, or anything to eat or drink without consulting a doctor. Patients should lie or sit comfortably; however, if moving around makes them feel better, it won't hurt them to do so.

Artificial respiration

A person who has stopped breathing—for whatever reason—will die within as few as 6 minutes if nothing is done. After only 4 minutes without oxygen, the brain can suffer irreversible damage. In such an emergency, it is urgent to get air into the lungs as quickly as possible.

A heart attack, stroke, drug overdose, shock, or poisoning can cause a person to stop breathing; so can a blockage in the windpipe, or trachea, which can occur for a variety of reasons. For example, an unconscious person's head may fall forward, narrowing the airway; his tongue may slip back in the throat, covering the airway; or a foreign object, vomit, or saliva may collect at the back of the throat, blocking air passage.

When breathing fails completely or is not strong or frequent enough to support life, the skin, including the lips and earlobes, takes on a bluish-gray tinge. However, it isn't always easy to tell if breathing has stopped. To find out, kneel down, put your ear beside the victim's mouth and nose, and look along the chest. If the person is breathing, you should be able to hear it and to see the chest rising and falling.

Simply opening the airway, as shown on the facing page, may allow breathing to start up again and is safe as long as there is no neck or back injury. When breathing has stabilized, put the victim in the recovery position (p. 425) until medical help arrives.

If opening the airway doesn't restore breathing, proceed with artificial respiration.

HOW TO RESTORE BREATHING

Administering artificial respiration is a simple but vital skill, best learned in a first-aid course. If you're giving artificial respiration, ask someone to call for an ambulance while you lay the victim face up on a firm surface. First clear the airway. If that doesn't restore breathing, begin artificial respiration.

CLEARING THE AIRWAY

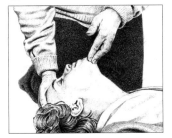 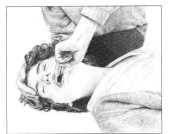 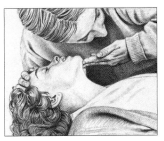

1. Tilt the head back by lifting the chin with one hand and pressing down on the forehead with the other. This opens the airway.

2. If breathing does not begin, turn the victim's head to the side and, with your fingers, clear the mouth of any foreign matter.

3. Listen for breathing. See if the chest rises and falls. Place your ear close to the nose and mouth and feel for exhaled air.

ARTIFICIAL RESPIRATION

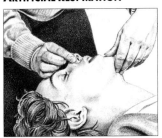 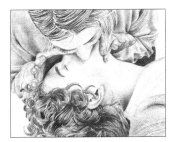 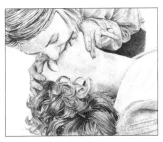

1. Open the airway as described above. Then pinch the nose shut with one hand and take a deep breath (you'll need to inhale yourself before each ventilation).

2. Seal your lips around the open mouth and deliver two full breaths (1 to 1½ seconds each). The victim's chest should rise and fall. If it does not, check for choking (p.435).

3. Remove your mouth to allow the victim to exhale between ventilations. After the first two breaths, check the pulse (see *Has the Heart Stopped Beating?*, p.428). If there is a pulse, continue giving ventilations every 5 seconds until the victim breathes alone, or help comes. If there is no pulse, the patient requires external chest compressions (pp.428–429).

INFANTS AND SMALL CHILDREN

1. When resuscitating an infant or small child, seal your lips around both mouth and nose.

2. Give two gentle puffs of air, then feel the pulse (p.428): check inside the upper arm in infants (under 1 year) and the neck pulse in small children (1–8 years).

3. If there is a pulse, continue giving gentle puffs of air—one every 3 seconds for an infant, one every 4 seconds for a child.

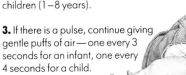

IF MOUTH-TO-MOUTH IS IMPOSSIBLE

Occasionally you can't use a victim's mouth because it is injured or it may contain a lethal poison. The alternative procedure is to hold the mouth shut with your hand and breathe into the patient's nose.

CARDIOPULMONARY RESUSCITATION (CPR)

When a person's heart stops beating, blood no longer carries oxygen to the brain and brain damage may begin within a matter of minutes. Artificial respiration (p.427) gets oxygen into the blood, but doesn't pump it throughout the body; you must also compress the victim's chest to force blood through the circulatory system. If the brain and heart continue to receive blood, the heart may spontaneously resume beating. The technique of cardiopulmonary resuscitation, or CPR, alternates artificial respiration and carefully timed chest compressions.

Caution. Chest compression can be dangerous. If the heart is compressed while it is still beating, even faintly, it may stop completely. Damage to the lungs, liver, spleen, and ribs can also occur. You can administer CPR safely only after establishing conclusively that the victim's heartbeat has stopped (see below). Administering CPR requires understanding, skill, and practice. *Use CPR only if you have been formally trained* (see *When Emergency Strikes*, p.424). Practice on a doll, never on a healthy person. The information given here is intended only as a memory aid for trained people.

HAS THE HEART STOPPED BEATING?

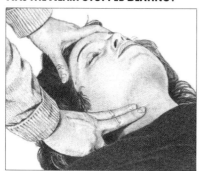

After giving the first two breaths of artificial respiration (p.427), feel the pulse of one of the carotid arteries on either side of the neck. (The wrist pulse is not a good indicator.) To feel the neck pulse, place your fingers gently in the hollow of the neck between the Adam's apple and neck muscle. If there is no pulse, begin chest compression (make sure someone is calling for emergency help). Check the pulse again after 1 min. and then after every 3 min. If the pulse returns, it means that the heart has started beating again. Don't perform any more chest compressions after the heart resumes beating.

CPR ON AN ADULT

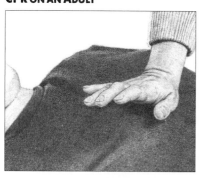

1. Kneeling beside the victim, place the heel of one hand on her chest, two finger widths up from the bottom of the breastbone. Keep your thumb and fingers raised, so that they do not press on the ribs.

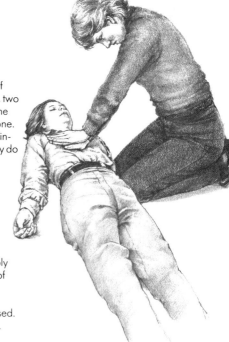

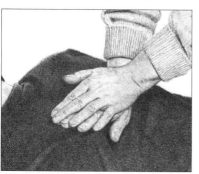

2.. With your second hand over the first, apply pressure with the heel of your hand. Press down 1½ in., keeping your thumbs and fingers raised. Let the chest rise again.

3. Give 15 presses at normal pulse rate (80 per min.), then inflate lungs twice by artificial respiration. Repeat the sequence four times per min. Check the neck pulse after 1 min., then every 3 min.

COMPRESSION ON A BABY

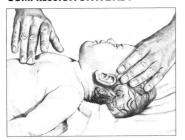

1. Put the baby on a firm surface such as a table, or hold him on your arm, cradling his head in your hand. Put your index finger on the breastbone at the level of the nipples. A finger width below this point—between the middle and the ring fingers—is the area of chest compression.

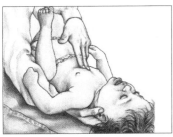

2. Administer chest compressions to a baby, using two fingers only, the index and middle finger of one hand. The depth of compression must be no more than 1 in. and the rate of compression 100 times per min. Pause to ventilate the baby with artificial respiration after each five compressions. Check the carotid (neck) pulse after 1 min., then every 3 min.

COMPRESSION ON A YOUNG CHILD

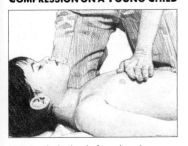

Using only the heel of one hand, press down the lower breastbone 1 to 1½ in. at a rate of 80 to 100 presses per min. Give 5 presses, then one breath using artificial respiration.

Bandages

A bandage is a strip of fabric that has three basic medical uses. It keeps a dressing in position over a wound (to prevent dirt and germs from getting in), it applies pressure to a wound (to absorb and stop bleeding), or it supports or immobilizes an injured part of the body. You can buy—and keep indefinitely in your medicine cabinet—muslin, gauze, crepe, or elastic bandages. But in an emergency it's possible to improvise bandages from sheets, pillowcases, stockings, scarves, shirts, dresses, or any other suitable material.

Packages of rolled bandages can be bought in different widths designed for different uses: the 1-inch size is good for fingers and toes; the 2-inch size, for hands; the 3-inch size, for arms and legs; the 4-inch or 6-inch size, for the trunk.

Dressings, which are used to absorb blood and prevent infection, are usually made of several layers of sterile material covered with gauze. In an emergency, a dressing can be made from a pad of any clean, dry, absorbent material. (Fluffy material such as absorbent cotton should never be applied directly on a wound because the fibers will stick.) The inside of a folded handkerchief, a towel, or a pillowcase—even a pad of paper tissues or toilet paper—can be used as dressings.

Sterile dressings sealed in protective wrapping can be bought from any drugstore and will keep indefinitely in a medicine cabinet.

Stretchy crepe or elastic bandages are the easiest to put on, and because they follow the contours of the body, the pressure they exert on the wound is more evenly distributed. No matter what type of bandage you use, however, take care not to wrap it too tight, because even bandages with give can cut off circulation. After applying a bandage, and again 10 minutes later, check for any of the following warning signals that the bandage has been wound too tight:

☐ The patient has a tingling feeling in the fingers or toes, or loses feeling altogether.
☐ The tips of the fingers or the toes are very cold.
☐ The patient is unable to move the fingers or toes.
☐ The beds of the fingernails or the toenails appear unusually pale or blue in color.
☐ The pulse of an injured arm is weak compared with the other arm's pulse, or you can't feel a pulse at all on the injured limb.

If any of these danger signs occurs, remove the bandage immediately and apply it again more loosely.

Triangular bandages
Triangular bandages can be purchased from most drugstores, or you can improvise one by cutting a piece of linen or cotton, about 3 feet square, in half diagonally.

Unfolded, triangular bandages are ideal for making slings to hold injured arms in place (see *Securing a Fractured Limb*, p.441). They can also be folded into broad bandages, suitable for strapping up a broken limb or tying a limb to a splint, or into narrow bandages, suitable for holding dressings in place.

To make a broad bandage, spread the triangular bandage out on a flat, clean surface. Fold the top of the triangle to the center of the base, and then fold it once more in the same direction.

To make a narrow bandage, make a third fold in the same direction as the first two.

A folded triangular bandage can also be used instead of rolled bandages to make a ring-pad (following page), which is used to dress a wound containing a for-

HOW TO USE ROLLED BANDAGES

Traditional nonstretch, open-weave gauze bandages should be included in every well-stocked home medicine cabinet. Sold in rolls of different widths, they are inexpensive, clean, and very convenient when first aid is needed in a hurry, but they do require a little practice to apply correctly. Basic techniques for using rolled bandages are shown below.

APPLYING A BANDAGE

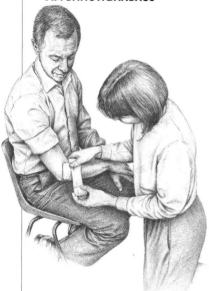

1. Start by putting the end of the bandage on the limb and making a firm turn to hold it in place. Apply the outer surface to the skin so that you can unroll it easily. Bandage a limb in the position in which it is to remain.

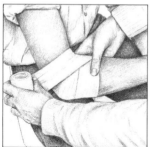

2. Bandage outward from the trunk, maintaining even pressure. Start two or three turns below the wound and finish two or three turns above it. Fold in the end, and fix it securely with a safety pin, adhesive tape, or a knot.

FINISHING IT WITH A KNOT

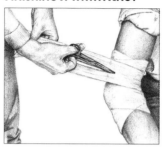

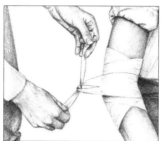

1. If you don't have a safety pin or adhesive tape, leave a piece of bandage free. The length will depend on the thickness of the area being bandaged. Cut the end of the bandage in half lengthwise (left).

2. Tie the two strips together with a single knot, pulling fairly tight at the bottom of the cut (lower left). This knot will keep the cut from tearing further when you tie off the bandage. Make sure that the knot doesn't press on the wound.

3. Take the two ends around the limb again and tie them off, preferably with a reef knot (right end over left end, then left end over right). Once again, make sure that the knot doesn't press on the wound. Tuck in the ends.

MAKING A RING-PAD

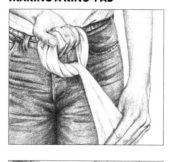

1. A ring-pad protects a wound that has glass or another foreign body in it from the pressure of a bandage. Wind one end of a narrow bandage once or twice around your fingers to make a loop. Bring the other end through the loop, under, and back through again to start a ring.

2. Continue winding the free end of the bandage around the ring loop until the bandage is almost used up. Finish off the end with a slip knot as shown.

eign object or to protect a fracture in which the bone juts through the skin.

Bites, animal

Bites from mammals (dogs, cats, rabbits, gerbils, and even human beings) are dangerous because germs from the animal's mouth enter the wound, and can cause infection (see *Rabies*, right). Report animal bites to your local animal control agency.

Any bite should be washed thoroughly, and if the skin has been broken, the victim should see a doctor. Serious wounds should be treated at a hospital emergency department.

SNAKEBITES

There are close to 9,000 cases of poisonous snakebite a year in the United States. Mortality from snakebites is low, but there is a high incidence of crippling injuries to the affected limbs.

All snakebite victims should be treated in a hospital. The snakebite kits sold in drugstores and camping stores are for situations where medical help can't be reached. The kits, which contain instruments for incising and drawing venom from a bite, should be used only by people trained to deal with snakebite.

Until you reach the hospital, keep the victim still, with the area of the bite resting below the level of the heart. Immobilize the bitten area with splints.

If you can safely kill the snake, bring it to the hospital. Otherwise, note its size, coloring, and skin pattern to help hospital staff identify it and chose a treatment.

The warning signs

☐ Sharp pain, bruising, or swelling around the bite.
☐ One sometimes, but usually two small puncture wounds.
☐ Blurry vision, nausea, vomit-

RABIES

Rabies is an extremely dangerous infectious disease caused by a virus carried by animals, particularly skunks, raccoons, foxes, bats, cattle, dogs, and cats. It is also known as hydrophobia (meaning "fear of water") because an aversion to water is one of its symptoms.

Rabies occurs in most parts of the world (Britain, Scandinavia, Australia, Japan, and Antarctica are exceptions) and has recently become quite prevalent in the northeastern United States. It is rare in North America for anyone to actually develop rabies, but over 25,000 people receive antirabies treatment each year because of known or suspected exposure to the virus.

The virus is transmitted to humans through the bite or scratch of an infected animal. From the site of the injury, the virus travels to the brain. The nearer the bite is to the brain (on the face or neck, for example) the less far the virus has to travel to attack the brain, and the sooner treatment must be started to prevent the disease.

The time between a bite and the onset of symptoms can range from 10 days to more than a year, but usually it's between 20 and 90 days. Before the symptoms appear, the bite usually heals but remains red and inflamed. Once symptoms have developed, treatment is ineffective and the patient usually dies within 4 days.

What you should do

☐ See a doctor immediately if you are bitten by a wild animal or a stray domestic animal. To be effective, treatment must begin before symptoms appear. Depending on the circumstances, the doctor may give antirabies treatment immediately, or if the culprit has been captured, the doctor may wait to see if the animal develops rabies symptoms.
☐ If possible, the animal should be captured (or in the case of a pet, its owner identified) so that the creature can be confined and observed by a veterinarian for 7 to 10 days for symptoms of rabies. Call your local health authorities if you need help.
☐ If the animal escapes, notify the police immediately.

Symptoms of rabies

☐ Fever, headache, sore throat, and muscle pains are followed by pain or numbness at the site of the healed bite.
☐ One or 2 days later, the patient becomes restless and agitated.
☐ Muscle spasms, stiffness of the neck and back, convulsions, and areas of paralysis may also develop.
☐ Excess saliva and difficulty in swallowing produce foaming at the mouth.
☐ Painful throat spasms develop, accompanied by an extreme difficulty in swallowing.
☐ Death usually occurs within 4 days of the onset of symptoms.

ing, diarrhea, slurred speech, difficulty in swallowing.
□ Breathing difficulties, convulsions, and the onset of paralysis.

What you should do
□ If medical help is more than 2 hours away, apply a constricting band 2 inches above the bite, or above the swelling if this has begun. Don't make the band too tight: you should be able to slip a finger underneath. As the swelling spreads, move the band to keep it always 2 inches above the swelling. If there is no swelling, loosen the band every 15 to 30 minutes for circulation.
□ Give a victim who can swallow fluids to drink, but no alcohol.
□ If the victim becomes unconscious, but is breathing normally, put the body in the recovery position (p.425) until help arrives.
□ If breathing stops, administer artificial respiration (p.427).
□ A victim who looks frightened and then becomes weak and pale may be in shock. For treatment of shock, see pages 445–446.

Bites, insect

Stings and bites from bees, wasps, and ants may be very painful, but they usually aren't dangerous unless they are multiple, unless you're bitten in the throat or mouth, or unless you have an allergic reaction, which can be life-threatening.

If you have been stung by a bee, the stinger may stay embedded in the skin. Remove it by gently scraping the skin with a clean knife blade. Don't squeeze the sting with tweezers. By compressing the stinger area, you may force more venom into the body. Wasps and ants do not leave stingers behind.

Allergic reaction
A massive allergic reaction to a sting (or to a drug such as peni-

cillin) is known as anaphylactic shock. It can occur within seconds or be delayed 30 minutes or more. The victim becomes very weak and feels sick. His chest feels tight and he has difficulty breathing. He may wheeze and his face may swell up, or he may lose consciousness and stop breathing.
□ Call for emergency medical help at once.
□ If an emergency kit for insect bites is available, follow instructions in the kit. If not, lay the victim on his back. Raise his feet on a cushion or folded coat or blanket. Keep the person's head low and turn it to one side in case he vomits. Be sure to keep his airway open and give artificial respiration (p.427) or CPR (pp.428–429) if necessary.
□ Keep the victim warm with a blanket or rug.
□ Loosen tight clothing around the neck and waist to make breathing easier.
□ Apply a cold compress to the injured area. Don't put ice right on the skin (it might cause frostbite).
□ Don't give the victim anything to eat or drink. Don't allow him to smoke, either.
□ You can give the victim an antihistamine.
□ If the victim becomes unconscious or breathing becomes very difficult, put him in the recovery position (p.425).

Stings in the mouth or throat
The danger of a sting in the mouth or throat is that the throat may swell rapidly and block the airway to the lungs.
□ Give the victim an ice cube to suck or cold water to swish around in the mouth and then spit out to lessen the swelling.
□ If the victim has difficulty breathing, forget the ice and liquids and start artificial respiration immediately (p.427). Call for professional help.

Bleeding

Although bleeding can be alarming and dramatic, most cases are not fatal, provided the injury is treated promptly.

Bleeding can usually be stopped by pressing down on the wound, which slows the flow of blood and facilitates clotting. The flow of blood can also be slowed by raising the injured area above the heart, but this is safe only if no fracture is involved.

If severe bleeding is left untreated, however, it can lead to the potentially fatal condition known as shock (p.445).

Stopping severe bleeding
□ Lay the victim down. Remove clothing from around the wound if you can without wasting time or causing distress. Press down hard on the wound with any absorbent material or your bare hands, unless something is embedded in the wound.
□ If possible, raise the wounded area above the level of the heart to reduce the flow of blood. When the bleeding stops, apply an absorbent sterile dressing or, if necessary, the inside of a clean, folded handkerchief.
□ If the blood seeps through the dressing, do not remove it. Put another dressing on top. Tie the dressing in place with a bandage or other material. Keep the victim as still as possible and do not give him food or drink.

A large wound
Squeeze the sides of a large wound together gently but firmly, and maintain the pressure for up to 10 minutes. Then treat as above and call an ambulance.

Large foreign object in wound
If a large object, such as a piece of glass, is embedded in a wound, do not try to remove it. Its removal may cause further

STOPPING BLOOD FLOW AT A PRESSURE POINT

If severe bleeding from an arm or leg cannot be stopped by elevation and direct pressure on the wound, it may be possible to stop the bleeding at one of the body's two main pressure points. These are places where an artery can be pressed against an underlying bone to stop the flow of blood.

Use this technique to reduce severe bleeding only as a last resort and with extreme care. Reduce pressure after 5 minutes and continue alternating 5 minutes maximum pressure with 5 minutes reduced pressure for as long as necessary.

THE FEMORAL PRESSURE POINT

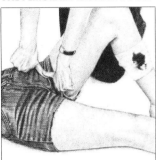

High inside the thigh the femoral artery can be pressed against the pelvis to stop blood flow. Lay the victim down and bend the injured leg at the knee. Press down firmly in the center of the fold of the groin, one thumb on top of the other, against the rim of the pelvis. Do not press forcefully for longer than 5 min.

THE BRACHIAL PRESSURE POINT

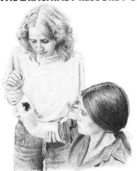

The brachial artery runs along the inner side of the upper arm and can be pressed against the humerus, or upper arm bone. To control bleeding from the lower arm, hold the victim's arm at right angles to the body as shown. Then put one hand under the upper arm and press your fingers hard against the bone.

damage to nerves, muscles, and other tissue. Also, the object may serve to plug the wound, helping to restrict bleeding.

Control the bleeding by pressing down on the sides of the wound. This may take time, so continue pressure on the way to the hospital. Bind up the wound, using a ring-pad (p. 430) to keep pressure off the object. Wind bandages diagonally so that strips don't go over the object.

When a varicose vein bursts

If a varicose vein in the leg bursts or is injured, severe blood loss can occur rapidly. Take these steps to stop the bleeding:

☐ Lay the victim down and press on the wound with a dressing (p. 429). If no dressing is available, press the wound with your bare fingers.

☐ Prop the leg up and maintain the pressure for up to 45 minutes to stop the bleeding.

☐ Put a clean dressing on the wound and tie it firmly in place with some sort of a bandage.

☐ If bleeding continues, place additional dressings and bandages over the first.

☐ Let the patient rest, and prop up the leg with pillows or on a chair seat.

If the bleeding is severe and does not stop with the application of pressure, call an ambulance.

Bleeding from the nose, mouth, or ears

If an injured person bleeds from the nose, mouth, or ears, she or he may be suffering from a severe internal injury to the head, the chest, or the abdomen.

A fractured skull may cause blood to trickle from the nose or ears. An injury to the lungs, such as a puncture caused by a fractured rib, may result in pink frothy blood dribbling from the mouth and nose.

First, call an ambulance. Then place the victim in a half-sitting position with the head tilted toward the side from which the blood is coming. Cover the bleeding point with a pad of material, but don't apply pressure. Don't give the patient anything to eat or drink.

Bleeding scalp

An injury to the scalp may look more threatening than it actually is because the scalp has a rich supply of blood and bleeds profusely, even from small cuts. And because the skin of the scalp is stretched tight over the head, a wound may also gape open, giving the impression of a much larger and more serious injury than might be the case.

However, if there is danger of a fracture to the skull, the victim should be examined by a doctor as soon as possible. In the meantime, don't clean the wound or remove any foreign matter; as long as there are no bone fragments or a skull depression, try to control the bleeding by holding your hand or a compress, such as the inside of a clean, folded handkerchief, on the wound. (For more on injuries to the skull, see *Facial Injuries,* p. 438, and *Head Injuries,* p. 443.)

Bruises

A bruise is the visual sign of bleeding beneath the skin. Swelling may be considerable whenever the bruise occurs on the head or shin or any place where the bone is just beneath the skin.

Before treating a minor bruise, check that there are no other injuries, especially fractures (pp. 439–442).

Applying a cold compress to a bruised area helps to limit the swelling. The compress can be a small towel, a piece of cloth soaked in cold water and wrung out, or a plastic bag of crushed ice wrapped in a towel or cloth.

Apply the compress as soon as possible and keep it on for at least 30 minutes. Instead of using a compress, you can also hold the bruised area under cold running water. If a bruise develops on an arm or a leg, elevate the limb above heart level to help alleviate the swelling.

A bruise requires consultation with your doctor under the following circumstances:
☐ If it has not started to fade within a few days.
☐ If the pain is severe, if there is difficulty in moving the bruised area 24 hours later, or if a bruise is large and occurs near the abdomen or on the back.
☐ If bruises occur without any apparent reason.
☐ If the lower leg is bruised in an elderly person or a person suffering from poor circulation.
☐ If vision is disturbed as the result of a black eye (p. 439).

Burns and scalds

First-degree burns redden the skin but only affect the surface. Second-degree burns cause blisters and deeper damage to the skin. Third-degree burns destroy the skin completely; the burned area will look charred or white. All but minor burns and scalds are potentially serious and should be seen by a doctor.

Do's and don'ts

Remove the victim as quickly as possible from the source of the heat that caused the burn. Don't put butter, oil, ointment, lotion, or ice on a burn. Don't touch a burn, don't break any blisters, and don't remove anything that is sticking to a burn (you can irritate it and cause an infection). Don't use cotton balls or adhesive bandages on a burn.

If the burn is caused by a dry chemical, such as caustic soda or dry lime, irrigate the burned area copiously with water. Wear gloves to protect your own hands while you help the burn victim. Remove the victim's contaminated clothing, which can continue to burn, and check that the patient isn't lying in the chemical.

Treating a minor burn

When a burn is extremely painful, it is usually superficial. If a burn is smaller than a 50-cent piece, hold it under a slow-running cold-water faucet or put it in cold water for at least 10 minutes. If no water is available, use some other cold liquid, such as milk or juice.

For minor burns and scalds in the mouth, give the patient cold water and tell him or her to rinse and spit.

Large superficial burns

If a superficial burn is larger than a 50-cent piece, there is a danger of infection. Cool the burn in cold water and cover it with a clean dressing, but take the victim to a doctor or a hospital as soon as possible.

Dealing with serious burns

If a burned area of skin appears gray and/or is peeling or charred, the burn may be deep. It may not be painful because the nerves in the area may have been destroyed. Whatever the size of a deep burn, do not immerse it in water, and do not apply water or ice to it. Cover the burned area with a clean, nonsticking dressing and get medical help immediately; there is a strong risk of serious infection.

Widespread burns

Burns covering a large area of the body, such as an arm, a thigh, or the chest, are medical emergencies that must be treated in a hospital as quickly as possible with minimum interference to the damaged skin.

Remove rings, a watch, or tight clothing before the area starts to swell. Remove scalding clothing as soon as you can handle it, and cover the burn with clean, nonsticking material. If burned clothing clings to the skin, don't remove it unless it is smoldering.

If the victim is unconscious but breathing, put him in the recovery position (p. 425) before calling for an ambulance.

When clothes catch fire

Keep the victim from running, which only feeds the fire. As you approach a person with burning clothing, hold a cotton or wool blanket, rug, or coat in front of you for protection (synthetic fabrics may melt). Wrap the victim with the material and lay him flat on the ground to keep the flames from rising to the head; then roll the victim to smother the fire. You can also douse the fire with water or any non-flammable liquid such as milk (but not alcoholic spirits such as whiskey or gin). If your own clothes catch fire, lie down and roll on the ground.

When the fire has been put out, remove any hot clothing that can be taken off the victim easily but leave fragments that have stuck to the skin. Depending on the extent of the burns, proceed as suggested above.

Choking

When a piece of food or some other object gets caught in your trachea, or windpipe, your breath is either partially or fully cut off and you choke. If the blockage is partial, you may be able to take in enough air to cough out the object yourself. If the blockage is complete, you can die of suffocation within minutes if something isn't done.

Not chewing food properly and laughing while you eat can cause choking; so can drinking too much alcohol, which dulls the nerves that control swallowing. Peanuts, hot dogs, and hard candies are a common cause of choking in very young children (and shouldn't be given to them). Children can also choke on small toys or pieces of toys that they put in their mouths, and adults can choke on dislodged dentures.

Instant action is vital if you are to save someone who is choking. The first signal that something is wrong with the victim may be a fit of coughing; then the skin, lips, tongue, fingernail beds, or earlobes turn blue and the veins on the head and neck swell. People who are choking instinctively clutch their throats, which has become a universal distress signal for choking.

Treating a conscious adult
Encourage the victim to cough; this may be enough to expel the obstruction. If the victim can't cough or speak, apply the Heimlich maneuver as shown at right.

If you are alone and start to choke, you can perform the Heimlich maneuver on yourself. Clench a fist and place it, thumb side against the stomach, slightly above the navel. With the other

THE HEIMLICH MANEUVER

1. Tell the choking victim what you are going to do. Stand behind the victim, who can be standing or sitting, and put both your arms around the waist.

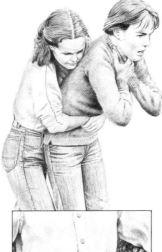

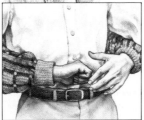

2. Make a fist with one hand and place the thumb side against the victim's abdomen, just above the navel but below the breastbone. Grasp the fist with the other hand and press it forcefully into the victim's abdomen with a quick inward-and-upward thrust. You are trying to push the upper abdomen against the bottom of the lungs to push out the remaining air, which in turn should force out the obstruction.
3. Repeat as often as necessary, but pause briefly between each thrust to see if the obstruction has been dislodged. Check the victim's mouth and remove anything that has come up.
4. Even after the obstruction is dislodged, the victim may be winded and unable to breathe for a few moments. When breathing begins again, encourage the victim to sit quietly and, if requested, offer a sip of water.

hand, jerk the fist firmly inward and upward. Repeat the thrust until the obstruction is dislodged and expelled.

Alternatively you can use the back of a chair, or stand at a sink or railing, and press your abdomen right above the navel firmly against the hard edge. Thrust yourself downward and forward.

For very obese people or pregnant women, the Heimlich maneuver is best performed higher on the torso. Clench your fist and hold it at the base of the breastbone just above the place where the bottom ribs are joined. Grasp your fist with the other hand and thrust upward into the chest.

Treating children and infants
Watch closely but don't interfere as long as the youngster can breathe, speak, or make sounds and is coughing. These are all signs that the child is getting some air in the windpipe and may be able to expel whatever is causing the partial blockage. Be ready, however, to act quickly the minute the youngster stops breathing or making sounds.

You can rescue a child, 12 months and older, by applying the Heimlich maneuver. If the child is small, do it gently. With small children, you may find it easier to administer the thrusts with the child lying down.

For babies under a year old, there is a different technique:
☐ Sit down, rest one forearm on your thigh, and straddle the child face down along this forearm with her head lower than her body and her chin and neck held firmly in your hand.
☐ Thump rapidly but firmly on the child's back between the shoulder blades with the heel of your free hand. Do this up to four times.
☐ If the blows fail to expel the object, turn the infant over on

her back and, using only the index and middle finger of one hand, compress the chest rapidly but gently four times. Use a point in the center of the chest, just below the nipples.

☐ Repeat this sequence of back blows and chest thrusts until the obstruction is dislodged.

☐ Be very careful when removing anything from a baby's mouth. Put your finger into the mouth only if you can actually see the object. Take care not to push it farther down the throat.

Treating an unconscious victim

First, get someone to call for an ambulance while you attend to the victim. Make the call yourself if no one else is around.

Put a choking victim who has passed out on his or her back immediately, and try to open the blocked airway by tilting the head back and lifting the chin (p. 427). Check for breathing. If there is still none, attempt a finger sweep of the mouth. With your thumb on the tongue and your fingers under the chin, lift the victim's lower jaw with one hand while you perform a sweeping movement with the index finger of your other hand along the cheeks and deep into the throat. Try to hook and remove the obstruction. Be careful not to push a foreign object deeper into the throat. Don't use this mouth sweep with infants or small children unless you can clearly see the obstruction.

If breathing still isn't restored, position the victim's head for artificial respiration (p. 427). If the lungs don't inflate with the first two breaths, retilt the head, give another two breaths, then check for a pulse. If there is none, CPR will be necessary to circulate blood to the brain (p. 428).

If the victim has a pulse but is not breathing, prepare to perform the Heimlich maneuver with the patient lying stretched out on the ground. To do this, first turn the victim face up. Kneel astride his hips and put the heel of one hand slightly above the navel and well below the bottom of the breastbone. Cover this hand with the other and, with your arms straight, give a quick, upward thrust. Repeat nine times.

After the first 10 thrusts, check the mouth again. If the object has not been expelled, try artificial respiration again. If the lungs don't expand after two breaths, repeat the sequence of thrusts, finger sweep of the mouth, and artificial respiration. Continue as long as necessary.

Anyone who has been revived by the Heimlich maneuver should see a doctor. Although applying the technique may be necesssary to restore a victim's breathing, abdominal thrusts can damage the liver and other internal organs. Also, some foreign material sucked in during choking may remain in the lungs.

Diabetes: insulin shock and diabetic coma

Insulin shock, or hypoglycemia, is the result of too little glucose (sugar) in the blood of a person with diabetes (pp. 342–345). In contrast, a diabetic coma, or hyperglycemia, is caused by too much sugar in a diabetic's blood.

INSULIN SHOCK

Low blood sugar affects the brain and leads to unconsciousness. Death can follow, sometimes in only 20 minutes.

The warning signs

☐ Confusion and sometimes aggressive, hostile behavior.

☐ Pale appearance, with sweating, rapid pulse, shallow breathing, and possibly trembling.

☐ Faintness and weakness, leading to unconsciousness in 15 to 20 minutes.

What you should do

If insulin shock comes on quickly, you can assume that the patient needs sugar at once. If the patient is conscious, administer 3 or 4 teaspoons of sugar, some cookies, honey, candy, juice, or a nondiet soft drink. But don't give anything to someone who cannot swallow. The patient may inhale the substance and suffocate.

If a diabetic in shock doesn't respond to first aid, call for emergency medical help. If the patient loses consciousness, and if glucagon (p. 345) is available and you know how to inject it, do so right away, then call for help.

DIABETIC COMA

Too much glucose in the blood, or hyperglycemia, can also lead to coma, but because the process is slower than in hypoglycemia, the diabetic usually becomes aware of the situation in time and can treat himself by taking insulin.

Put an unconscious diabetic in the recovery position (p. 425) and call for immediate medical attention. Encourage a conscious patient to check his glucose level and take insulin as directed.

What the patient should do

A person who is subject to hypoglycemic attacks should carry a card or wear a bracelet specifying his condition and giving instructions for emergencies. This protects the diabetic from being mistaken for a drunk when he suffers insulin shock and needs fast emergency care.

Diabetics on insulin should avoid driving or using dangerous machinery when they haven't eaten for 2 hours or more.

Drowning

In the United States each year there are more than 5,000 deaths from drowning. In many cases, the victim didn't know how to swim and didn't intend to go into the water. Some unexpected occurrence—a boat capsizing, a fall from a dock—is responsible for the drowning. Many drownings occur within 15 feet of shore. Oddly, more than 80 percent of victims are male.

Assume that anyone you see in the water fully clothed is a potential victim, and be ready to help. A swimmer who develops a cramp or becomes exhausted is less easy to recognize. The swimmer who is having breathing problems may not be able to draw attention by shouting.

Suspect a problem if the victim's body tends to sink until it is vertical and only his head shows above water, if his strokes become erratic and his movements in the water appear jerky or simply stop, or if the victim's lips and ears turn bluish.

Rescue methods
Never go into the water yourself unless you are trained in life saving and there's no alternative. A panicky victim can drag the rescuer under. If the victim is near a pier or the side of a pool, extend a life belt, pole, rope, towel, or something that the drowning person can hold onto while being pulled to safety.

If a person is drowning away from shore, use a boat to reach him and get someone to go with you. Take along a life belt or other device to throw to the victim. Tow him in, making certain that his face stays above water.

Be sure that someone has called for a medical emergency team. Then start revival procedures immediately while waiting for professional help.

Revival techniques
If the drowning person has stopped breathing, start artificial respiration as quickly as possible (p.427). Remove any debris from the mouth with your index finger, tilt the head back, and begin breathing into the mouth. Either press your cheek against the victim's nose to stop air from escaping or pinch the nose between your finger and thumb.

Victims of drowning sometimes swallow water, which may be brought up with food during artificial respiration. Turn the head to one side and regularly clear the mouth of any debris. Once breathing has restarted, place the victim in the recovery position (p.425). Cover the victim and treat any injuries while you wait for medical help. Even a victim who appears to have recovered from a near drowning should be examined by a doctor.

Electric shock

Electricity can kill or produce a wide range of injuries, including severe burns and asphyxiation.

Rescue methods
Never touch the victim of an electrical accident until you're sure that you aren't risking a shock yourself. If the victim is still touching the source of electricity, cut off the power at the main circuit-breaker panel or fuse box.

If the victim is in contact with an electrical source and you can't turn off the power, don't touch him directly. Instead, push him away with a piece of wood that you know to be completely dry, such as a broom handle. If you can, stand on insulating material such as a rubber mat.

Caution. Remember that water conducts electricity. If you touch the victim with anything that may be even slightly moist, you can electrocute yourself.

Once an unconscious victim is away from the electrical source, check for breathing and give artificial respiration (p.427) if necessary. Put a victim who is breathing in the recovery position (p.425). In either situation, call for emergency medical help.

Treat minor burns as described on page 434.

High-voltage electricity
Electricity from high-voltage sources, such as power lines and some industrial equipment, can give a fatal shock up to 20 feet away. Around electric railway, subway, or streetcar systems, 10 feet away is considered a safe distance for people.

When confronted with any emergency involving high-voltage electricity, call your local emergency number and stay clear of the power source yourself.

When lightning strikes
Lightning is another form of high-voltage electricity that can kill. If you are caught in a storm take these precautions:
☐ If possible, seek shelter in a large building.
☐ If you can't make it to shelter, sit or crouch (don't lie flat) in a low place away from water and metal fences. Avoid tall isolated objects such as trees.
☐ If you are driving, stay inside a car or truck (don't touch metal), but not in a convertible.
☐ Avoid open metal vehicles like golf carts or tractors.
☐ Do not use the telephone, television, electrical appliances, and any form of plumbing, all of which can conduct lightning.

Epileptic seizure

There are two main types of epileptic seizure. In a generalized seizure, the victim's whole body twitches and convulses and he or she loses consciousness. In a partial seizure, a more limited area of the brain and body is affected and the victim may retain consciousness throughout the episode. An absence seizure is a type of generalized seizure in which the victim blanks out for a moment. (For more on epilepsy, see pages 353–354.)

Symptoms of a generalized seizure

□ A few seconds before a generalized seizure, the victim may experience a strange sensation called an aura. This may take the form of an odd taste or smell or a feeling of fear or malaise. Or the epileptic may utter an involuntary scream before a seizure.
□ The victim loses consciousness.
□ Limbs and neck stiffen for a few seconds; then the whole body is overcome by rhythmic and often violent twitching.
□ The victim may bite his tongue, froth at the mouth, or urinate involuntarily.
□ Once the muscles relax, the victim may remain unconscious for some minutes longer.
□ When consciousness returns, the victim may be drowsy and confused for an hour or more.

What you should do

Do not try to restrain a person who is having a generalized seizure. You want only to keep the person from harm. Break or cushion the epileptic's fall to the ground, for example. Clear a space around him and remove furniture and other objects that his head may hit.

If possible, loosen the victim's clothing around the neck and place something soft under his head. Don't put anything in his mouth or try to force it open.

When convulsions end, place the victim in the recovery position (p. 425) and wait for consciousness to return. Don't leave a person who's just had a seizure alone until he is fully recovered.

Do not give the patient anything to eat or drink until you are sure that he is alert and completely recovered.

Call an ambulance if

□ A person not known to be epileptic has a seizure. (Epileptics often wear a medical ID bracelet.)
□ A person has a series of seizures without regaining consciousness in between.
□ A person is injured during the seizure, perhaps by a fall.
□ The active part of the seizure lasts longer than 15 minutes.
□ A woman who is pregnant has a seizure.

Facial injuries

Even when an injury to the face appears to be minor, always have the victim see a doctor as soon as possible. The face encompasses delicate organs like the eyes, ears, and nose that are vulnerable to injury.

EAR INJURIES

Damage to the middle or inner ear can be caused by injuries to the head, a very loud noise or explosion, diving into water, or probing in the ear—to remove a foreign object, for example.

Although a perforated eardrum is not necessarily serious, bleeding from the ear or discharge of watery, straw-colored fluid can be a sign of a fractured skull (p. 433) and should be checked without delay.

Symptoms of an ear injury include severe earache, dizziness and loss of balance, deafness in one ear following an accident, headache, loss of consciousness, and discharge of blood or fluid.

Stop the victim of an ear injury from hitting the side of the head to try to restore hearing; this will only make the damage worse.

Cover the injured ear with a piece of clean cotton or gauze as protection. Bandage it lightly.

Don't try to plug the ear canal; this can cause a buildup of pressure in the middle ear.

Sit the victim up with the head tilted over on the injured side so that blood or fluid can drain out.

If the victim is unconscious but breathing, put him in the recovery position (p. 425) with the injured ear downward and a clean pad underneath it to absorb fluids.

If the victim's breathing stops, begin administering artificial respiration (p. 427) immediately.

Foreign object in the ear

Children often stick things into their ears harmlessly, but when an object is pushed hard and deep into the ear canal, the eardrum may be perforated. The symptoms are variable:
□ There may be no symptoms at all except that the object has disappeared.
□ Discharge from the ear.
□ Pain or buzzing in the ear.
□ Deafness on the affected side.

Don't attempt to remove a foreign object from your own or your child's ear. Get medical help right away.

Insects in the ear

If an insect crawls or flies into an ear, its buzzing can sound frighteningly loud.

Calm and comfort the victim. Prevent the victim from putting a finger in the ear. If the insect has a stinger, the finger may provoke an attack.

Put several drops of mineral or vegetable oil into the ear to kill the insect. Hold the victim's head still with the affected ear angled toward the ground. Although the insect may still sting in a reflex reaction, its body should float out on the oil.

If all attempts to remove the insect fail, or if it stings while inside the ear, get medical help.

EYE INJURIES

Getting an eyelash or a piece of grit lodged in your eye is the most common mishap that eyes suffer. More serious injuries are caused by corrosive chemicals or sharp objects, such as flying fragments of glass or metal.

Injury can also occur if contact lenses get displaced or stuck to the eyeball. If you have any difficulty with a contact lens, get medical help rather than risk hurting your eye.

Foreign object in the eye

Don't let the victim rub the eye. Turn his or her face up to the light. With your thumb and forefinger, push the eyelids away from the eyeball. Ask the victim to look left, right, up, and down while you look for the foreign matter on the exposed eyeball.

If you can see the foreign object, try to wash it out. Tilt the victim's head to the injured side, and gently run cool or lukewarm water over the eye from a faucet or jug. Alternatively, encourage the victim to blink underwater.

If flushing proves to be ineffective, try to lift the object off the eye with a moistened piece of clean gauze or the corner of a clean handkerchief or a damp piece of cotton.

Chemical burns to the eye

If chemicals—either liquid or solid—get into the eye, tilt the victim's head, injured eye downward, over the sink. Flood the open eye with gently running water from a faucet or jug for at least 20 minutes. You may need to force the eyelids open if they are shut tight in a spasm of pain.

When you have thoroughly flushed the chemical from the eye, dry the face and put a clean dressing lightly over the eye. Get the victim to a hospital emergency room right away.

Object impaled in the eye

Don't try to remove any foreign matter that is embedded in the eye yourself. You might cause irreparable damage. Instead, pro-

tect the injured eye by covering it with a paper or plastic cup, taking great care not to touch or apply any pressure to the eye. Put a bandage over both eyes to keep them from moving and take the victim to a hospital emergency room immediately.

Treating a black eye

A blow to the eye socket often causes internal bleeding, which colors the skin dark blue or black and produces swelling.

☐ Put a cold compress over the eye to limit the swelling and relieve the pain. To make the compress, put crushed ice or ice cubes into a plastic bag, add some salt to encourage the ice to melt, seal the bag, and wrap it in a cloth. Or soak a small towel in iced water and wring it out.

☐ Cool the eye for at least 30 minutes, replacing the compress as it becomes warm.

☐ Take the victim to a doctor as soon as possible. A blow that is violent enough to blacken the eye socket could fracture the skull or cause serious damage to the eye itself.

Fainting

If the blood supply to the brain is suddenly and temporarily reduced, a person may faint. An emotional stimulus such as bad news or a fright can cause fainting. So can a stuffy room, a drop in blood sugar due to missed meals or dieting, standing still for a long time, or standing up suddenly. If fainting is caused by illness or injury, if it occurs often, or if the fainter is old or has a cardiac problem, a doctor should be consulted.

The warning signs

☐ A person who is about to faint becomes pale or greenish white.

☐ Frequent yawning may indicate a lack of oxygen.

☐ The skin becomes cold and clammy. Beads of sweat appear on the face, neck, and hands. The victim may complain of feeling very warm or hot.

☐ The victim may experience blurred vision, dizziness, nausea, or generalized weakness.

What you should do

When a person feels faint, sit him down right away. Loosen tight clothing at the neck and waist, and put his head down to his knees. Or stretch the person out flat on his back and prop up his legs 8 to 12 inches.

If the person actually faints, first make sure he is breathing. Then raise his feet above the level of his head to increase blood circulation to the brain. Resist putting a pillow under the patient's head; it could obstruct his breathing.

Don't pour water over the victim's head, but you can wave smelling salts under his nose. If the victim doesn't recover in minutes, get medical help.

Recovery from a faint is usually rapid and complete, but check for any injury that may have occurred during the patient's fall. If his head hit something hard enough to cause a cut or wound, for example, the victim should be examined by a doctor for a possible concussion (p. 443).

Don't give the victim anything to eat or drink until full consciousness returns, and then only sips of cold water. Don't give the victim any alcohol. An alcoholic drink acts as a depressant and may worsen whatever condition caused the fainting spell in the first place.

Fractures and sprains

A fracture is a crack or break in a bone. A sprain is a stretching or tearing of the ligaments that hold a joint together.

TYPES OF FRACTURE

☐ A closed fracture is a bone break that leaves the skin intact, although it may be heavily bruised from internal bleeding.

☐ A greenstick fracture is an incomplete break in a bone. It usually occurs in children, whose bones are still soft and pliable.

☐ In an open, or compound, fracture either a piece of bone protrudes through the skin or a deep gash leads down to the bone. In either case, germs may enter the wound, and there is a risk of serious infection.

The warning signs

Often a fracture victim will actually hear or feel the bone snap and be aware of the sensation of broken bone ends grating together, which sometimes makes a definite sound.

The victim most likely won't be able to use the injured part of the body and will feel pain when attempting to do so. Only occasionally can a broken bone still be moved, and then awkwardly.

A limb may be in an unnatural position, or it will look deformed when compared with the uninjured side. The area around the break may be tender to the touch, swollen, or bruised.

What you should do

All doubtful cases of injured bones should be considered fractures. The principles of treatment are the same in all cases.

☐ Don't move the victim unless he or she is in imminent danger.

☐ Deal first with any difficulty in breathing (p. 427), unconsciousness (p. 446), or any severe bleeding (p. 432) before treating the fracture.

☐ Make the victim as comfortable as possible and provide support for the injured limb with a rolled-up blanket or coat or with cushions.

☐ Don't move the fractured

bone unnecessarily and never try to push a bone back in position.

☐ For ways to limit the danger of shock, see pages 445–446.

☐ If it is essential to move the victim—and time allows—try to immobilize the injured limb. For ways to secure a fractured arm or leg until you can get the patient to a doctor or hospital, see facing page.

BROKEN KNEE

A fractured knee is extremely painful and may be bent in an unnatural way. Do not try to straighten it forcibly. Lay the victim down with the leg in the most comfortable position.

Support the knee by placing a cushion or a rolled-up piece of clothing underneath it; place rolled-up coats or rugs around the leg for further support. Don't tie a splint over the break.

BROKEN JAW

A person who has suffered a broken jaw will often have a wound inside the mouth. The victim may have difficulty speaking, and there may be an excessive flow of saliva, often tinged with blood and broken teeth.

On the way to the hospital, the patient can support his jaw by cupping it with his hands. In order to allow him to clear secretions effectively from his mouth or to vomit if he has to, it's better not to support the jaw by tying a bandage around the head. Watch the patient to make sure he is not having difficulty breathing.

RIB FRACTURES

A severe blow to the chest or a bad fall can fracture a rib, causing a sharp chest pain when the victim breathes deeply or coughs. A person who appears to have only a simple rib fracture can be taken to a hospital in a car, preferably in the back seat. However, call an ambulance at once if you

Slings. Drugstores sell ready-made slings and triangular bandages (p. 429) that can be used as slings.

A conventional arm sling supports the forearm across the chest, with the hand slightly higher than the elbow and the fingers exposed (facing page). It is used for arm and some rib injuries.

An elevation sling raises the arm so that the hand rests on the shoulder. It is used to control bleeding and for complicated chest injuries or a broken collarbone. It will support the arm of a victim who cannot stand or sit.

Splints. Sometimes a person with a fractured bone has to be moved. To minimize the chance of injuring the patient further during the move, you need to immobilize the fractured bone in the position in which you found it.

The simplest way to do this is to tie the damaged limb to an uninjured part of the body with bandages—a technique known as body splinting.

To immobilize an arm, put it in a sling and bandage it against the chest. Bandage a broken leg to the other leg (facing page).

If the injured person has to be carried to safety, the fractured limb can be given even greater support with a rigid splint, such as a tightly rolled blanket, a walking stick, or a board. Any splint must be long enough to extend well beyond the joints above and below the fracture.

Whatever type of splint you use, never manipulate the fractured bone. Don't remove clothes to apply a splint; add padding if possible between the splint and the limb.

SECURING A FRACTURED LIMB

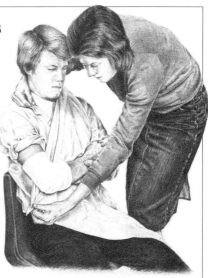

MAKING AN ARM SLING

1. Get the victim to support the injured arm with his hand. Place an open triangular bandage between the chest and forearm, its apex stretching well beyond the elbow. Take the upper end over the shoulder on the uninjured side, around the back of the neck to the front of the injured side.

2. Take the lower end of the bandage up over the hand and forearm, and tie it to the upper end in the hollow just above the collarbone. The tips of the fingers should just protrude from the side of the sling.

3. Pin the apex of the triangular bandage near the elbow, or twist and tuck it in. If the arm was bandaged before the sling went on, check that the nail beds are not turning blue, a signal that you need to loosen the bandage.

SECURING AN ARM THAT WILL BEND

Place the arm across the chest, with some padding between the fracture site and the body. Don't bend the arm by force. Put on an arm sling, then strap the arm to the body with a piece of wide material tied around the arm and chest.

SECURING AN UNBENDABLE ARM

Lay the victim down in the most comfortable position. Put padding between the injury and the body, and strap the arm to the body with three pieces of wide material spaced apart to avoid the immediate area of the fracture.

SPLINTING A BROKEN ELBOW

1. Sit the victim down and keep the arm straight. Fold a newspaper and place it along the arm.

2. Get the victim to support the splint while you tie it in place with two bandages, one at the top of the splint and the other at the bottom.

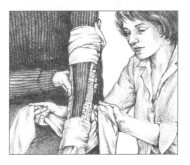

SECURING A FRACTURED LEG WITH BANDAGES

1. A broken leg is most easily immobilized by bandaging it to the other leg. Move the uninjured leg close to the injured one; put padding between the legs, especially at the knees and ankles.

2. Tie the feet together with a scarf or necktie in a figure eight. Knot it on the outer edge of the shoe on the uninjured leg.

3. Tie the knees together with a wide piece of material knotted on the uninjured side. Tie extra bandages above and below the fracture.

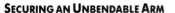

MAKING A BLANKET SPLINT FOR A FRACTURED LEG

1. If you have to transport a person with a broken leg on a stretcher or in an automobile, use a blanket to improvise a splint. Roll the blanket lengthwise as tightly as you can. Put one end of the blanket between the injured person's legs, starting at the crotch. Bring the blanket around the foot of the injured leg and along the outer side up to the thighs.

2. Tie the feet and ankles together with a bandage or other piece of material in a figure eight. Use a square knot to tie it off.

3. Tie a wide piece of material around the victim's knees, and knot the ends together on the uninjured side, again using a square knot.

4. Tie a third and fourth bandage above and below the fracture site.

5. Tie a fifth bandage around the thigh or calf, avoiding the fracture.

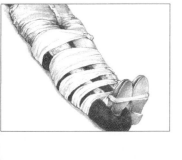

notice any of the following signs of a more serious chest injury:
☐ The victim can't breathe properly and seems to be suffocating.
☐ Red frothy blood issues from the mouth.
☐ The victim becomes restless and complains of thirst.

DISLOCATED JOINTS

A bone that is wrenched out of place at a joint is said to be dislocated. Shoulders, elbows, fingers, hips, kneecaps, and toes are the bones most likely to be dislocated. A dislocation is usually accompanied by torn ligaments (a sprain) and sometimes by a break in the bone as well.

The symptoms may include severe pain, swelling and bruising, deformity of the joint, and difficulty in moving the joint. Never try to push a dislocated bone back into place. Treat a dislocation as you would a fracture and get the victim to a hospital emergency room.

SPRAINS

Although the wrist, elbow, knee, hip, and shoulder can all suffer sprains, the ankle is the joint that people most often sprain. A fall or stumble that makes the ankle bend or twist excessively can sprain (or break) it.

A serious ankle sprain, in which the ligaments that hold the joint together are stretched or torn, can be hard to distinguish from a fracture. The symptoms of both include immediate, often severe pain, swelling, or bruising of the joint; pain when the ankle is moved; and inability to stand on the injured leg.

If there is any doubt, assume that the ankle is broken and get medical help right away.

Treating an injured ankle

If you think you've sustained a fracture or a sprain, remove the shoe and raise the foot above the heart. If you're near a source of ice or cold water, limit the swelling by applying a cold compress to the ankle for 20 to 30 minutes. Then bandage the ankle firmly and see a doctor as soon as possible.

A cold compress helps decrease swelling of the soft tissue surrounding the injury. Once started, it should be applied several times a day for 15 to 20 minutes at a time during the first 48 hours after the injury.

Don't apply heat to the ankle or soak it in hot water for the first 48 hours after the injury.

Don't put weight on a sprained or fractured ankle if you can help it. If you're caught away from help, support the ankle (see below) before using it.

Treating other sprains

If you sprain a wrist, elbow, or shoulder, apply compresses to the joint and bandage it firmly, then support it with a sling (p. 441). Have the injury checked by a doctor to make certain there is no fracture.

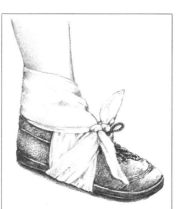

Support for a sprained ankle can be improvised if you injure the joint on a hike far from home. Leave your shoe and sock on. Using strips of bandage or cloth, bind the ankle in a figure-eight pattern under and over the instep and back around the heel of the shoe as shown. Then head for a haven where you can treat the sprain properly.

Frostbite

Exposed parts of the body, such as the nose, ears, cheeks, and chin, are susceptible to frostbite in freezing weather. Frostbite occurs when ice crystals form in the fluid of the skin and in the underlying tissue, constricting blood vessels and thereby cutting off the blood supply. Damage or death to the affected area follows. The hands and feet can also become frostbitten, even when they are enclosed in warm gloves and boots. Unless a frostbitten area is warmed up and circulation to it is restored, it may have to be amputated.

The warning signs

The frostbitten part of the body first feels cold and stiff, with an aching, sharp pain. The skin becomes hard, then turns white or grayish blue in fair-skinned people or becomes lighter in people with dark complexions. The area finally becomes numb, and the pain misleadingly disappears.

What you should do

☐ If possible, get the victim into a building for shelter.
☐ Don't thaw a frostbite if there is any danger of further injury from the cold.
☐ Remove clothing from the frostbitten area; take off jewelry from an affected hand.
☐ Warm the area with skin-to-skin contact. The victim can put a frostbitten foot into your armpit, for instance. Cover ears, nose, or cheeks with warm hands. Or immerse the frostbitten part in a basin of lukewarm water.
☐ Don't warm the area with dry or radiant heat. Slow thawing is essential because frostbitten parts can be burned before the victim's feeling returns.
☐ Don't rub or massage the frostbitten area; this increases tissue damage.

☐ When color and feeling return to the frostbitten area, wrap a towel or other cloth loosely around it and then cover that with a blanket or sleeping bag. Fingers and toes should be exercised to help restore circulation.

☐ To relieve swelling and pain, raise the affected area above the level of the victim's heart.

☐ As the area thaws, it may become blue and develop blood-filled blisters. Don't break the blisters or apply any medication.

☐ Put sterile gauze or a cloth between fingers and toes to keep them separated.

☐ Don't allow the victim to walk on a frostbitten foot.

☐ Seek medical attention if feeling does not return or if there is obvious tissue damage.

Head injuries

Traffic accidents and falls are among the most common causes of head injuries; sports such as cycling, hockey, and baseball are also a frequent source of head injuries. A blow to the head can damage the brain without any obvious sign, except perhaps for brief unconsciousness. Especially in the elderly, who are prone to falling, any slight knock to the head may cause internal bleeding, which, if not recognized and treated promptly, can result in permanent damage.

Anyone who has suffered a head injury should be taken to a doctor or to the emergency department of a hospital for examination—even if the injury does not appear to be serious.

If you suspect that someone has suffered a blow to the head, look for these symptoms:

☐ The pupils of the eyes are unequal in size, and the victim may have double vision.

☐ Cuts, bruises, and swellings are evident on the scalp, face, jaw, or behind the ear.

☐ Confusion or drowsiness, which may or may not be followed by unconsciousness.

☐ Headache.

☐ Loss of memory about the events just before or at the time of the accident.

☐ Weak pulse and shallow or noisy breathing.

☐ Clear fluids or blood flowing from the nose or ears; blood coming from the mouth.

☐ Vomiting, convulsions, or a change in pulse rate.

CONCUSSION

A blow to the head or a bad fall can cause a concussion, a brief period of unconsciousness lasting from a few seconds to minutes. Treat an unconscious patient as described on page 446.

After the spell of unconsciousness—however brief—the victim may experience nausea, vomiting, a severe headache, or he may fall into a deep sleep. The victim may remember nothing about the event that caused the injury. Any of these symptoms calls for prompt medical attention.

If a victim complains of feeling very weak after a blow to the head, treat as for shock (p.445).

Heart attack

Many conditions other than a heart attack can cause chest pains (p.214). But because early intervention can save lives and lessen damage to the heart, report chest pains to your doctor at once.

The classic sign of a heart attack is a crushing pain in the chest that often radiates to the jaw, neck, and arm. The victim may also become breathless, sweat profusely, and feel weak, nauseated, restless, and anxious.

For some days or weeks before a heart attack, the victim may experience unaccustomed indigestion, chest pain, fatigue, shortness of breath, and nausea.

What you should do

☐ Call for emergency help, making it clear that you suspect a heart attack. If there is a history of heart disease, tell the ambulance team when they arrive.

☐ If the patient is conscious, arrange him in a comfortable, half-sitting position, with head and shoulders supported by pillows and knees bent.

☐ Loosen the patient's clothing around the neck, chest, and waist to help circulation and breathing.

☐ Don't give the patient anything to eat or drink.

☐ Don't allow the patient to move unnecessarily; it will put extra strain on the heart.

☐ If the patient becomes unconscious, put her or him in the recovery position (p.425). Check frequently for breathing and pulse, and administer artificial respiration (p.427) and CPR (p.428) if necessary.

Heat exhaustion and heatstroke

People who exercise or otherwise exert themselves too much during hot, humid weather may suffer from heat exhaustion or from even more serious heatstroke. Both conditions can lead to unconsciousness, and both require medical treatment.

Profuse sweating on a hot day depletes the body of vital fluids and minerals. If the fluids and minerals aren't replaced, your muscles will cramp and you will feel a general weakness.

Symptoms of heat exhaustion include dizziness, headache, fatigue, and nausea. The victim's body temperature stays normal or rises very slightly. The skin feels moist; the face looks pale. Breathing is fast and shallow, and the pulse is fast and weak. The condition is made worse if the sufferer has recently had diarrhea or a bout of vomiting, causing the body to lose even greater amounts of fluid.

Those most vulnerable to the effects of extreme heat include the very young and the very old, the chronically ill, the overweight, and patients on certain psychotherapeutic drugs.

Heatstroke occurs suddenly and dramatically, with body temperature rising to 104°F or higher, possibly accompanied by a rapid and strong pulse. The victim's skin feels hot and may be dry. At first, the victim may complain of headache, dizziness, and nausea; later, as the condition worsens, he may become confused, irritable, and combative. Some people have a seizure or lapse into unconsciousness.

Treating heat exhaustion
☐ Place the victim in a cool area, preferably indoors, and have him drink cold (not iced) salted water (1 teaspoon of salt per quart of water), juice, or a sports drink.
☐ If the victim passes out, put him in the recovery position (p.425); call for medical help.

Treating heatstroke
Without quick treatment, a heatstroke victim risks dying.
☐ Call for medical help.
☐ Move the sufferer to a cool place. Remove the clothing, sponge the face, and cover the body with a wet sheet or spray it with cool water. Keep the victim wet and cool with cold water and fanning until the body temperature comes down to normal. Do not induce shivering.
☐ If the victim loses consciousness, put him in the recovery position (p.425) and continue the cooling treatment.

Hypothermia

Hypothermia is a serious condition in which the body's temperature drops below about 95°F

from the normal level of 98.6°F. Most at risk are babies, young children, and the very old. Alcoholics and people suffering from malnutrition and heart disease are also vulnerable.

If a baby in a cold room feels cold to the touch and refuses food, he may have hypothermia. Unless the drop in temperature is reversed, the baby could die in a few hours.

When an elderly person complains of the cold, take notice (p.408). If such complaints are ignored, the condition may grow worse until the victim becomes mentally confused and experiences such symptoms as fatigue, stiff muscles, uncontrollable shivering, and slurred speech. Without help, a hypothermia victim—young or old—eventually passes out; suffers heart, lung, and brain failure; and finally dies.

What you should do
If you suspect that someone is suffering from hypothermia, check for drowsiness, low body temperature, numb body parts, and a glassy stare. Call for medical help without delay, and take these steps to keep the condition from getting worse:
☐ Remove wet clothing.
☐ If a dry blanket or rug is readily available, wrap it around the victim, covering the body but not the face.
☐ Lay the victim down. Place an unconscious victim in the recovery position (p.425). Lie down beside the victim so that your body heat can help warm him.
☐ If possible, increase the temperature of the room, or move the victim to a warmer room.
☐ Give the victim—if conscious—hot, sweet drinks such as milk, tea, or hot chocolate. Do *not* give alcohol.
☐ Don't massage the victim's limbs or suggest exercise. Exercise will circulate cold blood from

the extremities throughout the body, thereby lowering the body's core temperature.
☐ Wrap a hot-water bottle or electric heating pad in a towel or cloth and put it on the victim's trunk, not on the arms or legs. Do not apply a heating device directly to the skin.

Poisoning

Many poisonings occur when a person—often a child—drinks some household or garden chemical. Adult gardeners have been known to accidentally drink insecticides that they had stored in soft drink bottles. Some common plants can be toxic if ingested (see *Houseplants: Hazardous to Your Health?*, p.313). Almost any nonfood substance is poisonous if taken in large doses. Aspirin poisons more children than any other household product.

To avoid poisoning, keep all medications and dangerous chemicals out of the reach of children, and never store unused weed killers or insecticides in unmarked bottles. Keep the local poison control center's number close by your telephone.

The warning signs
A person who has taken poison is likely to show some of the following symptoms:
☐ Stomach pain
☐ Vomiting and nausea
☐ Diarrhea
☐ Erratic behavior or excessive sleepiness
☐ Burns around the mouth if the poison was corrosive, and severe pain throughout the mouth, throat, and stomach
☐ Unusual breath or body odor
☐ Difficulty in breathing
☐ Unconsciousness.

What you should do
If the victim is conscious, try to find out what was swallowed.

Remember that the victim may become unconscious at any time.

Look around for a container or the remains of a poisonous plant that might be a clue. If the victim has vomited, collect samples. With this information in hand, call the poison center for instructions on what to do.

Also call for emergency medical help. If the victim is unconscious, place him in the recovery position (p. 425). If the victim's breathing stops, begin administering artificial respiration (p. 427), but take care not to get poison on your own mouth. Clean the victim's mouth, or use the mouth-to-nose technique.

If the victim is being hospitalized, be sure to give the ambulance attendants anything that will help identify the poison in question—pill containers, for example—and a sample of vomit.

ALCOHOL POISONING
After excessive drinking, the imbiber may lapse into a stupefied state, leading to coma. In severe cases, the drinker may stop breathing altogether.

Don't assume that someone who seems drunk is intoxicated. Other conditions—including stroke and diabetes—can produce similar symptoms, as can other drugs, legal and illegal.

How to treat an overdose
□ If the victim stops breathing, administer artificial respiration at once (p. 427).
□ If the victim is unconscious but still breathing, use your finger to clear any obstruction from the mouth and throat.
□ Don't, however, try to induce vomiting. Vomiting can kill an unconscious patient.
□ Put the victim in the recovery position (p. 425).
□ Loosen the victim's clothing at the neck and waist, and check that the airway is still clear.

□ Call an ambulance if the victim is unconscious or cannot be roused. Other danger signs that justify calling an ambulance include an uneven or slow pulse rate, pale color, continued difficulty in breathing, persistent vomiting, seizure, or a continued state of excitement or agitation.
□ You should also call for emergency medical help if the victim is a diabetic or if you suspect that he has taken drugs in combination with the alcohol.

DRUG OVERDOSE
Anyone who has taken a drug overdose requires immediate medical attention. This applies to an overdose of a prescribed medicine or an over-the-counter drug such as aspirin or ibuprofen as much as it does to an illegal drug such as heroin.

The warning signs
Symptoms depend on the size of the overdose and the type of drug, but they can include any of the following:
□ Vomiting
□ Difficulty in breathing
□ Unconsciousness
□ Sweating
□ Hallucinations
□ Dilation or contraction of the pupils of the eyes
□ Excessive sleepiness, confusion, and bizarre outbursts.

What you should do
Call the local poison control center while waiting for medical help to arrive. Generally, don't induce vomiting unless a doctor or the poison control center suggests it.

Don't try to keep the victim awake by giving him black coffee or walking him about. (Physical activity will only speed up the body's absorption of the drug.)

If the victim is unconscious, put the body in the recovery position (p. 425) until the ambulance team arrives.

GAS POISONING
Many gases are toxic. For example, ammonia, which is used in refrigeration plants and as a fertilizer; fumes from burning polyurethane foam, sometimes found in mattresses and upholstered furniture; and carbon monoxide from automobile exhausts can all cause poisoning.

The warning signs
The victim may demonstrate unsound judgment and may be difficult and uncooperative. He or she may also be confused, stupefied, or unconscious.

What you should do
□ With ammonia, which has a particularly strong smell, poisoning mostly occurs when people are trapped in an enclosed area. Don't enter the affected area without a face mask. Ventilation works very slowly.
□ The fire department should handle burning polyurethane foam. Be aware that fumes from this substance can kill in minutes.
□ If you suspect that a car or garage is filled with carbon monoxide, open the doors to ventilate the area. Get the victim into the open air as quickly as possible.

Shock

Severe injury or illness may produce shock, a dangerous reduction in the flow of blood throughout the body, which, if untreated, can cause the victim to collapse, fall into a coma, or die. Severe bleeding, heavy vomiting or diarrhea, and widespread burns can reduce blood or body fluid volume sufficiently to cause shock.

The warning signs
Faced with the lack of adequate blood supply, the body reacts by concentrating the remaining supply on the vital organs—the heart, brain, and kidneys. The

less important areas, such as the muscles and skin, go without adequate blood, and the victim weakens and becomes pale.

Other symptoms include:
☐ Fainting
☐ Anxiousness and restlessness
☐ Nausea and perhaps vomiting
☐ Pallor
☐ Thirst
☐ Sweating
☐ Shallow, rapid breathing, with yawning and sighing
☐ A weak pulse that is fast and may be irregular.

What you should do
☐ Call for an ambulance.
☐ Lay the victim down with his head low, and treat any obvious injury or condition that may be causing the shock.
☐ Comfort the victim.
☐ Loosen clothing at the neck, chest, and waist to assist breathing and blood circulation.
☐ If possible, raise the legs on a folded coat or cushion to direct the blood to the brain.
☐ Keep the victim warm with a coat or blanket. Don't use a hot-water bottle or an electric heating pad, as such devices will bring the blood to the skin and away from vital organs.
☐ If the victim is thirsty, wet his lips, but don't give him anything to eat or drink. If a person in shock is given food or drink, the hospital may have to delay giving him an anesthetic; food can also cause the victim to choke.
☐ Don't move the victim unnecessarily. Moving may increase the shock.
☐ Don't let the victim smoke.
☐ If the victim has difficulty

breathing, becomes nauseated, or loses consciousness, put him in the recovery position (p.425).
☐ If breathing stops, begin artificial respiration (p.427).

Stroke

The signs that someone is having a stroke include difficulty in speaking or swallowing, weakness or paralysis on one side of the body, impaired vision, sudden headache, confusion, drowsiness, involuntary urination, and loss of bowel control. Some of these symptoms can resemble drunkenness. A severe stroke may cause unconsciousness. If you suspect that someone is having a stroke, get him to a doctor or a hospital for treatment as soon as possible.

What you should do
Lay a conscious stroke victim down with head and shoulders slightly raised on pillows or cushions. Lay the victim on the weak side so that saliva can drain from the mouth. Loosen clothing at the neck, chest, and waist. If necessary, restore breathing by mouth-to-mouth resuscitation (p.427). Assure the victim that help is on the way, but don't offer anything to eat or drink.

If the patient becomes unconscious, put him in the recovery position (p.425).

Unconsciousness

There are three stages of unconsciousness, and a person may go through all three or remain in one. The three stages are:
☐ Drowsiness, in which the victim is easily roused for a few moments, but then passes back into a sleeplike state. The patient may be able to give reasonably

coherent answers to questions about his or her condition.
☐ Stupor, in which the victim doesn't react to questions easily or does so incoherently, giving the impression of being drunk.
☐ Coma, in which the victim cannot be roused at all, and is motionless and silent.

A person who has become unconscious needs to be checked immediately for any obstruction to the airway. If breathing has stopped, begin artificial respiration (p.427). If the victim is breathing normally, make sure the airway stays unclogged while you are waiting for medical assistance. Vomit, blood, or saliva may block the top of the windpipe, or the base of the tongue may slide back over it.

If the cause of unconsciousness is not apparent, always suspect a head, neck, or back injury. Take care not to move the neck. In fact, if an unconscious person is breathing normally and is in a safe place, don't disturb him at all. Moving the person could cause serious, even fatal injury.

Handle any serious wound gently. Injuries that can be treated and bleeding that can be stopped without moving the victim should be taken care of while you wait for the ambulance.

Whatever the circumstances, don't leave an unconscious person alone at any time, and don't give the victim anything to eat or drink, even if he or she regains consciousness.

Anyone who has been unconscious, even for a short time, should receive immediate medical treatment.

Appendix

The professional, government, and service organizations that are listed on the following pages offer information or support on a wide variety of health matters. (Check your telephone book for the addresses and telephone numbers of local chapters of national organizations.) The branches of the National Institutes of Health are grouped together below, along with the Centers for Disease Control. Other organizations are listed by chapter and page, in the order in which they are mentioned in this book.

NATIONAL INSTITUTES OF HEALTH

Consisting of 13 institutes and covering a broad spectrum of health issues, the National Institutes of Health is the major federal agency funding medical research in the United States. In addition to conducting research, the various institutes distribute health information to the public.

National Institute on Aging
301-496-1752

National Institute of Allergy and Infectious Diseases
301-496-5717

National Institute of Arthritis and Musculoskeletal and Skin Diseases
301-496-8188

National Cancer Institute
800-4-CANCER (800-422-6237)

National Institute of Child Health and Human Development
301-496-5133

National Institute on Deafness and Other Communications Disorders
301-496-7243

National Institute of Dental Research
301-496-4261

National Institute of Diabetes and Digestive and Kidney Diseases
301-496-3583

National Institute of Environmental Health Sciences
Information Office
P.O. Box 12233
Research Triangle Park, NC 27709
919-541-3345

National Eye Institute
301-496-5248

National Institute of General Medical Sciences
301-496-7301

National Heart, Lung, and Blood Institute
301-496-4236

National Institute of Neurological Disorders and Stroke
301-496-5751

Written inquiries to any of these institutes except *the National Institute of Environmental Health Sciences should be addressed to*
National Institutes of Health
Information Office/Public Inquiries
(Name of the institute to which you are writing)
Bethesda, MD 20892

CENTERS FOR DISEASE CONTROL

The Centers for Disease Control is a federal agency whose mission is "to prevent unnecessary disease, disability, and premature death and to promote healthy lifestyles." It also operates a health information hotline:
404-332-4555.
Address written inquiries to
Centers for Disease Control
Public Inquiries
1600 Clifton Rd. NE
Atlanta, GA 30333

For a referral to an organization that deals with a specific illness but that is not listed in this Appendix, call the National Health Information Center of the Office of Disease Prevention and Health Promotion:
800-336-4797
In 301 area code: 565-4167

Chapter 1
Eating Well to Stay Well

p.46

American Board of Allergy and Immunology
University City Science Center
3624 Market St.
Philadelphia, PA 19104-2675
215-349-9466

p.50

U.S. Department of Agriculture
Meat and Poultry Hotline
USDA-FSIS, Room 1165-S
Washington, DC 20250
800-535-4555
In 202 area code: 447-3333
These numbers are also TDD numbers.

National Fisheries Institute
1525 Wilson Blvd., Suite 500
Arlington, VA 22209
703-524-8881

p.61

The American Dietetic Association
National Center for Nutrition and Dietetics
216 West Jackson Blvd., Suite 800
Chicago, IL 60606-6995
800-366-1655

Chapter 2
Exercise and Physical Fitness

p.72

National Organization of Mall Walkers
P.O. Box 191
Hermann, MO 65041
314-486-3945

p.75

Achilles Track Club
9 East 89th St.
New York, NY 10128
212-967-9300

National Handicapped Sports
451 Hungerford Dr., Suite 100
Rockville, MD 20850
301-217-0960

Wheelchair Workout with Janet Reed
12275 Greenleaf Ave.
Potomac, MD 20854
301-279-2994
*Audio cassette tape and manual and video
workout are available.*

Paralyzed Veterans of America
Sports and Recreation Department
801 18th St. NW
Washington, DC 20006
800-424-8200
In 202 area code: 872-1300

p.77

American College of Sports Medicine
P.O. Box 1440
Indianapolis, IN 46206-1440
317-637-9200

Institute for Aerobics Research
12330 Preston Rd.
Dallas, TX 75230
800-635-7050
In 214 area code: 701-8001

American Council on Exercise
(formerly the IDEA Foundation)
6190 Cornerstone Ct. East, Suite 202
San Diego, CA 92121
800-825-3636
In 619 area code: 452-1223

p.96

Aquatic Exercise Association
1032 South Spring St.
Port Washington, WI 53074
414-284-3416

Council for National Cooperation in Aquatics
901 West New York St.
Indianapolis, IN 46202
317-638-4238

p.98

United States Rowing Association
201 South Capitol Ave., Suite 400
Indianapolis, IN 46225
317-237-5656

North American Telemark Organization
P.O. Box 44
Waitsfield, VT 05673
802-496-4387

p.99
Triathlon Federation/USA
3595 East Fountain Blvd., Suite F1
Colorado Springs, CO 80910
719-597-9090

p.100
Consumer Product Safety Commission
Attn.: FOI
Washington, DC 20207
800-638-2772
In 301 area code: 492-6800

National Recreation and Park Association
2775 South Quincy St., Suite 300
Arlington, VA 22206
703-820-4940

Playground Safety Clearinghouse
36 Sycamore Ln.
Phoenixville, PA 19460
215-935-1549

p.101
American College of Sports Medicine
P.O. Box 1440
Indianapolis, IN 46206-1440
317-637-9200

Chapter 3
You and Your Doctors

p.120
American Board of Medical Specialties
1 Rotary Ctr., Suite 805
Evanston, IL 60201
800-776-CERT (800-776-2378)
In 708 area code: 491-9091

p.124
American College of Radiology
1891 Preston White Dr.
Reston, VA 22091
703-648-8900

p.130
Centers for Disease Control
International Travelers' Hotline
404-332-4559
Address written inquiries to
Center for Prevention Services
Division of Quarantine (E-03)
Attn.: Travelers' Health Section
Centers for Disease Control
Atlanta, GA 30333

p.131
American Diabetes Association
Call your local chapter or contact
American Diabetes Association
1660 Duke St.
Alexandria, VA 22314
800-232-3472
In 703 area code: 549-1500

American Heart Association
Call your local chapter or contact
American Heart Association
7320 Greenville Ave.
Dallas, TX 75231

Arthritis Foundation
P.O. Box 19000
Atlanta, GA 30326
800-283-7800

See also Appendix listings for Chapter 8:
Managing Chronic Health Problems.

p.141
American Board of Medical Specialties
1 Rotary Ctr., Suite 805
Evanston, IL 60201
800-776-CERT (800-776-2378)
In 708 area code: 491-9091

p.149
Department of Health and Human Services
Health Care Financing Administration
6325 Security Blvd.
Baltimore, MD 21207
800-638-6833
In 301 area code: 966-3000

Chapter 4
Staying Mentally Healthy

*For information on mental health issues
in general contact*
National Institute of Mental Health
Public Inquiries
Parklawn Bldg. 15C-05
Rockville, MD 20857
301-443-4513

p.163
For help with an alcohol addiction contact
Al-Anon Family Group Headquarters
P.O. Box 862, Midtown Station
New York, NY 10018-0862
General Information: 212-302-7240
U.S. Meetings Information: 800-344-2666

Alcoholics Anonymous World Services
P.O. Box 459, Grand Central Station
New York, NY 10163
212-686-1100

National Association on Drug Abuse Problems
355 Lexington Ave.
New York, NY 10017
212-986-1170

National Council on Alcoholism and Drug
Dependence, Inc.
12 West 21st St.
New York, NY 10010
800-NCA-CALL (800-622-2255)

For help with a drug addiction problem contact
National Association on Drug Abuse Problems
355 Lexington Ave.
New York, NY 10017
212-986-1170

p.167
National Clearinghouse for Alcohol
and Drug Information
P.O. Box 2345
Rockville, MD 20852
800-729-6686

Chapter 5
Self-Care From Head to Toe

p.201
American Lung Association
Call your local chapter.

American Cancer Society
Call your local chapter or contact
American Cancer Society
1599 Clifton Rd. NE
Atlanta, GA 30329
404-320-3333
Cancer Response System: 800-ACS-2345
(800-227-2345)

General Conference of Seventh-Day Adventists
Health and Temperance Department
12501 Old Columbia Pike
Silver Spring, MD 20904-1608
301-680-6733
301-680-6718

p.207
Association for Applied Psychophysiology
and Biofeedback
10200 West 44th Ave., Suite 304
Wheat Ridge, CO 80033
*Include a stamped, addressed return envelope
with all inquiries.*

p.230
National Council Against Health Fraud
P.O. Box 1276
Loma Linda, CA 92354
714-824-4690

U.S. Food and Drug Administration
Office of Consumer Affairs and
Consumer Inquiries
HFE-88, Room 16-63
5600 Fishers Ln.
Rockville, MD 20857
301-443-3170

p.231
Centers for Disease Control
International Travelers' Hotline
404-332-4559
Address written inquiries to
Center for Prevention Services
Division of Quarantine (E-03)
Attn.: Travelers' Health Section
Centers for Disease Control
Atlanta, GA 30333

IAMAT: International Association for Medical
Assistance for Travellers
417 Center St.
Lewiston, NY 14092
716-754-4883

Chapter 6
Sex and Family Life

p.240

American Association of Sex Educators,
    Counselors and Therapists
435 North Michigan Ave., Suite 1717
Chicago, IL 60611
*Include a stamped, addressed return
envelope and $2.00 with your request.*

p.241

American Association for Marriage
    and Family Therapy
1100 17th St. NW, 10th Floor
Washington, DC 20036
800-374-2638

p.258

National Society of Genetic Counselors, Inc.
233 Canterbury Dr.
Wallingford, PA 19086
*The NSGC does not maintain or disseminate
information about specific genetic disorders.*

p.268

March of Dimes Birth Defects Foundation
1275 Mamaroneck Ave.
White Plains, NY 10605
914-428-7100

National Organization for Rare Disorders
P.O. Box 8923
New Fairfield, CT 06812-1783
800-999-NORD (800-999-6673)
In 203 area code: 746-6518

National Information Center for
    Children and Youth with Disabilities
P.O. Box 1492
Washington, DC 20013
800-999-5599
In 703 area code: 893-6061
TDD in 703 area code: 893-8614

p.277

*For information on workshops for parents
throughout the U.S., contact one of the following:*

Sex Information and Education Council of the U.S.
130 West 42nd St., Suite 2500
New York, NY 10036
212-819-9770

Planned Parenthood Federation of America
Call your local affiliate or contact
Planned Parenthood
810 Seventh Ave.
New York, NY 10017
212-541-7800

*Booklets for parents are available from the
following organizations:*

American Academy of Pediatrics
Attn.: Dept. C
141 Northwest Point Blvd.
P.O. Box 927
Elk Grove Village, IL 60009-0927
708-228-5005

National PTA — National Congress of Parents
    and Teachers
700 North Rush St.
Chicago, IL 60611
312-787-0977

Planned Parenthood Federation of America
Call your local affiliate or contact
Planned Parenthood
810 Seventh Ave.
New York, NY 10017
212-541-7800

p.281

Planned Parenthood Federation of America
(See previous entry.)

The Alan Guttmacher Institute
111 Fifth Ave., 11th Floor
New York, NY 10003
212-254-5656

Sex Information and Education Council of the U.S.
130 West 42nd St., Suite 2500
New York, NY 10036
212-819-9770

p.283

Stepfamily Association of America
215 Centennial Mall South, Suite 212
Lincoln, NE 68508
402-477-7837

Chapter 7
Health at Home and Work

p.291
Clean Water Action
1320 18th St. NW
Washington, DC 20036
202-457-1286

Citizens for a Better Environment
407 South Dearborn, Suite 1775
Chicago, IL 60605
312-939-1530
*Send a stamped, addressed return envelope and
50 cents with your request.*

p.292
International Bottled Water Association
113 North Henry St.
Alexandria, VA 22314

p.319
Environmental Protection Agency Hotlines:

National Radon Hotline
800-SOS-RADON (800-767-7236)

National Response Center
800-424-8802
*For information on accidental release of oil,
hazardous chemical, biological, and radiological
substances.*

Asbestos Ombudsman Clearinghouse/Hotline
800-368-5888

National Small Flows Clearinghouse
800-624-8301
*For information about sewage management in
small communities (under 10,000 people).*

Safe Drinking Water Hotline
800-426-4791

National Pesticides Telecommunications Network
800-858-PEST (800-858-7378)

Solid Waste Information Clearinghouse
P.O. Box 7219
Silver Spring, MD 20910
Fax 301-585-0204

*Department of Labor
Occupational Safety and Health Administration
Regional Offices:*

Region I (CT, MA, ME, NH, RI, VT)
133 Portland St., First Floor
Boston , MA 02114
617-565-7164

Region II (NJ, NY, PR, VI)
201 Varick St., Room 670
New York, NY 10014
212-337-2378

Region III (DC, DE, MD, PA, VA, WV)
Gateway Building, Suite 2100
3535 Market St.
Philadelphia, PA 19104
215-596-1201

Region IV (AL, FL, GA, KY, MS, NC, SC, TN)
1375 Peachtree St. NE, Suite 587
Atlanta, GA 30367
404-347-3573

Region V (IL, IN, MI, MN, OH, WI)
230 South Dearborn St., Room 3244
Chicago, IL 60604
312-353-2220

Region VI (AR, LA, NM, OK, TX)
525 Griffin St., Room 602
Dallas, TX 75202
214-767-4731

Region VII (IA, KS, MO, NE)
911 Walnut St.
Kansas City, MO 64106
816-426-5861

Region VIII (CO, MT, ND, SD, UT, WY)
Federal Building, Room 1576
1961 Stout St.
Denver, CO 80294
303-844-3061

Region IX (AZ, CA, HI, NV)
71 Stevenson St., Room 420
San Francisco, CA 94105
415-744-6670

Region X (AK, ID, OR, WA)
1111 Third Ave., Suite 715
Seattle, WA 98101
206-553-5930

Chapter 8
Managing Chronic Health Problems

p.335
American Cancer Society
Call your local chapter or contact
American Cancer Society
1599 Clifton Rd. NE
Atlanta, GA 30329
404-320-3333
Cancer Response System: 800-ACS-2345
(800-227-2345)

p.344
American Diabetes Association
1660 Duke St.
Alexandria, VA 22314
800-232-3472
In 703 area code: 549-1500

p.349
United Ostomy Association
36 Executive Park, Suite 120
Irvine, CA 92714
800-826-0826
In 714 area code: 660-8624

p.350
Comfortably Yours
Catalog Request
61 West Hunter Ave.
Maywood, NJ 07607
Send $1.00 with your catalog request.

Independence House, Inc.
400 North Main St.
Goshen, IN 46526
800-932-2120
Care at Home *catalog is available free of charge.*

Sears Telecatalog
P.O. Box 7012
Downers Grove, IL 60515-8012
800-326-1750
TDD 800-733-4833
Sears Home Health Care Catalog *is available free of charge.*

Arthritis Foundation
Attn.: PCS
P.O. Box 19000
Atlanta, GA 30326
800-283-7800
The Guide to Independent Living for People with
Arthritis, *a self-help manual, costs about $8.00.*

American Foundation for the Blind
15 West 16th St.
New York, NY 10011
800-AFBLIND (800-232-5463)
In 212 area code: 620-2147

p.354
American Parkinson Disease Association
60 Bay St.
Staten Island, NY 10301
800-223-APDA (800-223-2732)

Parkinson Support Groups of America
11376 Cherry Hill Rd., Apt. 204
Beltsville, MD 20705
301-937-1545

Parkinson's Disease Foundation
William Black Medical Research Building
    at Columbia-Presbyterian Medical Center
650 West 168th St.
New York, NY 10032
800-457-6676
In 212 area code: 923-4700

p.356
For a listing of local support groups contact
National Chronic Fatigue Syndrome Association
3521 Broadway, Suite 222
Kansas City, MO 64111
816-931-4777

For information on chronic fatigue syndrome write to
National Institute of Allergy and Infectious
    Diseases
Office of Communications
Building 31, Room 7A-32
9000 Rockville Pike
Bethesda, MD 20892

p.358
American Chronic Pain Association, Inc.
P.O. Box 850
Rocklin, CA 95677
916-632-0922

National Chronic Pain Outreach Association
7979 Old Georgetown Rd., Suite 100
Bethesda, MD 20814-2429
301-652-4948
Fax 301-907-0745

Chapter 9
Making the Most of Middle Age

p.365
National Association of Private Geriatric
    Care Managers
655 North Alvernon, Suite 108
Tucson, AZ 85711
602-881-8008

p.367
Choice in Dying
*(Formerly Concern for Dying/Society for
    the Right to Die)*
250 West 57th St.
New York, NY 10107
212-246-6973

p.371
American Society of Plastic and
    Reconstructive Surgeons
444 East Algonquin Rd.
Arlington Heights, IL 60005
800-635-0635

p.378
National Osteoporosis Foundation
2100 M St. NW, Suite 602
Washington, DC 20037

Chapter 10
Living Better in the Later Years

*For reliable and up-to-date information on many
concerns of older persons contact*
National Council on the Aging
409 Third St. SW
Washington, D.C. 20024
202-479-1200

p.395
*For sources of household and personal-care
aids for people with disabilities, see Appendix
listings for p.350.*

p.397
American Foundation for the Blind
15 West 16th St.
New York, NY 10011
800-AFBLIND (800-232-5463)
In 212 area code: 620-2147

National Association for Visually Handicapped
22 West 21st St.
New York, NY 10010
212-889-3141
*If you live in the 11 Western states (AZ, CA,
CO, ID, MT, NM, NV, OR, WA, WY, UT) or in
Alaska or Hawaii, contact*
National Association for Visually Handicapped
3201 Balboa St.
San Francisco, CA 94121
415-221-3201

p.406
Help for Incontinent People
P.O. Box 544
Union, SC 29379
*Send a legal-size, stamped, addressed return
envelope and $1.00 with your request.*

For *sources of household and personal-care
aids for people with disabilities, see Appendix
listings for p.350.*

p.410
Alzheimer's Association
919 North Michigan Ave., Suite 1000
Chicago, IL 60611-1676
800-272-3900
TDD in 312 area code: 335-8882

p.413
Women for Sobriety
P.O. Box 618
Quakertown, PA 18951
800-333-1606
In 215 area code: 536-8026
(See also Appendix listings for pp.163 and 167.)

pp.414–415
American Association of Homes for the Aging
Attn.: Publications
901 E St. NW, Suite 500
Washington, DC 20004-2039
*To receive one of the following brochures free
of charge, send a business-size, addressed
return stamped envelope; for all five brochures,
send $1.00:*
Choosing a Nursing Home: A Guide to Quality
    Care
The Continuing Care Consumer Brochure: A Life
    Style Offering Security and Independence
Living Independently: Housing Choices for
    Older People
Community Services for Older People
    Living at Home
The Nursing Home, Alzheimer's and You

American Health Care Association
1201 L St. NW
Washington, DC 29995-4014
202-842-4444
A booklet Thinking About a Nursing Home? *is
available free of charge; a video* Helping Hands:
The Right Way to Choose a Nursing Home *is
available for about $25.00.*

p.416
American Association of Retired Persons
Reminiscence Program
601 E St. NW
Washington, DC 20049

p.419
Health Insurance Association of America
P.O. Box 41455
Washington, DC 20018
A booklet entitled The Consumer's Guide to Long-
Term Care Insurance *is available free of charge.*

AARP Pharmacy Service Center
Attn.: Key 350600
7609 Energy Pkwy., Suite 1003
Baltimore, MD 21226-1755
Customer service and price information:
800-456-4636
Ordering:
800-456-2277

p.420
American Association of Retired Persons
Membership Communications
601 E St. NW
Washington, DC 20049

AARP Pharmacy Service Center
(See listing for p.419.)

ACTION
Attn.: Public Affairs Office
1100 Vermont Ave. NW
Washington, DC 20525
202-606-5108

Elderhostel
75 Federal St.
Boston, MA 02110
617-426-7788

Outward Bound USA
384 Field Point Rd.
Greenwich, CT 06830
800-243-8520
In 203 area code: 661-0797

National SCORE Office
409 Third St. SW, Suite 5900
Washington, DC 20024
202-205-6762

National Home Study Council
1601 18th St. NW, Suite 2
Washington, DC 20009
202-234-5100

p.421
National Hospice Organization
1901 North Moore St., Suite 901
Arlington, VA 22209
800-658-8898
In 703 area code: 243-5900

p.422
Continental Association of Funeral and Memorial
    Societies
6900 Lost Lake Rd.
Egg Harbor, WI 54209
800-458-5563
In 414 area code: 868-3136

Acknowledgments

The editors are especially grateful to the following individuals and organizations for their help in providing or reviewing information for this book.

American Academy of Allergy and Immunology
American Academy of Dermatology
American Academy of Family Physicians
American Academy of Ophthalmology
American Academy of Otolaryngology
American Academy of Pediatrics
American Academy of Periodontology
American Association for the Study of Headache
American Association of Naturopathic Physicians
American Cancer Society
American College of Emergency Physicians
American College of Obstetricians and Gynecologists
American College of Radiology
American College of Surgeons
American Dental Association
American Diabetes Association
American Heart Association
American Hospital Association
American Lung Association
American Medical Association
American Nurses' Association, Inc.
American Society of Plastic and Reconstructive
    Surgeons, Inc.
David Barad, M.D., Director, Division of Reproductive
    Endocrinology, Albert Einstein College of Medicine
Sally A. Barrett, Office of Scientific Information, National
    Institute of Mental Health
Stephen Barrett, M.D., National Council Against
    Health Fraud
Bicycle Institute of America
Katherine Bradley, American Nurses' Association, Inc.
Robin Brown, American Academy of Allergy and
    Immunology
Tom Celebrezze, American Academy of Ophthalmology
Center for Safety in the Arts
Centers for Disease Control
James Cleeman, M.D., Coordinator, National
    Cholesterol Education Program, National Heart, Lung,
    and Blood Institute
Consumer Product Safety Commission
Council on Chiropractic Education
Nick Croce, American College of Radiology

Susan Curzan, Food and Drug Administration
Elaine Leong Eng, M.D., New York, NY
Environmental Protection Agency
Food and Drug Administration
Marion Franz, M.S., R.D., C.D.E., International
    Diabetes Center
Gay Men's Health Crisis
Roberta W. Gershner, M.S., R.D., Consulting Nutritionist,
    Ossining, NY
Henry N. Ginsberg, M.D., College of Physicians and
    Surgeons of Columbia University
Diane Goetz, American Heart Association
Robert J. Guarino, R.Ph., Orlando, FL
Alan Guttmacher Institute
Karen Hein, M.D., Director, Adolescent AIDS Program,
    Montefiore Medical Center, New York, NY
Gregory L. Henry, M.D., Clinical Assistant Professor,
    University of Michigan Medical School
John Marks, M.D., New York, NY
Laurie Meyer, R.D., Consulting Nutritionist, Mequon, WI
Al Minor, Health Insurance Association of America
National Cancer Institute
National Heart, Lung, and Blood Institute
National Institute of Allergy and Infectious Diseases
National Institute of Mental Health
National Osteoporosis Foundation
National Safe Kids Campaign
National Safety Council
Renae Norton, Psy.D., Clinical Psychologist and Marriage
    Counselor, Cincinnati, OH
Dianne Odland, M.S., C.H.E., Human Nutrition
    Information Service, U.S. Department of Agriculture
Pennsylvania Reproductive Associates, Pennsylvania
    Hospital, Philadelphia, PA
Johna L. Pierce, Director, Public Affairs, Human Nutrition
    Information Service, U.S. Department of Agriculture
Planned Parenthood Federation of America
President's Council on Physical Fitness and Sports
Jill Maura Rabin, M.D., Assistant Professor, Obstetrics
    and Gynecology, Long Island Jewish Medical Center
    Campus for the Albert Einstein College of Medicine
Margaret R. Reinfeld, Gay Men's Health Crisis
Kate Ruddon, American College of Obstetricians and
    Gynecologists
Earl Schwartz, M.D., F.A.C.E.P., Chairman, Department
    of Emergency Medicine, Bowman Gray School of
    Medicine, Wake Forest University
James A. Simon, M.D., Chief, Division of Reproductive
    Endocrinology and Infertility, Georgetown University
Stepfamily Association of America, Inc.
U.S. Department of Agriculture
Kathy Wenzel, R.N., N.P., Hypertension Section,
    Department of Veterans Affairs Medical Center,
    St. Louis, MO
Joyce Zeitz, American Fertility Society

Credits

PHOTOGRAPHS

5 *top right* Marc Rosenthal; *bottom right* R.C. Eagle/Photo Researchers, Inc. **6** *middle right* © David Madison 1991; *middle left* Suzanne Arms-Wimberley. **7** *middle left* Comstock. **13** Marc Rosenthal. **19** Eric Roth. **24** USDA Photo. **30** James A. McInnis. **43** Julie Habel/H. Armstrong Roberts. **44–45** Marc Rosenthal. **51** James A. McInnis. **66** *left* H. Armstrong Roberts; *right* David Stoecklein/The Stock Market. **67** *left* Jon Feingersh/Tom Stack & Associates; *middle* Brian Payne/West Stock, Inc.; *right* Bob Winsett/Jeff Andrew/Tom Stack & Associates. **75** © David Madison 1990. **78** *top left* StairMaster Exercise Systems; *bottom left* Roy Morsch/The Stock Market; *center* NordicTrack; *top right and bottom right* Precor Incorporated/Burnside Photography. **82–83** © David Madison 1990. **84** *both* Art Zeller. **88–89** © David Madison 1990. **90** Jan Cobb. **91** Nike, Inc. **92** Joseph McNally. **97** Trek Bicycle Corporation, Waterloo, WI. **99** RollerBlade, Inc. **100** *all* SuperStock. **107** Ed Landrock/Rodale Press, Inc. **127** *top left* CNRI/Science Photo Library /Photo Researchers, Inc.; *middle left* Howard Sochurek; *bottom left* © Westwood/Custom Medical Stock; *top right* Howard Sochurek; *middle right* Dan McCoy/Rainbow; *bottom right* Howard Sochurek. **132** *top* John P. Endress/The Stock Market; *middle left* © John Dominis, 1990/Telephoto; *middle right* Berthoule/Explorer/Photo Researchers, Inc.; *bottom* Dave King/Dorling Kindersley Limited. **133** *top left* Bruce Coleman Inc.; *top right* Doug Plummer/Photo Researchers, Inc.; *bottom* Dave King/Dorling Kindersley Limited. **136** *top left* Custom Medical Stock Photo; *middle left* Walter Hodges/H. Armstrong Roberts; *bottom left* Sepp Seitz/Woodfin Camp & Associates; *center* R.C. Eagle/Photo Researchers, Inc. **157** Richard Hutchings/InfoEdit. **159** Philip Jones Griffiths/Magnum. **181** Steven E. Sutton/Duomo. **186** Ed Bock/The Stock Mar-

ket. **206** *top left* Geoffrey Clifford/Woodfin Camp & Associates; *top right* © 1984 Leonard E. Morgan, Inc.; *middle right* © David Madison 1991. **206–207** *bottom* © David Madison 1991. **207** *top* © David Madison 1991; *center* Dan McCoy/Rainbow; *bottom right* James A. McInnis. **218–219** *all* © David Madison 1991. **237** *left* © Marilyn Wood: Photo/NATS; *middle* Michel Viard/Peter Arnold, Inc.; *right* Charles Krebbs/The Stock Market. **246** *all* James A. McInnis. **261** Will & Deni McIntyre/Photo Researchers, Inc. **266** Suzanne Arms-Wimberley. **268** Mario Ruiz. **289** TreePeople. **299** David Scharf/Peter Arnold, Inc. **302** Thomas Kitchin/Tom Stack & Associates. **317** Chrysler Corporation. **321** James A. McInnis. **326** James A. McInnis. **329** *top* Custom Medical Stock Photo; *bottom* National Heart, Lung & Blood Institute. **331** © Biophoto Associates/Science Source/Photo Researchers, Inc. **332** James Prince/Photo Researchers, Inc. **336** Science Photo Library/Photo Researchers, Inc. **350** *top center and right* From *The Family Handyman*; *top left* From *Comfortably Yours*; *bottom* Enrichments®, © 1991 Bissell Healthcare Corporation. **351** *bottom right* From *Comfortably Yours*; *remainder* From *The Family Handyman*. **352** Photo Researchers, Inc. **372** *all* Permission of The Skin Cancer Foundation, New York, NY. **379** *top* Howard Sochurek; *middle and bottom* M.J. Klein, M.D. **387** Comstock. **391** Frank Fournier /Contact Press Images. **398** *all* The Lighthouse Inc. **401** *top* Miracle-Ear®; *bottom left and right* Courtesy of ENSONIQ Corp. **414** *top* Jeffrey Muir Hamilton; *bottom* Richard S. Allen. **415** *top* The Molly Hare Cooperative; *bottom* Mario Ruiz. **417** Nina Barnett. **418** © 1986 Dahlgren/The Stock Market.

TEXT

Grateful acknowledgment is made for permission to excerpt or adapt featured materials from the following works: **Brentwood Christian Communications Press.** "These Hands of Mine" from *Thoughts for Sharing* by Vicky Pope. Copyright © 1984 by Vicky Pope. Reprinted by permission of the author. **Health Letter Associates.** "Wearing the Wrong Glasses," excerpted from *The University of California, Berkeley, Wellness Letter.* Copyright © Health Letter Associates, 1991. Reprinted by permission. **National Sporting Goods Association.** Sports participation statistics for the years 1986 to 1989. Copyright © 1986 to 1989 by the National Sporting Goods Association. Reprinted by permission. **St. Martin's Press, Inc.** "Examples of One Day's Diary Under Weight-Loss Program" from *The Mount Sinai School of Medicine Complete Book of Nutrition,* copyright © 1990 by the Mount Sinai School of Medicine. Reprinted by permission of St. Martin's Press.

Index

Reader's Digest Fund for the Blind is
publisher of the Large-Type Edition
of *Reader's Digest*. For subscription
information about this magazine,
please contact Reader's Digest
Fund for the Blind, Inc., Dept. 250,
Pleasantville, N.Y. 10570.